AF631264

Utilisation and Management of Medicinal Plants

Utilisation and Management of Medicinal Plants

– Editor-in-Chief –

V.K. Gupta

– Editors –

Anil K. Verma

Sushma Koul

2010

DAYA PUBLISHING HOUSE

Delhi - 110 035

© 2010 EDITORS
ISBN 81-7035-625-3
ISBN 978-81-7035-625-7

All rights reserved. Including the right to translate or to reproduce this book or parts thereof except for brief quotations in critical reviews.

Published by : **Daya Publishing House**
1123/74, Deva Ram Park
Tri Nagar, Delhi - 110 035
Phone: 27383999
Fax: (011) 23260116
e-mail : dayabooks@vsnl.com
website : www.dayabooks.com

Showroom : 4760-61/23, Ansari Road, Darya Ganj,
New Delhi - 110 002
Phone: 23245578, 23244987

Laser Typesetting : **Classic Computer Services**
Delhi - 110 035

Printed at : **Chawla Offset Printers**
Delhi - 110 052

PRINTED IN INDIA

Dedicated to

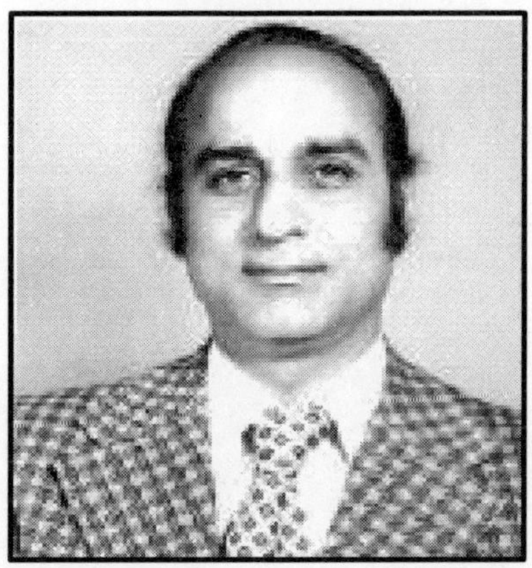

Prof. C. K. Atal

Former Director, Indian Institute of Integrative Medicine, Jammu
(Erstwhile, Regional Research Laboratory, Jammu)

AMITY
We nurture talent

AMITY INSTITUTE FOR HERBAL AND BIOTECH PRODUCTS DEVELOPMENT

– An Institution of Ritnand Balved Education Foundation –
Thiruvananthapuram

Prof. (Dr.) P. PUSHPANGADAN
M.Sc, M.Phil, Ph.D., FBRS, FES, FNRS, FNSE, FNESA, FNAASc, FNASc., (UN Equator Initiative Laureate)
Director General & Senior Vice President, RBEF
(Former Director, NBRI, Lucknow)

Foreword

With the growing demand and popularity of herbal drugs and the wide use of plant derived phyto-molecules in modern medicine, in recent times, there has been great demand for medicinal plants in the drug industry.

The gap between demand and supply are widening in the herbal drug industry. Until recently, the demands for raw materials were mostly met from wild naturally growing plants. Owing to various reasons, particularly because of habitat destruction and shrinking of forest area, it is no longer possible to meet the requirement of medicinal plants from wild or natural sources. This book–*Utilisation and Management of Medicinal Plants* edited by Dr. Anil K. Verma and Dr. Sushma Koul with Dr. V.K. Gupta as Editor-in-chief is a valuable and timely attempt to bring together expert opinions and ideas for the Utilisation and Management of Medicinal Plants in a single volume.

There are twenty one chapters in this book. The editors have invited eminent scientists from all over the world to contribute chapters for the book. The contributed chapters cover a wide range of subjects related to the management and utilisation of medicinal plants such as biotechnology, phytochemistry, plant-physiology, fungal metabolites, bioactivity of secondary metabolites, anti-bacterial and anti-fungal activity of secondary metabolites, bio-prospecting etc. Each chapter in the book is contributed by eminent scientists who have been working in the relevant areas for a considerable period.

No. 3, Ravi Nagar, Ambalamukku
Peroorkada P.O
Thiruvananthapuram - 695 005
Kerala

Tel: (0471) 3269772, 2432138, 2432148
Mob: 0-98950 66816
E-mail: palpuprakulam@yahoo.co.in

This book, I am glad to see, is dedicated to Dr. C.K. Atal, a towering figure in the study of medicinal plants and their bioactive secondary metabolites. As Director of Regional Research Laboratory, Jammu which is now known as Indian Institute of Integrative Medicine, Dr. Atal inspired a generation of young scientists to devote their life in the study of medicinal and aromatic plants. Under his leadership and guidance, several scientific discoveries in natural sciences, especially discovery of a large number of bioactive molecules, novel mechanisms of drug action etc were carried out. He instilled confidence and inspiration in his colleagues, co-workers and students. Being a visionary with a brilliant, intuitive and analytical mind, Dr. Atal, encouraged his co-workers to tread untravelled paths which yielded great dividends in terms of research publications, discovery of novel bioactivities, molecules, new drugs and perfumery products, patents and recognition. Prof. Atal has been known to me from 1969 onwards. I had the privilege of working in his team from 1969 to 1989 at IIIM. All these years, I had very close association with Prof. (Dr.) C.K. Atal. It is with his blessings and good wishes that I have grown up in the scientific ladder. Hence I have immense pleasure in writing this foreword to a publication dedicated to Dr. C.K.Atal.

I complement the editors as well as the authors for their valuable contribution. This book will be of immense value and use to students, researchers and professionals engaged in the study and utilisation of medicinal and aromatic plants.

P. Pushpangadan

Preface

Nature has provided mankind with products for good health since the beginning of time. For thousands of years medicine and natural products have been closely linked through the use of traditional medicines and natural poisons (Newman *et al.*, 2000). Plants hold a prominent position in the available sources of natural bioactive molecules. Clinical, pharmacological, and chemical studies of traditional medicines, derived predominantly from plants, were the basis of most early medicines such as aspirin, digitoxin, morphine, quinine, emetine, and pilocarpine. Approximately 25 per cent of the drugs prescribed worldwide come from plants, whereas 11 per cent of the 252 drugs considered as basic and essential by the World Health Organization (WHO) derive their origin exclusively from plants. Prescription drugs containing phytochemicals were valued at more than US$ 30 billion in 2002 in the US alone.

Eighty percent of the people in developing countries rely on traditional medicines for primary health care. Development of phyto-therapeutic during last few decades has evolved into a science itself and is undergoing further change. The traditional, complementary and the alternative medicine is attracting more and more attention within the context of health care provision and health sector reforms. Many of the Botanicals as ingredients have histories of prior human. These components are already being used in food as dietary ingredients, in traditional system of medicine for different ailments or as food and medicine both. Obliviously the food substances are considered to be safe and nourishing, for those which are having medicinal properties and are described for treatment of specific alignments, proper procedure to eliminate adulteration, contamination and toxic side effects are needed. Worldwide need of alternative medicine and growth of natural product inserts the traditional systems of medicine into markets. The traditional medicines are slowly being integrated into modern medicine in the form of dietary and nutritional supplements and the scientific community is challenged to address the issues of utility, safety, quality efficacy and standardization.

During the last few decades, public interest in natural therapies has increased tremendously around the world and natural bioresource as therapeutic has evolved into a science and is undergoing faster changes. The challenge today is transforming the long history of experience-based medicine in evidence based medicine. Indeed, the lack of readily accessible information on how much of what medicinal plant biodiversity occurs where has become a limiting factor in conservation planning and converting our biowealth into economic wealth. Over harvesting from forests, deforestation and other anthropogenic factors have already placed several species at risk.

Since new diseases as well as drug-resistant strains of known pathogens continue to emerge, the search for novel compounds in combating many diseases and conditions is continuing globally. The scientific integration of herbal medicinal into modern medical practices must take into account the interrelated issues of quantitative and qualitative assessment of bioresource, mass production and its appropriate use. The current worldwide trend towards the utilisation of natural remedied has created an enormous need for information about the properties and uses of natural resources.

In the present book *"Utilisation and Management of Medicinal Plants"* an attempt has been made to encapsulate scientific information pertaining to modern-day drug research and this effort is likely to serve as a catalyst for the development of innovative methodologies and approaches for further studies, paving the way for discovery of novel drug for various human ailments.

The topics have been contributed by the experts in the field with exhaustive, relevant and up-to-date information. It is hoped the book be a useful resource of knowledge for ethnobotanists, pharmacologists, biochemists, physiologists, agronomists, medicinal researchers, pharmaceutical scientists and people of allied disciplines engaged in research new drugs of plant origin. We are greatly indebted to the scientists and researchers who have contributed for this volume.

V. K. Gupta

Anil K. Verma

Sushma Koul

Contents

Utilisation and Management of Medicinal Plants (2010) *Pages 1–31*
Editors: **V.K. Gupta, Anil K. Verma and Sushma Koul**
Published by: **DAYA PUBLISHING HOUSE, NEW DELHI**

Chapter 1

Biotechnological Interventions for Enhancing the Availability of High Value Medicinal Plants

Nishritha Bopana[1] and Sanjay Saxena[2*]
[1]TERI University, Darbari Seth Block, Habitat Place, Lodhi Road, New Delhi – 110 003, India
[2]The Energy and Resources Institute (TERI), Darbari Seth Block, Habitat Place, Lodhi Road, New Delhi – 110 003, India

ABSTRACT

The indiscriminate harvesting of medicinal plants from the wild and the problems associated with conventional methods of propagation have pushed several species to the brink of extinction. This could translate into a tremendous loss to the world of modern as well as traditional systems of medicine. Bearing in mind the threat of extinction that looms large on this important natural resource, it has now become prudent to undertake germplasm conservation of medicinal plants. In addition, a large number of plant species are yet to be screened for active compounds highlighting the fact that the importance of medicinal plants as a resource would only grow further in the future.

This article attempts to review the various biotechnological interventions that have contributed in enhancing the availability of various economically important plant material for *e.g.* medicinal plants. For good quality produce, consistency in quality and quantity of planting material assumes paramount importance. This can be ensured by identifying elites through the application of molecular marker techniques and chemoprofiling followed by mass multiplication

* Corresponding Author: Tel: 91-11-24682100; Fax: 91-11-24682144; E-mail sanjays@teri.res.in.

using both conventional and biotechnological approaches. Furthermore, optimization of climatic conditions and development of appropriate agro-techniques would enhance the overall produce thereby assuring a higher remuneration to the growers. This in turn would encourage farmers to undertake commercial cultivation thus curbing the overexploitation of these plants from wild, and thereby complement the conservation process.

Keywords: *Agrobacterium, Conservation, Elites, Medicinal plants, Micropropagation, Secondary metabolites.*

Introduction

The use of plants as medicines has been well documented in the history of all civilizations. In the recent past, there has been a renewed public interest in complementary and alternative medicines as a result of increased side effects observed in the allopathic system of medicine. In addition, lack of curative treatments for several chronic diseases, high cost of new drugs and microbial resistance have caused a tremendous increase in the demand for plant-based medicines (Patwardhan *et al.*, 2005).

The international market for medicinal plants is to the tune of US$ 60 billion with an annual growth rate of 7 per cent (Belt *et al.*, 2003). According to the World Bank report of 1998, world trade in medicinal plants and related products is expected to touch US$ 5 trillion by AD 2050 (cited in Tewari, 2000). Indiscriminate harvesting of medicinal plants from the wild to meet the ever-increasing demand, and the problems associated with conventional methods of propagation have pushed several species to the brink of extinction. The IUCN Red list of threatened plants published by the World Conservation Union includes 12,043 species, of which 87 are extinct, 27 are extinct in the wild, 4,600 are critically endangered, endangered or vulnerable and the rest near-threatened or conservation dependent (IUCN, 2007). This could translate into a tremendous loss to the world of modern as well as traditional systems of medicine. Bearing in mind the threat of extinction that looms large on this important natural resource, germplasm conservation of medicinal plants has become necessary for preventing genetic erosion. According to the International Board for Plant Genetic Resources (IBPGR), medicinal plant species figure high in the priority list for *in vitro* conservation (Staritsky, 1997). In addition, a large number of plant species are yet to be screened for active compounds highlighting the fact that the importance of medicinal plants as a resource would only grow further in the future.

In India, medicinal plants as a group comprise approximately 8000 species and account for around 50 per cent of all the higher flowering plant species. In terms of the volume and value of medicinal plants exported, India ranks second in the world, next only to China, which tops the list of exporting countries. Projections of global trade in medicinal plants indicate a steep upward trend for the future. Also, in India there is a substantial volume of internal trade in medicinal plants, a large part of which is in the informal unorganized sector and hence it is virtually impossible to assess the current volume of trade in the domestic market. There are 7800 medicinal drug-manufacturing units in India consuming about 2000 tonnes of herbs annually (Singh, 2001). 95 per cent of medicinal plant collection to meet the demands of the pharmaceutical industry is from the wild, 70 per cent of the times by destructive harvesting which leads to depletion of the valuable genetic resources base (Tewari, 2000). Pharmaceutical companies too contribute to inefficient, imperfect and opportunistic marketing of medicinal plants. Since the prices paid to the gatherers (generally villagers) are low; they often 'mine' the plant resources rather than 'manage' them as their main objective is to generate a higher income. As a result, several medicinal plants have been assessed as endangered, vulnerable and threatened due to over or improper harvesting. Habitat destruction on account of deforestation is an added danger. As per IUCN guidelines, there are around 200 species of medicinal plants that are rare, endangered and threatened in the northern and southern parts of India (Shankar, 1998).

Since the value of medicinal plants lies in the amount of the active principle present in it, it is desirable to undertake cultivation of superior clones (recognized as 'elite') containing higher amount of active principle. This can be ensured by identifying elites through chemoprofiling followed by mass multiplication using both conventional and biotechnological approaches. Various chromatographic techniques have been applied for identification and quantification of secondary metabolites in medicinal plants. Thin Layer Chromatography was used for the detection of secondary metabolites from *Camptotheca acuminata* (Hengel *et al.*, 1992), *Ruta* species (Baumert *et al.*, 1992) and *Hypericum perforatum* (Smith *et al.*, 2002). High Performance Liquid Chromatography (HPLC) with photodiode array detector has been used to screen secondary metabolites in *Catharanthus roseus* (Tikhomiroff *et al.*, 2002). It has also been used by several workers (Chen *et al.*, 1999; Xie *et al.*, 2000) to identify and quantify artemisinin from *Artemisia annua* which is a high value, potent anti-malarial. Reverse-phase HPLC has been used in detecting five major kavapyrones in *Piper methysticum* (Smith *et al.*, 2002).

Furthermore, optimization of climatic conditions and development of appropriate agro-techniques would enhance the overall produce thereby assuring a higher remuneration to the growers. This in turn would encourage farmers to undertake commercial cultivation thus reducing the overexploitation of these plants from wild, and thereby complement the conservation process. A multi-pronged approach for conservation as has been diagrammatically represented in Figure 1.1 could well provide a practical solution.

Biotechnological Approaches

The use of biotechnological approaches that include micropropagation, cell culture and transgenic technology, would greatly facilitate conservation and sustainable utilization of genetic diversity of medicinal plants.

Micropropagation

Micropropagation is a viable alternative for species which are difficult to regenerate by conventional methods; where populations have shrunken due to over-exploitation by destructive harvesting; where there is a lot of variability in terms of the active principles present, and, where elites have been identified based on their potential for yielding higher amount of active principle.

The success of micropropagation greatly depends upon the selection of the stock or mother plant and therefore, this aspect should be carefully looked into before starting with any tissue culture work. Since the value of medicinal plants lies in the amount of the active principle present in it, the choice of the donor plant is particularly important. Therefore, elites should be identified by chemo-profiling prior to beginning the micropropagation process. In addition, the age of the plant, the season in which the explants are collected, the surface sterilization procedures etc. need to be optimized for best results.

There are three main approaches for the multiplication of medicinal plants through tissue culture. The first is induction from explants having a pre-existing meristem (axillary proliferation); the second approach involves initiation of adventitious shoots (organogenesis); and, the third system of propagation is somatic embryogenesis.

Axillary Shoot Proliferation

Axillary shoot proliferation is a method involving induction of shoots from explants having a pre-existing meristem and thus is less prone to genetic variations (somaclonal variations) that might

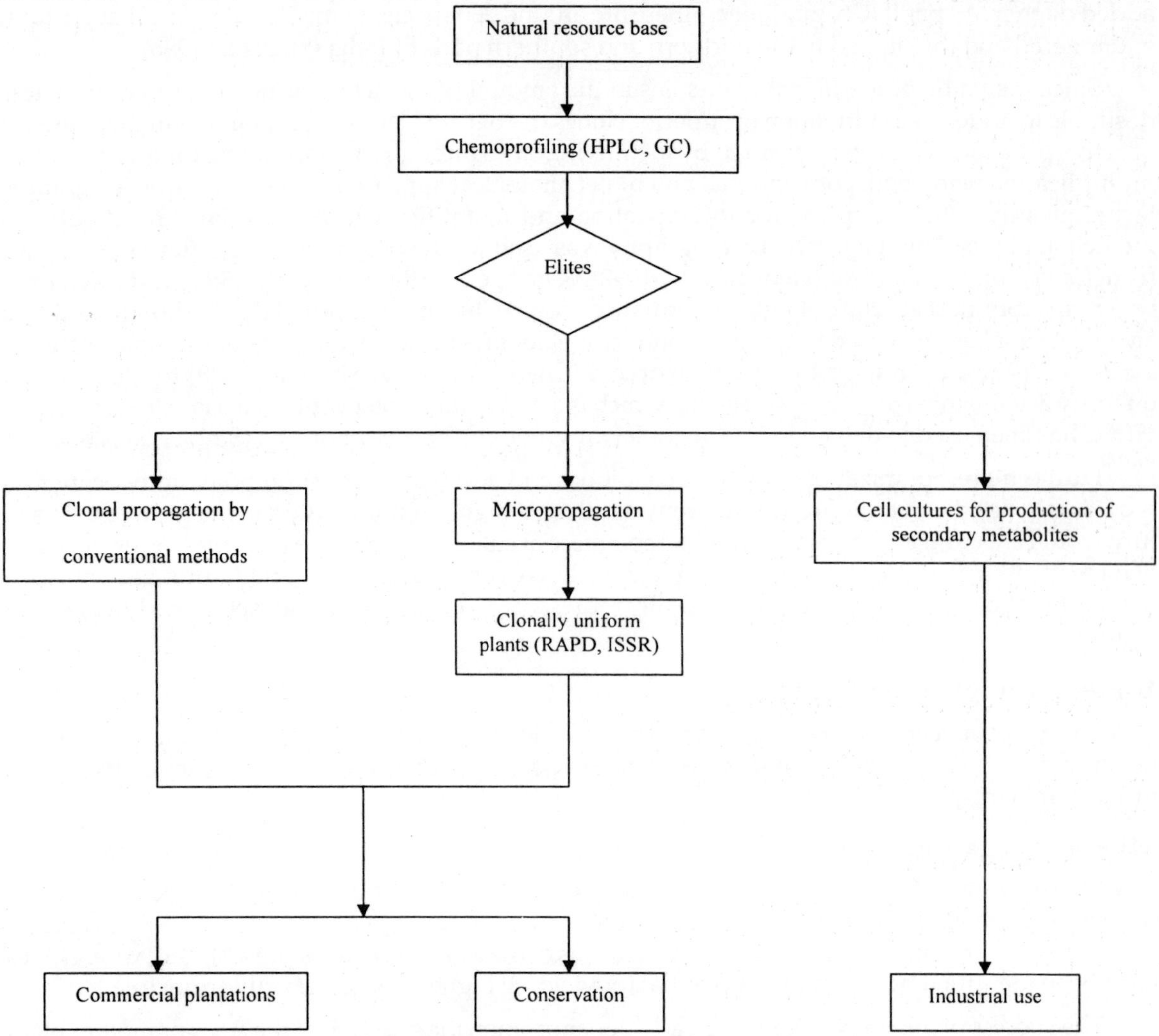

Figure 1.1: Multifaceted Strategy for the Conservation and Sustainable Utilization of Medicinal Plants (Bopana and Saxena, 2007)

occur during cell division or differentiation under *in vitro* conditions (Shenoy and Vasil, 1992). For this reason, this is the most preferred method for micropropagation.

Each axillary bud present in the axil of the leaf has the potential to develop into a shoot. In nature, these axillary buds remain dormant for various periods depending upon the growth pattern of the plant. In species with strong apical dominance, the removal or injury of the terminal bud is necessary to stimulate the lateral axillary buds to grow out into shoots. In culture, the rate of shoot multiplication by axillary branching can be substantially enhanced by culturing shoots in a medium containing suitable cytokinin/s with or without an auxin at appropriate concentrations. Initially, the multiplication rates achieved by this method may be low but with each passage the number of shoots increases logarithmically.

The type of explant used is one of the major factors affecting the multiplication rate. Nodal explants were found to be superior to apical shoot buds in *Melia azedarach* (Thakur *et al.*, 1998), *Rauwolfia micrantha* (Sudha and Seeni, 1996) and *Woodfordia fruticosa* (Krishnan and Seeni, 1994). Kumar *et al.* (2005) observed an improved morphogenic response when explants from seedling raised *in vitro* shoots were employed instead of mature trees in *Holarrhena antidysenterica*. Explant orientation is another factor that was found to be important in achieving optimal shoot multiplication in certain species such as *Rauwolfia micrantha* (Sudha and Seeni, 1996). In *Lilium nepalense* and *Allium wallichi*, Wawrosch *et al.* (2001a, 2001b) observed that longitudinally split shoot halves gave a better response as compared to whole shoot explants. In *Adathoda beddomei* too, Sudha and Seeni (1994) had observed that vertical halves of pre-cultured nodes yielded a larger aggregate number of shoots as compared to the intact pre-cultured node.

Under the influence of growth hormones, the *in vitro* formed shoots give rise to additional axillary shoots. In literature, benzyl amino purine (BAP) has been reported to be the most effective hormone in inducing multiplication, and hence has been used in the micropropagation of several species such as *Holarrhena antidysenterica* (Kumar *et al.*, 2005), *Chlorophytum borivilianum* (Dave *et al.*, 2003), *Ocimum americanum* and *O. canum* (Pattnaik and Chand, 1996). BAP was found to be better than Kinetin (Kn) and 2-isopentenyl adenine (2ip) in *Crataeva magna* (Benniamin *et al.*, 2004), *Orthosiphon stamineus* (LaiKeng and WaiLeng, 2004) and *Picrorhiza kurroa* (Upadhyay *et al.*, 1989).

Tiwari *et al.* (2001) studied the effect of four cytokinins namely, BAP, thidiazuron (TDZ), Kn and 2ip on multiple shoot induction in *Bacopa monniera* and found TDZ to be best for optimal shoot bud formation. In certain cases, a combination of two or more cytokinins yielded higher multiplication rates as compared to individual cytokinins. In *Eclipta alba*, a combination of BAP, Kn and 2ip was found to be essential for shoot proliferation (Baskaran and Jayabalan, 2005). Studies have demonstrated a synergistic effect between auxins and cytokinins on shoot multiplication in various species. Chueh *et al.* (2001) achieved multiple shoot formation in *Gentiana davidii* on MS (Murashige and Skoog, 1962) medium supplemented with BAP and 1-naphthalene acetic acid (NAA). In *Withania somnifera*, maximum shoots were obtained when 2,4-dichlorophenoxyacetic acid (2,4D) or indole 3-butyric acid (IBA) was added to the medium containing BAP during shoot multiplication (Sen and Sharma, 1991). Sudha and Seeni (1994) observed shoot multiplication of *Adathoda beddomei* to be a function of cytokinin activity but found sustained growth of shoots to be dependent on the combined influence of BAP with indole 3-acetic acid (IAA). Similar observations have also been made in *Saussurea obvallata* (Joshi and Dhar, 2003), *Aegle marmelos* (Ajithkumar and Seeni, 1998), *Acacia catechu* (Kaur *et al.*, 1998), *Alpinia galanga* (Anand and Hariharan, 1997), *Rauwolfia micrantha* (Sudha and Seeni, 1996) and *Valeriana wallichi* (Mathur *et al.*, 1988).

In order to improve the shoot multiplication rate, the use of additives has been attempted in several studies. Addition of ascorbic acid was found to be necessary to induce sprouting of axillary buds of *Tylophora indica*. MS medium supplemented with IBA and adenine sulphate ($AdSO_4$) was found to be essential for bud-break and shoot development in *Plumbago zeylenica* (Selvakumar *et al.*, 2001). Gibberellic acid (GA_3) along with coconut water in the multiplication medium containing BAP, Kn and 2ip was found to enhance both shoot number and shoot length in *Eclipta alba* (Baskaran and Jayabalan, 2005). Barve and Mehta (1993) observed highest shoot multiplication in *Commiphora wightii* on MS medium supplemented with BAP, Kn, glutamine, thiamine, HCl and 0.3 per cent activated charcoal (AC). Kumar *et al.* (2005) found that silver nitrate significantly improved shoot multiplication of *Holarrhena antidysenterica* in the presence of BAP. The nature of gelling agent too was observed to play an important role in shoot proliferation. In most studies agar (0.6 per cent–0.8 per cent; a complex mixture of related polysaccharides built up from galactose) is used as the gelling agent. Dave *et al.* (2003) observed that Phytagel™ (a linear polysaccharide produced by the bacterium *Pseudomonas elodea*) at 0.2 per cent gave a marginally better response in *Chlorophytum borivilianum* than BDH™ agar in terms of shoot multiplication but the latter was more cost effective. In certain plant species, liquid medium has been found to be more responsive for shoot multiplication as compared to semi-solid medium. Use of floating membrane rafts for micropropagation of *Aconitum napellus* resulted in 45 per cent higher shoot proliferation than on semi-solid medium (Watad *et al.*, 1995). Similar responses have been reported in *Isoplexis isabelliana* (Arrebola and Verpoorte, 2002) and *Rheum emodi* (Lal and Ahuja, 1989).

Organogenesis

Buds arising from any place other than the leaf axil or shoot apex are termed as 'adventitious' buds. Adventitious shoot regeneration has been well documented in several medicinal plants. However, it is known to affect genetic uniformity and gives rise to somaclonal variants due to genome re-arrangements. At the same time somaclonal variation provides an additional source of genetic variability, useful in improvement and selection programmes.

Adventitious shoot regeneration can take place either directly from a plant organ (direct organogenesis) or a piece thereof, or through an intervening callus phase (indirect organogenesis). Direct regeneration has been accomplished from leaf in *Plumbago* species, *Pothomorphe umbellata* and *Aristolochia indica* (Vanegas *et al.*, 2002; Das and Rout, 2002a; Pereira *et al.*, 2000; Manjula *et al.*, 1997), shoot tip and inflorescence in *Limonium wrightii* (Huang *et al.*, 2000), petiole in *Thapsia garganica* (Makunga *et al.*, 2003) and root explants in *Tylophora indica* (Chaudhuri *et al.*, 2004). Indirect regeneration has also been achieved from different explants such as shoot tips in *Limonium wrightii* and *Rheum emodi* (Huang *et al.*, 2000; Lal and Ahuja, 1989), hypocotyls in *Acacia sinuata* and *Echinacea purpurea* (Vengadesan *et al.*, 2000; Coker and Camper, 2000), roots in *Saussurea obvallata*, *Tylophora indica*, *Withania somnifera* and *Swertia chirata* (Dhar and Joshi, 2005; Chaudhuri *et al.*, 2004; Rani and Grover, 1999; Wawrosch *et al.*, 1999), leaf in *Echinacea pallida*, *Tylophora indica*, *Echinacea purpurea*, *Plumbago* species, *Plumbago zeylanica*, *Centella asiatica* and *Aristolochia indica* (Koroch *et al.*, 2003; Faisal and Anis, 2003; Koroch *et al.*, 2002; Rout, 2002; Rout *et al.*, 1999; Patra *et al.*, 1998; Manjula *et al.*, 1997), internode in *Centella asiatica* and *Aristolochia indica* (Patra *et al.*, 1998; Manjula *et al.*, 1997), immature zygotic embryo cotyledons in *Salvia sclarea* (Liu *et al.*, 2000), leaf bases in *Curcuma longa* (Salvi *et al.*, 2001), anther in *Azadirachta indica* (Gautam *et al.*, 1993), seeds in *Hybanthus enneaspermus* (Prakash *et al.*, 1999) and inflorescence in *Ocimum sanctum* (Singh and Sehgal, 1999).

The explant used for the initiation of callus exhibits a significant influence on organogenesis. Dhar and Joshi (2005) studied the effect of different explants such as root, hypocotyl, cotyledon and leaf on callus formation and plant regeneration in *Saussurea obvallata*. They observed 100 per cent callusing and 100 per cent differentiation using leaf explants. Joshi *et al.* (2004) found that the cotyledonary explants of *Heracleum candicans* responded better than cotyledonary node explants for organogenesis. Martin *et al.* (2002) found that callus from basal cut ends of nodes of *Holostemma ada-kodien* gave a larger number of shoots as compared to callus from internodal explants. Leaf-derived callus on the other hand did not undergo organogenesis. Li *et al.* (2000) observed more regenerants along hypocotyls of intact seedlings as against excised hypocotyls of *Scutellaria baicalensis*. Thengane *et al.* (2001) found that leaf explants of *Nothapodytes foetida* formed more adventitious shoots followed by hypocotyls and cotyledons. *In vitro* derived leaves were found to be better explants than those obtained from field-grown plants for shoot regeneration in *Bacopa monnieri* (Shrivastava and Rajani,

1999). Rani and Grover (1999) found that axillary shoot base-derived callus gave best shoot differentiation as compared to callus initiated from leaves, hypocotyls and root segments in *Withania somnifera*. Wawrosch *et al.* (1999) however, found the adventitious shoot regeneration in *Swertia chirata* to be best from root explants.

The type of growth regulators used significantly influence adventitious shoot formation. For callus formation, auxins such as 2,4D and NAA have been commonly used with or without cytokinins such as BAP and Kn. 2,4D in combination with BAP has been used for callus formation in *Acacia sinuata* (Vengadesan *et al.*, 2000) and *Hypericum perforatum* (Pretto and Santarém, 2000); NAA with BAP has been used to obtain callus from leaf tissue of *Echinacea purpurea* (Koroch *et al.*, 2002) and *Hybanthus enneaspermus* (Prakash *et al.*, 1999); while NAA in combination with Kn has been used in *Centella asiatica* (Patra *et al.*, 1998). Phloroglucinol (PG) has been used in combination with auxins and cytokinins in *Aristolochia indica* to avoid phenolic accumulation during callus formation (Manjula *et al.*, 1997). Salvi *et al.* (2001) initiated callus cultures from leaf bases of turmeric on MS medium supplemented with picloram, dicamba or NAA in combination with BAP. Bonfill *et al.* (2002) found that 2,4D inhibited the organogenic capacity of *Panax ginseng* calli while IBA and IAA enhanced it. Rout *et al.* (1999) used BAP and IAA to initiate callus in *Plumbago zeylanica,* while Faisal and Anis (2003) used 2,4,5 Trichlorophenoxyacetic acid (2,4,5T) for the same purpose in *Tylophora indica*. In the presence of IAA and BAP, the percentage of callus obtained from anthers of *Azadirachta indica* was higher on Nitsch medium than on MS medium (Gautam *et al.*, 1993).

For shoot differentiation either directly or through calli, various growth regulators have been used. Nin *et al.* (1996) observed that the initiation of shoot and root primordia of *Artemisia annua* occurred directly on 2,4D medium but adventitious shoot formation from callus was observed when BAP was added to the medium along with IAA. Kn in combination with 2,4D has been used in *Hypericum perforatum* (Pretto and Santarém, 2000) and with NAA in *Echinacea purpurea* (Coker and Camper, 2000) for differentiation purposes. Several additives too have been used to improve the regeneration frequencies. Vengadesan *et al.* (2000) used 10 per cent coconut water with BAP and IAA for inducing regeneration in *Acacia sinuata* while Subbaiah *et al.* (2003) used 5 per cent coconut milk with BAP in *Echinacea purpurea*. $AdSO_4$ was added to medium containing BAP, Kn and NAA for regeneration in *Centella asiatica* (Patra *et al.*, 1998) and in *Plumbago rosea* (Das and Rout, 2002a). Murch *et al.* (2000) reported TDZ-induced plant regeneration from hypocotyls of *Hypericum perforatum*. TDZ has also been used in *Nothapodytes foetida* by Thengane *et al.* (2001). In *Hybanthus enneaspermus,* Prakash *et al.* (1999) found the addition of casein hydrolysate (CH) and potassium phosphate to enhance shoot differentiation from callus.

Somatic Embryogenesis

Somatic embryogenesis is the process of embryo initiation and development from vegetative and non-gametic cells (Bhojwani and Razdan, 1996). Since the first observation of *in vitro* somatic embryogenesis in *Daucus carota* (Reinert, 1958; Steward *et al.*, 1958), it has been attempted in several other species as well. Somatic embryos can arise either directly from the cells of the explant as in *Eleutherococcus senticosus* (Choi *et al.*, 1999), *Bupleurum scorzonerifolium* (Guang-min *et al.*, 1992), *Panax ginseng* (Arya *et al.*, 1993) and *Acanthopanax senticosus* (Gui *et al.*, 1991); or through an intervening callus phase as in the case of *Holostemma ada-kodien* (Martin, 2003a), *Bacopa monniera* (Tiwari *et al.*, 1998), *Panax notoginseng* (Shoyama *et al.*, 1997) to name a few.

Somatic embryogenesis has several advantages over organogenesis. Since somatic embryos are bipolar structures, a separate rooting stage gets eliminated. Their small and uniform size makes them more amenable to automation at the multiplication stage and for field planting as synthetic seeds. Also unlike microcuttings, somatic embryos can be cryopreserved or desiccated for long-term storage. In addition, these plants are derived from meristematic cells that are genetically stable by nature and, therefore, there is a strong selection pressure in favour of generating clonal populations.

Explant selection plays a vital role in initiation (raising embryogenic cultures) and multiplication of somatic embryos in medicinal plants. This process of *in vitro* regeneration has been attempted using a variety of explants such as leaf in *Centella asiatica, Holostemma ada-kodien, Gymnema sylvestre, Plumbago rosea, Tylophora indica* and *Bacopa monniera* (Paramageetham *et al.*, 2004; Martin, 2003a; Kumar *et al.*, 2002; Das and Rout, 2002b; Manjula 2000; Tiwari *et al.*, 1998), cotyledon in *Gymnema sylvestre* and *Eleutherococcus senticosus* (Kumar *et al.*, 2002; Choi *et al.*, 1999), seeds in *Eschscholzia californica* and *Azadirachta indica* (Park and Facchini, 2004; Murthy *et al.*, 1998), hypocotyls in siberian ginseng and *Gymnema sylvestre* (Choi *et al.*, 2002; Kumar *et al.*, 2002), root in *Holostemma ada-kodien*, siberian ginseng and *Psoralea corylifolia* (Martin, 2003a; Choi *et al.*, 2002; Chand and Sahrawat, 2002), immature zygotic embryos in *Serenoa repens, Ginkgo biloba* and *Panax ginseng* (Gallo-Meagher and Green, 2002; Laurain *et al.*, 1996; Arya *et al.*, 1993), anthers in *Aconitum carmichaeli* (Hatano *et al.*, 1987) and protoplasts in *Bupleurum scorzonerifolium* and *Panax ginseng* (Guang-min *et al.*, 1992; Arya *et al.*, 1991). Choi *et al.* (1999) found that in *Eleutherococcus senticosus*, the frequency of somatic embryo formation was highest in the hypocotyl segments (75 per cent) as compared to cotyledon (56 per cent) or root segments (12 per cent). 93 per cent somatic embryos obtained from explants (zygotic embryos) are in the fused state, while 89 per cent somatic embryos from more developed seedlings were in the single state. Fereol *et al.* (2002) found that although root sections of *Allium sativum* produced the maximum amount of callus, however, it was the callus obtained from young leaves that expressed higher embryogenic potential. Zobayed and Saxena (2003a) found that exposing the abaxial surface of the leaves to media increased the number of somatic embryos formed in *Echinacea purpurea*.

Although in majority of the cases, MS medium has been used for somatic embryogenesis; success has also been reported on White's medium (Sata *et al.*, 2000), B5 medium (Fereol *et al.*, 2002) and Linsmaier and Skoog medium (Ignacimuthu *et al.*, 1999).

Almost all of the systems studied for somatic embryogenesis required a synthetic auxin for somatic embryo induction and 2,4D has been most commonly used for this purpose (Martin, 2003a; Manjula, 2001; Choi *et al.*, 1999; Wakhlu and Sharma, 1998; Gui *et al.*, 1991). Culturing explants in the presence of auxins results in the formation of more than one type of callus and it is important to select and separate the embryogenic callus from other tissues including the non-embryogenic callus at an early stage. Embryogenic callus is usually nodular in appearance as in *Psoralea corylifolia* (Chand and Sahrawat, 2002). On an auxin-rich medium, the callus differentiates localized clusters of meristematic cells termed 'proembryogenic masses' (PEMs). Therefore, an auxin rich medium is favoured for induction of somatic embryogenesis. Auxins other than 2,4D, such as IAA (Choffe *et al.*, 2000b), IBA (Zobayed and Saxena, 2003a) and NAA (Chand and Sahrawat, 2002) have also been used for induction purposes. Laurain *et al.* (1996) observed direct embryogenesis on cotyledons of *Gingko biloba* in the presence of only BAP in the induction medium. The addition of NAA to this BAP containing medium led to indirect embryogenesis. However, in *Corydalis yanhusuo*, Sagare *et al.* (2000) demonstrated cytokinin-induced somatic embryogenesis on MS medium containing BAP, Kn or zeatin. Murthy *et al.* (1998) induced somatic embryogenesis by using TDZ in *Azadirachta indica*. In *Eleutherococcus senticosus*, Choi *et al.* (1999) produced somatic embryos from cotyledon explants directly on medium without growth regulators.

ABA was added for somatic embryo induction in *Taxus brevifolia* (Chee, 1996). Rao and Bahadur (1990) found ascorbic acid to promote somatic embryo induction in *Oldenlandia umbellata* and AC had a similar action in *Taxus brevifolia* (Chee, 1996). Das (Pal) and Raychaudhuri (2001) found that CH and coconut water promoted the growth of embryogenic cultures of *Plantago ovata* but at supra-optimal doses caused eventual death of embryos.

For embryo development to occur, the PEMs need to be transferred to a low auxin or basal medium. Subsequent conversion of somatic embryos into plantlets occurred on media supplemented with GA_3, BAP and IBA in *Psoralea corylifolia*, *Eryngium foetidum* and *Aconitum carmichaeli* (Chand and Sahrawat, 2002; Ignacimuthu *et al.*, 1999; Hatano *et al.*, 1987). Addition of $AgNO_3$ to half strength MS medium significantly improved embryo maturation in *Andrographis paniculata* (Martin, 2004). A similar promotory effect was observed in the presence of ABA in *Heracleum candicans* (Wakhlu and Sharma, 1998). Maturation and germination of embryos was also found to be influenced by the sucrose concentration of the medium as in *Eleutherococcus sessiliflorus* (Choi *et al.*, 2002). In the presence of 1 per cent sucrose, maturation and germination of embryos occurred readily while at over 6 per cent, somatic embryos did not germinate. However, this could be overcome by GA_3 treatment. In *Corydalis yanhusuo*, Sagare *et al.* (2000) used 6 per cent sucrose for conversion of somatic embryos to plantlets and tuber formation. A reduction in sucrose concentration from 3 per cent to 1.5 per cent was essential for somatic embryo formation in *Piper nigrum* (Joseph *et al.*, 1996) while on the other hand a sucrose concentration of 10 per cent was necessary in *Panax ginseng* (Asaka *et al.*, 1994). Jung *et al.* (2004) observed that Siberian ginseng embryos encapsulated with 2 per cent sucrose and 1 per cent starch powder enhanced the post-germinative growth of encapsulated embryos. Choi and Jeong (2002) demonstrated induced dormancy in Siberian ginseng embryos under high osmotic stress in 9 per cent sucrose. Langhansova *et al.* (2004) found that *Panax ginseng* somatic embryos treated with ABA and polyethylene glycol showed 70 per cent shoot regeneration as against a mere 31 per cent in untreated somatic embryos. Also, 75 per cent plants regenerated from PEG and ABA treated embryos formed roots while non-treated embryos did not.

Since the multiplication of embryogenic cells and the subsequent development of somatic embryos can occur in liquid medium, somatic embryogenesis offers a potential system for large-scale plant propagation in automated bioreactors (Bhojwani and Razdan, 1996). The first attempt to scale up somatic embryogenesis was done with carrot cells by Backs-Husemann and Reinert (1970). Choi *et al.* (2002) described a process for the mass production of Siberian ginseng plants by large-scale tank cultures. Using the same protocol, about 12,000 embryos were produced per 500ml flask after 4 weeks of culture. Park *et al.* (2005) established large-scale bioreactor cultures for somatic embryo production of *Eleutherococcus koreanum*.

Once the shoots have been multiplied, for rooting, in certain medicinal plants such as *Tylophora indica* (Chaudhuri *et al.*, 2004), *Scopolia parviflora* (Kang *et al.*, 2004), *Ochreinauclea missionis* (Dalal and Rai, 2001) and *Alpinia galanga* (Borthakur *et al.*, 1998), elongation of regenerated shoots was performed on hormone free MS medium. However, in *Gymnema elegans* (Komalavalli and Rao, 1997), *Ocimum americanum* and *O. sanctum* (Pattnaik and Chand, 1996) shoot elongation was obtained by the use of additives such as GA_3, $AdSO_4$, ascorbic acid, coconut milk and calcium pantothenate, biotin etc. prior to being placed on rooting medium.

It is a common practice to transfer shoots from a high to low strength media in order to induce rooting. Half-strength MS medium without growth regulators has been attempted for rooting purposes in several medicinal plants such as *Crataeva nurvala* (Walia *et al.*, 2007; Benniamin *et al.*, 2004), *Echinacea purpurea* (Koroch *et al.*, 2002), *Decalepsis hamiltonii* (Reddy *et al.*, 2001), turmeric (Salvi *et al.*, 2001), *Hypericum perforatum* (Pretto and Santarém, 2000), *Swertia chirata* (Wawrosch *et al.*, 1999) and *Artemisia pallens* (Benjamin *et al.*, 1990). In many species such as *Lavandula vera* (Andrade *et al.*, 1999) and *Chlorophytum borivilianum* (Purohit *et al.*, 1994), root formation was found to be better when shoots were rooted on low strength MS medium.

For *in vitro* rooting of regenerated shoots, different auxins have been attempted such as IBA in *Artemisia judaica* (Liu *et al.*, 2003), *Tylophora indica* (Faisal and Anis, 2003), *Holostemma ada-kodien* (Martin, 2002), *Plumbago* (Das and Rout, 2002a) and *Hybanthus enneaspermus* (Prakash *et al.*, 1999); NAA in *Rotula aquatica* (Martin, 2003b) and *Saussurea lappa* (Arora and Bhojwani, 1989), and, IAA in *Tylophora indica* (Chaudhuri *et al.*, 2004), *Plumbago zeylanica* (Rout *et al.*, 1999) and *Centella asiatica* (Patra *et al.*, 1998).

Dipping of rootable shoots in high concentrations of auxins (pulse treatment) such as NAA and IBA is widely used for root initiation in many medicinal plants such as *Rauwolfia tetraphylla* (Sharma *et al.*, 1999) and *Swertia chirata* (Wawrosch *et al.*, 1999).

The concept of *ex vitro* rooting was conceived in the early eighties, when Debergh and Maene (1981) described the advantages of *ex vitro* rooting as compared to *in vitro* rooting. *Ex vitro* rooting combines both the rooting as well as acclimatization stages and thus reduces aseptic handling, labour costs and production time. As a result it has been widely used for different medicinal plant species including *Picrorhiza kurroa* (Wawrosch *et al.*, 2003) and *Bacopa monniera* (Tiwari *et al.*, 1998).

For acclimatization purposes, a sequential hardening procedure involving the transfer of plants to greenhouse, polyhouse, shade area and finally to the field has usually been followed. Krishnan *et al.* (1995) observed that 80 per cent of *Trichopus zeylanicus* plants directly transferred to the nursery failed to survive while those hardened for 4 weeks in humidity chambers showed 85 per cent survival. Dave *et al.* (2003) observed that *Chlorophytum borivilianum* plants hardened under agro-shadenet during the monsoon months of high humidity showed a better rate of survival and growth compared to plantlets hardened *in vitro* and subsequently transferred to the greenhouse for acclimatization. Rate of plantlet survival was 87 and 90 per cent under open field and agro-shadenet conditions, respectively. Low temperature conditions were found essential during acclimatization of high-altitude medicinal plants such as *Aconitum napellus* (Watad *et al.*, 1995), *Swertia chirata* (Wawrosch *et al.*, 1999) and *Valeriana wallichi* (Mathur *et al.*, 1988). The plant survival was optimal between 17 to 20°C while most of the plantlets died at 25°C.

Molecular Characterization for Clonal Fidelity Analysis

Howsoever small, the possibility of getting somaclonal variants even by axillary method cannot be ruled out. Since the occurrence of somaclonal variations in the micropropagated plants can seriously limit the broader utility of *in vitro* propagation systems, it is always advisable to test the clonal fidelity of tissue-cultured plants under *in vitro* conditions at regular intervals and prior to their release for field plantation.

Somaclonal variations can be associated with different types of changes such as chromosomal changes (numerical and structural), amplification or deamplification of the genes, activation of transposable elements, changes in DNA methylation patterns and single base changes (Phillips *et al.*, 1994 and Scowcroft, 1985). Among these, chromosomal re-arrangements are considered to be most prevalent and are a result of late or delayed replication of heterochromatin (Rani and Raina, 2000).

It however, cannot be said that *in vitro* culture will always give rise to variation. In fact, there are a number of factors that influence the frequency and extent of variation produced. Some of these factors are as follows:

1. The degree of departure from organized meristematic growth *i.e.* whether the growth is from already established meristems or through an intervening callus phase.
2. The culture environment especially the choice and concentration of growth regulators in the medium, has a significant influence on somaclonal variations.
3. The tissue source also affects the frequency and nature of somaclonal variation. Generally, the older and/or the more specially, howsoever small, the possibility of getting somaclonal variants even by axillary method cannot be ruled out. Since the occurrence of somaclonal variations in the micropropagated plants can seriously limit the broader utility of in vitro propagation systems, it is always advisable to test the clonal fidelity of tissue-cultured plants under in vitro conditions at regular intervals and prior to their release for field plantation.

Rani *et al.* (1995) reported tissue culture-induced mutations in micropropagated plants of *Populus deltoides* raised through axillary proliferation of nodal cuttings. The detection of genetic stability through the use of molecular markers has been amply demonstrated in micropropagated *Swertia chirayita* (Joshi and Dhawan, 2007), *Eucalyptus* (Rani and Raina, 1998) etc. (Table 1.1). Desirably, markers should show highly polymorphic behaviour, co-dominant inheritance, frequent occurrence and even distribution throughout the genome, easy and fast assay and high reproducibility. Of all the markers used (morphological markers, cytological markers, protein markers and molecular markers *i.e.* DNA-based markers), DNA-based molecular markers are known to be the most reliable because they are heritable, easy to score, free from developmental and environmental influence, insensitive to epistatic and pleiotropic interactions and provide a choice of co-dominant and dominant markers.

Cell Culture

Besides micropropagation, cell suspension culture systems could be used for large scale production of plant cells from which secondary metabolites could be extracted. This method could function as a continuous and reliable source for the production of medicinally important compounds. Cell culture systems have several major advantages over the conventional cultivation of whole plants as it is independent of geographical and seasonal variations; it offers a defined production system ensuring a continuous supply of good quality products of high yield; it is independent of space constraints; it is possible to produce novel compounds not found in the parent plant; it allows for automated control of cell growth and regulation of metabolite processes which in turn will reduce labour costs and in the process improve productivity; and, it enables efficient downstream recovery of the product. In addition, at times the amount of secondary metabolites produced in cell cultures is considerably higher than in the natural plant system. Secondary metabolites can be used as starting compounds for further chemical modification and enhancement for *e.g.* the use of podophyllotoxin for the development of anti-tumour agents etoposide and teniposide (Gordaliza *et al.*, 2000).

Biochemical analysis helps in estimating the amount of active principle present in a particular individual, thereby ensuring the multiplication of only the superior clones (recognized as 'elite') by tissue culture. Once elites have been identified, it is essential to ensure that the amount of active principle produced in wild plants is replicated under *in vitro* conditions as well. The degree of accumulation of secondary metabolites is dependent on the cellular differentiation and organisation of the tissue as well as the developmental and physiological condition of the plant (Verpoorte and Memelink, 2002).

Table 1.1: Genetic Fidelity Analysis in Medicinal Plants Using Molecular Markers

Plant	*Molecular Assay*	*Observations*	*Reference*
Azadiracta indica	AFLP	No somaclonal variations were observed	Singh *et al.*, 2002
Chlorophytum arundinaceum	RAPD	Banding profile was identical among all micro-propagated plants and *in vivo* explant donor	Lattoo *et al.*, 2006
Codonopsis lanceolata	ISSR and RAPD	Variation was detected in the 63 regenerants analysed; percentages of polymorphic bands in the ISSR and RAPD analysis were 15.7 per cent and 24.9 per cent respectively	Guo *et al.*, 2006
Curcuma anada	RAPD	10 primers produced 103 bands, including nine which were absent in the control	Prakash *et al.*, 2004
Curcuma longa	RAPD	8 regenerants were analyzed using 14 primers produced 38 novel bands indicating somaclonal variation	Salvi *et al.*, 2001
Digitalis obscura	RAPD	Variations were observed in banding profile regenerants vis-à-vis the mother plants derived from cryo-preserved tissue	Sales *et al.*, 2001
Dioscorea floribunda	RAPD	10 primers generated 5120 bands of which only one was polymorphic indicating clonal fidelity	Ahuja *et al.*, 2002
Eucalyptus tereticornis and *E. camaldulensis*	RFLP, RAPD, Oligo-nucleotide fingerprinting	Analysis of shoots regenerated by axillary branching method	Rani and Raina, 1998
Mentha arvensis	RAPD	Regenerants showed 99.9 per cent homo-geneity w.r.t mother plant	Shasany *et al.*, 1998
Panax notoginseng	RAPD	Somaclonal variation among somatic embryos	Shoyama *et al.*, 1997
Plumbago zeylanica	RAPD	20 primers were employed and all bands scored were monomorphic	Rout, 2002
Swertia chirayata	ISSR	16 ISSR primers generated 102 monomorphic amplicons	Joshi and Dhawan, 2007
Tylophora indica	RAPD	20 arbitrary oligo-nucleotides were used and the amplification products were monomorphic among all the regenerants	Jayanthi and Mandal, 2001
Zingiber officinales	RAPD	15 primers were employed to screen shoots derived from axillary branching and no variation was detected	Rout *et al.*, 1998

Franca *et al.* (1995) observed that micropropagated plantlets of *Eclipta alba* cultured on basal medium did not produce the active principle wedelolactone, while those cultured on medium supplemented with cytokinin did. Studies conducted in *Coleus forskohlii* indicated that the forskolin content in tubers of plants obtained by micropropagation was the same as that found in wild plants (Sharma *et al.*, 1991). Similarly in another study, the valepotriate content in *in vitro* cultures was found to be similar to that in the roots and rhizomes of wild plants of *Valeriana edulis* (Castillo *et al.*, 2002). Lisowska and Wysokinska (2000) found micropropagated plants of *Catalpa ovata* to exhibit an irridoid pattern similar to the leaves of wild plants. In *Corydalis ambigua*, different genotypes showed variable metabolite profile, however, they were not significantly different from the corresponding alkaloid content in wild plants (Hiraoka *et al.*, 2001). Le veille and Wilson (2002) on analysis of tuber tissue of micropropagated *Harpagophytum procumbens* detected iridoids at concentrations comparable with those found in wild plant material.

Chueh *et al.* (2001) conducted HPLC analysis to reveal that gentiopicroside and swertiamarin content in the aerial and underground parts of micropropagated *Gentiana davidii* was higher than the crude drug available in the market and also varied with the age of the plant. Similar observations were made by Sagare *et al.* (2001) in *Scrophularia yoshimurae* (for harpagoside content) and Lee *et al.* (2001) in *Corydalis yanhusuo* (for D,L-tetrahydropalmaline and D-corydaline). Sreekumar (2000) observed that in *Hemidesmus indicus*, the concentration of the root specific compound, 2-hydroxy 4-methoxy benzaldehyde, was 2-3 folds higher in micropropagated plants as compared to plants raised from conventional stem cuttings.

Khanam *et al.* (2000) detected hyoscyamine and scopolamine in 11 week old callus cultures of *Duboisia myoporoides* induced by BAP and NAA and in 6 and 9 week old shoots regenerated from callus on semisolid medium. However, no tropane alkaloids were detected in the shoots regenerated in liquid medium. In *Hyoscyamus niger*, hyoscyamine and scopolamine was found in the roots of the whole plant, however in callus cultures only hyoscyamine was detected (Ee May *et al.*, 2003). Kang *et al.* (2004) quantified hyoscyamine and scopolamine contents in different parts of *in vivo* and *in vitro* grown plants and found that the contents of both to be two to three-fold higher in roots than in the leaf and stems. They also found the levels of tropane alkaloids in *in vitro* propagated plants to be comparable to the concentrations found in the native field growing plants.

Low productivity is the main hindrance towards commercial application of the production of secondary metabolites by plant cells in suspension culture. The factors determining productivity include the specific growth rate, product formation rate and biomass concentration during the production phase. To increase productivity, these three factors need to be optimized (Hoopen *et al.*, 1994). There are several strategies that have been applied to improve the production of secondary metabolites in plant cell cultures. Culture conditions play a very important role in secondary metabolite accumulation. A low concentration of 2,4D has been used for anthraquinone accumulation in *Morinda citrifolia* (Hagendoorn *et al.*, 1994). Addition of 6 per cent sucrose to cell suspension cultures of *Forsythia* resulted in an increase in accumulation of pinoresinol and matairesinol. In *Catharanthus roseus*, light was found to influence the ajmalicine/serpentine accumulation ratio (Moreno *et al.*, 1995). At low dissolved oxygen concentrations, ajmalicine production in *Catharanthus roseus* appeared to be replaced by tryptamine production (Hoopen *et al.*, 1994). Thymol levels were highest in *Thymus vulgaris* cultures grown under 10 per cent to 21 per cent oxygen and they progressively decreased in amount under either higher or lower oxygen levels (Tisserat *et al.*, 2002).

The productivity of a heterogenous culture would be an average of the productivities of its high and low yielding lines. Selection and cloning of high yielding cells from such cultures is, therefore, an effective method to improve the *in vitro* production of secondary metabolites. The breeding of pure line cultivars for dual exploitation of the roots and the leaves for their alkaloids has been attempted in *Catharanthus roseus* (Levy *et al.*, 1983).

Another biological aspect of critical importance in the production of secondary metabolites is the role of elicitors. Elicitors are signals triggering the formation of secondary metabolites. Elicitors of fungal, bacterial and yeast origin have been used for production of various secondary metabolites

(Lu *et al.*, 2001; Pereira *et al.*, 2000). Seitz *et al.* (1989) used preparations from *Pythium aphanidermatum* for accumulation of phenols and indole alkaloids in *Catharanthus roseus* cell suspension cultures. *Aspergillus* application increased the accumulation of ajmalicine in *Catharanthus roseus* (Vázquez-Flota *et al.*, 1994). The addition of homogenate derived from an isolate of *Botrytis* species resulted in a 26-fold increase in sanguinarine content of *Papaver sominiferum* cell cultures (Eilert *et al.*, 1985). MeJA increased the production of valepotriates by transformed root cultures of *Valeriana* (Kittipongpatana *et al.*, 2002) and increased catharanthine and ajmalicine synthesis in hairy roots of *Catharanthus roseus* (Vázquez-Flota *et al.*, 1994). Late exponential phase hairy root cultures of *Catharanthus roseus* were elicited with pectinase and JA and an increase of 150 per cent in tabersonine was observed (Rijhwani *et al.*, 1998). Use of abiotic elicitors, such as the treatment of root cultures of *Datura stramonium* with copper and cadmium salts has been found to induce the rapid accumulation of high levels of sesquiterpenoid defensive compounds (Furze *et al.*, 1991). $AgNO_3$ was found to significantly increase scopolamine release (3-fold) in *Brugmansia candida* (Pitta–Alvarez *et al.*, 2000). A low accumulation of secondary compounds in cell cultures in a number of cases may not be due to a lack of key biosynthetic enzymes, but rather due to feedback inhibition, enzymatic or non-enzymatic degradation of the product in the medium or volatility of substances produced. Therefore, it is important that the secreted products are removed from the medium. Amberlite XAD-7 was used to adsorb terpenoid indole alkaloids ajmalicine and serpentine from the culture medium of *Catharanthus roseus* (Payne *et al.*, 1988). The camptothecin content in the medium of hairy root cultures of *Ophiorrhiza pumila* was increased by the presence of a polystyrene resin (diaion HP-20) that adsorbed camptothecin (Saito *et al.*, 2001).

A list of secondary metabolites produced by medicinal plant tissue cultures have been detailed in Table 1.2.

Organ Culture

It has been observed that the production of secondary metabolites is higher in differentiated tissues and therefore, several attempts have been made to generate shoot and root cultures for the production of secondary metabolites from medicinal plants. Shoot cultures have been developed in several medicinal plants such as *Withania somnifera* for withaferin A (Ray and Jha, 2001), *Decentra pergrina* for alkaloids (Konishi *et al.*, 1998), *Polygonum tinctorium* for indirubin (Shim *et al.*, 1998), *Stevia rebaudiana* for stevioside (Akita *et al.*, 1994), *Picrorrhiza kurroa* for kutkin (Upadhyay *et al.*, 1989) etc. Similarly, root cultures have been developed for the production of ginsenosides from *Panax ginseng* (Yu *et al.*, 2002), saikosaponins from *Bupleurum falcatum* (Kusakari *et al.*, 2000), indirubin from *Polygonum tinctorium* (Shim *et al.*, 1998), 2-hydroxy-4-methoxybenzaldehyde from *Hemidesmus indicus* (Sreekumar *et al.*, 1998) etc.

Transgenic Technology

The application of transgenic technology to pharmacognosy for biotransformation and increased production of secondary metabolites has great potential (Table 1.3). *Agrobacterium* mediated transformation offers several advantages over direct gene transfer methods such as the possibility for the transfer of only one or a few copies of DNA fragments carrying the genes of interest and transfer of very large DNA fragments with least re-arrangements (Tripathi and Tripathi, 2003).

Agrobacterium tumefaciens and *A. rhizogenes* are gram-negative soil bacteria that cause crown gall tumour and hairy root disease respectively in plants. The interaction between *Agrobacterium* and the plant involves a complex series of chemical signals communicated between the pathogen and the host, which includes neutral and acidic sugars, phenolic compounds, opines, vir proteins and the

Table 1.2: Secondary Metabolites Found in Medicinal Plants Produced by Tissue Cultures

Plant Name	*Secondary Metabolite*	*Culture Type*	*Reference*
Bupleurum falcatum	Saikosaponin	Callus	Wang and Huang, 1982
Catharanthus roseus	Indole alkaloids	Suspension	Moreno *et al.*, 1993
Catharanthus roseus	Catharanthine	Suspension	Zhao *et al.*, 2001
Cinchona robusta	Robustaquinones	Suspension	Schripsema *et al.*, 1999
Cinchona sp.	Anthraquinones	Suspension	Wijnsma *et al.*, 1985
Cinchona sp.	Alkaloids	Suspension	Koblitz *et al.*, 1983
Digitalis purpurea	Cardenolides	Suspension	Hagimori *et al.*, 1982
Dioscorea deltoidea	Diosgenin	Suspension	Heble and Staba, 1980.
Dioscorea doryophora Hance	Diosgenin	Suspension	Huang *et al.*, 1993
Ephedra spp.	Ephedrine	Suspension	O'Dowd *et al.*, 1993
Eucalyptus tereticornis SM.	Sterols and Phenolic compounds	Callus	Venkateswara *et al.*, 1986
Eucommia ulmoides	Chlorogenic acid	Suspension	Wang *et al.*, 2003
Fumaria capreolata	Isoquinoline alkaloids	Suspension	Tanahashi and Zenk, 1985
Gentiana sp.	Secoiridoid glucosides	Callus	Skrzypczak *et al.*, 1993
Ginkgo biloba	Ginkgolide A	Suspension	Carrier *et al.*, 1991
Glehnia littoralis	Furanocoumarin	Suspension	Kitamura *et al.*, 1998
Glycyrrhiza echinata	Flavanoids	Callus	Ayabe *et al.*, 1986
Glycyrrhiza glabra var. glandulifera	Triterpenes	Callus	Ayabe *et al.*, 1990
Hyoscyamus niger	Tropane alkaloids	Callus	Yamada and Hashimoto, 1982
Isoplexis isabellina	Anthraquinones	Suspension	Arrebola *et al.*, 1999
Morinda citrifolia	Anthraquinones	Suspension	Bassetti *et al.*, 1995; Zenk *et al.*, 1975
Nothapodytes foetida	Camptothecin	Callus	Thengane *et al.*, 2003
Ophiorrhiza pumila	Camptothecin related alkaloids	Callus	Kitajima *et al.*, 1998
Panax ginseng	Saponins and Sapogenins	Callus	Furuya *et al.*, 1973
Panax notoginseng	Ginsenosides	Suspension	Zhong and Zhu, 1995
Papaver bracteatum	Thebaine	Callus	Day *et al.*, 1986
Papaver somniferum	Alkaloids	Callus	Furuya *et al.*, 1972
Papaver somniferum	Morphine, Codeine	Suspension	Siah and Doran, 1991
Podophyllum hexandrum royle	Podophyllotoxin	Suspension	Uden *et al.*, 1989; Chattopadhyay *et al.*, 2002
Rauwolfia sellowii	Alkaloids	Suspension	Rech *et al.*, 1998
Rauwolfia serpentina Benth.	Reserpine	Suspension	Yamamoto and Yamada, 1986
Taxus sp.	Taxol	Suspension	Wu *et al.*, 2001
Taxus baccata	Taxol, baccatin III	Suspension	Cusido *et al.*, 1999
Taxus cuspidata	Taxoids	Suspension	Ketchum *et al.*, 2003

Table 3: Secondary metabolites produced by transgenic medicinal plants

Plant Name	*Secondary Metabolite*	*Reference*
Aconitum heterophyllum	Aconitine	Giri *et al.*, 1997
Artemisia annua	Artemisinin	Souret *et al.*, 2002; Vergauwe *et al.*, 1996; Cai *et al.*, 1995; Jaziri *et al.*, 1995
Atropa belladonna	Tropane alkaloids	Bonhomme *et al.*, 2000; Aoki *et al.*, 1997
Atropa belladonna	Alkaloid	Yun *et al.*, 1992
Digitalis lanata	Anthraquinones and flavonoids	Pradel *et al.*, 1997
Hyoscyamus muticus	Scopolamine	Jouhikainen *et al.*, 1999
Ophiorrhiza pumila	Camptothecin	Saito *et al.*, 2001
Panax ginseng	Phytosterol	Lee *at al.*, 2004
Papaver sominiferum	Codeine	Park and Facchini, 2000
Rauvolfia micrantha	Ajmalicine and ajmaline	Sudha *et al.*, 2003
Solanum aviculare	Solasodine	Argolo *et al.*, 2000
Taraxacum platycarpum	Sesquiterpenoids	Bae *et al.*, 2005
Taxus	Taxol	Han *et al.*, 1994

T-DNA (Transfer-DNA) that is ultimately transferred from the bacterium to the plant cell. Infection of the plant with *A. rhizogenes* causes development of hairy roots at the site of the infection. The bacterium contains a single copy of a large Ri (Root inducing) plasmid. The Ri plasmid T-DNA is referred to as left T-DNA (TL-DNA) and right T-DNA (TR-DNA). TR-DNA contains genes for agropine synthesis and genes homologous to Ti (Tumour inducing) plasmid tumour inducing genes. Genes of Ri TL-DNA direct the synthesis of a substance that recruits the cells to differentiate into roots under the influence of endogenous auxin synthesis. Virulence genes of the *vir* region of the Ri plasmid and *chv* genes found on the bacterial chromosomes mediate the transfer of T-DNA. Various phenolic compounds such as acetosyringone released by wounded plant cells induce transcription of the *vir* region. Hairy roots obtained by infection with different bacterial strains exhibit different morphologies. The hairy roots are highly branched roots covered densely with root hairs. The capacity of hairy roots to synthesize opines is often used as confirmative evidence for the process of genetic transformation since plants do not synthesize these opines.

Hairy roots are unique in their genetic and biosynthetic stability with an additional advantage of fast growth, which makes them a continuous source for the production of valuable secondary metabolites. Moreover, transformed roots are able to regenerate whole viable plants while maintaining clonal fidelity through subculturing and regeneration. Use of hairy root cultures has revolutionized the role of plant tissue culture for secondary metabolite synthesis. Hairy root cultures are characterized by fast growth, low doubling time, ease of maintenance and the ability to synthesize a range of chemical compounds. These roots can also synthesize more than a single metabolite, and therefore, prove economical for commercial production purposes. They also possess the capacity to produce secondary metabolites over successive generations without losing genetic or biosynthetic stability. In *Datura stramonium*, hairy roots were found to have a hyoscyamine and scopolamine bioproductivity two times higher than mother plants (Maldonado-Mendoza *et al.*, 1993). Baíza *et al.* (1998) observed that the differences in growth pattern and alkaloid accumulation in hairy roots and untransformed root cultures of *Datura stramonium* were not due to the different cell division rates, nor due to the presence of large meristems, but were a result of the development and growth of lateral roots and the presence of active intercalary meristematic zones in each line. Hairy root cultures for increased secondary metabolite production were also established in *Ophiorrhiza pumila* (Saito *et al.*, 2001), *Catharanthus roseus* (Toivonen *et al.*, 1989) and *Hyssopus officinalis* (Murakami *et al.*, 1998). Auxins in the presence of low levels of Kn induce the rapid disorganization of transformed roots of *Nicotiana rustica* ultimately to form suspension cultures of transformed cells and this process is associated with a decrease in nicotine content of the cells. In contrast, exogenously supplied GA_3 enhanced branching in two transformed root clones of the tropane alkaloid producing species *Brugmansia candida* (Rhodes *et al.*, 1994). Artemisinin and stigmasterol were isolated from hairy roots of *Artemisia annua* (Xie *et al.*, 2000). HPLC was done to identify glucotropaeolin from glucosinolate extract obtained from hairy root cultures of *Tropaeolum majus* (Wielanek *et al.*, 1999) and it was found to be highest in hairy roots as compared to callus and suspension cultures. As an alternative means of producing metabolites normally produced in plant shoots, the teratomas induced by *Agrobacterium tumefaciens* have been used for the *de novo* biosynthesis and biotransformation of some specific secondary products. Using the HPTLC system Asmari *et al.* (2004) showed that in *A. racemosus*, the highest amount of sarsasapogenin (0.133 per cent) was present in shoot tumour followed by root callus (0.127 per cent) and these levels were 2.59 and 2.5 times higher than the natural roots respectively. Hairy root cultures have also been used for biotransformation which is defined as stereo–or region-specific modification of the functional groups of organic compounds by living cultures in order to produce a chemically different product. This has been demonstrated in *Atropa belladonna* wherein hyoscyamine was converted to scopolamine (Subroto *et al.*, 1996), in *Panax ginseng* where glycyrrhetinic acid was transformed to glucosides (Asada *et al.*, 1993), in *Cinchona ledgeriana* where tryptophan was converted to quinine (Hay *et al.*, 1986).

Conclusion

Keeping in view the tremendous economic importance of medicinal plants, it is imperative to ensure good quality produce. For this, consistency in quality and quantity of planting material assumes paramount importance and several different strategies can be followed to facilitate conservation and for optimizing the product yield. In this study, we have reviewed some of the most widely used biotechnological tools for enhancing the availability of high value medicinal plants. Tissue culture protocols have been developed for many plants but there are several other over-exploited species that need to be worked upon. Techniques such as hairy root cultures offer good prospects for the development of commercial biotechnological approaches for the production of valuable secondary plant products. They are also useful models to study diverse secondary metabolite pathways. Another long-term potential source for natural products is to use plant cell cultures that can be standardized to optimize the production of the desired compound.

References

Ahuja, S., Mandal, B.B., Dixit, S., and Srivastava, P.S. (2002) Molecular, phenotypic and biosynthetic stability in *Dioscorea floribunda* plants derived from cryopreserved shoot tips. *Plant Science*, 163(5): 971-977.

Ajithkumar, D., and Seeni, S. (1998) Rapid clonal multiplication through *in vitro* axillary shoot proliferation of *Aegle marmelos* (L.) Corr., a medicinal tree. *Plant Cell Reports*, 17(5): 422-426.

Anand, P.N.M., and Hariharan, M. (1997) *In vitro* multiplication of *Alpinia galanga* (L.) Wild.: a medicinal plant. *Phytomorphology*, 47: 45-50.

Andrade, L.B., Echeverrigaray, S., Fracaro, F., Pauletti, G.F., and Rota, L. (1999) The effect of growth regulators on shoot propagation and rooting of common lavender (*Lavandula vera* DC.). *Plant Cell, Tissue and Organ Culture*, 56(2): 79-83.

Aoki, T., Matsumoto, H., Asako, Y., Matsunaga, Y., and Shimomura, K. (1997) Variation of alkaloid productivity among several clones of hairy roots and regenerated plants of *Atropa belladonna* transformed with *Agrobacterium rhizogenes* 15834. *Plant Cell Reports*, 16(5): 282-286.

Argolo, A.C., Charlwood, B.V., and Pletsch, M. (2000) The regulation of solasodine production by *Agrobacterium rhizogenes*-transformed roots of *Solanum aviculare*. *Planta Medica*, 66: 448-451.

Arora, R., and Bhojwani, S.S. (1989) *In vitro* propagation and low temperature storage of *Saussurea lappa* C.B. Clarke–an endangered, medicinal plant. *Plant Cell Reports*, 8(1): 44-47.

Arrebola, M.L., and Verpoorte, R. (2002) Micropropagation of *Isoplexis isabelliana* (Webb and Berth.) Masf., a threatened medicinal plant. *Journal of Herbs, Spices and Medicinal Plants*, 10(2): 89-94.

Arrebola, M.L., Ringbom, T., and Verpoorte, R. (1999) Anthraquinones from *Isoplexis isabelliana* cell suspension cultures. *Phytochemistry*, 52: 1283-1286.

Arya, S., Arya, I.D., and Eriksson, T. (1993) Rapid multiplication of adventitious somatic embryos of *Panax ginseng*. *Plant Cell, Tissue and Organ Culture*, 34(2): 157-162.

Arya, S., Liu, J.R., and Eriksson, T. (1991) Plant regeneration from protoplasts of *Panax ginseng* (C.A. Meyer) through somatic embryogenesis. *Plant Cell Reports*, 10(6-7): 277-281.

Asaka, I., Hirotani, M., Asada, Y., and Furuya, T. (1994) Ginsenoside contents of plantlets regenerated from *Panax ginseng* embryoids. *Phytochemistry*, 36(1): 61-63.

Asmari, S., Zafar, R., Ahmad, S. (2004) Production of sarsasapogenin from tissue culture of *Asparagus racemosus* and its quantification by HPTLC. *Iranian Journal of Pharmaceutical Research Supplement*, 2: 66-67.

Ayabe, S., Iida, K., and Furuya, T. (1986) Induction of stress metabolites in immobilized *Glycyrrhiza echinata* cultured cells. Plant Cell Reports, 3: 186-189.

Ayabe, S., Takano, H., Fujita, T., Hirota, H., and Takahashi, T. (1990) Triterpenoid biosynthesis in tissue cultures of *Glycyrrhiza glabra* var. *glandulifera*. *Plant Cell Reports*, 9: 181-184.

Backs-Hüsemann, D., and Reinert, J. (1970) Embryobildung durch isolierte einzelzellen aus gewebekulturen von *Daucus carota*. *Protoplasma*, 70(1): 49-60.

Bae, T.W., Park, H.R., Kwak, Y.S., Lee, H.Y., and Ryu, S.B. (2005) *Agrobacterium tumefaciens*-mediated transformation of a medicinal plant Taraxacum platycarpum. *Plant Cell, Tissue and Organ Culture*, 80(1): 51-57.

Baíza, A.M., Quiroz, A., Ruíz, J.A., Mendonza, I.M., and Vargas, V.M.L. (1998) Growth patterns and alkaloid accumulation in hairy root and untransformed root cultures of *Datura stramonium*. *Plant Cell, Tissue and Organ Culture*, 54: 123-130.

Barve, D.M., and Mehta, A.R. (1993) Clonal propagation of mature elite trees of *Commiphora wightii*. *Plant Cell, Tissue and Organ Culture*, 35(3): 237-244.

Baskaran, P., and Jayabalan, N. (2005) An efficient micropropagation system for *Eclipta alba*–A valuable medicinal herb. *In Vitro Cellular and Developmental Biology–Plant*, 41(4): 532-539.

Bassetti, L., Hagendoorn, M., and Johannes, T. (1995) Surfactant-induced non-lethal release of anthraquinones from suspension cultures of *Morinda citrifolia*. *Journal of Biotechnology*, 39: 149-155.

Baumert, A., Gröger, D., Kuzovkina, I.N., and Reisch, J. (1992) Secondary metabolites produced by callus cultures of various *Ruta* species. *Plant Cell, Tissue and Organ Culture*, 28:159-162.

Belt, J., Lengkeek, A., and Van der Zant, J. (2003) Cultivating a healthy enterprise–developing a sustainable medicinal plant chain in Uttaranchal–India. *Bulletin–Royal Tropical Institute No. 350*, KIT Publishers, Netherlands p. 19

Benjamin, B.D., Sipahimalani, A.T., and Heble, M.R. (1990) Tissue cultures of *Artemisia pallens*: Organogenesis, terpenoid production. *Plant Cell, Tissue and Organ Culture*, 21(2): 159-164.

Benniamin, A., Manickam, V.S., Johnson, M., and Joseph, L.H. (2004) Micropropagation of *Crataeva magna* (Lour.) DC.–A medicinal plant. *Indian Journal of Biotechnology*, 3: 136-138.

Bhojwani, S.S., and Razdan, M.K. (1996) Plant tissue culture: theory and practice, a revised edition. Elsevier Science, The Netherlands, pp. 49-51.

Bonfill, M., Cusidó, R.M., Palazón, J., Piñol, M.T., and Morales, C. (2002) Influence of auxins on organogenesis and ginsenoside production in *Panax ginseng* calluses. *Plant Cell, Tissue and Organ Culture*, 68(1): 73-78.

Bonhomme, V., Laurain-Mattar, D., Lacoux, J., Fliniaux, M., and Jacquin-Dubreuil, A. (2000) Tropane alkaloid production by hairy roots of *Atropa belladonna* obtained after transformation with *Agrobacterium rhizogenes* 15834 and *Agrobacterium tumefaciens* containing rol A, B, C genes only. *Journal of Biotechnology*, 81:151-158.

Borthakur, M., Hazarika, J., and Singh, R.S. (1998) A protocol for micropropagation of *Alpinia galanga*. *Plant Cell, Tissue and Organ Culture*, 55(3): 231-233.

Cai, G., Li, G., Ye, H., and Li, G. (1995) Hairy root culture of *Artemisia annua* L. by Ri plasmid transformation and biosynthesis of artemisinin. *Chinese Journal of Biotechnology*, 11: 227-235.

Carrier, D., Chauret, N., Mancini, M., Coulombe, P., Neufeld, R., Weber, M., and Archambault, J. (1991) Detection of ginkgolide A in *Ginkgo biloba* cell cultures. *Plant Cell Reports*, 10: 256-259.

Castillo, P., Zamilpa, A., Marquez, J., Hernandez, G., Lara, M., and Alvarez, L. (2002) Comparative study of differentiation levels and valepotriate content of *in vitro* cultures and regenerated and wild plants of *Valeriana edulis* ssp. *procera*. *Journal of Natural Products*, 65(4): 573-575.

Chand, S., and Sahrawat, A.K. (2002) Somatic embryogenesis and plant regeneration from root segments of *Psoralea corylifolia* L., an endangered medicinally important plant. *In Vitro Cellular and Developmental Biology–Plant*, 38(1): 33-38.

Chattopadhyay, S., Srivastava, A. K., Bhojwani, S. S., and Bisaria, V. S. (2002) Production of podophyllotoxin by plant cell cultures of *Podophyllum hexandrum* in bioreactor. *Journal of Bioscience and Bioengineering*, 93(2): 215-220.

Chaudhuri, K.N., Ghosh, B., and Jha, S. (2004) The root: a potential new source of competent cells for high-frequency regeneration in *Tylophora indica*. *Plant Cell Reports*, 22(10): 731-740.

Chee, P.P. (1996) Plant regeneration from somatic embryos of *Taxus brevifolia*. *Plant Cell Reports*, 16(3-4): 184-187.

Choi, Y.E., and Jeong, J. (2002) Dormancy induction of somatic embryos of Siberian ginseng by high sucrose concentrations enhances the conservation of hydrated artificial seeds and dehydration resistance. *Plant Cell Reports*, 20(12): 1112-1116.

Choi, Y.E., Ko, S.K., Lee, K.S., and Yoon, E.S. (2002) Production of plantlets of *Eleutherococcus sessiliflorus* via somatic embryogenesis and successful transfer to soil. *Plant Cell, Tissue and Organ Culture*, 69(2): 201-204.

Choi, Y.E., Yang, D.C., and Yoon, E.S. (1999) Rapid propagation of *Eleutherococcus senticosus* via direct somatic embryogenesis from explants of seedlings. *Plant Cell, Tissue and Organ Culture*, 58(2): 93-97.

Chueh, F.S., Chen, C.C., Sagare, A.P., and Tsay, H.S. (2001) Quantitative determination of secoiridoid glucosides in *in vitro* propagated plants of *Gentiana davidii* var. *formosana* by high performance liquid chromatography. *Planta Medica*, 67: 70-73.

Coker, P.S., and Camper, N.D. (2000) *In vitro* culture of *Echinacea purpurea* L. *Journal of Herbs, Spices and Medicinal Plants*, 7(4): 1-7.

Cusido, R.M., Palazon, J., Navia-Osorio, A., Mallol, A., Bonfill, M., Morales, C., and Pinol, M.T. (1999) Production of taxol and baccatin III by a selected *Taxus baccata* callus line and its derived cell suspension culture. *Plant Science*, 146: 101-107.

Dalal, N.V., and Rai, V.R. (2004) *In vitro* propagation of *Oroxylum indicum* Vent., a medicinally important forest tree. *Journal of Forest Research*, 9(1): 61-65.

Das (Pal), M., and Raychaudhuri, S.S. (2001) Enhanced development of somatic embryos of *Plantago ovata* Forsk. by additives. *In Vitro Cellular and Developmental Biology–Plant*, 37(5): 568-571.

Das, G., and Rout, G.R. (2002 a) Direct plant regeneration from leaf explants of *Plumbago* species. *Plant Cell, Tissue and Organ Culture*, 68(3): 311-314.

Das, G., and Rout, G.R. (2002 b) Plant regeneration through somatic embryogenesis in derived callus of *Plumbago rosea*. *Biologia Plantarum*, 45(2): 299-302.

Dave, A., Bilochi, G., and Purohit, S.D. (2003) Scaling-up production and field performance of micropropagated medicinal herb 'Safed Musli' (*Chlorophytum borivilianum*). *In vitro Cellular and Developmental Biology–Plant*, 39(4): 419-424.

Day, K.B., Draper, J, and Smith, H. (1986) Plant regeneration and thebaine content of plants derived from callus culture of *Papaver bracteatum*. *Plant Cell Reports*, 5: 471-474.

Debergh, P.C., and Maene, L.J. (1981) A scheme for commercial propagation of ornamental plants by tissue culture. *Scientia Horticulturae*, 14: 335-345.

Dhar, U., and Joshi, M. (2005) Efficient plant regeneration protocol through callus for *Saussurea obvallata* (DC.) Edgew. (Asteraceae): effect of explant type, age and plant growth regulators. *Plant Cell Reports*, 24(4): 195-200.

EeMay, L., LaiKeng, C., and Boey, P.L. (2003) Tropane alkaloids in micropropagated plantlets and callus of *Hyoscyamus niger*. *Journal of Tropical Medicinal Plants*, 4(1): 103-108.

Eilert, U., Kurz, W.G.W., and Constabel, F. (1985) Stimulation of sanguinarine accumulation in *Papaver somniferum* cell cultures by fungal elicitors. *Journal of Plant Physiology*, 119(1): 65-76.

Faisal, M., and Anis, M. (2003) Rapid mass propagation of *Tylophora indica* Merrill via leaf callus culture. *Plant Cell, Tissue and Organ Culture*, 75(2): 125-129.

Fereol, L., Chovelon, V., Causse, S., Michaux-Ferriere, N., and Kahane, R. (2002) Evidence of a somatic embryogenesis process for plant regeneration in garlic (*Allium sativum* L.). *Plant Cell Reports*, 21(3): 197-203.

Franca, S.C., Bertoni, B.W., and Pereira, A.M.S. (1995) Antihepatotoxic agent in micropropagated plantlets of *Eclipta alba*. *Plant Cell, Tissue and Organ Culture*, 40(3): 297-299.

Furuya, T., Ikuta, A., and Syono, K. (1972) Alkaloids from callus cultures of *Papaver somniferum*. *Phytochemistry*, 11: 3041-3044.

Furuya, T., Kojima, H., Syono, K., Ishi, T., Uotani, K., and Nishio, M. (1973) Isolation of saponin and sapogenins from callus tissue of *Panax ginseng*. *Chemical and Pharmaceutical Bulletin*, 21: 98-101.

Furze, J.M., Rhodes, M.J.C., Parr, A.J., Robins, R.J., Withehead, I.M., and Threlfall, D.R. (1991) Abiotic factors elicit sesquiterpenoid phytoalexin production but not alkaloid production in transformed root cultures of *Datura stramonium*. *Plant Cell Reports*, 10(3): 111-114.

Gallo-Meagher, M., and Green, J. (2002) Somatic embryogenesis and plant regeneration from immature embryos of saw palmetto, an important landscape and medicinal plant. *Plant Cell, Tissue and Organ Culture* 68(3): 253-256.

Gautam, V.K., Nanda, K., and Gupta, S.C. (1993) Development of shoots and roots in anther-derived callus of *Azadirachta indica* A. Juss.–a medicinal tree. *Plant Cell, Tissue and Organ Culture*, 34(1): 13-18.

Giri, A., Banerjee, S., Ahuja, P.S., and Giri, C.C. (1997) Production of hairy roots in *Aconitum heterophyllum* Wall. using *Agrobacterium rhizogenes*. *In vitro Cellular and Developmental Biology–Plant*, 33: 293-306.

Gordaliza, M., Castro, M.A., Miguel del Corral, J.M., and Feliciano, A.S. (2000) Antitumor properties of podophyllotoxin and related compounds. *Current Pharmaceutical Design*, 6(18):1811-1839.

Guang-min, X., Zhongyi, L., Guang-qin, G., and Hui-min, C. (1992) Direct somatic embryogenesis and plant regeneration from protoplasts of *Bupleurum scorzonerifolium* Willd. *Plant Cell Reports*, 11(3): 155-158.

Gui, Y., Guo, Z., Ke, S., and Skirvin, R.M. (1991) Somatic embryogenesis and plant regeneration in *Acanthopanax senticosus*. *Plant Cell Reports*, 9(9): 514-516.

Guo, W.L., Gong, L., Ding, Z.F., Li, Y.D., Li, F.X., Zhao, S.P., and Liu, B. (2006) Genomic instability in phenotypically normal regenerants of medicinal plant *Codonopsis lanceolata* Benth. et Hook. f., as revealed by ISSR and RAPD markers. *Plant Cell Reports*, 25(9): 896-906.

Hagendoorn, M.J.M., Plas, L.H.W.V.D., and Segers, G.J. (1994) Accumulation of anthraquinones in *Morinda citrifolia* cell suspensions. *Plant Cell, Tissue and Organ Culture*, 38: 227-234.

Hagimori, M., Matsumoto, T., and Obi, Y. (1982) Studies on the production of Digitalis cardenolides by plant tissue culture. III. Effects of nutrients on digitoxin formation by shootforming cultures of *Digitalis purpurea* L. grown in liquid media. *Plant Cell Physiology*, 23(7): 1205-1211.

Han, K.H., Fleming, P., Walker, K., Loper, M., Chilton, W.S., Mocek, U., Gordon, M.P., and Floss, H.G. (1994) Genetic transformation of mature *Taxus*: an approach to genetically control the *in vitro* production of the anticancer drug, taxol. *Plant Science*, 92(2): 187-196.

Hatano, K., Shoyama, Y., and Nishioka, I. (1987) Somatic embryogenesis and plant regeneration from the anther of *Aconitum carmichaeli* Debx. *Plant Cell Reports*, 6(6): 446-448.

Heble, M.R. and Staba, E. (1980) Steroid metabolism in stationary phase cell suspensions of *Dioscorea deltoidea*. *Planta Medica* Supplement, pp. 124-128.

Hengel, A.J.V., Harkes, M.P., Wichers, H.J., Hesselink, P.G.M., and Buitelaar, R.M. (1992) Characterization of callus formation and camptothecin production by cell lines of *Camptotheca acuminata*. *Plant Cell, Tissue and Organ Culture*, 28:11-18.

Hiraoka, N., Kato, Y., Kawaguchi, Y., and Chang, J.I. (2001) Micropropagation of *Corydalis ambigua* through embryogenesis of tuber sections and chemical evaluation of the ramets. *Plant Cell, Tissue and Organ Culture*, 67: 243-249.

Hoopen, H.J.G.T., Gulik, W.M.V., Schlatmann, J.E., Moreno, P.R.H., Vinke, H., Heijnen, J.J., and Verpoorte, R. (1994) Ajmalicine production by cell cultures of *Catharanthus roseus*: from shake flask to bioreactor. *Plant Cell, Tissue and Organ Culture*, 38: 85-91.

Huang, C.L., Hsieh, M.T., Hsieh, W.C., Sagare, A.P., and Tsay, H.S. (2000) *In vitro* propagation of *Limonium wrightii* (Hance) Ktze. (Plumbaginaceae), an ethnomedicinal plant, from shoot-tip, leaf– and inflorescence-node explants. *In Vitro Cellular and Developmental Biology–Plant*, 36(3): 220-224.

Huang, W.W., Cheng, C.C., Yeh, F.T., and Tsay, H.S. (1993) Tissue culture of *Dioscorea doryophora* HANCE 1. Callus organs and the measurement of diosgenin content. Chin. Med. Coll. J. 2(2): 151-160.

Ignacimuthu, S., Arockiasamy, S., Antonysamy, M., and Ravichandran, P. (1999) Plant regeneration through somatic embryogenesis from mature leaf explants of *Eryngium foetidum*, a condiment. *Plant Cell, Tissue and Organ Culture*, 56(2): 131-137.

IUCN. (2007) The World Conservation Union Species Survival Commission. <http://www.iucnredlist.org/info/tables/table3b>

Jayanthi, M., and Mandal, P.K. (2001) Plant regeneration through somatic embryogenesis and rapid analysis of regenerated plants in *Tylophora indica* (Burm. F. Merrill.). *In Vitro Cellular and Developmental Biology–Plant*, 37(5): 576-580.

Jaziri, M., Shimomura, K., Yoshimatsu, K., Fauconnier, M.L., Marlier M., Homes, J. (1995) Establishment of normal and transformed root cultures of *Artemisia annua* L. for artemisinin production. *Journal of Plant Physiology*, 145(1-2): 175-177.

Joseph, B., Joseph, D., and Philip, V.J. (1996) Plant regeneration from somatic embryos in black pepper. *Plant Cell, Tissue and Organ Culture*, 47(1): 87-90.

Joshi, K., Chavan, P., Warude, D., and Patwardhan, B. (2004) Molecular markers in herbal drug technology. *Current Science*, 87(2): 159-165.

Joshi, M., and Dhar, U. (2003) *In vitro* propagation of *Saussurea obvallata* (DC.) Edgew.–an endangered ethnoreligious medicinal herb of Himalaya. *Plant Cell Reports*, 21(10): 933-939.

Joshi, P., and Dhawan, V. (2007) Assessment of genetic fidelity of micropropagated *Swertia chirayita* plantlets by ISSR marker assay. *Biologia Plantarum*, 51(1): 22-26.

Jouhikainen, K., Lindgren, L., Jokelainen, T., Hiltunen, R., Teeri, T.H., and Oksman-Caldentey, K.M. (1999) Enhancement of scopolamine production in *Hyoscyamus muticus* L. hairy root cultures by genetic engineering. *Planta*, 208(4): 545-551.

Jung, S.J., Yoon, E.S., Jeong, J.H., and Choi, Y.E. (2004) Enhanced post-germinative growth of encapsulated somatic embryos of Siberian ginseng by carbohydrate addition to the encapsulation matrix. *Plant Cell Reports*, 23(6): 365-370.

Kang, Y.M., Min, J.Y., Moon, H.S., Kaigar, C.S., Prasad, D.T., Lee, C.H., and Choi, M.S. (2004) Rapid *in vitro* adventitious shoot propagation of *Scopolia parviflora* through rhizome cultures for enhanced production of tropane alkaloids. *Plant Cell Reports*, 23(3): 128-133.

Kaur, K., Verma, B., and Kant, U. (1998) Plants obtained from the Khair tree (*Acacia catechu* Willd.) using mature nodal segments. *Plant Cell Reports*, 17(5): 427-429.

Ketchum, R.E.B., Rithner, C.D., Qiu, D., Kim, Y.S., Williams, R.M., and Croteau, R.B. (2003) *Taxus* metabolomics: Methyl jasmonate preferentially induces production of taxoids oxygenated at C-13 in *Taxus* x media cell cultures. *Phytochemistry*, 62: 901-909.

Khanam, N., Khoo, C., and Khan, A.G. (2000) Effects of cytokinin/auxin combinations on organogenesis shoot regeneration and tropane alkaloid production in *Duboisia myoporoides*. *Plant Cell, Tissue and Organ Culture*, 62(2): 125-133.

Kitajima, M., Fischer, U., Nakamura, M., Ohsawa, M., Ueno, M., Takayama, H., Unger, M., Stockigt, J., and Aimi, N. (1998) Anthraquinone from *Ophiorrhiza pumila* tissue and cell cultures. *Phytochemistry*, 48(1): 107-111.

Kitamura, Y., Ikenaga, T., Ooe, Y., Hiraoka, N., and Mizukami, H. (1998) Induction of furanocoumarin biosynthesis in *Glehnia littoralis* cell suspension cultures by elicitor treatment. *Phytochemistry* 48(1): 113-117.

Kittipongpatana, N., Davis, D.L., and Porter, J.R. (2002) Methyl jasmonateincreases the production of valepotriates by transformed root cultures of *Valerianella locusta*. *Plant Cell, Tissue and Organ Culture*, 71: 65-75.

Koblitz, H., Koblitz, D., Schmauder, H.P., and Groger, D. (1983) Studies on tissue cultures of the genus *Cinchona* L. alkaloid production in cell suspension cultures. *Plant Cell Reports*, 2: 122-125.

Komalavalli, N., and Rao, M.V. (1997) *In vitro* micropropagation of *Gymnema elegans* W&A-a rare medicinal plant. *Indian Journal of Experimental Biology*, 35: 1088-1092.

Koroch, A., Juliani, H.R., Kapteyn, J., and Simon, J.E. (2002) *In vitro* regeneration of *Echinacea purpurea* from leaf explants. *Plant Cell, Tissue and Organ Culture*, 69(1): 79-83.

Koroch, A.R., Kapteyn, J., Juliani, H.R., and Simon, J.E. (2003) *In vitro* regeneration of *Echinacea pallida* from leaf explants. *In Vitro Cellular and Developmental Biology–Plant*, 39(4): 415-418.

Krishnan, P.N., and Seeni, S. (1994) Rapid micropropagation of *Woodfordia fruticosa* (L.) Kurz (Lythraceae), a rare medicinal plant. *Plant Cell Reports*, 14(1): 55-58.

Krishnan, P.N., Sudha, C.G., and Seeni, S. (1995) Rapid propagation through shoot tip culture of *Trichopus zeylanicus* Gaertn., a rare ethnomedicinal plant. *Plant Cell Reports*, 14(11): 708-711.

Kumar, H.G.A., Murthy, H.N., and Paek, K.Y. (2002) Somatic embryogenesis and plant regeneration in *Gymnema sylvestre*. *Plant Cell, Tissue and Organ Culture*, 71(1): 85-88.

Kumar, R., Sharma, K., and Agrawal, V. (2005) *In vitro* clonal propagation of *Holarrhena antidysenterica* (L.) Wall. through nodal explants from mature trees. *In Vitro Cellular and Developmental Biology–Plant*, 41(2): 137-144.

LaiKeng, C., and WaiLeng, L. (2004) Establishment of *Orthosiphon stamineus* cell suspension culture for cell growth. *Plant Cell, Tissue and Organ Culture*, 78(2): 101-106.

Lal, N., and Ahuja, P.S. (1989) Propagation of Indian rhubarh (*Rheum emodi* Wall.) using shoot-tip and leaf explant culture. *Plant Cell Reports*, 8(8): 493-496.

Langhansová, L., Konrádová, H., and Vank, T. (2004) Polyethylene glycol and abscisic acid improve maturation and regeneration of *Panax ginseng* somatic embryos. *Plant Cell Reports*, 22(10): 725-730.

Lattoo, S.K., Bamotra, S., Dhar, R.S., Khan, S., and Dhar, A.K. (2006) Rapid plant regeneration and analysis of genetic fidelity of *in vitro* derived plants *of Chlorophytum arundinaceum* Baker–an endangered medicinal herb. *Plant Cell Reports*, 25(6): 499-506.

Laurain, D., Chénieux, J.C., and Trémouillaux-Guiller, J. (1996) Somatic embryogenesis from immature zygotic embryos of *Ginkgo biloba*. *Plant Cell, Tissue and Organ Culture*, 44(1): 19-24.

Lee, M.H., Jeong, J.H., Seo, J.W., Shin, C.G., Kim, Y.S., In, J.G., Yang, D.C., Yi, J.S., and Choi, Y.E. (2004) Enhanced triterpene and phytosterol biosynthesis in *Panax ginseng* overexpressing squalene synthase gene. *Plant and Cell Physiology*, 45(8):976-984.

Lee, Y.L., Sagare, A.P., Lee, C.Y., Feng, H.T., Ko, Y.C., Shaw, J.F., and Tsay, H.S. (2001) Formation of protoberberine-type alkaloids by the tubers of somatic embryo-derived plants of *Corydalis yanhusuo*. *Planta Medica*, 67: 839-842.

Levieille, G., and Wilson, G. (2002) *In vitro* propagation and iridoid analysis of the medicinal species *Harpagophytum procumbens* and *H. zeyheri*. *Plant Cell Reports*, 21(3): 220-225.

Levy, A., Milo, J., Ashri, A., and Palevitch, D. (1983) Heterosis and correlation analysis of the vegetative components and ajmalicine content in the roots of the medicinal plant-*Catharanthus roseus* (L.) G. Don. *Euphytica* 32(2): 557-564.

Li, H., Murch, S.J., and Saxena, P.K. (2000) Thidiazuron-induced *de novo* shoot organogenesis on seedlings, etiolated hypocotyls and stem segments of Huang-qin. *Plant Cell, Tissue and Organ Culture*, 62(3): 169-173.

Li, S-L., Lin, G., Chan, S-W., and Li, P. (2001) Determination of the major isosteroidal alkaloids in bulbs of *Fritillaria* by high-performance liquid chromatography coupled with evaporative light scattering detection. *Journal of Chromatography A*, 909 (2): 207-214.

Lisowska, K., and Wysokinska, H. (2000) *In vitro* propagation of *Catalpa ovata* G. Don. *Plant Cell, Tissue and Organ Culture*, 60(3): 171-176.

Liu, C.Z., Murch, S.J., EL-Demerdash, M., and Saxena, P.K. (2003) Regeneration of the Egyptian medicinal plant *Artemisia judaica* L. *Plant Cell Reports*, 21(6): 525-530.

Liu, W., Chilcott, C.E., Reich, R.C., and Hellmann, G.M. (2000) Regeneration of *Salvia sclarea* via organogenesis. *In Vitro Cellular and Developmental Biology–Plant*, 36(3): 201-206.

Lu, M.B., Wong, H.L., and Teng, W.L. (2001) Effects of elicitation on the production of saponin in cell culture of *Panax ginseng*. *Plant Cell Reports*, 20: 674-677.

Makunga, N.P., Jäger, A.K., and Van Staden, J. (2003) Micropropagation of *Thapsia garganica*–a medicinal plant. *Plant Cell Reports*, 21(10): 967-973.

Maldonado-Mendonza, *I.E.*, Ayora-Talavera, T., and Loyola-Vargas, V.M. (1993) Establishment of hairy root cultures of *Datura Stramonium*. *Plant Cell, Tissue and Organ Culture*, 333: 21-329.

Manjula, S., Job, A., and Nair, G.M. (2000) Somatic embryogenesis from leaf derived callus of *Tylophora indica* (Burm. f.) Merrill. *Indian Journal of Experimental Biology*, 38(10): 1069-1072.

Manjula, S., Thomas, A., Daniel, B., and Nair, G.M. (1997) *In vitro* plant regeneration of *Aristolochia indica* through axillary shoot multiplication and organogenesis. *Plant Cell, Tissue and Organ Culture*, 51(2): 145-148.

Martin, K. (2002) Rapid propagation of *Holostemma ada-kodien* Schult., a rare medicinal plant, through axillary bud multiplication and indirect organogenesis. *Plant Cell Reports*, 21(2): 112-117.

Martin, K. (2002) Rapid propagation of *Holostemma ada-kodien* Schult., a rare medicinal plant, through axillary bud multiplication and indirect organogenesis. *Plant Cell Reports*, 21(2): 112-117.

Martin, K.P. (2003 a) Plant regeneration through somatic embryogenesis on *Holostemma ada-kodien*, a rare medicinal plant. *Plant Cell, Tissue and Organ Culture*, 72(1): 79-82.

Martin, K. (2003 b) Rapid *in vitro* multiplication and ex vitro rooting of *Rotula aquatica* Lour., a rare rhoeophytic woody medicinal plant. *Plant Cell Reports*, 21(5): 415-420.

Martin, K.P. (2004) Plant regeneration protocol of medicinally important *Andrographis paniculata* (Burm. F.) Wallich ex Nees via somatic embryogenesis. *In Vitro Cellular and Developmental Biology–Plant*, 40(2): 204-209.

Mathur, J., Ahuja, P.S., Mathur, A., Kukreja, A.K., and Shah, N.C. (1988) *In vitro* propagation of *Valeriana wallichi. Planta Medica*, 54: 82-83.

Moreno, P.R.H., van der Heijden, R., and Verpoorte, R. (1993) Effect of terpenoid precursor feeding and elicitation on formation of indole alkaloids in cell suspension cultures of *Catharanthus roseus. Plant Cell Reports*, 12: 702-705.

Moreno, P.R.H., van der Heijden, R., and Verpoorte, R. (1995) Cell and tissue cultures of *Catharanthus roseus*: A literature survey. *Plant Cell, Tissue and Organ Culture*, 42(1): 1-25.

Murakami, Y., Omoto, T., Asai, I., Shimomura, K., Yoshihira, K., and Ishimaru, K. (1998) Rosmarinic acid and related phenolics in transformed root cultures of *Hyssopus officinalis. Plant Cell, Tissue and Organ Culture*, 53(1): 75-78.

Murashige, T., and Skoog, F. (1962) A revised medium for rapid growth and bio-assays with tobacco tissue cultures. *Physiologia Plantarum*, 15: 473-497.

Murch, S.J., Choffe, K.L., Victor, J.M.R., Slimmon, T.Y., Raj, S.K., and Saxena, P.K. (2000) Thidiazuron-induced plant regeneration from hypocotyl cultures of St. John's wort (*Hypericum perforatum*. cv 'Anthos'). *Plant Cell Reports*, 19(6): 576-581.

Murthy, B.N.S., and Saxena, P.K. (1998) Somatic embryogenesis and plant regeneration of neem (*Azadirachta indica* A. Juss.). *Plant Cell Reports*, 17(6-7): 469-475.

Nin, S., Morosi, E., Schiff, S., and Bennici, A. (1996) Callus cultures of *Artemisia absinthium* L.: initiation, growth optimization and organogenesis. *Plant Cell, Tissue and Organ Culture*, 45(1): 67-72.

O'Dowd, N., McCauley, P.G., Richardson, D.H.S., and Wilson, G. (1993) Callus production, suspension culture and *in vitro* alkaloid yields of *Ephedra*. *Plant Cell Tissue and Organ Culture*, 34: 149-155.

Paramageetham, C., Babu, G.P., and Rao, J.V.S. (2004) Somatic embryogenesis in *Centella asiatica* L. an important medicinal and neutraceutical plant of India. *Plant Cell, Tissue and Organ Culture*, 79(1): 19-24.

Park, S.U. and Facchini, P.J. (2000) *Agrobacterium*-mediated transformation of opium poppy, *Papaver somniferum* L., via shoot organogenesis. *Journal of Plant Physiology*, 157: 207-214.

Park, S.U., and Facchini, P.J. (2004) High-efficiency somatic embryogenesis and plant regeneration in California poppy, *Eschscholzia californica* Cham. *Plant Cell Reports*, 19(4): 421-426.

Park, S.Y., Ahn, J.K., Lee, W.Y., Murthy, H.N., and Paek, K. (2005) Mass production of *Eleutherococcus koreanum* plantlets via somatic embryogenesis from root cultures and accumulation of eleutherosides in regenerants. *Plant Science*, 168(5): 1221-1225.

Patra, A., Rai, B., Rout, G.R., and Das, P. (1998) Successful plant regeneration from callus cultures of *Centella asiatica* (Linn.) Urban. *Plant Growth Regulation*, 24(1): 13-16.

Pattnaik, S., and Chand, P.K. (1996) *In vitro* propagation of the medicinal herbs *Ocimum americanum* L. syn. *O. canum* Sims. (hoary basil) and *Ocimum sanctum* L. (holy basil). *Plant Cell Reports*, 15(11): 846-850.

Patwardhan, B., Warude, D., Pushpangadan, P., and Bhatt, N. (2005) Ayurveda and traditional chinese medicine: a comparative overview. *Evidence Based Complementary Alternative Medicine*, 2(4): 465–473.

Payne, G.F., Payne, N.N., Shuler, M.L., and Asada, M. (1988) *In situ* adsorption for enhanced alkaloid production by *Catharanthus roseus*. *Biotechnology Letters*, 10(3): 187-192.

Pereira, A.M.S., Bertoni, B.W., Appezzato-da-Glória, B., Araujo, A.R.B., Januário, A.H., Lourenço, M.V., and França, S.C. (2000) Micropropagation of *Pothomorphe umbellata* via direct organogenesis from leaf explants. *Plant Cell, Tissue and Organ Culture*, 60(1): 47-53.

Pereira, A.M.S., Bertoni, B.W., Câmara, F.L.A., Duarte, I.B., Queiroz, M.E.C., Leite, V.G.M., Moraes, R.M., Carvalho, D., and França, S.C. (2000) Co-cultivation of plant cells as a technique for the elicitation of secondary metabolite production. *Plant Cell, Tissue and Organ Culture*, 60: 165-169.

Pitta–Alvarez, S.I., Spollansky, T.C., and Giulietti. (2000) The influence of different biotic and abiotic elicitors on the production and profile of tropane alkaloids in hairy root cultures of *Brugmansia candida*. Enzyme and Microbial Technology, 26(2-4): 252-258.

Pradel, H., Dumkelehmann, U., Diettrich, B., and Luckner, M. (1997) Hairy root cultures of *Digitalis lanata*. Secondary metabolism and plant regeneration. *Journal of Plant Physiology*, 51:209–215.

Prakash, E., Khan, P.S.S.V., Reddy, P.S., and Rao, K.R. (1999) Regeneration of plants from seed-derived callus of *Hybanthus enneaspermus* L. Muell., a rare ethnobotanical herb. *Plant Cell Reports*, 18(10): 873-878.

Prakash, S., Elangomathavan, R., Seshadri, S., Kathiravan, K., and Ignacimuthu, S. (2004) Efficient regeneration of *Curcuma amada* Roxb. plantlets from rhizome and leaf sheath explants *Plant Cell, Tissue and Organ Culture*, 78(2): 159-165.

Pretto, F.R., and Santarém, E.R. (2000) Callus formation and plant regeneration from *Hypericum perforatum* leaves. *Plant Cell, Tissue and Organ Culture*, 62(2): 107-113.

Purohit, S.D., Dave, A., and Kukda, G. (1994) Micropropagation of safed musli (*Chlorophytum borivilianum*), a rare Indian medicinal herb. *Plant Cell, Tissue and Organ Culture*, 39(1): 93-96.

Rani, G., and Grover, I.S. (1999) *In vitro* callus induction and regeneration studies in *Withania somnifera*. *Plant Cell, Tissue and Organ Culture*, 57(1): 23-27.

Rani, V., and Raina, S.N. (1998) Genetic analysis of enhanced-axillary-branching-derived *Eucalyptus tereticornis* Smith and *E. camaldulensis* Dehn. plants. *Plant Cell Reports*, 17: 236-242.

Rao, G.P., and Bahadur, B. (1990) Somatic embryogenesis and plant regeneration in self-incompatible *Oldenlandia umbellata* L. *Phytomorphology*, 40: 95-102.

Rech, S.B., Batista, C.V.F., Schripsema, J., Verpoorte, R., and Henriques, A. T. (1998) Cell cultures of *Rauwolfia sellowii*: growth and alkaloid production. *Plant Cell, Tissue and Organ Culture*, 54: 61-63.

Reddy, B.O., Giridhar, P., and Ravishankar, G.A. (2001) *In vitro* rooting of *Decalepsis hamiltonii* Wight and Arn., an endangered shrub, by auxins and root-promoting agents. *Current Science*, 81(11): 1479-1481.

Reinert, J. (1958) Morphogenese und ihre kontrolle an gewebekulturen aus carotten. *Naturwissenschaft*, 45: 344-345.

Rhodes, M.J.C., Parr, A.J., Giulietti, A., and Aird, E.L.H. (1994) Influence of exogenous hormones on the growth and secondary metabolite formation in transformed root cultures. *Plant Cell, Tissue and Organ Culture*, 38:143-151.

Rijhwani, S.K., and Shanks, J.V. (1998) Effect of elicitor dosage and exposure time on biosynthesis of indole alkaloids by *Catharanthus roseus* hairy root cultures. *Biotechnol. Prog.*, 14: 442-449.

Rout, G.R. (2002) Direct plant regeneration from leaf explants of *Plumbago* species and its genetic fidelity through RAPD markers. *Annals of Applied Biology*, 140 (3): 305–313.

Rout, G.R., Das, P., Goel, S., and Raina, S.N. (1998) Determination of genetic stability of micropropagated plants of ginger using Random Amplified Polymorphic DNA (RAPD) markers. *Botanical Bulletin of Academia Sinica*, 39: 23-27.

Rout, G.R., Saxena, C., Samantaray, S., and Das, P. (1999) Rapid plant regeneration from callus cultures of *Plumbago zeylanica*. *Plant Cell, Tissue and Organ Culture*, 56(1): 47-51.

Sagare, A.P., Kuo, C.L., Chueh, F.S., and Tsay, H.S. (2001) *De novo* regeneration of *Scrophularia yoshimurae* Yamazaki (Scrophulariaceae) and quantitative analysis of harpagoside, an iridoid glucoside, formed in aerial and underground parts of *in vitro* propagated and wild plants by HPLC. *Biological and Pharmaceutical Bulletin*, 24(11): 1311-1315.

Sagare, A.P., Lee, Y.L., Lin, T.C., Chen, C.C., and Tsay, H.S. (2000) Cytokinin-induced somatic embryogenesis and plant regeneration in *Corydalis yanhusuo* (Fumariaceae)–a medicinal plant. *Plant Science*, 160(1): 139-147.

Saito, K., Sudo, H., Yamazaki, M., Koseki-Nakamura, M., Kitajima, H., and Aimi, N. (2001) Feasible production of camptothecin by hairy root culture of *Ophiorrhiza pumila*. *Plant Cell Reports*, 20:267-271.

Sales, E., Nebauer, S.G., Arrillaga, I., and Segura, J. (2001) Cryopreservation of *Digitalis obscura* selected genotypes by encapsulation-dehydration. *Planta Medica*, 67: 833-838.

Salvi, N.D., George, L., and Eapen, S. (2001) Plant regeneration from leaf base callus of turmeric and random amplified polymorphic DNA analysis of regenerated plants. *Plant Cell, Tissue and Organ Culture*, 66(2): 113-119.

Sata, S.J., Bagatharia, S.B., and Thaker, V.S. (2000) Induction of direct somatic embryogenesis in garlic (*Allium sativum*). *Methods in Cell Science*, 22(4): 299-304.

Schripsema, J., Ramos-Valdivia, A., and Verpoorte, R. (1999) Robustaquinones, novel anthraquinones from an elicited *Cinchona robusta* suspension culture. *Phytochemistry* 51: 55-60.

Seitz, H.U., Eilert, U., De Luca, V., and Kurz, W.G.W. (1989) Elicitor-mediated induction of phenylalaine ammonia lyase and tryptophan decarboxylase: accumulation of phenols and indole alkaloids in cell suspension cultures of *Catharanthus roseus*. *Plant Cell, Tissue and Organ Culture*, 18: 71-78.

Selvakumar, V., Anbudurai, P.R., and Balakumar, T. (2001) *In vitro* propagation of the medicinal plant *Plumbago zeylanica* L. through nodal explants. *In Vitro Cellular and Developmental Biology–Plant*, 37(2): 280-284.

Sen, J., and Sharma, A.K. (1991) Micropropagation of *Withania somnifera* from germinating seeds and shoot tips. *Plant Cell, Tissue and Organ Culture*, 26(2): 71-73.

Shankar, D. (1998) Medicinal plants: A global heritage. *Proceedings of the International Conference on Medicinal Plants for Survival*, 16-19 February 1998, IDRC, New Delhi, India.

Sharma, D., Sharma, S., and Baruah, A. (1999) Micropropagation and *in vitro* flowering of *Rauvolfia tetraphylla*; a potent source of antihypertensive drug. *Planta Medica*, 72: 961–965.

Sharma, N., Chandel, K.P.S., and Srivastava, V.K. (1991) *In vitro* propagation of *Coleus forskohlii* Briq., a threatened medicinal plant. *Plant Cell Reports* 10(2): 67-70.

Sharma, V., and Padhya, M.A. (1996) *In vitro* rapid multiplication and propagation of *Crataeva nurvala*. *Indian Journal of Experimental Biology*, 34: 243-246.

Shasany, A.K., Khanuja, S.P.S., Dhawan, S., Yadav, U., Sharma, S., and Kumar, S. (1998) High regenerative nature of *Mentha arvensis* internodes. *Journal of Biosciences*, 23(5): 641-646.

Shenoy, V.B., and Vasil, I.K. (1992) Biochemical and molecular analysis of plants derived from embryogenic tissue cultures of napiergrass (*Pannisetum purpureum* K. Schum).*Theoretical and Applied Genetics*, 83: 947-955.

Shoyama, Y., Zhu, X.X., Nakai, R., Shiraishi, S., and Kohda, H. (1997) Micropropagation of *Panax notoginseng* by somatic embryogenesis and RAPD analysis of regenerated plantlets. *Plant Cell Reports*, 16(7): 450-453

Shrivastava, N., and Rajani, M. (1999) Multiple shoot regeneration and tissue culture studies on *Bacopa monnieri* (L.) Pennell. *Plant Cell Reports*, 18(11): 919-923.

Siah, C.L. and Doran, P.M. (1991) Enhanced codeine and morphine production in suspended *Papaver somniferum* cultures after removal of exogenous hormones. *Plant Cell Reports*, 10: 349-353.

Singh, H.P. (2001) National perspective on development of medicinal and aromatic plants. *Technical report*, Agri Watch.

Singh, N.K., and Sehgal, C.B. (1999) Micropropagation of 'Holy Basil' (*Ocimum sanctum* Linn.) from young inflorescences of mature plants. *Plant Growth Regulation*, 29(3): 161-166.

Sivakumar, L., and Mukundan, U. (2003) *In vitro* culture studies on *Stevia rebaudiana*. *In Vitro Cellular and Developmental Biology-Plant*, 39: 520-523.

Skrzypczak, L., Wesolowska, M., and Skrzypczak, E. (1993) *Gentiana* species XII: *In vitro* culture, regeneration, and production of secoirridoid glucosides. In Y.P.S. Bajaj (ed.), Biotechnology in agriculture and forestry, Vol. 21, Medicinal and aromatic plants IV. Berlin, Heidelberg: Springer-Verlag, pp. 172-186.

Smith, M.A.L., Kobayashi, H., Gawienowski, M., and Briskin, D.P. (2002) An *in vitro* approach to investigate medical chemical synthesis by three herbal plants. *Plant Cell, Tissue and Organ Culture*, 70:105-111.

Souret, F.F., Weathers, P.J., and Wobbe, K.K. (2002) The mevalonate-independent pathway is expressed in transformed roots of *Artemisia annua* and regulated by light and culture age. *In vitro Cellular and Developmental Biology Plant*, 38: 581-588.

Sreekumar, S., Seeni, S., and Pushpangadan, P. (2000) Micropropagation of *Hemidesmus indicus* for cultivation and production of 2-hydroxy 4-methoxy benzaldehyde. *Plant Cell, Tissue and Organ Culture*, 62(3): 211-218.

Staritsky, G. (1997) Backgrounds and principles of *in vitro* conservation of plant genetic resources. Volume 1: General aspects. In: *Conservation of Plant Genetic Resources in vitro*. Razdan MK and Cocking EC (Eds.) Science Publishers Inc., USA pp. 26-49

Steward, F.C., Mapes, M.O., and Smith, J. (1958) Growth and organized development of cultured cells. *American Journal of Botany*, 45: 693-703.

Subbaiah, M.M., Baum, B.R., Johnson, D.A., and Arnason, J.T. (2003) Direct shoot regeneration from leaf segments of mature plants of *Echinacea purpurea* (L.) Moench. *In Vitro Cellular and Developmental Biology–Plant*, 39(5): 505–509.

Sudha, C.G., and Seeni, S. (1994) *In vitro* multiplication and field establishment of *Adhatoda beddomei* C. B. Clarke, a rare medicinal plant. *Plant Cell Reports*, 13(3-4): 203-207.

Sudha, C.G., Reddy, B.O., Ravishankar, G.A., and Seeni, S. (2003) Production of ajmalicine and ajmaline in hairy root cultures of *Rauvolfia micrantha* Hook F., a rare and endemic medicinal plant. *Biotechnology Letters*, 25(8): 631-636.

Sudha, G.G., and Seeni, S. (1996) *In vitro* propagation of *Rauwolfia micrantha*, a rare medicinal plant. *Plant Cell, Tissue and Organ Culture*, 44(3): 243-248.

Tanahashi, T., and Zenk, M.H. (1985) Isoquinoline alkaloids from cell suspension cultures of *Fumaria capreolata*. *Plant Cell Reports*, 4: 96-99.

Tewari, D.N. (2000) Report of the task force on conservation and sustainable use of medicinal plants. Government of India, Planning commission p. 90

Thakur, R., Rao, P. S., and Bapat, M. (1998) *In vitro* plant regeneration in *Melia azedarach* L. *Plant Cell Reports*, 18: 127–131.

Thengane, S.R., Kulkarni, D.K., Shrikhande, V.A., and Krishnamurthy, K.V. (2001) Effect of thidiazuron on adventitious shoot regeneration from seedling explants of *Nothapodytes foetida*. *In Vitro Cellular and Developmental Biology–Plant*, 37(2): 206-210.

Tikhomiroff, C., and Jolicoeur, M. (2002) Screening of *Catharanthus roseus* secondary metabolites by high-performance liquid chromatography. *Journal of chromatography A*, 955(1): 87-93.

Tisserat, B., Vaughn, S.F., and Silman, R. (2002) Influence of modified oxygen and carbon dioxide atmospheres on mint and thyme on plant growth, morphogenesis and secondary metabolism *in vitro*. *Plant Cell Reports*, 20: 912-916.

Tiwari, V., Singh, B.D., and Tiwari, K.N. (1998) Shoot regeneration and somatic embryogenesis from different explants of Brahmi [*Bacopa monniera* (L.) Wettst.]. *Plant Cell Reports*, 17(6-7): 538-543.

Tiwari. V., Tiwari, K.N., and Singh, B.D. (2001) Comparative studies of cytokinins on *in vitro* propagation of *Bacopa monniera*. *Plant Cell, Tissue and Organ Culture*, 66(1): 9-16.

Toivonen, L., Balsevich, J., and Kurz, W.G.W. (1989) Indole alkaloid production by hairy root cultures of *Catharanthus roseus*. *Plant Cell, Tissue and Organ Culture*, 18: 79-93.

Uden, W., Pras, N.N, Visser, J.F., and Malingre, T.M. (1989) Detection and identification of Podophyllotoxin produced by cell cultures derived from *Podophyllum hexandrum* royle. *Plant Cell Reports*, 8: 165-168.

Upadhyay, R., Arumugam, N., and Bhojwani, S.S. (1989) *In vitro* propagation of *Picrorhiza kurrooa*. Royle ex Benth.–an endangered species of medicinal importance. *Phytomorphology*, 39: 235–242.

Vanegas, P.E., Cruz–Hernández, A., Valverde, M.A., and Paredes–López, O. (2002) Plant regeneration via organogenesis in marigold. *Plant Cell, Tissue and Organ Culture*. 69(3): 279-283.

Vázquez-Flota, F., Moreno-Valenzuela, O., Miranda-Ham, M.L., Coello-Coello, and Loyola-Vargas, V.M. (1994) Catharanthine and ajmalicine synthesis in *Catharanthus roseus* hairy root cultures. *Plant Cell, Tissue and Organ Culture*, 38: 273-279.

Vengadesan, G., Ganapathi, A., Anand, R.P., and Anbazhagan, V.R. (2000) *In vitro* organogenesis and plant formation in *Acacia sinuate*. *Plant Cell, Tissue and Organ Culture*, 61(1): 23-28.

Venkateswara, R., Sankara Rao, S., and Vaidyanathan, C.S. (1986) Phytochemical constituents of cultured cells of *Eucalyptus tereticornis* SM. *Plant Cell Reports*, 3: 231-233.

Vergauwe, A., Cammaert, R., Vandenberghe, D., Genetello, C., Inze, D., Montagu, M.V., and Eeckhout, E.V. (1996) *Agrobacterium tumefaciens*-mediated transformation of *Artemisia annua* L. and regeneration of transgenic plants. Plant Cell Reports, 15(12): 929-933.

Wakhlu, A.K., and Sharma, R.K. (1998) Somatic embryogenesis and plant regeneration in *Heracleum candicans* Wall. *Plant Cell Reports*, 17(11): 866-869.

Walia, N., Kaur, A., and Babbar, S.B. (2007) An efficient, *in vitro* cyclic production of shoots from adult trees of *Crataeva nurvala* Buch. Ham. *Plant Cell Reports*, 26(3): 277-284.

Wang, J., Liao, X., Zhang, H., Du, J, and Chen, P. (2003) Accumulation of chlorogenic acid in cell suspension cultures of *Eucommia ulmoides*. *Plant Cell Tissue and Organ Culture*, 74: 193-195.

Wang, P.J., and Huang, C.I. (1982) Production of saikosaponins by callus and redifferentiated organs of *Bupleurum falatum* L. In A. Fujiwara (Ed.), Plant Tissue Culture. Maruzen, Tokyo. pp. 71-72.

Watad, A.A., Kochba, M., Nissim, A., and Gaba, V. (1995) Improvements of *Aconitum napellus* micropropagation by liquid culture on floating membrane rafts. *Plant Cell Reports*. 14: 345-348.

Watad, A.A., Kochba, M., Nissim, A., and Gaba, V. (1995) Improvements of *Aconitum napellus* micropropagation by liquid culture on floating membrane rafts. *Plant Cell Reports* 14: 345-348

Wawrosch, C., Malla, P.R., and Kopp, B. (2001 a) Clonal propagation of *Lilium nepalense* D. Don, a threatened medicinal plant of Nepal. *Plant Cell Reports*, 20(4): 285-288.

Wawrosch, C., Malla, P.R., and Kopp, B. (2001 b) Micropropagation of *Allium wallichii* kunth, a threatened medicinal plant of Nepal. *In Vitro Cellular and Developmental Biology–Plant*, 37(5): 555-557.

Wawrosch, C., Maskay, N., and Kopp, B. (1999) Micropropagation of the threatened Nepalese medicinal plant *Swertia chirata* Buch.-Ham. ex Wall. *Plant Cell Reports*, 18(12): 997-1001.

Wawrosch, C., Zeitlhofer, P., Grauwald, B., and Kopp, B. (2003) Rooting chemicals on the establishment of micropropagated *Picrorhiza kurroa* plantlets in the greenhouse. *Acta Horticulturae*, 616:271-274.

Wielanek, M., and Urbanek, H. (1999) Glucotropaeolin and myrosinase production in hairy root cultures of *Tropaeolum majus*. *Plant Cell, Tissue and Organ Culture*, 57:39-45.

Wijnsma, R., Go, J.T.K.A., Weerden, van I.N., Harkes, P.A.A., Verpoorte, R., and Svendsen, A.B. (1985) Anthraquinones as phytolexins in cell and tissue cultures of *Cinchona* sp. *Plant Cell Reports*, 4: 241-244.

Wu, J., Wang, C., and Mei, X. (2001) Stimulation of taxol production and excretion in *Taxus* spp cell cultures by rare earth chemical lanthanum. Journal of Biotechnology 85: 67-73.

Xie, D., Wang, L., Ye, H., and Li, G. (2000) Isolation and production of artemesinin and stigmasterol in hairy root cultures of *Artemisia annua*. *Plant Cell, Tissue and Organ Culture*, 63: 161-166.

Yamada, Y., and Hashimoto, T. (1982) Production of tropane alkaloids in cultured cells of *Hyoscyamus niger*. *Plant Cell Reports*, 1: 101-103.

Yamamoto, O. and Yamada, Y. (1986) Production of reserpine and its optimization in cultured *Rauwolfia serpentina* Benth. cells. *Plant Cell Reports*, 5: 50-53.

Yua, K.W., Gaob, W., Hahna, E.J., and Paek, K.Y. (2002) Jasmonic acid improves ginsenoside accumulation in adventitious root culture of *Panax ginseng* C.A. Meyer. *Biochemical Engineering Journal*, 11(2-3): 211-215.

Yun, D.J., Hashimoto, T., and Yamada, Y. (1992) Metabolic engineering of medicinal plants: transgenic *Atropa belladonna* with an improved alkaloid composition. *Proceedings of the National Academy of Sciences USA*, 89: 11799-803.

Zenk, M.H., El-Shagi, H., and Schulte, U. (1975) Anthraquinone production by cell suspension cultures of *Morinda citrifolia*. *Planta Medica Supplement*, pp. 79-101.

Zhao, J., Hu, Q., Guo, Q., and Zhu, W.H. (2001) Effects of stress factors, bioregulators, and synthetic precursor on indole alkaloid production in compact callus clusters cultures of *Catharanthus roseus*. *Applied Microbial Biotechnology*, 55: 693-698

Zhong, J.J. and Zhu, Q.X. (1995) Effect of initial phosphate concentration on cell growth and ginsenoside saponin production by suspended cultures of *Panax notoginseng*. *Applied Biochemistry and Biotechnology*, 55: 241-246.

Zobayed, S.M.A., and Saxena, P.K. (2003 a) *In vitro* regeneration of *Echinacea purpurea* L.: enhancement of somatic embryogenesis by indole butyric acid and dark pre-incubation. *In Vitro Cellular and Developmental Biology–Plant*, 39(6): 605-612.

Utilisation and Management of Medicinal Plants (2010) *Pages 32–47*
Editors: V.K. Gupta, Anil K. Verma and Sushma Koul
Published by: DAYA PUBLISHING HOUSE, NEW DELHI

Chapter 2

Environmental Regulation of Secondary Metabolite Accumulation in Aromatic Crops: A Review

K. Ramesh* and Virendra Singh
Natural Plant Products Division, Institute of Himalayan Bioresource Technology, P.O. Box No. 6, Palampur – 176 061, Himachal Pradesh, India

ABSTRACT

Essential oils from aromatic plant species are widely used for flavouring of pharmaceuticals, confectionery, and alcoholic liquors and are valued in medicine for both internal and external uses. The essential oils are composed of terpenoids. Aromatic plants are grown in different parts of the world at different periods depending on the agro-climatic conditions. Seasonal changes in essential oil content and composition have been shown to exist in 2different species (Mastelic, 1995). Local climate influences a successful crop production in a particular region and it is one that evolved its physiological mechanisms to be effective in that region. Therefore, better understanding of the response of aromatic crops to ecological factors is one of the primary factors regulating plant growth and will give a better in sight in to the genotype environment interactions, which ultimately decide the performance of the crop in a given situation. The rapidly changing world climatic regime also prompts to examine the spectrum of variation in oil production and its composition due to temperature, humidity, day length and light intensity. More emphasis was given for mints because of the moderately high literature available for these species. This brief review in the light of the past researches and about current understanding on these relationships is an attempt towards this end.

Keywords: Mint, Light, Photoperiod, Menthol.

* Corresponding Author: E-mail: ramechek@yahoo.co.in.

Introduction

Climatic factors, rates of plant metabolism, differentiation and secretary activity of glandular hairs affect synthesis and secretion of essential oils (Jerovic *et al.*, 2001). Essential oil bearing plants have been valued since ages for their aroma (fragrance), medicinal and culinary properties, which include members of the genus *Mentha* (mint), belonging to family Lamiaceae. They represent one among the most popular essential oil yielding plants and are very widely cultivated. They are considered today the most important commercial essential oil bearing plants from the standpoint of worldwide production, with peppermint (*Mentha piperita*), menthol mint (*M. arvensis*), spearmint (*M. spicata*) and corn mint (*M. citrata*) essences being the most valued for their use in the food, cosmetics and pharmaceutical industries (Lawrence, 1972, 1985). The largest mint oil-producing countries are Bulgaria, Italy, China and the USA, which contribute about 90 per cent of total peppermint oil production of the world. Among different species yielding essential oil, *M. arvensis*, *M. piperita*, *M. citrata* and *M. cardiaca* have made economically important production systems in temperate, mediterranean and sub-tropical parts of the world (Farooqi *et al.*, 1999). Significant work on mint oil has been carried out in different parts of the world, particularly in peppermint, a hybrid between *M. spicata* and *M. aquatica*, which has received maximum attention. Thus peppermint is the most studied species among all (Giachetti *et al.*, 1988; Kokkini, 1991; Stengele and Stahl-Biskup, 1993; Katasawa *et al.*, 1995; Sternberg and Duke, 1996; Shahi *et al.*, 1999; Fuchs *et al.*, 2000). It has been found that the oil composition is modified by various external factors, like geographical area (Smith and Levi, 1961; Clark and Menary, 1979), agro-climatic requirements of the crop (Gupta *et al.*, 1971; Ghosh and Chatterjee, 1976), plant development (Clark and Menary, 1979; Lawrence, 1980), and environmental conditions like day length, temperature (Grahle and Holtzel, 1963; Burbott and Loomis, 1967a; Clark and Menary, 1981; Voirin *et al.*, 1990).

The essential oil of mint is biosynthesized and stored in specialized anatomical structures, termed as peltate glandular trichomes, on leaf surfaces (Amelunxen *et al.*, 1969; Gershenzon *et al.*, 2000). This is extracted by hydro-distillation of the flowering herbs. Given the commercial value of these oils, the processes involved in their biosynthesis and secretion, are attractive targets for genetic engineering (Lange *et al.*, 2000), while the relationship of these processes to the field management are of greater concern for successful crop cultivation. The study of environmental relationship with mint production contributes to understanding of plant responses to these variables. Additionally given that the environmental conditions may limit production of certain compounds, its study may also lead to ways and means of manipulating environment for commercial applications. In this review our focus will be made on (*i*) Quality of mint oils, (*ii*) Plant development on essential oil composition and (*iii*) Response to selected variables *viz.*, irrigation, light, photoperiod and temperature.

Plant Development on Essential Oil Composition

Mints produce high levels of *p*-menthane monoterpenes in glandular trichomes found on the surfaces of leaves, young stems, and parts of the inflorescence (Amelunxen, 1965). Oil accumulation in aromatic plants has been observed to depend on the growth stage of plant as well as plant part where oil is synthesised. Besides growth stage, the position of leaf also determines oil quality. Burbott and Loomis (1969), Croteau and Martinkus (1979) noticed that during leaf development, total content of monoterpenes increased with age and the composition was significantly altered. Monoterpene accumulation was found to be restricted to leaves of 12 to 20 days of age, the period of maximal leaf expansion. The developmental changes in monoterpene accumulation in peppermint were accompanied by alterations in monoterpene composition. Limonene and menthone were the major monoterpenes present in the youngest leaves. Proportion of limonene declined rapidly with plant development, while menthone increased rapidly and declined only at later stages and thereafter menthol became dominant (Burbott and Loomis, 1969; Croteau and Martinkus, 1979; Brun and Voirin, 1991). Singh *et al.* (1994) found that with advancement of crop age, menthol content increased while menthone and menthyl acetate contents were reduced. Proportions of menthofuran and pulegone declined, while those of 1,8-cineole, menthol, and neomenthol increased substantially upon leaf ageing. The major constituent, menthone, which was present in 5 days old leaves at 36 per cent of total monoterpenes, increased to nearly 75 per cent at 15 days and then declined to 10 per cent by the end of a study. Among the minor constituents, alpha pinene, myrcene, and linalool increased during development (Gershenzon *et al.*, 2000). Some of these compositional changes have been documented in detail in some studies (Brun and Voirin, 1991; Court *et al.*, 1993; Voirin and Bayet, 1996; Rohloff, 1999). But in most cases the position of leaf and the time/season of sampling were not clear and it is difficult to derive valid conclusions.

Environmental Factors

Seasonal changes in essential oil content and composition have been shown to exist in 2different species (Mastelic, 1995). Mints are grown in different parts of the world at different periods depending on the local agro-climatic conditions. The cause of concern here was that the essential oil production in mints, a physiologically programmed process and was subjected to several environmental cues. These environmental cues include, as discussed by Mahmoud and Croteau (2003), season, temperature, duration and intensity of solar irradiation, and related climatic and rhizospheric situations. They had a profound bearing on the performance of plants including oil composition. Local climate exerted selective influences on oil yield and oil composition and thus a successful production in particular region was one which could harness maximum potential of physiological mechanisms in that region. Therefore, better understanding of the response of mints to these factors is necessary to have a better insight into the genotype-environment interactions, which ultimately decide the production performance of the crop in a given agro-climatic situation. These factors vary with geographical areas, and it had been reported that peppermint oils of acceptable commercial quality can be produced only in certain geographic locations (Clark and Menary, 1981). Among the various agronomic factors responsible for producing maximum yield, planting time, which primarily depends on the prevailing climatic conditions, was considered as the most important (Singh *et al.*, 1997). It was shown that there was marked alteration in essential oil components *viz.*, a–pinene, b–pinene, 1,8-cineole, menthofuran, menthol, pulegone, menthyl acetate and b–caryophyllene due to environmental factors (Ozel and Ozguven, 2002). This underpinned the above said factors.

The main environmental difference between various locations is the length of day and the temperature. On the other hand, the seasonal gradient during the growing period is also associated with alterations in environmental parameters like photoperiod and air temperature. Kothari *et al.* (2000) opined that soil and climatic factors affected the essential oil composition mostly through altering leaf production, leaf growth and development, shedding of mature leaves in menthol mint.

These environmental cues may accelerate production of a specific type of compounds by directing the pathway at a specific direction to yield such compounds either desirable or undesirable. For example, oil yield and menthol content increased with leaf (and thus oil gland) maturity, and a range of stress conditions (related to light, temperature and moisture status) tended to promote accumulation of pulegone and menthofuran (Burbott and Loomis, 1967a; Clark and Menary, 1980; Voirin *et al.*, 1990). Content of menthofuran could reach industrially unacceptable levels in plants raised under stressful environmental conditions (high temperature, drought, low light intensity) (Burbott and Loomis, 1967a; Clark and Menary, 1980), over which commercial mint growers had very limited control.

Some researchers (Clark and Menary, 1979; Murray *et al.*, 1986; Voirin *et al.*, 1990) claimed that environmental factors (*i.e.* temperature and photoperiod) influenced pulegone levels in mint essential oils. Murray *et al.* (1986) found that b-pinene content was altered by the ecological factors. The metabolism of monoterpenes of *M. piperita* was also strongly influenced by environmental factors (Shahi *et al.*, 1999).

Shahi *et al.* (1999) demonstrated that menthol and menthyl acetate were strongly influenced by the environmental factors. Later developments in mint suggested that (+)-pulegone, the central intermediate in the biosynthesis of (-)-menthol and the most significant component of peppermint essential oil is the turning point in Mint quality pertaining to the ecological conditions. Depending on the environmental conditions, this branch point metabolite might be reduced to (-)-menthone en route to menthol, by pulegone reductase (PR), or oxidized to (+)-menthofuran, by menthofuran synthase (MFS) (Mahmoud and Croteau, 2003). Among the environmental cues water, light, photoperiod and temperature are the major factors that mediate essential oil regulation in many ecosystems.

Despite important information provided by many experimental results, it is still unclear that in most cases, the means by which these factors influence pathway flux or the specific steps of monoterpene metabolism were not understood (Mahmoud and Croteau, 2001).

Irrigation

Earliest systematic studies on irrigation needs of *Mentha* were carried out by Chopra *et al.* (1958) at the Regional Research Laboratory, Jammu, India and concluded that being a leafy crop; its irrigation requirement was very high. Later, studies conducted by Schroder (1963) revealed that when soil moisture was maintained at 80-90 per cent of field capacity, peppermint leaves were largest, herb and oil yield were highest whereas essential oil contents were highest at medium soil moisture level (60 per cent field capacity). However, he could not notice any clear trend/relation between leaf size and oil gland with oil content. Not withstanding to this fact, node number and internodes length were positively correlated with essential oil content. Roitsema (1958) opined that at higher moisture supply menthol was esterified to menthyl acetate or oxidized to menthone and the assertion was confirmed by Nelson *et al.* (1971) indicating that irrigated crop contained more of menthol and menthyl acetate, less menthone and menthofuran.

Later, Loomis (1977) suggested that in peppermints water stress and other associated factors determined whether photosynthate was to be directed towards growth, flowering or synthesis and maturation of essential oil. Therefore, maintaining higher water status on the plant was also essential for desirable oil composition. This view was strengthened by the studies conducted by Croteau (1977), who observed that sprinkler irrigated plants contained more menthol and less menthone than that of furrow irrigated ones, apparently due to wetting of foliage. This resulted in hydration of cuticle and oil glands. Consequently the permeability of the cuticular membrane might be altered towards more rapid evaporation of the volatile oil. Further studies, made by Duhan *et al.* (1977) also confirmed that menthol, menthofuran and menthyl acetate decreased and menthone increased by increasing level of irrigation in Japanese mint.

In contrast to the discussions made in the previous paragraphs, experiments conducted by Charles *et al.* (1990), who analysed the effect of osmotic stress on growth and oil content of peppermint revealed that oil content increased under water stress conditions since secondary metabolites were enhanced under such conditions through higher oil gland density due to stress induced reduction in leaf area. Menthone and menthyl acetate increased with increase in irrigation. Menthone levels tended to increase at the expense of menthol under higher moisture supply. High moisture level decreased the rate of reduction of menthone to menthol and increased the conversion of menthol to hydrocarbon terpenes and ultimately decreases menthol and increases the menthone content (Singh 1994). In brief, an assured supply of irrigation is a must for high yield and good quality of essential oil of *Mentha* (Vasyutev and Pyshnev, 1982; Mehra, 1992).

Altitude

The altitudinal gradient along a mountain is associated with alterations in a number of environmental factors, such as air temperature, wind exposure, light intensity, UV-B radiation, partial CO_2 pressure, etc. The combination of all these factors exert a pressure on plants, which becomes expressed as changes in morphology, physiology and productivity. This pressure is more pronounced in herbaceous plants like mints rather than in woody plants. An investigation on Indian peppermint oils reported that oils produced at higher altitudes contained higher concentrations of menthol, whereas larger amounts of menthofuran were found in oils from lower altitudes (Gupta *et al.*, 1971). This difference in the essential oil composition must be due to change in geographic location (Lawrence and Shu, 1989). When considering the altitudinal effect on *Mentha* quality, an increase in menthol and relative decrease in menthyl acetate has been demonstrated by Shahi *et al.* (1999) from high to low altitudinal belts.

Light

Light is obviously a key factor in the ultimate production of many compounds because it supplies the energy needed to fix carbon. Light can stimulate the synthesis of some secondary products, *e.g.* phenols, serpentine, procyanidins and diosgenin (Forrest, 1969; Schrall and Becker, 1977; Doller, 1978), hut inhibits nicotine synthesis (Ohta and Yatazawa, 1978). Higher interception of solar energy and higher crop growth in peppermint due to closer spacing was observed (Prasad and Saxena, 1980). Indeed, mutual shading of leaves in *M. arvensis* reduced oil content (Nijjar, 1990). Leela and Angadi (1993) obtained maximum mint oil yield and menthol content during July harvest at Bangalore, India apparently due to higher light intensity. Light intensity plays an important role in the biosynthesis of medically important metabolites. Here, photons trigger the enzymatic conversion of protochlorophyllide and phytol to chlorophyll a and b, and then, to chlorophyll-protein complexes in chloroplast (Mohr and Schopfer, 1995). Higher penetration of sunlight down the canopy before menthol mint maturity has been shown to improve l-menthol in oil (Kothari *et al.*, 1996).

Photoperiod

Quantification of plant growth responses to photoperiod facilitates an understanding of important facets of crop productivity linked genotype-environment interactions (Ezekiel and Bhargava, 1993). Photoperiod triggers responses ranging from altered plant growth to changes in plant metabolism and even oil components. Many factors affect mint responses to photoperiod, including the duration and magnitude of day length in terms of growth, biomass, oil yield and oil composition.

Growth and Flowering

Among the environmental factors, the prominent operative factor day length assumes paramount importance due to its marked modulating effect on growth and development of mints. Pioneering studies done by Allard (1941) and Crane (1951) have indicated that peppermint flowered and produced maximum growth under conditions of long days, suggesting mints are long day plants. Allard (1941) observed only few flowers on mint in a 14 hour day. Virtually, every aspect of plant growth and development is influenced by the photoperiod. Further, peppermint remained vegetative in day lengths of 10 hours and flowered when it was extended to 18 hours. Obviously, this resulted in higher leaf/stem ratio. Further studies carried out by Langston and Leopold (1954), indicated that very low light intensities would bring about photo induction of pepper mint. Although floral initiation was independent on a wide range of light intensities, floral development was dependent on the light intensity. Further, short day conditions gave rise to pepper mint plants that do not flower and form many stolons with small leaves. In contrast, pepper mint plants grown under long day conditions formed erect upright lateral shoots and produced large leaves and flowers (Crane and Steward, 1962b; Steward, 1962). Recent observations made by Farooqi *et al.* (1999) confirmed that photoperiod had strong influence on *Mentha* species (*M. arvensis*, *M. citrata* and *M. cardiaca*) since these are long day plants, exhibiting higher aerial growth under long day conditions, whilst the reverse for short day conditions. The leaf/stem ratio observations showed that reduced leafy plant canopy under short day conditions enhanced the ratio, as compared to those observed with normal and long-day conditions. These observations made them to conclude that photoperiod has a strong effect on plant performance and has direct relevance to essential oils obtained from the foliage of mint without any jeopardy. This had direct impact on mint since essential oils are obtained from the foliage. The varying day length might have direct influence through modulation of relevant metabolic pathways, from photosynthetic assimilate production and its reallocation to the Rohmer pathway, thus leading further to generation of essential oil terpenoids (Lichtenthaler *et al.*, 1997). However, little work has been done concerning photoperiodic effects on volatile oil biogenesis in aromatic plants. Farooqi *et al.* (1999) noticed that long day treatment to the plant induced emergence of inflorescences bearing normally developed flowers. Differences in the oil content among the plants raised under different day length conditions were striking. The short day plants of all the species had substantially higher concentrations of oil in their tissues compared to long-and normal-day plants, which had a similar amount of accumulated essential oil. The short-day response was quantitatively greater (about 3 fold enhancement) in *M. citrata* and *M. cardiaca*, compared to *M. arvensis* which had only a 35 per cent increase. They further suggested that since the leaves constitute the main plant part involved in essential oil biogenesis and accumulation, the response could be due partially to the higher leaf mass per unit weight of sampled plant biomass. However, higher trichome density and lack of physiological maturity in the leaves under short day conditions could also be contributing factors. These discussions suggested that photoperiod had a strong effect on mint through vegetative as well as the reproductive growth.

Biomass/Oil Yield

It was realized since a long time back that the greatest production of *M. piperita* oil was associated with long days (Guenther, 1949; Howe, 1956; Grahle and Holtzel, 1963). In the early periods of studies by Burbott and Loomis (1967a), Franz *et al.* (1984) and Lawrence (1986), revealing that extrinsic factors like long days (>14 h) and cool nights (<15°C) are strongly causative of maintaining high levels of respiratory substrates and reduced metabolic conditions in the glandular trichomes of peppermint.

Based on results obtained with time and number of harvests, Clark and Menary (1979) found that there is an increase in 1,8-cineole level depending upon cutting numbers. They suggested that this resulted from the fact that the photoperiod affected the essential oils and the 1,8-cineole levels increased with the increase in light intensity.

In an attempt to exactly quantify the study of photoperiod on oil yield, it was reported that *M. piperita* has minimum requirement of mid summer day-length of 15 h to flower and produce a good yield of oil with an acceptable quality (Clark and Menary, 1979; Voirin *et al.*, 1990; Lawrence, 1992). However, Burbott and Loomis (1967a) associated greater oil production under long days due to its effect on plant growth. This assertion was strengthened by Farooqi *et al.* (1999) stating that short day condition had substantially increased concentration of oil in mint due to the fact that the leaves constitute the main plant part involved in essential oil biogenesis and accumulation, and so the photoperiod response could be due partially to the higher leaf plant biomass ratio. Besides, higher trichome density and lack of physiological maturity in the leaves under short day conditions could also be other contributing factors. Since, trichomes or oil glands, the sites of essential oil synthesis, are unalterable by management/environmental conditions owing to its genetic make up (Ascensao and Pais 1987), it was presumed that their density was higher in short day plants due to reduced leaf area (Farooqi *et al.*, 1999).

Oil Synthesis and Composition

Photoperiod may exert a direct influence on plant metabolism, from photosynthetic carbon production and its partitioning to the Rohmer route leading further to generation of essential oil terpenoids (Lichtenthaler *et al.*, 1997). This might prove true for mints also.

Photoperiod has a pronounced effect on amino acid production too. It was observed that glutamine accumulated under long day whereas asparagine under short day photoperiods in *M. piperita* (Crane and Steward, 1962a). Accumulation of other amino acids like a-ketoglutaric and pyruvic acid were also influenced by the length of day and night temperature (Rabson and Steward, 1962). Further they showed that a-keto organic acid metabolism of mint was also to be partially photocontrolled.

Grahle and Holtzel (1963) found that proportions of individual monoterpenes in peppermint oil are strongly influenced by day length. The leaves of *Mentha piperita* grown at 20°C constant temperature subjected to long days (18:6) contained relatively small amounts of menthofuran and large amounts of menthol and menthone. In contrast, plants subjected to short days (12:12), in fact, contained very small quantities of menthol and menthone and large amounts of menthofuran. In turn, a large change in ratio of limonene to cineole (initial compounds produced in the pathway), a ratio deciding authenticity of mint oil, due to photoperiod was noticed (Clark and Menary, 1979).

These findings made strong foundation for further studies by many researchers and the results claimed that the difference in quality of mint oils were dependent on environmental factors that affect the biosynthesis (Franz *et al.*, 1984; Murray *et al.*, 1986, Brun *et al.*, 1990 and Voirin *et al.*, 1990) and plant metabolism too. Change in essential oil composition might be due to the fact that photoperiod influenced directly the oil composition of young leaves since essential oil biogenetic capacity is much higher in young and immature leaves (Shanker *et al.*, 1999) and the monoterpene composition; it induced the production of pulegone either through the oxidative or the reductive pathway. Therefore, oil rich menthone or menthol can not be produced if the plants are continuously subjected to short photoperiod (Farooqi *et al.*, 1998). In contrast to the above assertion that photoperiod directly affects oil composition in young leaves, Burbott and Loomis (1967a) reported that photoperiod as such is not directly influencing the composition of terpene in peppermint. But environmental effects of monoterpenes in peppermint were observable only in new leaves as soon as they have been developed. They suggested that oxidation-reduction levels of the monoterpenes reflects the oxidation-reduction state of the respiratory co-enzymes of the terpene producing cells, and that this, in turn, depends on the concentration of respiratory substrates in the cells. This was determined by night temperature and photosynthetic period which would affect terpene composition to a greater extent. Overall oil production under natural conditions was markedly affected by growth during the whole season (Singh and Singh, 1969). Not with standing to the above, Clark and Menary (1979) reiterated that photoperiodic treatments had profound direct influence on monoterpene composition of peppermint oil.

Later in 1980s, the strong influence of photoperiod on oil composition in peppermint was confirmed. In particular, Clark and Menary (1980) found alterations in mono and sesquiterpene composition, Croteau *et al.* (1991) found that long days promoted the proportion of menthone, menthol and some monoterpene hydrocarbons (like pinene, sabinene etc.) and reduced the level of undesirable components like menthofuran, pulegone and menthyl acetate.

In contrast with long days, which blocked menthofuran as described in previous paragraphs, short days promoted it. Mint grown under short day and high temperature conditions had a lower menthole ratio (Franz *et al.*, 1984). However, short day conditions caused a reduction in the menthofuran contents at the end of the growing season only and the menthone content was high in younger leaves (Clark and Menary, 1984), which was a major component of mint oil (Brun *et al.*, 1990). Besides, menthofuran accumulation occurs in non-photosynthetic organs, such as flowers and in very young leaves and its occurrence depends on the reducing state of tissue where monoterpenes synthesis takes place. Increased menthofuran content in the proceeding harvests might thus depend upon increased oxidizing conditions (Rohloff, 1999).

The menthol ratio was dependent on the direct or indirect effects of environmental factors, which led to changes in the components of oil, from pulegone to menthone, from menthone to menthole and from menthole to menthyl acetate (Murray *et al.*, 1986). Formation of the major monoterpene component in peppermint young leaves, L-menthone, was enhanced under either cool or short nights, and the associated oxidised substances, menthofuran and pulegone, were depressed. During plant maturity the L-menthone was metabolised to L-menthol which is accumulated in the peppermint oil. Further, young apical leaves contained monoterpene constituents that were more oxidized (*e.g.* menthone) and basal senescent leaves were richer in more reduced and esterified compounds (*e.g.* menthol and menthyl acetate), thus indicating a biosynthetic transformation as the pathway to menthol proceeds via menthone (Kokkini, 1991).

Menthone, menthofuran (Court *et al.*, 1993), menthol and menthyl acetate (Fahlen *et al.*, 1997) were greatly affected by changes in the growing seasons and environmental conditions as discussed above. Menthol content significantly correlated to the day length and relative humidity during the growing period of peppermint (Shahi *et al.*, 1998).

The oil composition of young leaves grown under long day conditions changed from menthofuran to menthone and menthole, and menthone was a major component of the oil of the leaves grown under short day conditions (Voirin *et al.*, 1990). This suggested that the enzyme menthofuran synthase was stimulated under short day environment while pulegone reducatse was stimulated under long day conditions. Some metabolic steps could be important in the responses to the varied day length conditions. Therefore, understanding activities of the limonene hydroxylases under photoperiodic regimes (Farooqi *et al.*, 1999) is a need.

Temperature

The influence of temperature on different species of mint has been studied (Allard, 1941; Langston and Leopold, 1954; Biggs and Leopold, 1955; Singh and Singh, 1969). As such temperature could not be separated from photoperiod effect and both act together, since it may affect the critical day length for flowering in pepper mint leaves (Biggs and Leopold, 1955). There are indications that low temperatures can stimulate secondary product formation, such as anthocyanin synthesis in carrot cells (de Capite, 1955). Low temperature stimulated the synthesis of celery flavour and also the synthesis of other terpenoids, especially limonene (Watts *et al.*, 1984). The literature is rich in data concerning temperature effect on conventional crops but analogous reports on mints are very scarce.

Growth and Yield

Temperature had effects on growth through its direct effects on leaf size; internode lengths, frequency of lateral break and dry weight in mints. A temperature of 70° F enhanced leaf development, lateral branching, floral primordial initiation and flower development. Floral initiation was greatly affected by temperature. In low day temperature, high night temperature promoted flowering and vice versa. The time required for floral initiation at temperatures *viz.*, 60, 70, 80 and 90° F was 86, 33, 35 and 84 respectively. Besides growth, temperature had pronounced effect on density of oil glands also. As the temperature increased either day or night, the oil gland count per unit area was increased. This suggested that peppermint is strikingly influenced by small temperature changes which would be common over most fields of commercially grown mint (Biggs and Leopold, 1955). Oil glands in the adaxial surface were greater at 35°C than those at 20°C, whereas the abaxial surface did not do so in Japanese mint *M. arvensis* (Duriyaprapan *et al.*, 1986). Reduced plant height of peppermint was observed due to low temperature in north India (Singh *et al.*, 1997). Not withstanding to the above Fahlen *et al.* (1997) could not detect any obvious change in leaf growth pattern of various *Mentha* spp. Poor oil yield in *M. arvensis* was noticed due to low temperature (18°C) prevailing during maturity at semi raid conditions of Hyderabad, India (Singh *et al.*, 1999).

Oil Composition

Rabak (1916), while studying the effects of frost on pepper mint, reported that cold temperatures increased the content of free menthol and the esters of menthol in the oil. This made the speculation that essential oil content of mint might be influenced by temperature although it is not the only factor associated with it. The higher temperature may be presumed to cause greater rate of volatilization of oil from the plant; that is the oil may be lost by distillation under natural conditions.

Moreover, it has been also shown that the diurnal change in temperature between day and night is an important factor of influence for the oil composition (Burbott and Loomis, 1967a; Clark and Menary, 1980).

Storage of higher soluble nitrogen in peppermint and Japanese mint has been reported under short day and low atmospheric temperature as compared to long day and high temperature (Crane and Steward, 1962a; Singh and Garg, 1976).

Oil content of Japanese mint is a function of mean daily temperature during the growing season (Baslas 1970). This was further confirmed by Duriyaprapan *et al.* (1986), by constructing a linear relationship between oil content of Japanese mint to mean daily temperature. Not withstanding to this fact, synthesis and accumulation of essential oils in Japanese mint are less affected by extremely high temperature than was the plant growth. There was increase in menthone with increase in higher day temperature. The combination of low day and night temperature tended to reduce menthol content, which is one of the important components of Japanese mint oil. Piperitone content tended to decline with increasing day temperature with a sharp decline between 30 and 35°C (Duriyaprapan *et al.*, 1986).

Franz *et al.* (1984) and Duriyaprapan *et al.* (1986) found that high temperature and the combination of low day and night temperature caused a decrease in the menthole level. For higher oil and menthol content, maximum and minimum temperature should range between 36-37°C and 14-16°C for *M. arvensis* (Singh *et al.*, 1988), a-pinene levels increased with increase in daily temperature (Duriyaprapan *et al.*, 1986; Ozel and Ozguven, 2002).

However, it was demonstrated by Fahlen *et al.* (1997) that night temperature had little effect on menthol levels at 21 hour photoperiod (day) regime. This suggested that higher the day length lower would be the effect of temperature. A detailed study on temperature was carried out by Shahi *et al.* (1998). Based on base temperature concept, it was shown that mint crop requires more than 2100 degree days for optimal production of menthol (45 per cent) in a growing season under optimum day length conditions. Further, they concluded that the phenomenon of accumulation of menthol is complex, but the final resultant of interaction of cropage of prevailing ambient temperature during the growing period.

Conclusion and Outlook

The knowledge of crop-weather relationship from a variety of plants, in combination with quality determinants, is particularly important not only to understand plant development and how plants are regulated by the environmental variables, but also to improve crop yields quantitatively and qualitatively. In this review, we have analysed the potential role of environmental variables underlying the differences in mint oil quality. We have highlighted the significance of specific environmental variables *viz.*, light, photoperiod and temperature on growth, oil yield and oil composition. This information based on crop-weather-physiology-field management can be readily integrated with farming practices to add new dimensions to crop production management. These are powerful tools to draw a broader picture of how plants alter biochemical processes in response to environmental stimuli. Despite evidences suggesting a role for environmental variables in essential oil regulation in mints, the exact means by which these factors influence path way flux or the specific steps of monoterpene metabolism are not understood (Mahmoud and Croteau, 2001)

However, the crop-weather relationship studied till now is in a piece meal approach in different parts of the world, it is still unclear what the exact role of the weather elements is in the biosynthetic pathway. There is scope for identifying particular enzymes in the path way that is triggered in the process of biomolecule production. This area needs further research to understand fully the plant-environment interactions in a better way.

References

Allard, H.A. (1941). Further studies of the photoperiodic behaviour of some mints (Labiatae). *Journal of Agricultural Research*, 63: 55-64.

Amelunxen, F. (1965). Elektronenmikroskopische Untersuchungen an den Drüsenschuppen von *Mentha piperita* L. *Planta Medica*, 13: 457-473

Amelunxen,F., Wahlig, T. and Arbeiter, H. (1969). Über den Nachweis des atherischen Öls in isolierten Drüsenhaaren und Drüsenschuppen von *Mentha piperita* L. *Z. Pflanzenphysiol.*, 61: 68–72.

Ascensao, L. and Pais, M.S.S. (1987). Glandular trichomes of Airtimes campestral: ontogeny and histochemistry of the secretary product. *Botanical Gazette*, 148: 221–227

Baslas, R.K. (1970). Studies on the influence of various factors on the essential oil from the plants of *Mentha arvensis* (Japanese mint). *The flavour industry*, 1:188-189.

Bertea, C.M., Maffei, M., Schalk, M., Karp, F. and Croteau, R. (2001). Demonstration that menthofuran synthase of mint (*Mentha*) is a cytochrome P450 monoxygenase: cloning, functional expression, and characterization of the responsible gene. *Arch. Biochem. Biophys.*, 390: 279–286.

Biggs, R.H. and Leopold, A.C. (1955). The effect of temperature on pepper mint (*Mentha piperita*). *Proceedings of American Society of Horticultural Science*, 66: 315-321.

Brun, N. and Voirin, B. (1991) Chemical and morphological studies of the effects of aging on monoterpene composition in *Mentha* × *piperita* leaves. *Canadian Journal of Botany*, 69: 2271-2278.

Brun, N.M., Colson, A., Perrin, B. and Voirin, B. (1990). Chemical and morphological studies on the effect of ageing on monoterpene composition in *Mentha piperita* leaves. *Canadian Journal of Botany*, 69: 2271–2278.

Burbott, A.J. and Loomis, W.D. (1967a). Effect of light and temperature on the monoterpenes of peppermint. *Plant Physiology*, 42: 20-28.

Burbott, A.J. and Loomis, W.D. (1969). Evidence for metabolic turnover of monoterpenes in peppermint. *Plant Physiology*, 44: 173-179

Charles, D.J., Jolly, R.J. and James, E. (1990) effect of osmotic stress on the essential oil content and composition of peppermint. *Phytochemistry*, 29: 2837-2840.

Chopra, R.N., Chopra, I.C., Handa, K.L. and Kapoor, L.D. (1958). Chopra's indigenous drug of India. 2nd Ed., pp.196-200 and 697-720.

Clark, R.J. and Menary, R.C. (1979). Effects of photoperiod on the yield and composition of pepper mint oil. *Journal of American Society of Horticultural Science*, 104: 699-702.

Clark, R.J. and Menary, R.C. (1980). Environmental effects on peppermint (*M. piperita* L.). I. Effect of day length, photon flux, density, night temperature and day temperature on yield and composition of pepper mint oil. *Australian Journal of Plant Physiology*, 7: 685-692.

Clark, R.J. and Menary, R.C. (1981). Variation in composition of peppermint oil in relation to production areas. *Economic Botany*, 35: 59-69.

Clark, R.J. and Menary, R.C. (1984). The effect of two harvests per year on the yield and composition of Tasmanian peppermint oil (*Mentha piperita* L.). *Journal of Science Food and Agriculture*, 35: 1191-1195.

Court, W.A., Roy, R.C. and Pocs, R. (1993). Effect of harvest date on the yield and quality of the essential oil of peppermint. *Canadian Journal of Plant Science* 73, 815-824.

Crane, F.A. (1951). Interaction between mineral nutrient, growth and development and metabolism with special reference to M piperita. Doctoral thesis, The University of Rochester, Rochester, New York.

Crane, S.F. and Steward, F.C. (1962a). Growth, nutrition and metabolism of *Mentha piperita*. IV. Effect of day length and Ca and K on nitrogenous metabolites of *Mentha piperita*. Cornell University, *Agricultural Experiment Station Menoir*, No. 379: 63-90.

Crane, S.F. and Steward, F.C. (1962b). Growth and nutrition of *Mentha piperita* under experimental conditions. In: Growth, nutrition and metabolism of *Mentha piperita*. Part-III, Cornell University *Agricultural Experiment Station Menoir*. No. 379: 91

Croteau, R. (1977). Effect of irrigation method on essential oil yield and rate of oil evaporation in mint grown under controlled conditions. *Horticultural Science*, 12: 563-565

Croteau, R., Karp, F., Wagaschal, K.C., Satterwhite, D.M., Hyatt,D.C. and Scotland, C.B. (1991). Biochemical characteristics of a spearmint mutant that resembles peppermint in monoterpenoids. *Plant Physiology*, 96: 589–593

Croteau, R. and Martinkus, C. (1979). Metabolism of monoterpenes: demonstration of (+)-neomenthyl-D-glucoside as a major metabolite of menthone in peppermint (*Mentha piperita*). *Plant Physiology*, 64: 169-175

DE Capite, L. (1955). Action of light and temperature on growth of plant tissue cultures *in vitro*. *American Journal of Botany*, 42: 869-873.

Doller, G. (1978). Influence of the medium on the production of serpentine by suspension cultures of *Catharanthus roseus CL.)*. In: *Production of Natural Compounds by Cell Culture Methods* (Ed. by G. Don), pp. 109-116. Gesselschaft fur Strahlen und Umweltforschung mbh Bereich Projekttragerschaften.

Duhan, S.P.S., Bhatachraya, A.K. and Husain, A. (1977). Effect of nitrogen and its method of application on the herb and oil yield and quality of Japanese mint. *Indian Perfumer*, 21: 47-50

Duriyaprapan, S., Britten, E.J. and Basford, K.E. (1986). The effect of temperature on growth, oil yield and oil quality of Japanese mint. *Annals of Botany*, 58: 729-736.

Ezekiel, R. and Bhargava, S.C. (1993). The influence of photoperiod on the growth and development of potato (*Solanum tuberosum* L.)–A review. *Plant Physiology Biochemistry* 20, 63–72

Fahlen, A., Welander, M. and Wennersten, R. (1997) Effects of Light–Temperature Regimes on Plant Growth and Essential Oil Yield of Selected Aromatic Plants. *Journal of Science Food Agriculture*, 73:111-119

Farooqi, A.H.A., Sangwan, N.S. and Sangwan, R.S. (1999). Effect of different photoperiodic regimes on growth, flowering and essential oil in *Mentha* species. *Plant Growth Regulation*, 29: 181–187.

Forrest, G. (1969). Studies of polyphenol metabolism of tissue cultures derived from tea plant *(Camellia sinensis). Biochemical Journa,,* 113: 765-772.

Franz, C., Ceylan, A., Holzl, J. and Vomel, A. (1984). Influence of the growing site on the quality of *Mentha piperita* L. oil. *Acta Horticulturae*,144: 145-150.

Fuchs, S., Gross, A., Beck, T. and Mosandl, A. (2000). Monoterpene biosynthesis in *Mentha piperita*: bioconversion of piperitone and piperitenone. *Flavour Fragrance Journal*, 15: 84–90.

Gershenzon, J., McConkey, M.E. and Croteau, R.B. (2000). Regulation of Monoterpene Accumulation in Leaves of Peppermint. *Plant Physiology*, 122: 205-214.

Ghosh, M.L. and Chatterjee, S.K. (1976). *Indian Journal of Experimental Biology*, 14: 366.

Giachetti, T.D., Taddi, F., Mantovani, P. and Bianchi, E. (1988). *Fitoterapia*, LIX: 463–468.

Grahle, A. and Holtzel, C. (1963). Photoperiodische Abhangigkeit der Bildung des atherischen ols bei *Mentha piperita*. *Naturwissen Schaften*, 50: 552.

Guenther, E. (1949). The essential oils. Vol III, D van Nostrand Co. Inc. Princeton, NJ.

Guenther, E. (1961). *Perfume Essential Oil Research*, 632–642.

Gupta, R., Gulati, B.C., Duhan, S.P.S. and Bhattacharya, A.K. (1971). *Agriculture Agroind. Journal*, 4: 33

Howe, K.J. (1956). Factors affecting the growth and development of *Mentha piperita* with special reference to the formation of essential oils. *Dissertation Abstracts*, 17: 730-731.

Jerkovic, I. J., Mastelic,Â. and Milos, M. (2001). The impact of both the season of collection and drying on the volatile constituents of *Origanum vulgare* L. ssp. hirtum grown wild in Croatia. *International Journal of Food Science and Technology*, 36: 649–654

Katasawa, D., Shatar, S. and Erdenechimeg, A. (1995). *Journal of Essential Oil Research*, 7: 255–260.

Kokkini, S. (1991). Chemical races within the genus *Mentha* L. In: Essential Oils and Waxes. Modern Methods of Plant Analysis (no 12), Eds Linskens, H. F. and Jackson, J. F. Springer–Verlag, Berlin, Germany, pp 63-75.

Kothari, S.K., Singh, C.P., Singh, K. and Sushil Kumar (2000). Physiological considerations for higher yield of good quality oil of menthol mint (M arvensis). *Indian Perfumer*, 44: 123-128.

Kothari, S.K., Singh, V.P. and Singh, U.B. (1996). The effect of row spacing and nitrogen fertilization on the growth and oil yield composition of Japanese mint. *Journal of Medicinal Aromatic Plant Sciences*, 18: 17-21.

Lange, B.M., Mark, R., Wildung, Stauber E.J. Christopher Sanchez, Derek Pouchnik and Rodney Croteau (2000). Probing essential oil biosynthesis and secretion by functional evaluation of expressed sequence tags from mint glandular trichomes. *PNAS*, 97: 2934-2939.

Langston, R.G. and Leopold, A.C. (1954). Photoperiodic responses of pepper mint. *Proceedings of American Society of Horticultural Science*, 63:347-352

Lawrence, B.M., Hogg, J.W. and Stuart, J.T. (1972). *Flavour Industry*, 3: 467.

Lawrence, B.M (1980). In: Essential oils: Monoterpene interrelationships *in the Mentha Genus: A Biosynthetic Discussion*, Mookherjee BD,Mussinan CJ (eds). Allured: Carol Stream, IL, 1.

Lawrence, B.M Lawrence BM (1985). *Perfumes and Flavours* 13, 2.

Lawrence,B.M (1986) Essential oil production–A discussion of influencing factors. In: Symposium Series 317, Biogeneration of Aromas. American Chemical Society, Washington, DC, USA, pp 363-369.

Lawrence,B.M 1992). In: Compte rendu des 3eÁmes rencontres techniques et economiques plantes aromatiques et medicinales, p. 59, (Ed). N. Verlet, Les Mimosas, Nyons.

Lawrence, B.M and Shu, C.K.(1989*). Perfum. Flav.*, 14, 21.

Leela, N.K. and Angadi, S.P. (1993) Yield and quality of peppermint as influenced by time of harvest. *Indian Perfumer*, 37: 324-326.

Lichtenthaler, H.K., Rohmer, M. and Schwender, J. (1997). Two independent biochemical pathways for isopentenyl diphosphate and isoprenoid biosynthesis in higher plants. *Physiologica Plantarum*, 101: 643–652

Loomis, W.D. (1977). Physiology of essential oil production in mint. Proceedings of 28th annual meeting Crog. Essential oil growers league, Jan 13-14.

Maffei, M. and Sacco, T. (1987). Chemical and morphometrical comparison between two peppermint notomorphs. *Planta Medica*, 53: 214–216.

Mahmoud, S.S. and Croteau, R.B. (2001). Metabolic engineering of essential oil yield and composition in mint by altering expression of deoxyxylulose phosphate reductoisomerase and menthofuran synthase. *Proceedings of National Academy of Science*, 98: 8915–8920.

Mahmoud, S.S. and Croteau, R.B. (2003). Menthofuran regulates essential oil biosynthesis in peppermint by controlling a downstream monoterpene reductase. *Proceedings of National Academy of Science*, 100: 14481-14486.

Mastelic, J. (1995). A study of the relations of terpenes and terpene glycosides of the aromatic plants belonging to the family Lamiaceae, PhD Thesis. Zagreb: University of Zagreb

Mehra, B.K. (1992). *Mentha* oil and menthol production in India–Past, present and future. In: Cultivation and utilization of aromatic plants. (Eds.) Atal,CK and Kapur, BM pp. 241-272.

Mohr, H. and Schopfer, P. (1995). Biosynthetic metabolism, In: Plant physiology, Springer Verlag, New York, Chap.18.

Murray, M.J., Marble, P., Lincoln, D. and Mefendehl, F.W. (1986). Peppermint oil quality differences and the reason for them. Flavours and Fragrances: A World Perspective, Proceeding on the 10th International Congress of Essential Oils, Washington DC, USA, 16–20 November.

Murray, M.J., Marble, P., Lincoln, D. and Mefendehl, F.W. (1988). Peppermint oil quality differences and the reasons for them. In: Flavors and Fragrances: A World Perspective. Proceedings of 10th International Congress of Essential Oils, Fragrances and Flavors, Eds Lawrence B M, Mookerje B D and Willis B J. pp 189-210.

Nelson, C.E., Mortenson, M.A. and Early, R.E. (1971). Evaporation cooling of peppermint by sprinkling. Circular Washington Agricultural experiment Station No 539:12

Nijjar, G.S. (1990). Optimising *Mentha* oil yield from Shivalik-88 variety of *M. arvensis*. *Indian Perfumer*, 34:189-189.

Ohta, S. and Yatazawa, M, (1978). Effect of ligbt and nicotine production in tobacco tissue culture. *Agricultural and Biological Chemistry*, 42: 873-877.

Ozel, A. and Ozguven, M. (2002). Effect of different planting times on essential oil composition of different mint varieties. *Turkish Journal of Agriculture and Forestry*, 26: 289-294.

Prasad, S. and Saxena, M.C. (1980). Effect of date of planting and row spacing on the growth and development of Peppermint in Tarai. *Indian Journal of Plant Physiology*, 23: 119-126.

Rabak, F. (1916). The effect of cultural and climatic conditions on the yield and quality of pepper mint oil. US Dept of Agriculture Professional Paper, 454.

Rabson, R. and Steward, F.C. (1962). Growth, nutrition, and metabolism of *Mentha piperita* L. VI. The keto and amino acids of mint plants: Interacting effects due to day length and night temperature. *Cornell University Agricultural Experiment Station Memoir*, 379: 130-140.

Rohloff, J. (1999). Monoterpene composition of essential oil from peppermint (*Mentha* X *piperita* L.) with regard to leaf position using solid-phase micro extraction and gas chromatography/mass spectrometry analysis. *Journal of Agriculture and Food Chemistry*, 47: 3782-3786

Roitsema, R.H. (1958). A biogenetic agreement of mint species. *Journal of American Pharma Association Science Ed.*, 47: 267-269.

Schball, R. and Beckeh, H. (1977). Production of catechins and oligomeric proanthocyanidins in tissue and suspension cultures of Crataegus *monogyna, C. oxycanthazndGingko biloba. Planta Medica,* 32: 297

Schroder, H. (1963). Studies on the influence of various water regimes on yields, contents of essential oils, transpiration quotients, leaf size and relative oil gland densities in the several species of the family Labiatae. *Pharmazie*, 18: 47-58.

Shahi, A.K., Chandra, S., Dutt, P., Kaul, B.L., Tava, A. and Avato, P, (1999). Essential oil composition of *Mentha piperita* L. from different environments of north India. *Flavour Fragrance,* 14: 5-8.

Shahi, A.K., Chandra, S. and Kaul, B.L. (1998). Accumulation of menthol in M piperita–A biometeorological approach. *Indian Perfumer,* 42: 206-210.

Shanker, S., Ajaya Kumar, P.V., Sangwan, N.S., Kumar, S. and Sangwan, R.S. (1999). Essential oil gland number and ultra structure during *M. arvensis* L. leaf ontogeny. *Biologia Plantarum.*

Singh, A., Naqvi, A.A., Singh, K. and Thakur, R.S. (1988). Transformation of menthol, menthone and menthyl acetate in M arvensis with relation to age of the plant. *Current Science,* 57: 480-481.

Singh, B.P. and Garg, O.K. (1976). Relative growth and development in *Mentha arvensis* during summer and winter seasons. *Indian Journal of Agricultural Research,* 10: 91-96.

Singh, J.N. and Singh, D.P. (1969). Effect of phosphorus deficiency and seasonal variation on growth and essential oil contents of Japanese mint (*Mentha arvensis* var. *piperascens*). *Soil Science and Plant Nutrition,* 15: 67-74.

Singh, K., Kaul, P.N., Bhattacharya, A.K. and Singh, C.P. (1999). Effect of planting dates and spacing on performance of M arvensis in semiarid climate of Hyderabad. *Indian Perfumer,* 43: 29-34.

Singh, V. (1994). Response of Japanese mint to nitrogen in relation to irrigation schedules. Ph.D Thesis, Meerut University, Meerut.

Singh, V.P., Singh, M. and Singh, D.V.(1997). Growth, yield and quality of peppermint as influenced by planting time. *Journal of Herbs, Spices and Medicinal Plants,* 5: 33-39.

Smith, D.M. and Levi, L. (1961). Treatment of compositional data for the characterization of essential oils. Determination of geographic origins of peppermint oils by gas chromatographic analysis. *Journal of Agriculture and Food Chemistry,* 9:230-244.

Stengele, M. and Stahl-Biskup, E. (1993). *Journal of Essential Oil Research,* 5: 13–19.

Sternberg, B.S.M. and Duke, J.A. (1996). In: *CRC Handbook of Medicinal Mints (Aromathematics): Phytochemicals and Biological Activities,* Beckstrom-Sternberg SM, Duke JA (eds). CRC Press: New York, 92–128.

Steward, F.C.(1962). *Mentha* as a plant for physiological investigations. In: Growth, nutrition and metabolism of *Mentha piperita*. Part–1, *Cornell University Agricultural Experiment Station, Menoir No.* 379.

USDA (1999). Risk Management Agency–Mint. Excerpt in *The Australian New Crops Newsletter*. No. 12, July. http://www.newcrops.uq.edu.au/newslett/ncnl1220e.htm

Vasyutev, G.C. and Pyshnev, V.M. (1982) Characteristics of the development of mint root system under irrigation. *Horticultural Abstracts,* 53: 7329

Voirin, B. and Bayet, C. (1996). Developmental changes in the monoterpene composition of *Mentha piperita* leaves from individual peltate trichomes. *Phytochemistry*, 43: 573-580

Voirin, B., Brun, N. and Bayte, C. (1990). Effects of day length on monoterpene composition of leaves of *Mentha* Í *piperita*. *Phytochemistry*, 29: 749-755.

Watts, M.J., Galpin, I.J. and Collin, H.A.(1984). The effect of growth regulators, light and temperature on flavour production in celery tissue cultures. *New Phytol.*,98: 583-591

Weller S, Green Jr R, Janssen C, Whitford F (2000). Mint Production and Pest Management in Indiana. Purdue University Extension. PPP-103. http: / / www. btny. purdue. edu / Pubs / PPP / PPP-103.pdf

White, J.G.H., Iskandar, S.H. and Barnes, M.F. (1987). Peppermint: effect of time of harvest on yield and quality of oil. *New Zealand Journal of Experimental Agriculture*, 15: 73-79.

Utilisation and Management of Medicinal Plants (2010) *Pages 48–54*
Editors: V.K. Gupta, Anil K. Verma and Sushma Koul
Published by: DAYA PUBLISHING HOUSE, NEW DELHI

Chapter 3

Search for Useful Substances in Papyrus *Cyperus papyrus* L.

Nariaki Wakiuchi[1], Hajime Tamaki[2], Takashi Nishino[3] and Yukihiro Sugimoto[1]*

[1]Graduate School of Agricultural Science, [3]Graduate School of Engineering, Kobe University, Rokkodai, Nada, Kobe 657-8501, Japan

[2]Graduate School of Agricultural Sciences, University of the Ryukyus, Nakagami-gun, Okinawa 903-0213, Japan

ABSTRACT

Papyrus plant is a macrophyte with thick stems and can grow in polluted water, extensively absorb the pollutants, *e.g.* nitrogen and phosphate, as nutrients, and thereby ameliorate quality of water in which it grows. In order to make efficient use of aerial parts of the plant, ingredients were extracted and analyzed. Methanol extracts of the aerial parts were subjected to liquid-liquid partitioning and silica gel column chromatography. Tricin and *p*-coumaric acid were isolated as phenolics. Pectic substances were extracted from alcohol-insoluble solids (AIS) with hot water (HW) or EDTA solution (ChSS). The residue of the ChSS extraction was further treated with alkaline solution (ASS). Each of these extracts were concentrated, dialyzed against water, lyophilized and hydrolyzed by trifluoroacetic acid. GLC and HPLC analyses revealed that the HW and ASS extracts consisted of galacturonic acid, glucose, arabinose, galactose, and xylose, while the ChSS extract contained galacturonic acid and arabinose. The cellulose fractions were also prepared from papyrus piths. Treatment of the AIS with hot water and acetone gave the

* Corresponding Author: E-mail: yukihiro@kobe-u.ac.jp;Tel. and Fax: +81-78-803-5884.

holocellulose fraction, which was sequentially fractionated to hemicellulose A, hemicellulose B and α-cellulose fractions. The ratio in weight of hemicellulose A : hemicellulose B : α-cellulose was 23 : 10 : 40. X-ray diffraction measurement indicated that the α-cellulose possessed cellulose I structure.

Keywords: *Cellulose, p-coumaric acid, Papyrus, Pectin, Tricin.*

Introduction

Papyrus (*Cyperus papyrus* L.) is a macrophyte with thick stalks. The C_4 plant is distributed in tropical freshwater (Jones and Milburn, 1978). Papyrus paper made from the piths of the stalks was used for writing and drawing in ancient Egypt. However, current utilization of the plant is limited. Roots of the plant are used as fuel, whereas the stalks are used as food and raw materials to produce mats, baskets, ropes and cordages (Allen, 1996). In natural papyrus habitat in Uganda, the average productivity is as high as about 40 g plant dry weight $m^{-2} d^{-1}$ (Westlake, 1975). Moreover, the plant can grow in polluted water, extensively absorb the pollutants, *e.g.* nitrogen and phosphate, as nutrients, and thereby ameliorate quality of water in which it grows (Abe *et al.*, 1999). Identification of economically important substances and/or development of extensive applications of papyrus will promote cultivation of the plant with high ability of carbon fixation and pollutant absorption. Recently, Nishino *et al.* (2007) reported that poly (L–lactic acid) resin was reinforced mechanically by mixing papyrus stem-milled particles. In the present study, various ingredients contained in aerial parts of papyrus were extracted and analyzed in order to probe potential value of the plant.

Materials and Methods

Plant Material

Papyrus seedlings were obtained from Kobe Papyrus Institute. The plants were grown in the experimental field of Kobe University, Japan. The aerial parts of the plants were air-dried, and pulverized.

Extraction, Isolation and Identification of Phenolics

The plant sample (1 kg) was soaked in methanol (2 L), sonicated and filtered. Methanol extraction was repeated four times, and the combined filtrates (8 L) were evaporated *in vacuo* to dryness at 40°C. The residue (76.4 g) was suspended in water (1L), and partitioned with hexane (1L), chloroform (1L), and then ethyl acetate (1 L). Chloroform extracts were dried over Na_2SO_4 and concentrated *in vacuo* to dryness. The residue (10.8 g) was dissolved in a small amount of chloroform and chromatographed on a silica gel column (200 x 48 mm) using mixed solvent of hexane and ethyl acetate. The proportion of ethyl acetate was increased stepwise, 9:1, 8:2, 7:3, 6:4, 5:5, 2:8, and 0:10 in 200 ml each of the solvents. Fractions were collected every 10 ml and solid substance obtained in the fractions was eluted with the solvents of 6:4 and 5:5. The substrate was further purified by TLC using ethyl acetate as a developing solvent. A purified chemical recovered from the major spot (Rf 0.8) was crystallized from a mixed solvent of ethyl acetate and hexane. A crystalline compound (6.9 m g) was obtained and subjected to NMR and MS analyses. ^1H NMR spectra were recorded in $CDCl_3$ on a JEOL Lambda 400 spectrometer. MS spectra were obtained on a Hitachi M-2500 mass spectrometer in the EI mode.

The ethyl acetate extracts were applied to a short column of ODS and eluted with aqueous methanol solutions with increasing methanol concentrations. After concentrating *in vacuo*, the residue (132.5 mg) of 80 per cent methanol eluate was dissolved in a small amount of methanol, and chromatographed on an ODS column (Yamazen) using 66 per cent methanol. The fractions rich in a chemical were collected and concentrated, and the residue was further purified with HPLC. The column was 5C18-AR (Nacalai Tesque), the solvent 45 per cent methanol, and the flow rate 4 ml/min. The most abundant chemical eluted at 32 min was collected and subjected to NMR and MS analyses.

Preparation of Pectin Fractions

Papyrus stalks (10 g) were treated with 200 ml of 80 per cent ethanol repeatedly. The residue, referred to as alcohol-insoluble solids (AIS, 5 g), was treated with 300 ml of 50 mM sodium acetate buffer (pH 5.2) containing 50 mM EDTA and 50 mM ammonium oxalate at 70°C for 30min, according to Ros *et al.* (1996). The extraction was repeated three times and the filtrates were combined. The residual stalks were then treated with 300 ml of 50 mM sodium hydroxide at 0°C three times and filtered. Each of the combined filtrates were dialyzed and lyophilized to yield pectin soluble in chelating agents (ChSS) and pectin soluble in diluted alkali (ASS). In a separate experiment, AIS was treated for 12 h with hot water to obtain pectin soluble in water, which was also dialyzed and lyophilized (HW).

The lyophilized pectin fractions were hydrolyzed by 2 N trifluoroacetic acid (2 h, 121°C) in sealed glass tubes, according to Baig *et al.* (1982). The hydrolysates were analyzed for sugar composition using HPLC (L-6000, Hitachi) equipped with Aminex HPX-87H column (Bio-Rad) at 80°C. The mobile phase was 0.01 N sulfuric acid at a flow rate of 0.7 ml/min. The detector was a RI monitor (Shodex RI-72). Galactose and xylose were determined using Cosmosil 5NH_2-MS column with acetonitril-H_2O (80:20). In addition, ChSS was treated with silblender (Nacalai Tesque) and analyzed by GLC (K23, Hitachi) equipped with 2 per cent silicone OV-1 Uniport HP glass column.

Preparation of Cellulose Fraction

The holocellulose fraction was obtained from AIS (4 g) by successive extraction with hot water (500 ml) and then with acetone (500 ml). After removing the solvents, the residue (3g) was dissolved in 1 N KOH (100 ml) and filtered. Ethanol (1,300 ml) was added to the filtrate to precipitate hemicellulose A fraction, which was collected by filtration and dried *in vacuo* (0.92 g). The hemicellulose B was extracted with 4 N KOH from the insoluble materials and precipitated in the same manner (0.4 g). The residue after the extraction with 4N KOH was washed with organic solvents (ethanol, acetone and diethyl ether) and dried (1.6 g). The α-cellulose fraction was analyzed with X-ray diffractometer (RAD-B, Rigaku, Japan) to investigate the structure.

Results and Discussion

Alcoholic extracts from papyrus stalks were subjected to liquid-liquid partitioning and silica gel column chromatography for phenolics. A compound (0.007 per cent) was isolated as crystals. Based on NMR (Table 3.1) and MS spectra (m/e 330), the compound was identified as tricin (1), which has been identified in wheat and Japanese barnyard millet (Watanabe, 1999). The flavonoid was reported to inhibit colon cancer cell growth (Cai *et al.*, 2005). Chloroform extracts were fractionated by solid phase extraction and chromatographed on a ODS column. Further purification by HPLC led to isolation of a chemical (0.006 per cent), which was identified as *p*-coumaric acid (2) on the basis of NMR data (Table 3.2). The phenylpropanoid was reported to be found in *Cyperus papyrus* as far back as 40 years ago (Bate-Smith, 1968). *p*-Coumaric acid is an important intermediate of lignin biosynthesis. Besides the phenolics we isolated in this study, sinapic acid and El-Hamidi and El-Gengaihi (1975) described the presence of b-amyrin, a pentacyclic triterpene, in the sap of papyrus stems.

Table 3.1: NMR Spectral Data of Tricin (1) Isolated from Papyrus Stalks

Position	*^1H (δ ppm)*	*^{13}C (δ ppm)*
2		164.1
3	6.97	103.5
4		181.8
5		157.3
6	6.19	98.8
7		164.1
8	6.55	94.2
9		161.4
10		103.7
1'		120.4
2'	7.32	104.4
3'		148.2
4'		139.9
5'		148.2
6'	7.32	104.4
OCH_3	3.87	56.3

Table 3.2: NMR Spectral Data of *p*-coumaric Acid Isolated from Papyrus Stalks

Position	*^1H (δ ppm)*	*^{13}C (δ ppm)*
1	7.46	143.9
2	6.27	115.8
3		168.1
1'		159.6
2'	6.77	115.8
3'	7.48	130.1
4'		125.3
5'	7.48	130.1
6'	6.77	115.8

There have been controversial questions about an adhesive of the paper because papyrus paper was manufactured without any additional adhesives (Allen, 1996). Based on an idea that the most probable candidate of an adhesive is pectic substance originally contained in papyrus tissues, we analyzed pectin fractions of the stalks. Pectin fractions, extracted from AIS, were hydrolyzed by trifluoroacetic acid, and subjected to analyses of carbohydrate compositions by GLC and HPLC. As shown in Table 3.3, galacturonic acid and arabinose were major components of the ChSS fraction. The pectin fraction was further separated into three fractions, HW, ChSS, and ASS. Contents of the fractions were 5.8, 8.8, and 1.6 per cent, respectively. The HW and ASS fractions were consisted of galacturonic acid, glucose, arabinose, galactose, and xylose. Pectin is consisted of 1→4-α-D-galactopyranosyl uronic acid as a main chain with branch-points containing different degrees of α-L-rhamnosyl residue. The fact that the papyrus pectin contained only small amount of rhamnose demonstrated that there are limited branch-points. Methylation of uronic acid was not detected in the papyrus pectin fractions, suggesting that pectic substances are involved in adhesive effect of papyrus strips in the process of paper-manufacturing.

Table 3.3: Carbohydrate Composition of the Pectic Fractions Extracted from Papyrus Stalks

	Carbohydrate Composition							
	GalA	*Glc*	*Ara*	*Gal*	*Xyl*	*Rha*	*Man*	*GlcA*
ChSS	97.0* (12.3) **	tr.	3.0 (0.3)	tr.	tr.	tr.	0 (0)	0 (0)
ASS	42.8 (15.7)	4.3 (1.5)	10.8 (3.1)	24.2 (8.2)	16.0 (4.5)	tr.	tr.	1.8 (0.7)
HW	51.0 (30.1)	21.2 (11.6)	17.1 (7.8)	1.2 (0.7)	5.7 (2.6)	2.3 (1.2)	0 (0)	1.4 (0.7)

*: Mol per cent, **: Wt per cent.

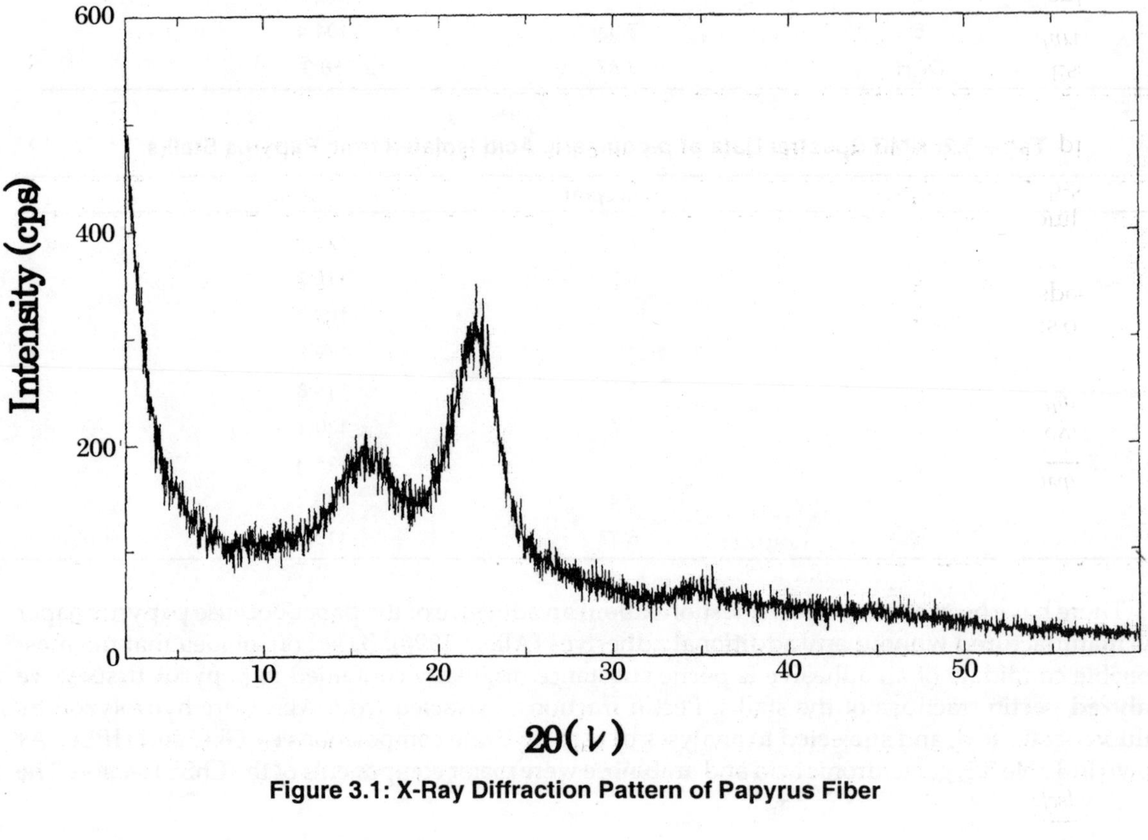

Figure 3.1: X-Ray Diffraction Pattern of Papyrus Fiber

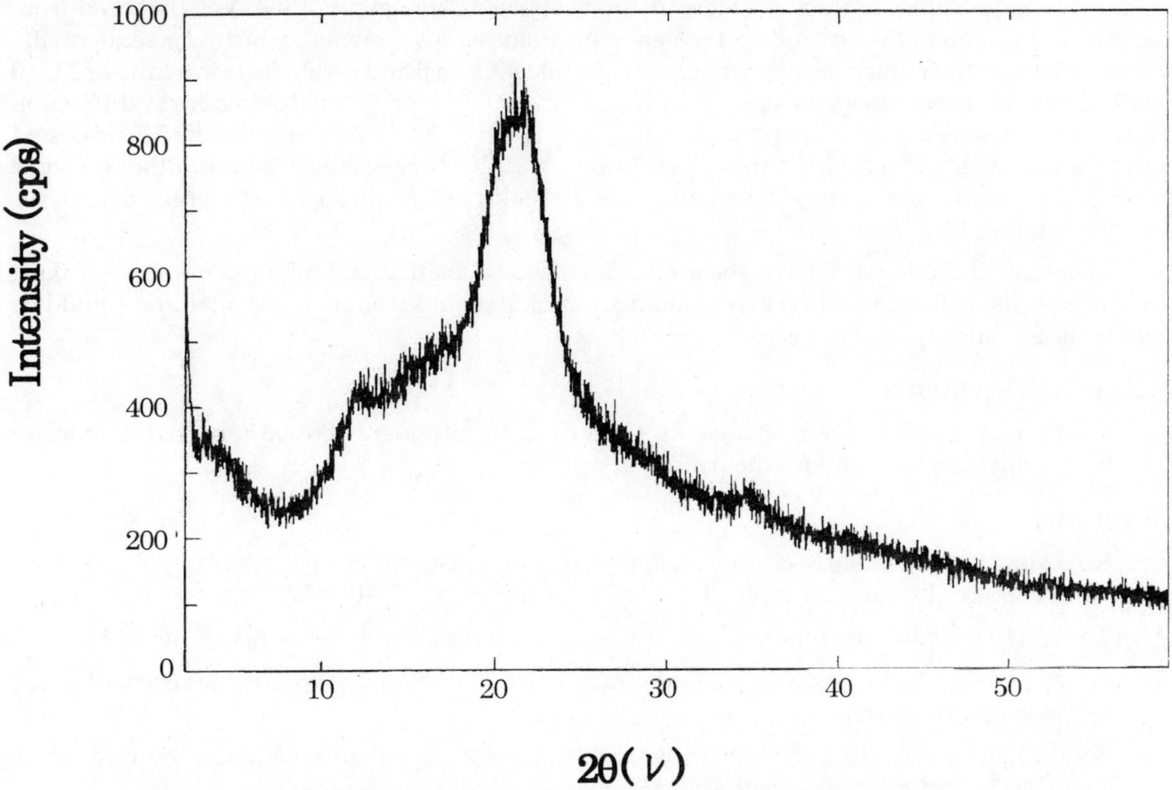

Figure 3.2: X-ray Diffraction Pattern of α-cellulose Prepared from Papyrus Stalks

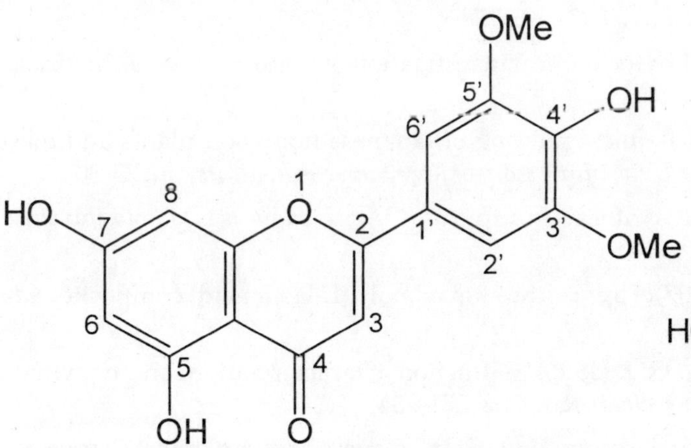

1

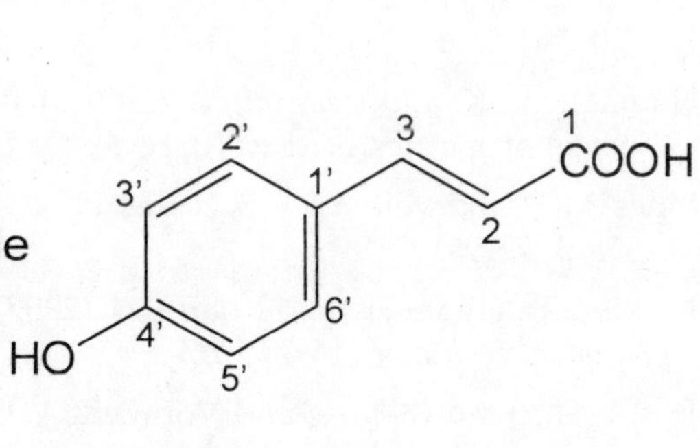

2

Figure 3.3: Chemical Formulae

Properties of cellulose fractions were also investigated. Treatment of the AIS, prepared from papyrus piths, with hot water and acetone gave the holocellulose fraction, which was sequentially fractionated into three fractions hemicellulose A, hemicellulose B and α-cellulose, in a ratio of 23 : 10 : 40. The ratio indicates that papyrus plant is useful as a material for paper-making. X-ray diffraction measurement revealed that both papyrus fiber (Figure 3.1) and α-cellulose fraction (Figure 3.2) possessed cellulose I structure, typical for natural plant fiber, and their crystallinity is poor although some crystalline structures may coexist. Hamaguchi and Iwasaki (2001) indicated the potential of papyrus for chemical pulping.

As described above, papyrus can be used as medicinal, adhesive, and cellulose resources. Taking into account its high ability of carbon fixation and pollutant absorption, more attention should be paid to the advanced use of papyrus.

Acknowledgements

The authors gratefully acknowledge Ms. H. Katsuta, the president of Kobe Papyrus Institute, for supplying papyrus plants and for the fruitful discussion.

References

Abe, K., Ozaki, Y. and Mizuta, K. (1999). Evaluation of useful plants for the treatment of polluted pond water with low N and P concentrations. *Soil Sci. Plant Nutr.*, 45: 409-417.

Allen, K. W. (1996). Papyrus–some ancient problems in bonding. *Int. J. Adhes. Adhes.*, 16: 47-51.

Baig, M. M., Burgin C. W. and Cerda, J. J. (1982). Fractionation and study of chemistry of pectic polysaccharides. *J. Agric. Food Chem.*, 30: 768-770.

Bate-Smith, E. C. (1968). The phenolic constituents of plants and their taxonomic significance. II. Monocotyledons. *J. Linn. Soc. (Bet.)*, 60: 325-356.

Cai, H., Al-Fayez, M., Tunstall, R. G., Platton, S., Greaves, P., Steward, W. P. and Gescher, A. J. (2005). The rice bran constituent tricin potently inhibits cyclooxygenase enzymes and interferes with intestinal carcinogenesis in *Apc*^{Min} mice. *Mol. Cancaer Ther.*, 4: 1287-1292.

El-Hamidi, A. and El-Gengaihi, S. (1975). Phytochemical investigation of *Cyperus papyrus*. *Pharmazie*, 30: 541-542.

Hamaguchi, K. and Iwasaki, M. (2001). Chemical pulping of Japanese nonwood plants and these sheet properties. *Selected Papers for the 10th Anniversary of Kobe Papyrus Institute*, pp. 75-80.

Jones, M. B. and Milburn T. R. (1978). Photosynthesis in papyrus (*Cyperus papyrus* L.) *Photosynthetica*, 13: 197-199.

Nishino, T., Hirano, K. and Kotera, M. (2007). Papyrus reinforced poly (L-lactic acid) composite. *Adv. Composite Mater.*, 16: 259-267.

Ros, J. M., Schols, H. A., and Voragen, A. G. J. (1996). Extraction, characterization, and enzymatic degradation of lemon peel pectins. *Carbohydr Res.*, 282: 271-284.

Watanabe M.£˙(1999)£© Antioxidative phenolic compounds from Japanese barnyard millet (*Echinochloa utilis*) grains. *J. Agric. Food Chem.*, 47: 4500–4505.

Westlake, D. F. (1975) Primary production of freshwater macrophyte. In Photosynthesis and productivity in different environments (Cooper, J.P. ed.) Cambridge University Press, London, pp. 189-206

Utilisation and Management of Medicinal Plants (2010) *Pages 55–106*
Editors: V.K. Gupta, Anil K. Verma and Sushma Koul
Published by: DAYA PUBLISHING HOUSE, NEW DELHI

Chapter 4

Secondary Plant Products and their Biopotentials

S.C. Jain[1]*, R. Singh[1] and R. Jain[2]
[1]Department of Botany, [2]Department of Chemistry, University of Rajasthan, Jaipur – 302 004, India

ABSTRACT

Nature produces a large number of chemical compounds whose structures and properties are of great interest and fascinating for the majority. These are organic compounds formed by the living systems and are emerging from the cocoon of organic chemistry. The term 'natural products' is applied to materials derived from plants, microorganisms, invertebrates and vertebrates, which are fine biochemical factories for biosynthesis of both, primary and secondary metabolites. The former class comprises molecules that are essential for life; principally proteins, carbohydrates, fats and nucleic acids, and these molecules are produced by metabolic pathways in most of the organisms. In contrast, secondary metabolites are usually of relatively limited occurrence and are often unique to a particular species. Secondary metabolites, such as phenolics, alkaloids, terpenoids, steroids and miscellaneous (vitamins, rotenoids, pyrethrins, polyacetylenes, etc.) are produced from a few key intermediates of primary metabolites on the basis of their biogenesis and utility to the plants. They are often restricted to a narrow set of species within a phylogenetic group. Phytochemical surveys can reveal natural products that are "markers" for botanical and evolutionary relationship. Due to tremendous researches in this field, a large number of these products have been demonstrated to be bioactive agents of many medicines, vitamins, food, flavor, fragrances, dyes-coloring agents, agro-chemicals and as plant protectants.

Further, these provide a new dimension to science for having pharmacologically active natural products, which not only give medicines but also carry nutraceutical values. Secondary

* Corresponding Author: E-mail: jainnatpro3@rediffmail.com.

metabolites have attracted interest due to their biological effect on other organisms and usually referred as 'biologically active constituents' of medicinal, commercial and poisonous plants, a subject which has developed in organic chemistry. Over 40 per cent of medicines have origin from this class of compounds. It is known that the secondary metabolites have greater diversity not only in structures but also in their bioefficacies and that particular structural characteristics arise from the way in which they are biosynthesized in nature. A number of screening programmes for bioactive compounds exist and have led to new drugs, *e.g.*, taxol, which is used for the treatment of various cancers.

Keywords: *Secondary plant products, Phenolics, Alkaloids, Terpenoids, Steroids.*

Introduction

During the course of evolution millions of secondary products have been synthesized from time to time by different species of plants and when the presence of a particular secondary product has conferred a selectionary advantage on the plant containing it, then the chances of survival of that plant, its offspring, and the secondary product itself will have been enhanced. The great majority of secondary products thrown up during the course of evolution probably proved to be of no advantage to the plants which synthesized them and neither the plants nor the compounds are likely to have survived. It is also possible that secondary products may have survived in a plant, not because it conferred an advantage on that plant, but rather because the gene or genes controlling its synthesis were closely associated on the same chromosome with genes determining another character which proved to be major selective advantage. More usually the role of secondary compounds in defence is related to their irritant, toxic, or unpalatable characteristics. In addition to their involvement in plant-animal relations, secondary compounds are also concerned in plant-plant relationships.

Secondary metabolites are chemicals produced by plants for which no role has yet been found in growth, photosynthesis, reproduction, or other "primary" functions. These chemicals are extremely diverse; many thousands have been identified in several major classes. Each plant family, genus, and species produces a characteristic mix of these chemicals, and they can sometimes be used as taxonomic characters in classifying plants. Many secondary metabolites are toxic or repellant to herbivores and microbes and help defend plants producing them. Recent research is identifying more and more primary roles for these chemicals in plants as signals, antioxidants, and other functions, so "secondary" may not be an accurate description in the future. Secondary plant products are equally important in use by humans. Most pharmaceuticals are based on plant chemical structures, and secondary metabolites are widely used for secretion and stimulation (the alkaloids nicotine and cocaine; the terpene cannabinol). The study of such plant use is called "ethnopharmacology". Psychoactive plant chemicals are central to some religions, and flavors of secondary compounds shape our food preferences. The characteristic flavors and aroma of cabbage and relatives are caused by nitrogen–and sulfur-containing chemicals, glucosinolates, which protect these plants from many enemies. The astringency of wine and chocolate derivatives from tannins, and the use of spices and other seasonings developed from their combined uses as preservatives (since they are antibiotic) and flavorings (Bell and Charlwood, 1980).

The chemical differentiation of cells or tissues allows an insight into the enormous chemical potential contained in the genetic material. The coordinated gene expression in secondary metabolism under the influence of intrinsic and extrinsic factors reflects a general phenomenon of the developmental biology. As the occurrence of particular secondary products may be restricted to few species or even to a single chemical race, as they are sometimes formed at certain stages of the individual's development.

Earlier, secondary products used to mean that these compounds are derivatives of primary products. This is surely valid for most of the true alkaloids whose N–and C–atoms are usually derived from protein amino acids, the basic ring system being modified by methyl, acetyl, isoprene or other groups. This concept is also valid for cyanogenic compounds, tannins, etc. However, it is essential to note that many secondary products (including some alkaloids) have their own biosynthetic pathways which are not directly related to primary metabolism (Misra *et al.*, 1999).

To define the role of secondary products within the framework of general metabolism the term 'excrete' has been used several times. Excretory products in plants are frequently formed in large excess. This kind of "energy waste" is evidently restricted to photoautotrophic organisms. Synthesis of secondary products in most instances required multistep reactions. The complexity of the whole process called 'secondary metabolism' therefore, becomes apparent because numerous enzymes or multienzyme complexes involved the regulated synthesis of these compounds, and the necessity of their spatial organization.

Classification

Secondary metabolites can be classified on the basis of chemical structure (*e.g.*, having rings or contain sugar), composition (containing nitrogen or not), their solubility in various solvents, or the pathway by which they are synthesized (*e.g.*, phenolics, which produces tannins). A simple classification includes three main groups: phenolics (made from simple sugars, containing benzene rings, hydrogen, and oxygen), and nitrogen-containing compounds (extremely diverse and formed from amino acids, may also contain sulfur) and the terpenes (made from mevalonic acid, composed almost entirely of carbon and hydrogen).

Biosynthesis

During the process of biogenesis of natural products, initiating from photosynthesis accompanied by respiration, a large number of metabolites are generated where several biochemical reactions commonly take place. Most of these are enzyme catalyzed and basically same as other organic reactions.

There are various types of reactions such as oxidation and reduction reactions, dehydration, dehydrogenations, carboxylations, decarboxylations, isomerizations, tautomerisation, interconversions, glycosylations, alkylations, eliminations, substitutions, Claisen and Michael type reactions and Wagner-Meerwein rearrangements which are commonly observed (Dewick, 2002). As a result of several individual and/or related chemical reactions a large number of secondary plant products of different class are synthesized (Figure 4.1).

Types of Secnodary Metabolites

There are several types of secondary metabolites, out of which more important classes have been included in this chapter having their exemplary molecules with biopotentials.

Phenolics

This class of compounds encompasses a broad range of plant substances having in common an aromatic ring with one or more hydroxyl group(s). Many phenolics occur as derivatives formed by condensation or addition reactions. These substances are water-soluble, since these occur combined with sugar as glycosides and thus, usually located in the cell vacuole. Over a thousand structures of

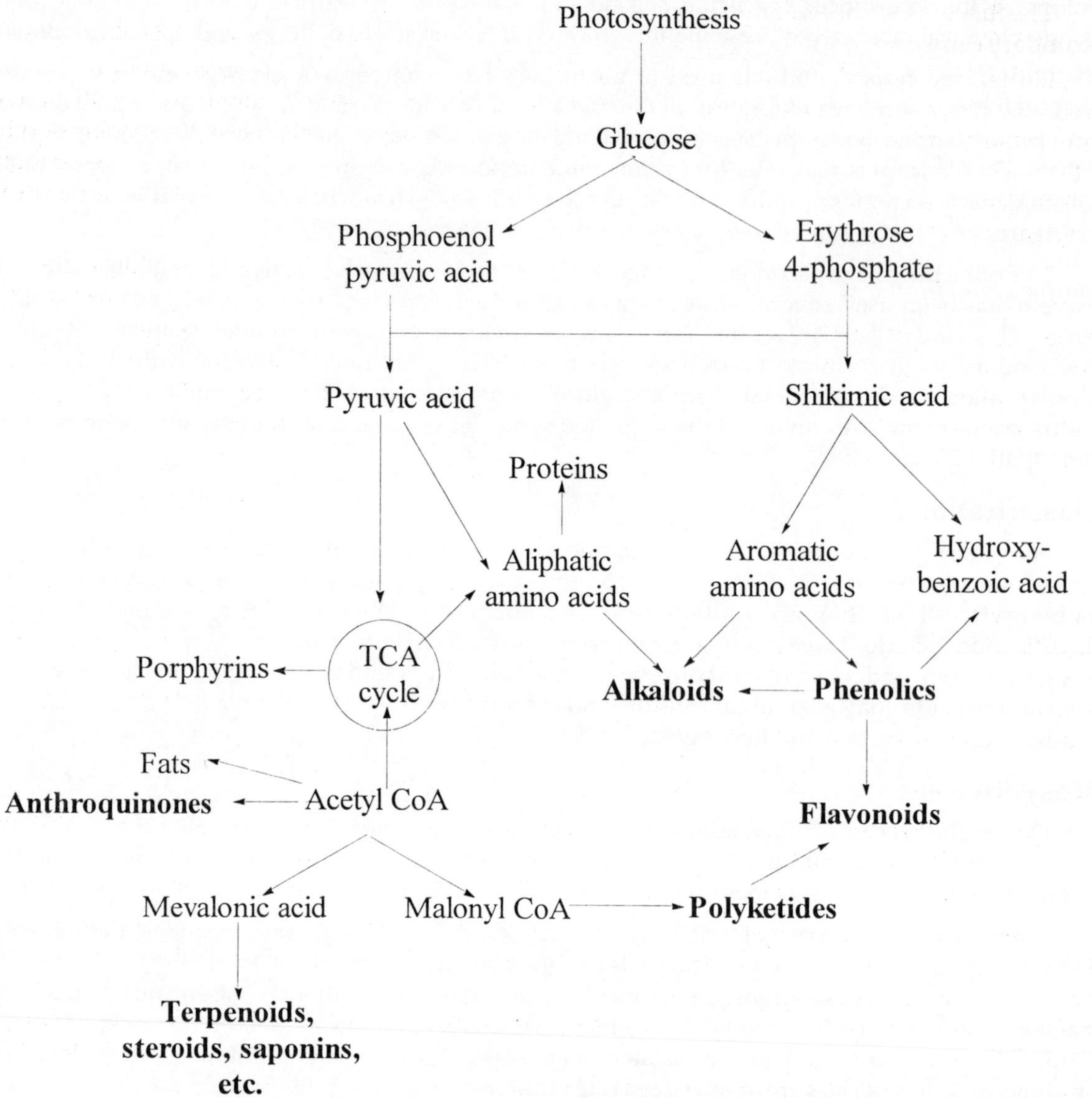

Figure 4.1: Concise Schematic Presentation of Biosynthesis of Secondary Plant Products

natural phenolic compounds are known today where the flavonoids form the largest group. Besides these, simple monocyclic phenols, phenylpropanoids and phenolic quinones also exist in appreciable amount. There are several other important polymeric phenolic compounds *viz.* lignins, melanins and tannins. Occasionally, phenolic units are also associated among proteins, alkaloids and terpenoids. Lignins after cellulose are the second most abundant organic metabolites on earth, as these build rigid structures in the form of woody stems and help in conducting water transport. However, due to the complexity of their molecules and biogenetic routes, phenols have been classified into five classes *i.e.*, phenols and phenolic acids, phenylpropanoids, flavonoids, quinones and phenolic polymers.

The functional aspects of phenolics are diverse and used in differentiation between primary and secondary compounds. Many phenolics are valuable storage vehicles and indispensable elements in anatomical and morphological structures. Primarily phenolics are of great importance as cellular support material because they form the integral part of cell wall structure by polymeric phenolics, *e.g.*, lignins and suberins, which provide protection against microbial invasion. Phenolic compounds especially anthocyanins, with flavones and flavonols as pigments are responsible for colour(s) in various flowers and fruits for attracting animals to make pollination and seed dispersal easy. Several plants used as folk medicines are rich source of phenolics and therefore, used as pharmacoactive drugs. The phenolics-rich plants were used for centuries in leather-making due to tannins forming complex with proteins. Polyphenols because of their astringent taste are important in foodstuffs and nutrition. Their toxic nature may protect plants from predators. As a result of microbial attack, low-molecular weight phenolic compounds formed in low concentrations are known as 'phytoalexins'.

There are several toxic, water-soluble simple phenols *viz.* hydroxyquinones, hydroxybenzoates and others as allelopathic compounds lead to competition among plants, a phenomenon called 'allelopathy'. Besides these, some phenolics in root exudates are toxic to the plant itself (autotoxic). There are a large number of such compounds which have demonstrated diverse biopotentialities (Table 4.1).

Table 4.1: Chemical Structure, Example Source and Biopotentials of Some Important Phenolics

Sl.No.	*Bioactive Molecules*	*Chemical Structures*	*Example Sources*	*Biopotentials*	*References*
1.	Afzalechin	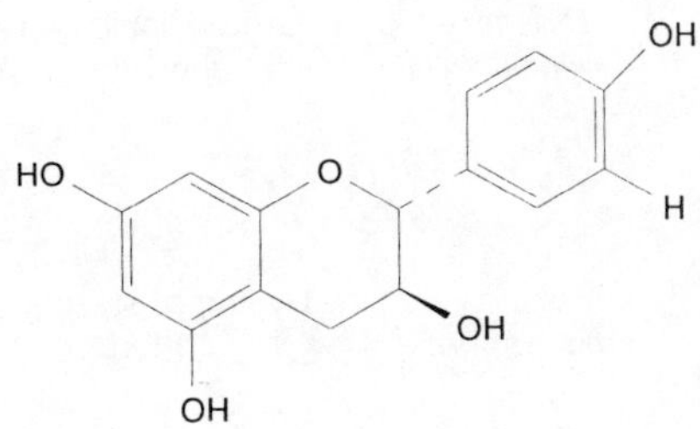	*Hovenia dulcis*	Neuroprotective, free radical scavenging activities	Dewick, 2002
2.	Alizarin	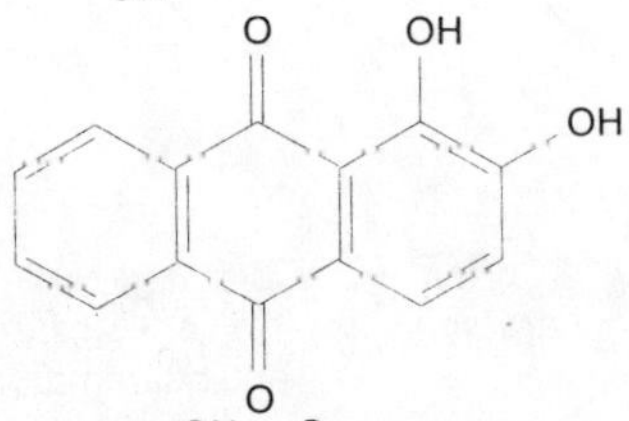	*Rubia tinctoria*	Oldest commercially valuable red dye, in snake-bite	Scott and Mercer, 1997
3.	Amentoflavone	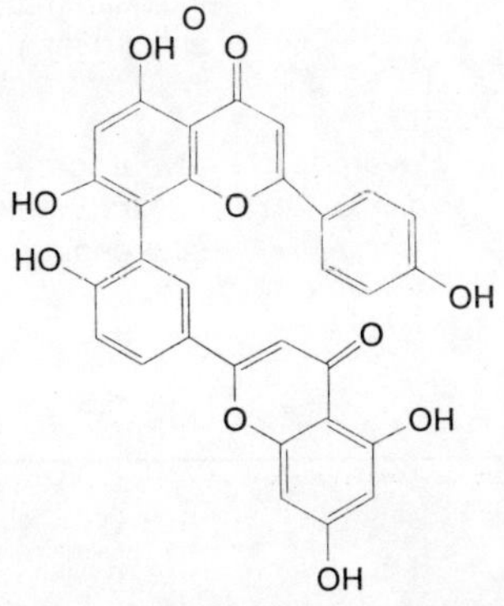	*Alchornea glandulosa*	Antiulcer, anti-fungal effect, vasorelaxant	Kang *et al.*, 2004

Contd...

Table 4.1–Contd...

Sl.No.	*Bioactive Molecules*	*Chemical Structures*	*Example Sources*	*Biopotentials*	*References*
4.	Anethole	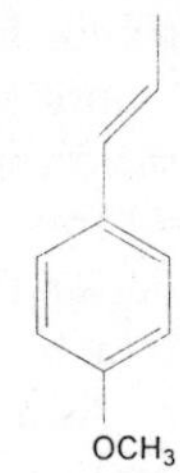	*Pimpinella anisum*	Diuretic, flavor, antimicrobial activity, carminative	Khanna *et al.*, 1998
5.	Arbutin	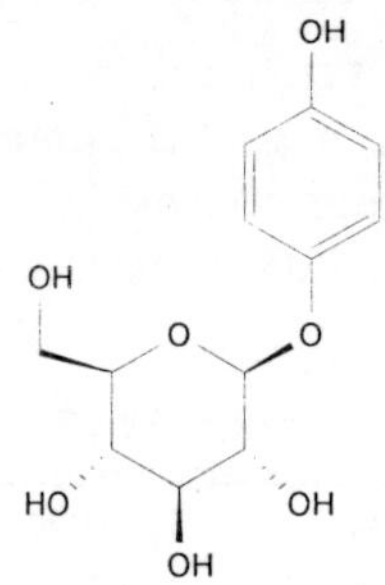	*Arctostaphylos uva-ursi*	Diuretic and antiseptic activity	O'Donoghue, 2006
6.	Batatasins	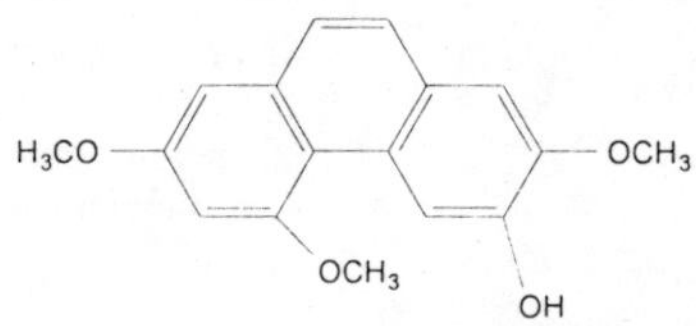	*Dioscorea oppositifolia*	Growth inhibitors phenolic	Hasegawa and Hashimoto, 1973
7.	Butrin	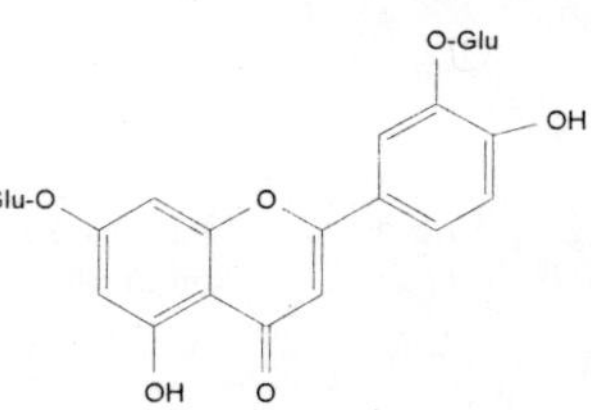	*Butea monosperma*	Dyeing of silk and cotton	Wagner *et al.*, 2006
8.	Caffeic acid	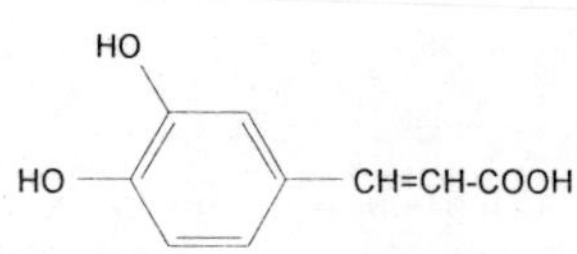	*Coffea arabica*	Carcinogenic inhibitor, antioxidant, antiinflammatory and anticancer property	Lee and Zhu, 2006
9.	Catechin	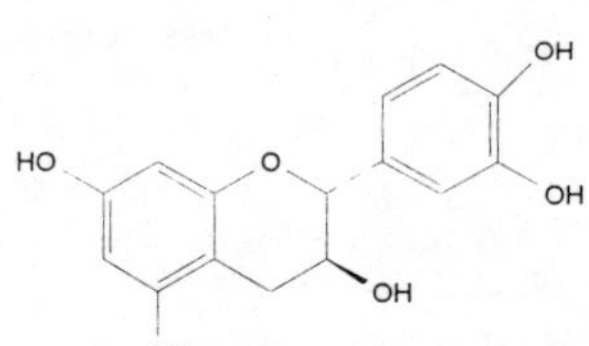	*Hovenia dulcis*	Neuroprotective, free radical scavenging activity	Ruidavets *et al.*, 2006

Contd...

Table 4.1–Contd...

Sl.No.	Bioactive Molecules	Chemical Structures	Example Sources	Biopotentials	References
10.	Catechol	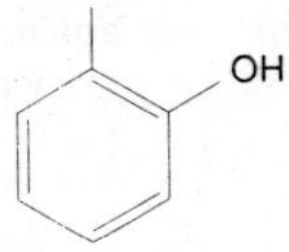	*Acacia catechu*	Photographic developer, in fur dyes, intermediate for antioxidants, in lubricating oils	Barner, 2004
11.	Cinnamal-dehyde	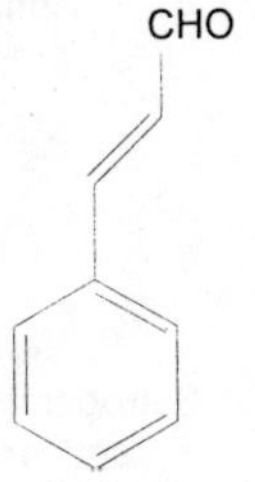	*Cinnamomum zeylanidum*	As spice and flavouring	Fischer, 1948
12.	Coumarin	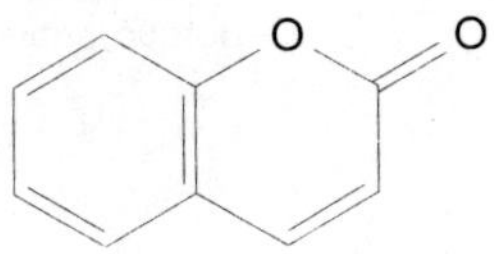	*Melilotus* sps.	Insecticidal agent, contributes to smell of new-mown hay	Dewick, 2002
13.	Coumesterol	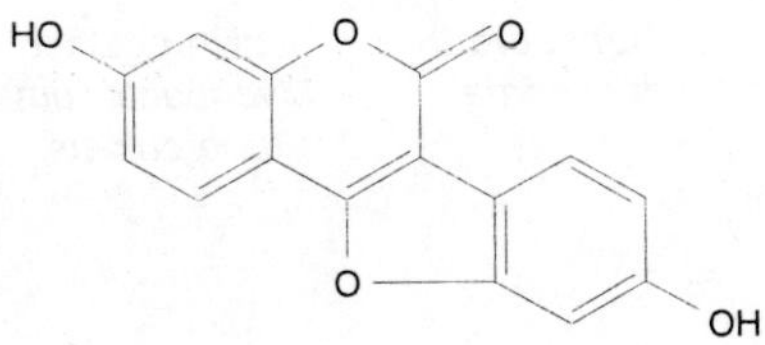	*Medicago sativa*	Oestrogenic activity	Dewick, 2002
14.	Daidzein	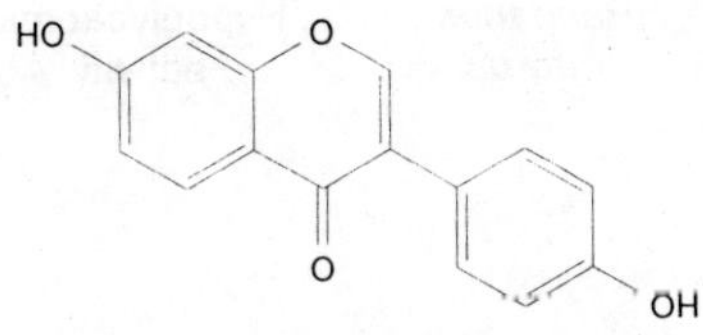	*Trifolium* sps.	Oestrogenic activity	Bayer *et al.*, 2001
15.	Ellagic acid	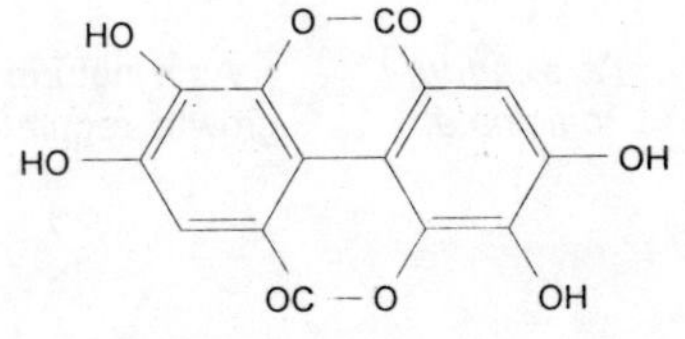	*Caesalpinia ferrea*	As an aldose reductase inihibitor	Lee and Talcott, 2002
16.	Emodin	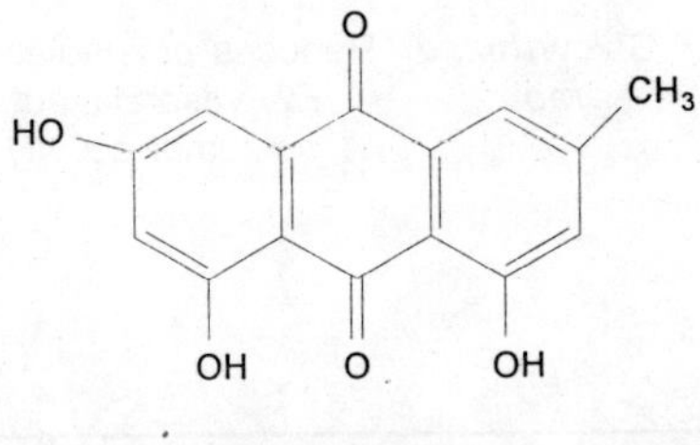	*Rheum* sps.	Laxative, as potential anticancer agent	Kurobane *et al.*, 1979

Contd...

Table 4.1–Contd...

Sl.No.	*Bioactive Molecules*	*Chemical Structures*	*Example Sources*	*Biopotentials*	*References*
17.	Eugenin	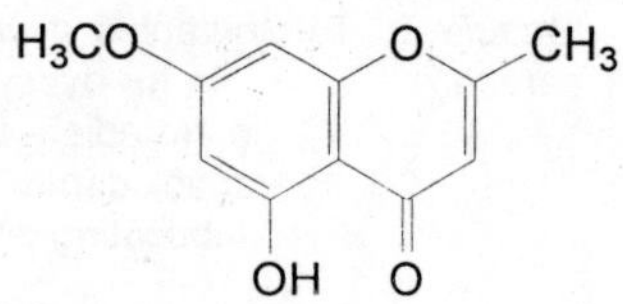	*Syzygium aromaticum*	Antiviral activity against Herpes viruses	Dewick, 2002
18.	Ferulic acid	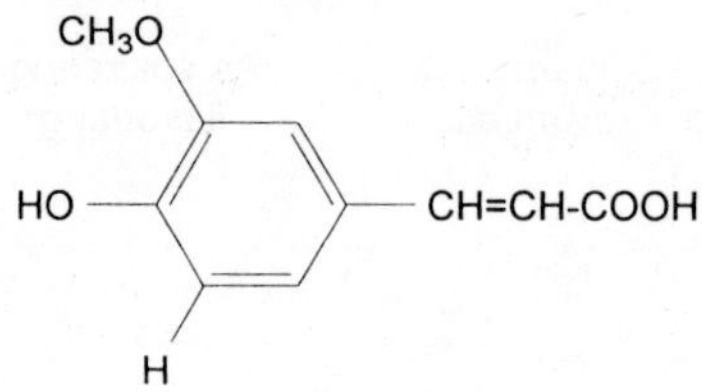	*Cyperus esculentus*	Antioxidant properties	Fereidoon and Marian, 2004
19.	Genistein	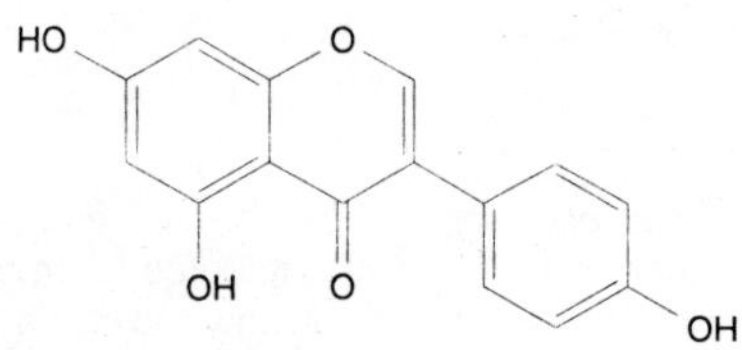	*Glycine max*	Estrogenic, antioxidant, anticarcinogenic and antiosteo-porotic activities	Kumi-Diaka *et al.*, 1998
20.	7-Hydroxy-xanthone	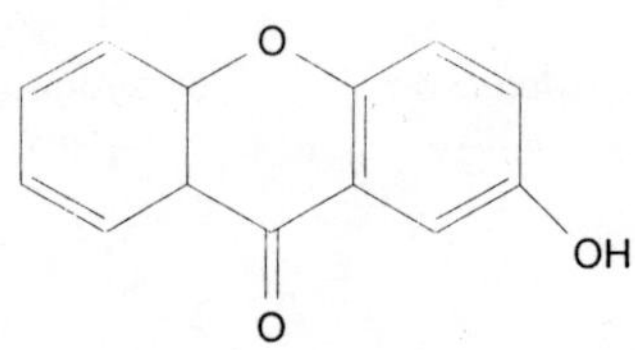	*Canscora decussata*	Active against *Mycobacterium tuberculosis*	Ignatushchenko *et al.*, 1997
21.	4–Hydroxy-benzoic acid	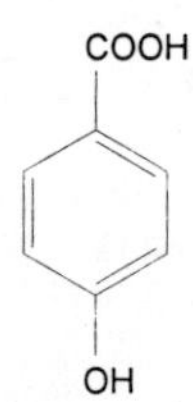	*Pandanus odorus*	Hypoglycaemic activity	Klaschka, 1964
22.	3–Hydroxy-phenylacetic acid	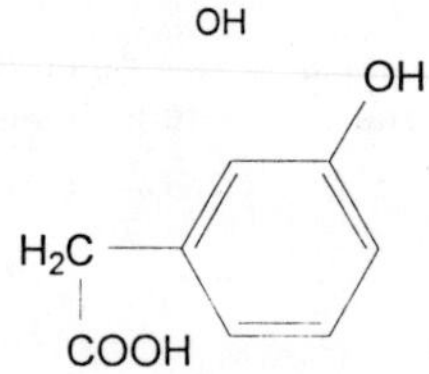	*Taraxacum officinale*	As a natural growth regulator	Dewick, 2002
23.	Isoliquiritigenin	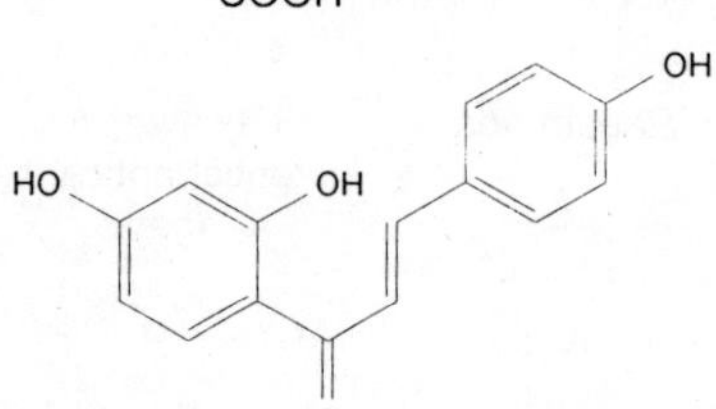	*Glycyrrhizae radix*	Reduces prostaglandin E2, vasorelaxant, antitumor activity	Kanazawa *et al.*, 2003

Contd...

Table 4.1–Contd...

Sl.No.	Bioactive Molecules	Chemical Structures	Example Sources	Biopotentials	References
24.	Juglone	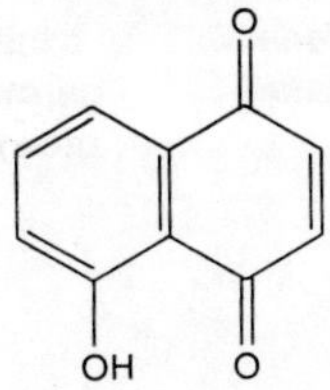	*Juglans nigra*	Colouring agent for food, as hair dyes, herbicide, in rheumatism	Hock and Elstner, 2004
25.	Kaempferol	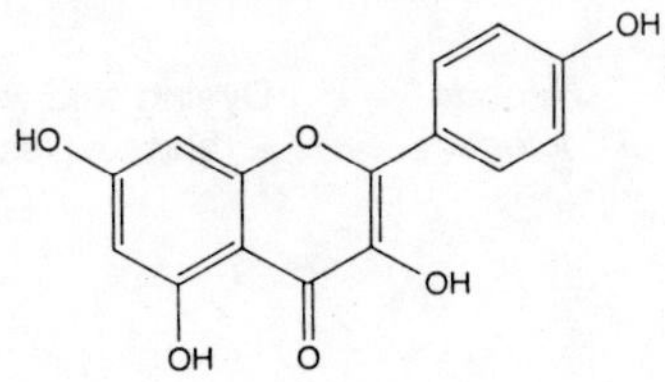	*Euphorbia peplus*	Spasmogenic, astringent, stimulant and diuretic	Park *et al.*, 2006
26.	Khellin	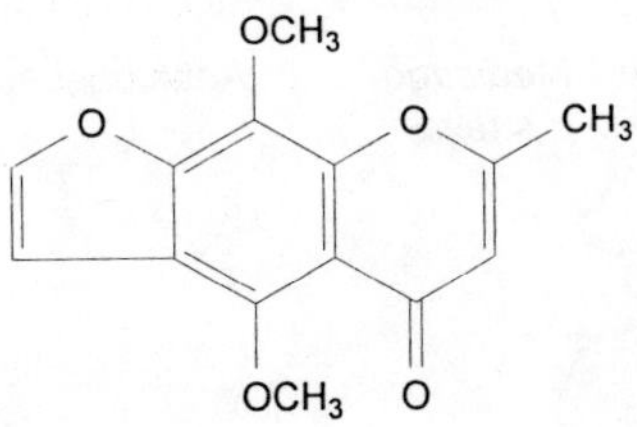	*Ammi visnaga*	As a vasodilator, treatment of angina, asthma and antispasmodic	Prokopenko *et al.*, 1968
27.	Leucocyanidin	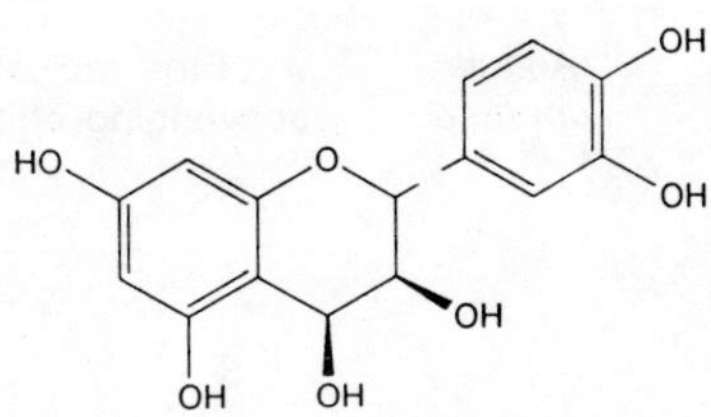	*Euphorbia peplus*	Antioxidant effect, insulin sparing action	Kumar and Rangaswamy, 1985
28.	Leucopelar-gonidin	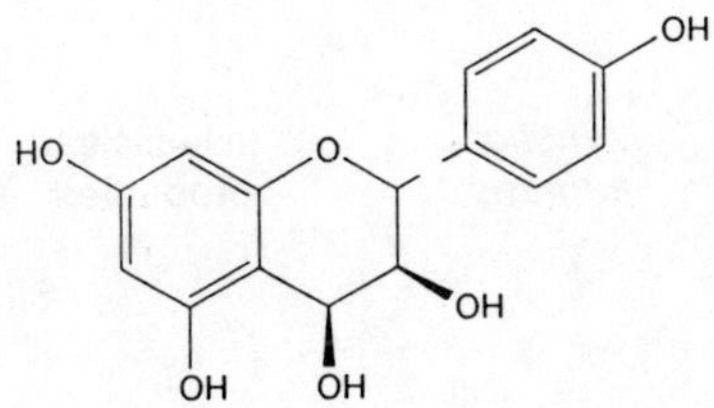	*Ficus benghalensis*	Decrease fasting blood sugar, antioxidant	Cherian and Augusti , 1993
29.	Liquiritigenin	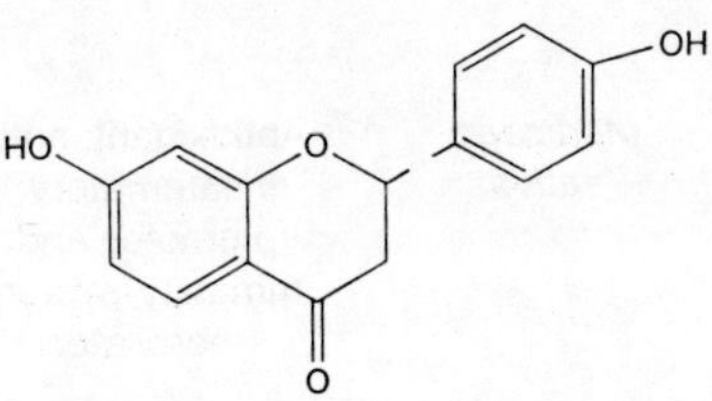	*Sinofranchetia chinensis*	Prevents allergy and liver injury	Young *et al.*, 2006

Contd...

Table 4.1–Contd...

Sl.No.	*Bioactive Molecules*	*Chemical Structures*	*Example Sources*	*Biopotentials*	*References*
30.	Lunularic acid	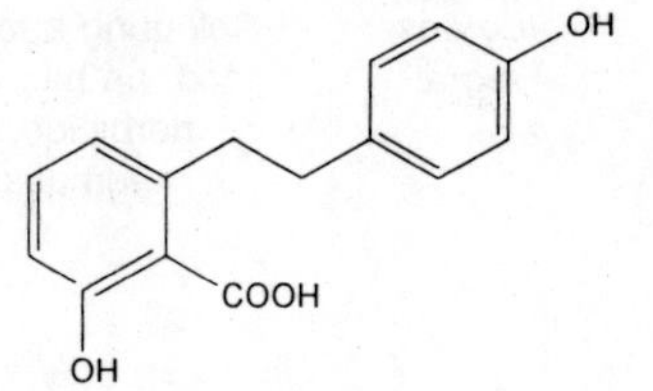	*Lunularia cruciata*	Inhibits the germination and growth of cress	Pryce, 1971
31.	Luteolin	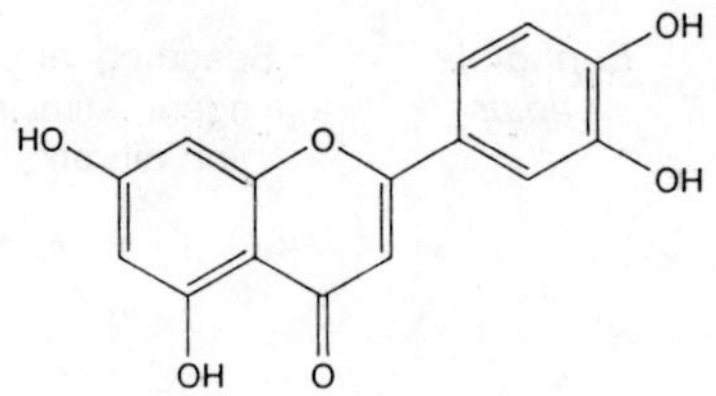	*Reseda luteola*	Dyeing silk, wool and textiles	Mann, 1992
32.	Medicarpin	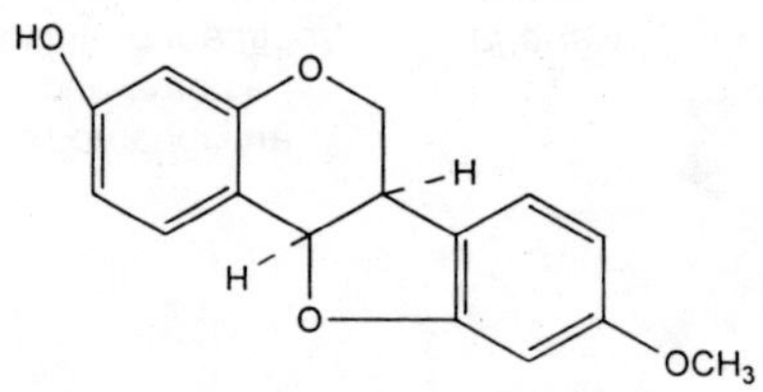	*Medicago sativa*	Antifungal activity	Hargreaves *et al.*, 1976
33.	Myricetin	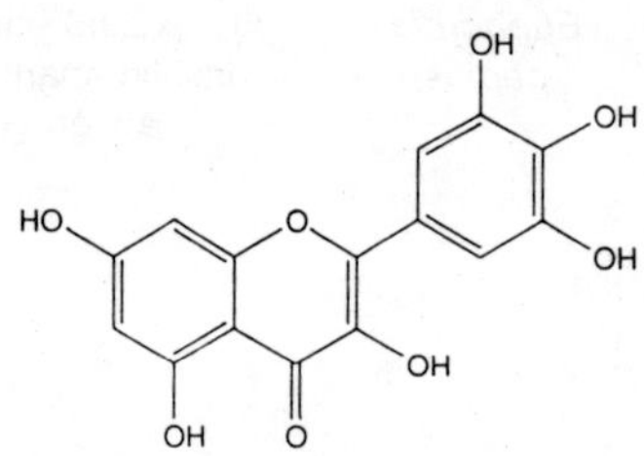	*Acacia confuse*	Free radical scavenging efficacy	Geahlen *et al.*, 1989
34.	Myristicin	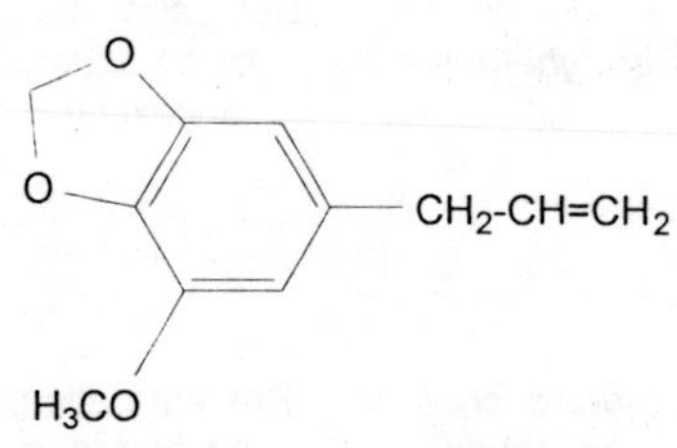	*Myristica fragrans*	Insecticidal properties	Truitt *et al.*, 1963
35.	Naringenin	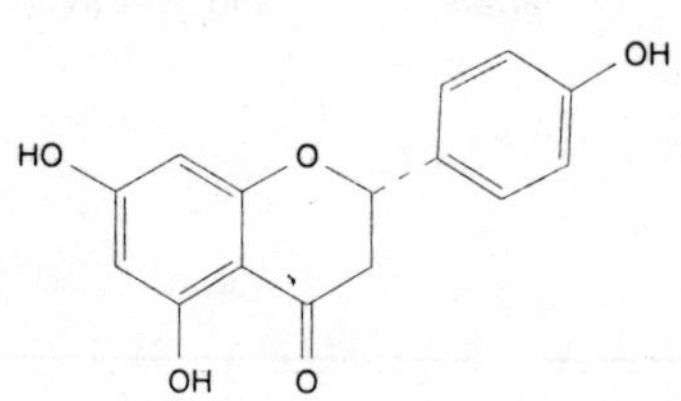	*Medicago sativa*	Antioxidant, anti-inflammatory, promoter and immunity system modulator	Edwards and Bernier, 1996

Contd...

Table 4.1–Contd...

Sl.No.	Bioactive Molecules	Chemical Structures	Example Sources	Biopotentials	References
36.	Phloroglucinol	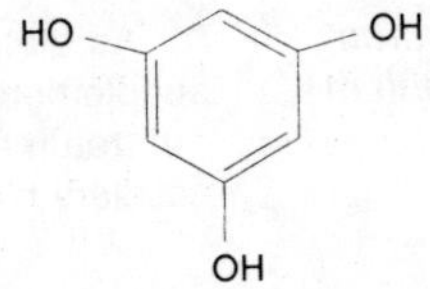	*Eucalyptus kino*	Smooth muscle relaxant properties, antispasmodic agent	Jafri *et al.*, 2006
37.	Podophyllotoxin	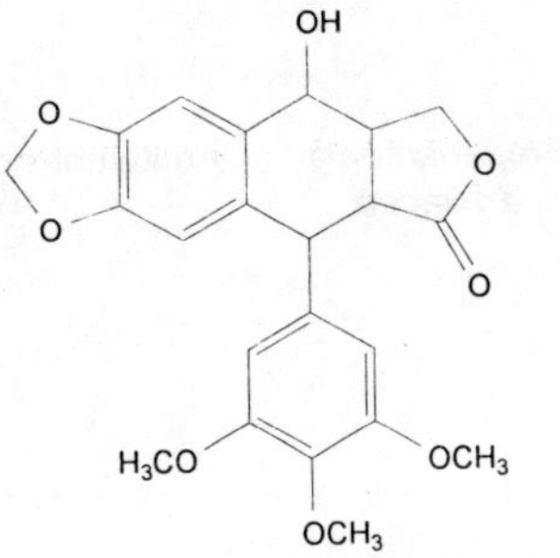	*Podophyllum hexandrum*	Purgative, cytotoxic	Hartwell and Schrecker, 1951
38.	Protocatechuic acid	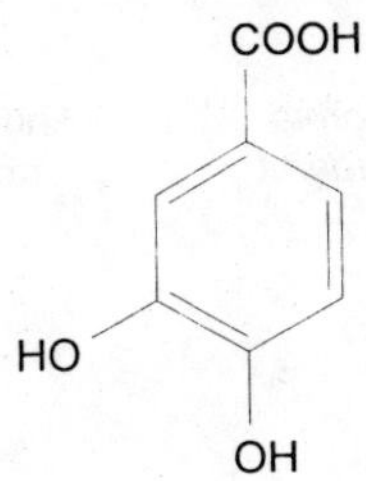	*Acacia catechu*	Antispasmodic action on smooth muscle	Babich *et al.*, 2002
39.	Psoralen	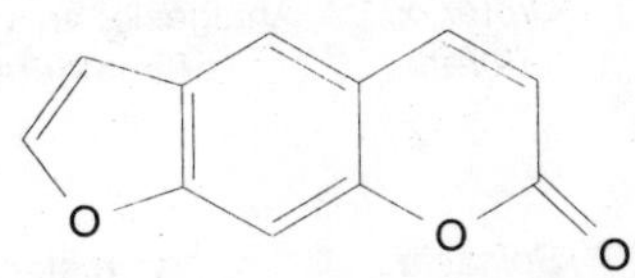	*Psoralea corylifolia*	Purgative, cytotoxic	Autier *et al.*, 1997
40.	Quercetin	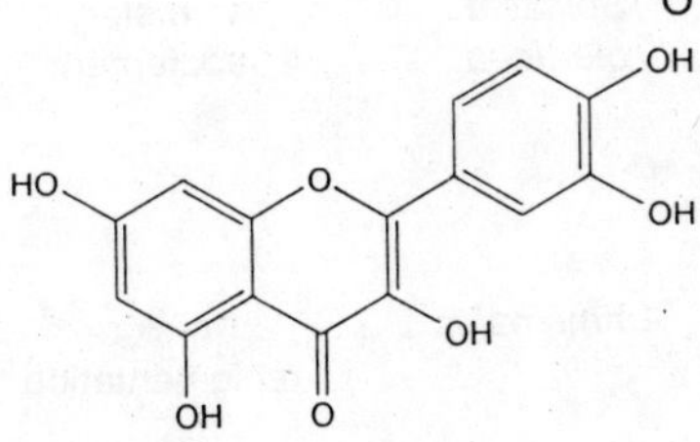	*Camellia sinensis*	Astringent, stimulant and diuretic	Geahlen *et al.*, 1989
41.	Resveratrol	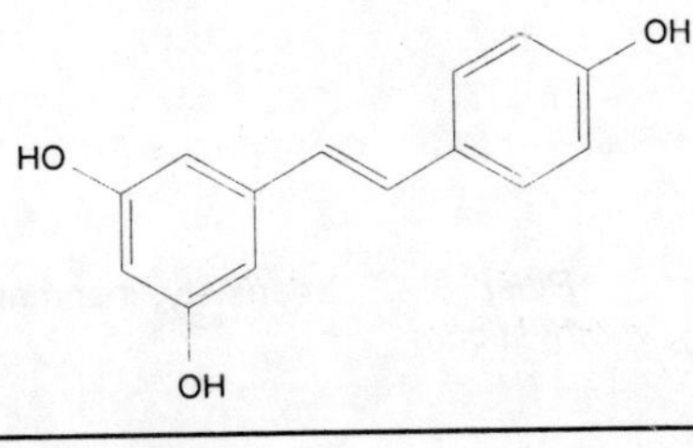	*Vitis vinifera*	Antioxidant, anti-inflammatory and antiplatelet activity	Farina *et al.*, 2006

Contd...

Table 4.1–Contd...

Sl.No.	Bioactive Molecules	Chemical Structures	Example Sources	Biopotentials	References
42.	Rutin	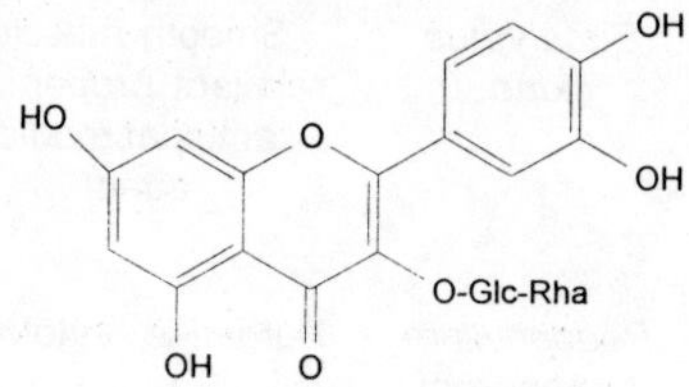	*Fagopurum esculentum*	As dietary supplements, and in treatment of capillary bleeding	Addae-mensah and Munenge, 1989
43.	Steganacin	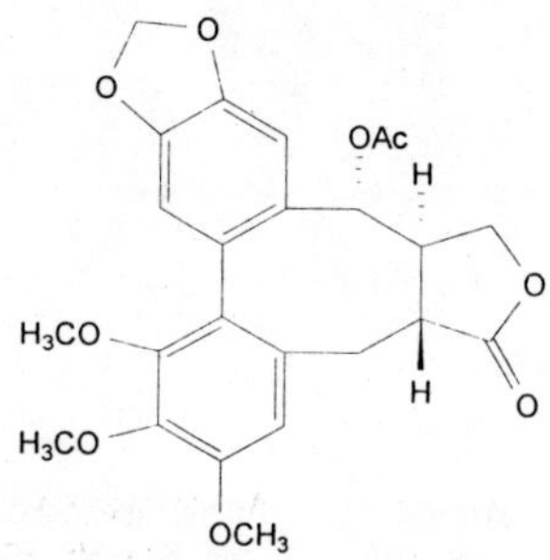	*Steganataenia araliacea*	Antitumor activity	Wang *et al.*, 1977
44.	Syringic acid	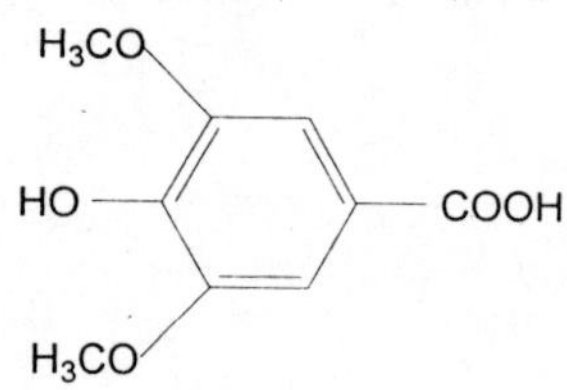	*Euphorbia heteradena*	Antioxidant activity	Jogia *et al.*, 1985
45.	Umbelliferone	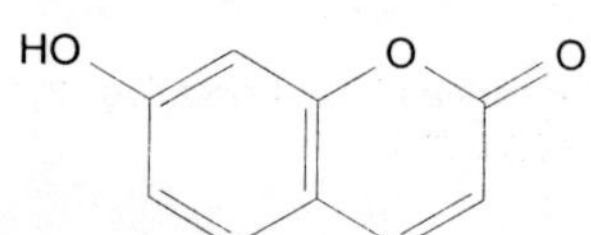	*Dipteryx odorata*	Analgesic, antioxidant, aromatherapy	Mikaberidze and Moniava, 1975
46.	Vitamin K (Phylloquinone)	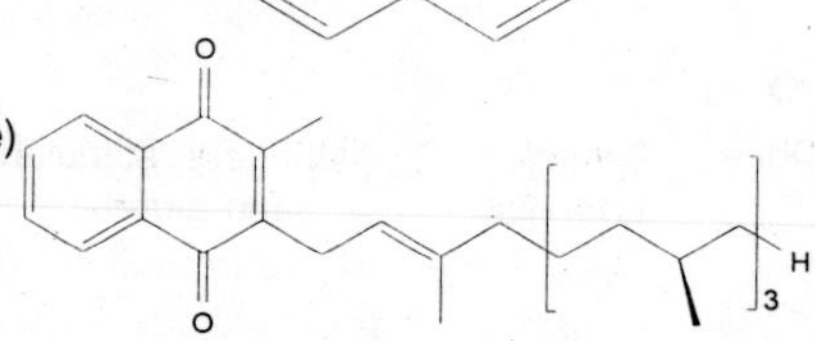	*Spinacia oleracea*	As dietary supplement	Ferland and Sadowski, 1992
47.	Xanthotoxin	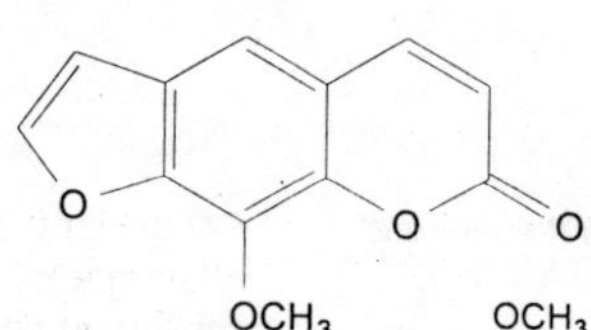	*Ammi majus*	In skin repigmentation	Wu *et al.*, 1972
48.	Yanogenin	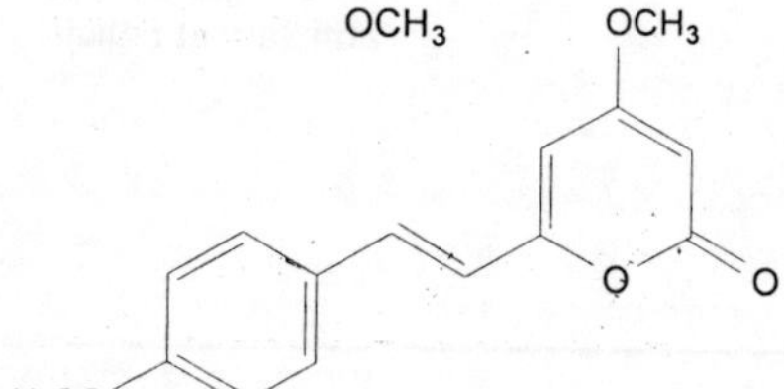	*Piper methysticum*	In anxiety, insomnia	Iwu, 1993

Alkaloids

The name is derived from the word 'alkaline', are naturally occurring chemical compounds containing basic nitrogen atoms. These are produced by a large variety of organisms, including bacteria, fungi, plants, and animals and are part of the group of natural products. Some alkaloids have a bitter taste while many are toxic to other organisms. Many alkaloids can be purified from crude extracts by acid-base extraction. Furthermore, not all protein amino acids give rise to specific alkaloids. Amongst those which frequently do, however, are: the aromatic amino acids phenylalanine, tyrosine, and tryptophan, the basic amino acids arginine, ornithine and lysine and the branched chain amino acids leucine and valine. They often have pharmacological effects and are used as medicines and recreational drugs, *e.g.*, the local anesthetic and stimulant cocaine, the stimulant caffeine, nicotine, the analgesic morphine, or the antimalarial drug quinine (Table 4.2).

Table 4.2: Chemical Structure, Example Source and Biopotentials of Some Important Alkaloids

Sl.No.	*Bioactive Molecules*	*Chemical Structures*	*Example Sources*	*Biopotentials*	*References*
1.	Acetyl-intermedine	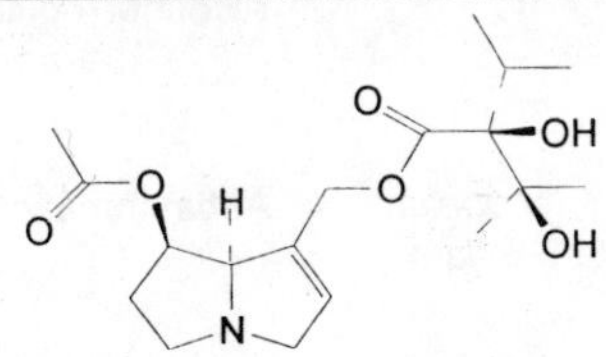	*Symphytum officinale*	In inflammatory, rheumatic and gastrointestinal disorders	Hartmann, 1999
2.	Acetyl-lycopsamine	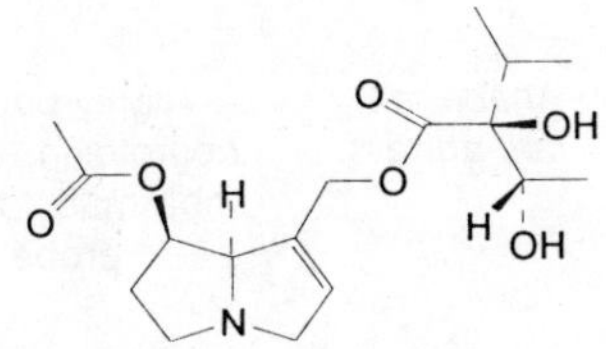	*Symphytum officinale*	In inflammatory, rheumatic and gastrointestinal disorders	Liddell, 2000
3.	Acronycine	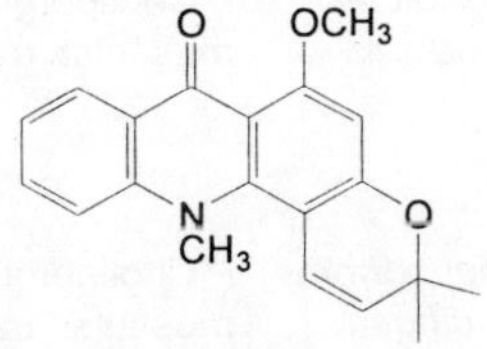	*Acronychia baueri*	Cytotoxicity against murine leukemia and human epidermoid carcinoma cell lines	Tillequin and Skaltsounis, 1998
4.	Actinidine	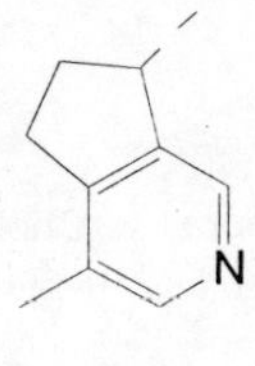	*Actinidia polygama*	Cat attractant, with similar effects as nepetalactone, the active compound found in catnip	Janot *et al.*, 1979
5.	Ajmalicine	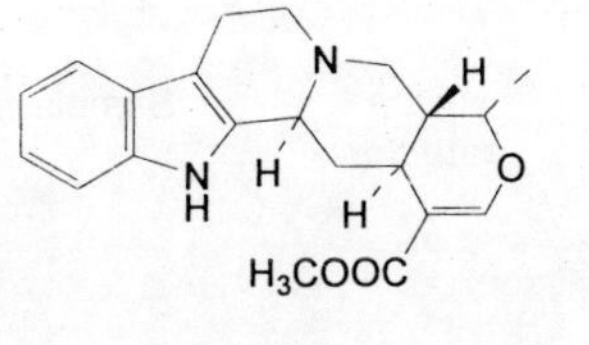	*Rauwolfia serpentina*	Antihypertensive, antiadrenergic	Dewick, 2002

Contd...

Table 4.1–Contd...

Sl.No.	*Bioactive Molecules*	*Chemical Structures*	*Example Sources*	*Biopotentials*	*References*
6.	Akuammicine	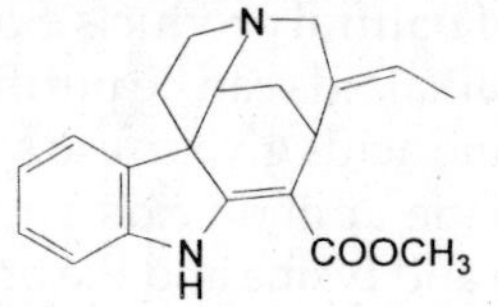	*Vinca major*	Hypotensive, antihistaminic, antiinflammatory, antiobesity, antipyretic	Dewick, 2002
7.	Anabasine	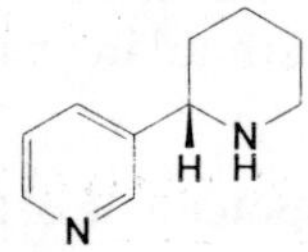	*Nicotiana tabacum*	Insecticidal activity	Jacob *et al.*, 1999
8.	Anatabine	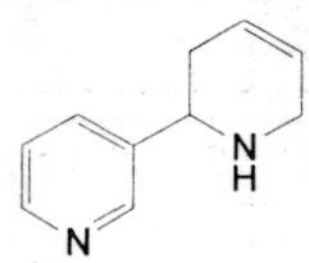	*Nicotiana tabacum*	Biomarkers for tobacco use during nicotine replacement therapy	Dewick, 2002
9.	Anaferine	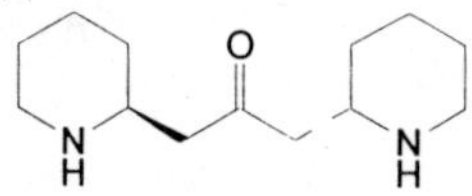	*Lobelia inflata*	Antiasthmatic activity	Dewick, 2002
10.	Anatoxin-a	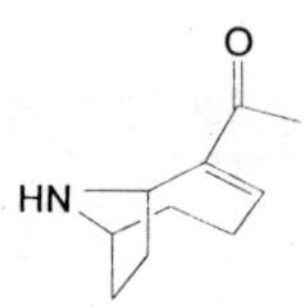	*Anabaena flos-aquae*	Highly potent neurotoxin, useful pharmacological probe	Wood *et al.*, 2007
11.	Anhalamine	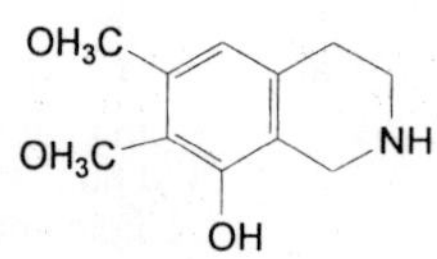	*Acacia rigidula*	Cholinergic, neuro-muscular transmission	Dewick, 2002
12.	Anhalonine	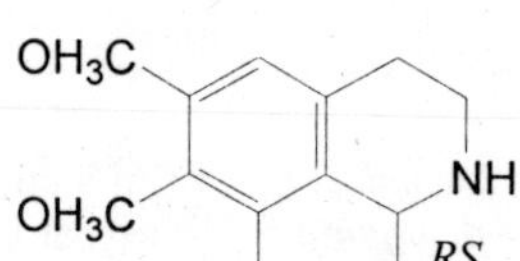	*Lophophora diffusa*	Cholinergic, neuro-muscular transmission	Dewick, 2002
13.	Anhalonidine	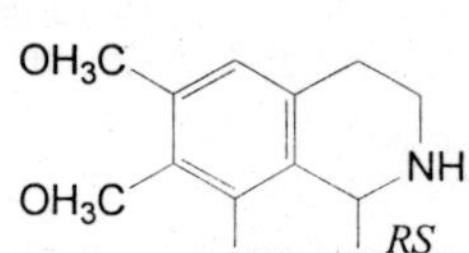	*Lophophora diffusa*	Cholinergic, neuro-muscular transmission	Dewick, 2002
14.	Arecoline	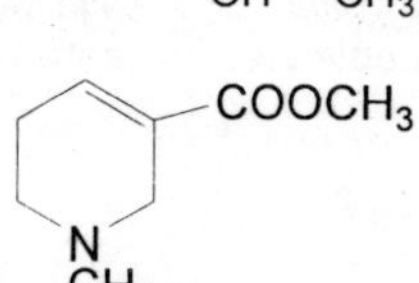	*Areca catechu*	Stimulant effect	Christie *et al.*, 1981

Contd...

Table 4.2–Contd...

Sl.No.	Bioactive Molecules	Chemical Structures	Example Sources	Biopotentials	References
15.	Aristolochic acid	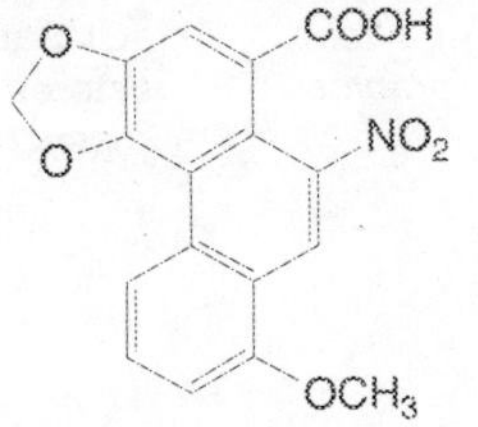	*Aristolochia* sps.	Used in traditional system of medicine	Dewick, 2002
16.	Atisine	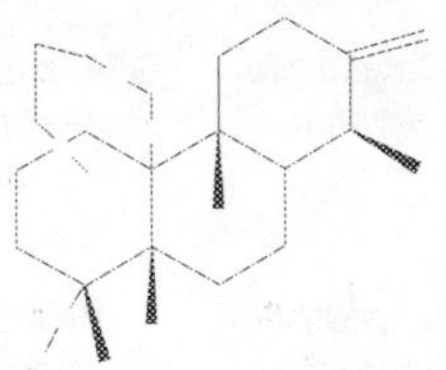	*Delphinium* sps.	Used in diarrhoea, dysentry, acute inflammation	Bhat *et al.*, 2005
17.	Atropine	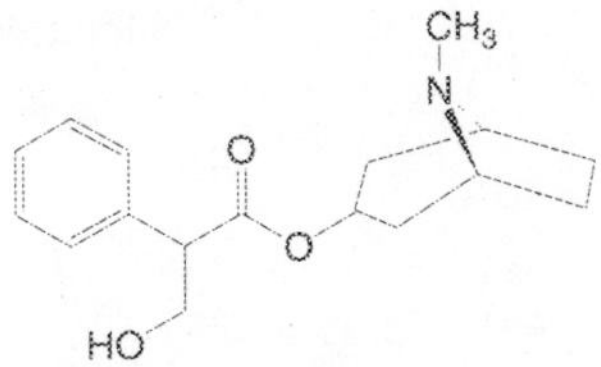	*Atropa belladonna*	Competitive antagonist of the muscarinic acetylcholine receptors, used as an antidote against nerve agents	Thomas *et al.*, 2008
18.	Autumnaline	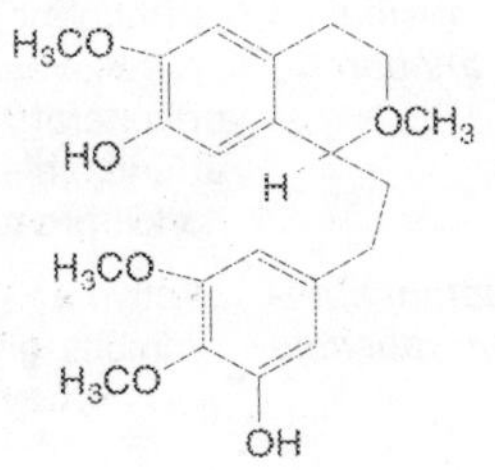	*Colchicum autumnale*	Efficient precursor for *Homoapophine* alkaloids	Dewick, 2002
19.	Berberine	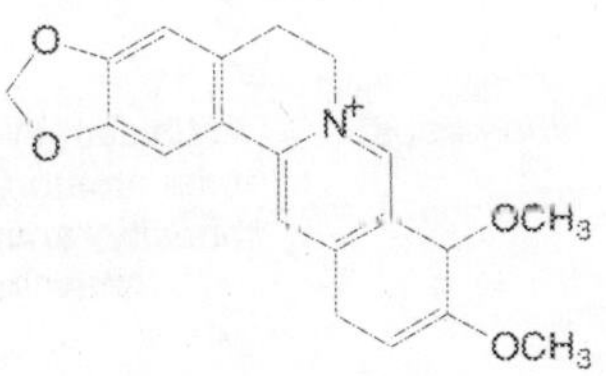	*Berberis* sps.	Antiamoeblc, anti-bacterial and anti-inflammatory activities	Qiming and Mingzhi, 1987
20.	Biscuculline	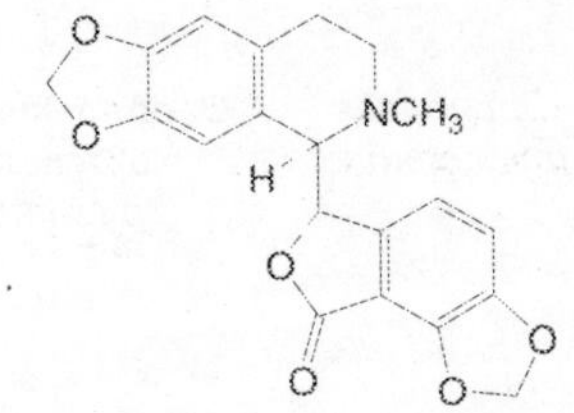	*Corydalis* sps.	Potent GABA (α-aminobutyric acid) antagonists	Khawaled *et al.*, 1999

Contd...

Table 4.2–Contd...

Sl.No.	Bioactive Molecules	Chemical Structures	Example Sources	Biopotentials	References
21.	Caffeine	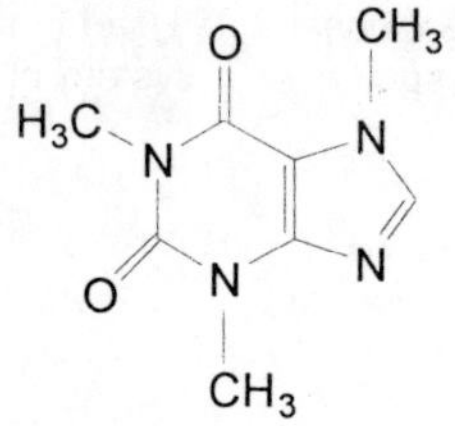	*Coffea arabica*	CNS stimulant, restores alertness, psychoactive	Wills, 1994
22.	Calystegines	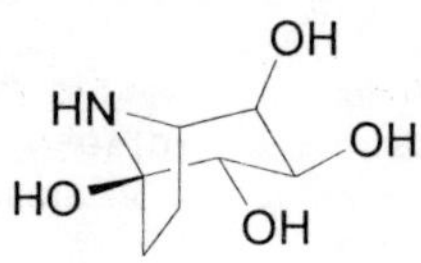	*Calystegia sepium*	Glycosidase inhibitor, active against AIDS and HIV	Molyneux *et al.*, 1996
23.	Camptothecin	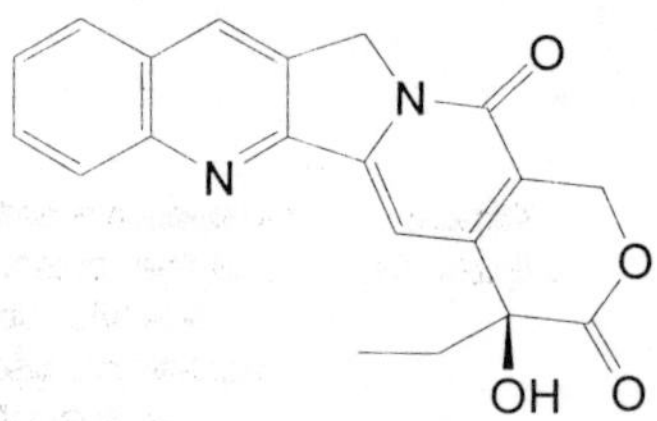	*Camptotheca acuminata*	Broad spectrum anticancer activity with toxicity	Wall and Wani, 1998
24.	Capsaicin	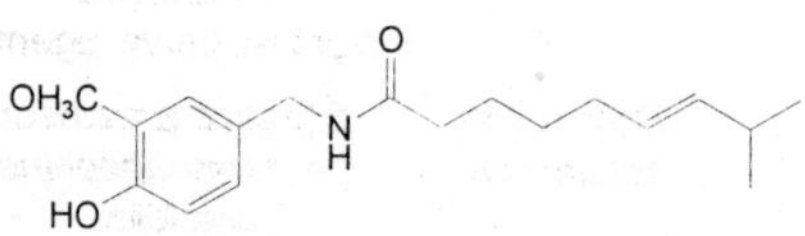	*Capsicum annuum*	Pungent principle, relieves pain of peripheral neuropathy, arthritis, diabetes, able to kill prostate cancer	Mitsubichi, 1982
25.	Castano-spermine	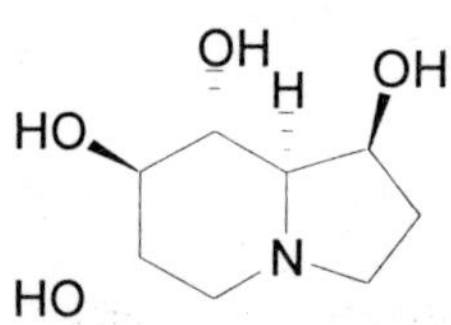	*Castanospermum australe*	Active against AIDS, inhibits glycosidase enzymes	Nash *et al.*, 1996
26.	Catharanthine	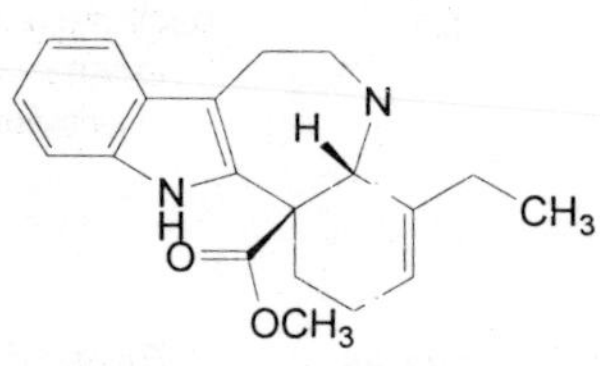	*Iboga* sps.	Antihistaminic, anti-inflammatory, anti-obesity, antipyretic activities	Kutney *et al.*, 1965
27.	Cephaeline	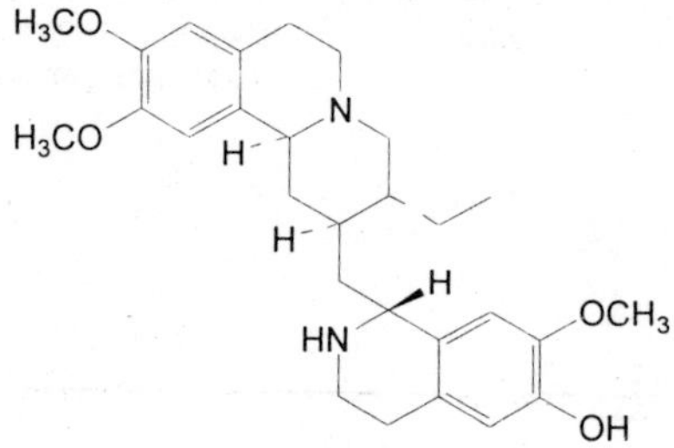	*Cepahaelis ipecacuanha*	Used for treatment of amoebic dysentery	Garcia *et al.*, 2005

Contd...

Table 4.2–Contd...

Sl.No.	Bioactive Molecules	Chemical Structures	Example Sources	Biopotentials	References
28.	Chelidonine	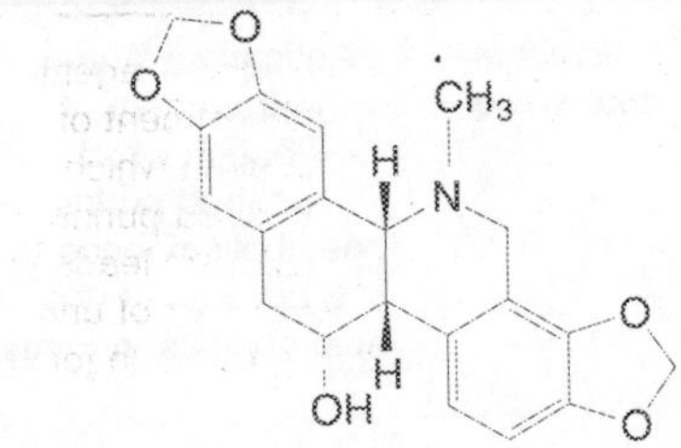	*Chelidonium majus*	Antimicrobial activity	Debska, 1958
29.	Chimonanthine	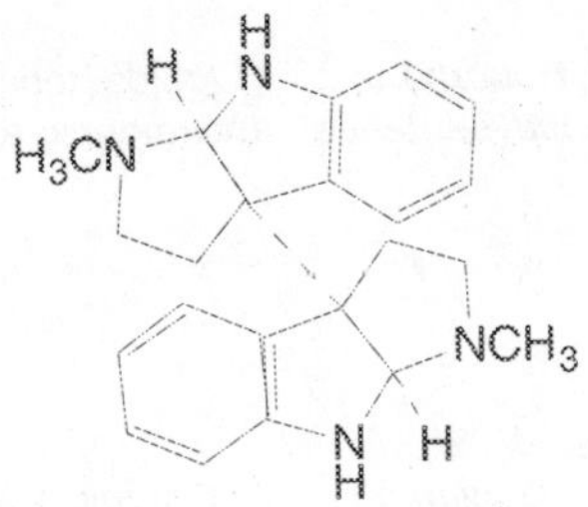	*Chimonanthus fragrans*	Low anti-nociceptive activity/analgesic	Grant *et al.*, 1965
30.	Cinchonidine	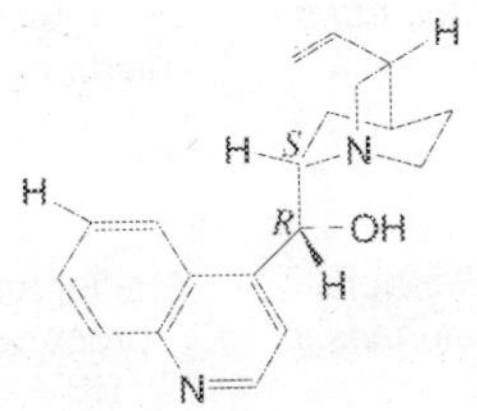	*Cinchona* sps.	Antitumor activity	Evans, 1989
31.	Cinchonine	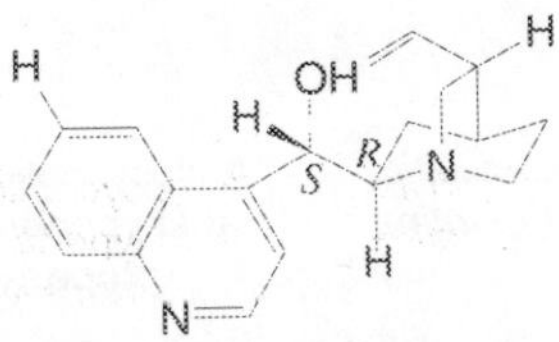	*Cinchona* sps.	Treatment of malaria	Evans, 1989
32.	Cocaine	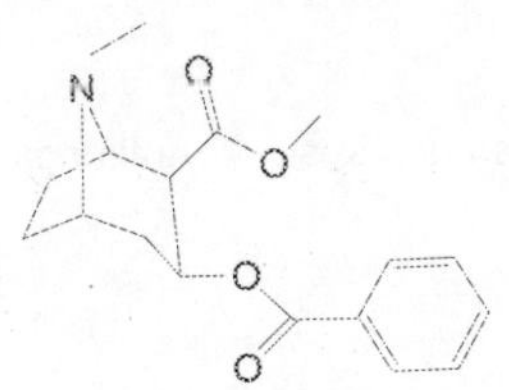	*Erythroxylon coca*	Local anesthetic, illicit drug for its euphoric properties	Johnson and Emcho, 1994
33.	Codeine	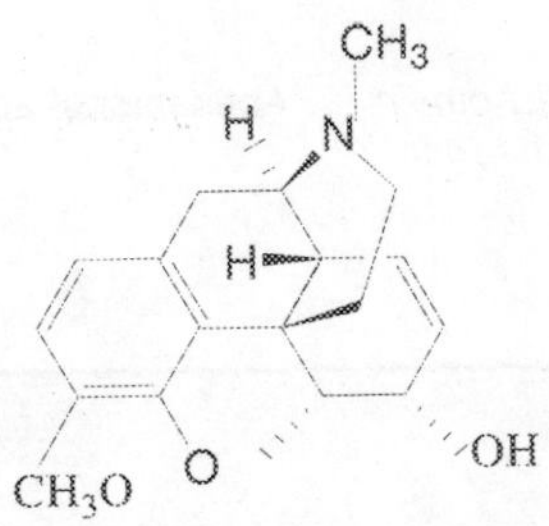	*Papaver sominiferum*	Analgesic, diarrhoea, mild to severe pain, irritable bowel syndrome	Bhat *et al.*, 2005

Contd...

Table 4.2–Contd...

Sl.No.	*Bioactive Molecules*	*Chemical Structures*	*Example Sources*	*Biopotentials*	*References*
34.	Colchicine	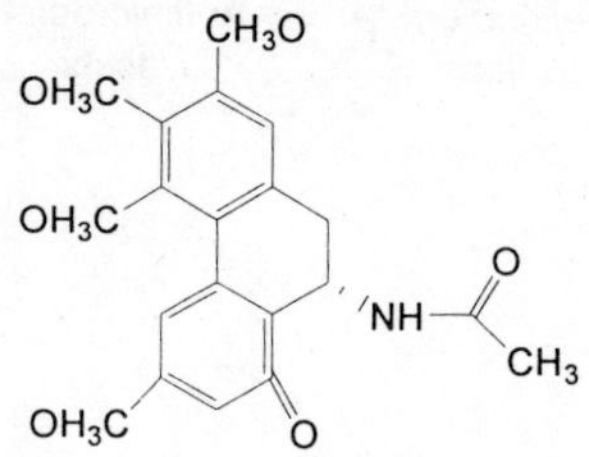	*Colchicum autumnale*	Anticancer agent, in treatment of gout, in which impaired purine metabolism leads to a build up of uric acid crystals in joints	Boye and Brossi, 1992
35.	Conessine	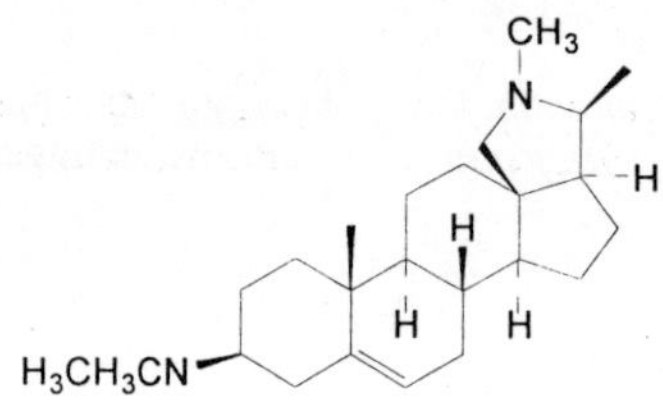	*Holarrhena antidysenterica*	Antibacterial and antiamoebic activities	Bhat *et al.*, 2005
36.	Coniine	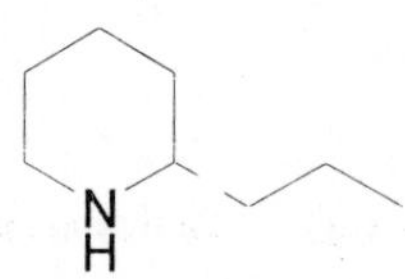	*Coninum maculatum*	Chronic toxicity neurotoxic-disrupts the CNS	Dewick, 2002
37.	Cytisine	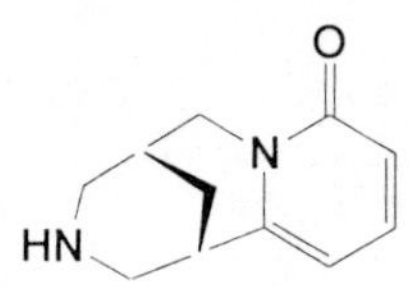	*Sophora tonkinensis*	Antidepressant like properties, anti HBV activity	Etter, 2006
38.	Deserpidine	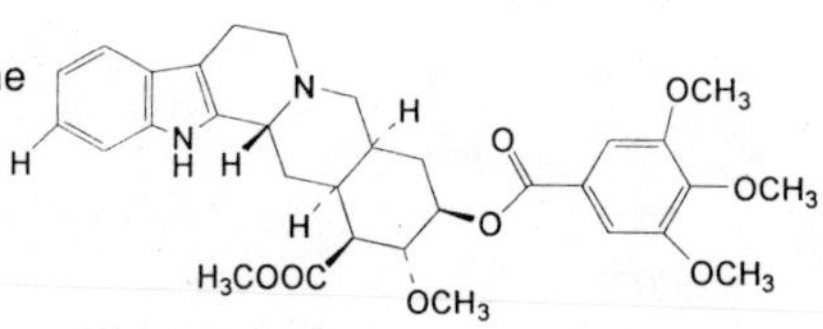	*Rauwolfia serpentina*	Antipsychotic and antihypertensive property	Huebner *et al.*, 1955
39.	Dictamnine	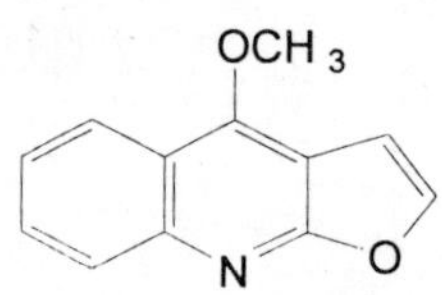	*Dictamnus* sps.	Antifungal agent	Dewick, 2002
40.	Dolichotheline	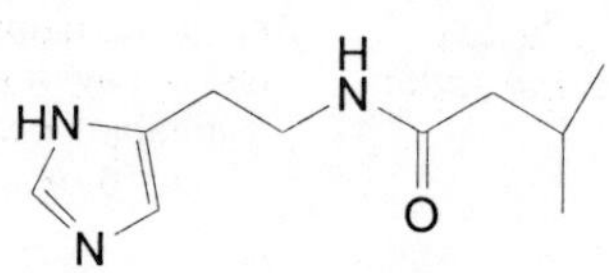	*Dolichothele sphaerica*	Antibacterial activity	Dewick, 2002

Contd...

Table 4.2–Contd...

Sl.No.	*Bioactive Molecules*	*Chemical Structures*	*Example Sources*	*Biopotentials*	*References*
41.	Emetine	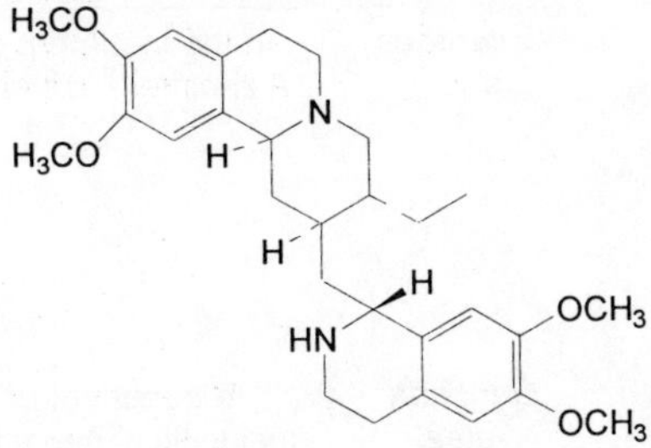	*Cepahaelis ipecacuanha*	Antiamoebic activity	Bhat *et al.*, 2005
42.	Ephedrine	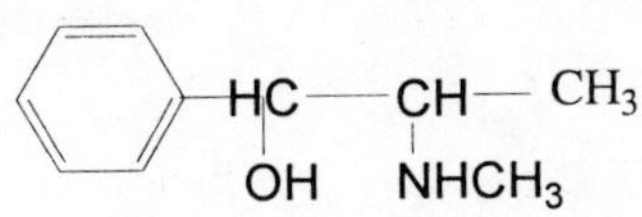	*Ephedra* sps.	A valuable nasal decongestant and bronchial dilator	Pugsley, 1994
43.	Epibatidine	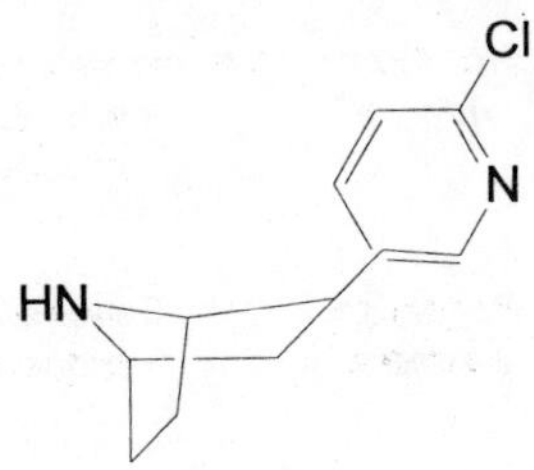	*Epipedobates tricolor*	Analgesic drug	Daly *et al.*, 2000
44.	Ergine	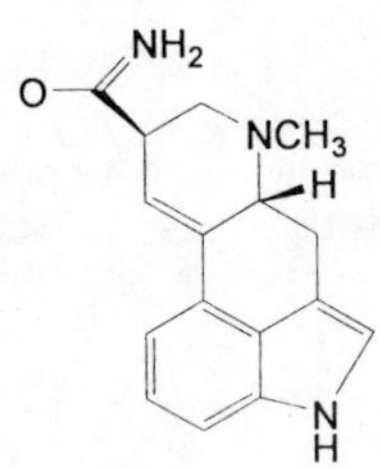	*Rivea* sps.	Cause vascular constriction	Smith and Timmis, 1932
45.	Ergotamine	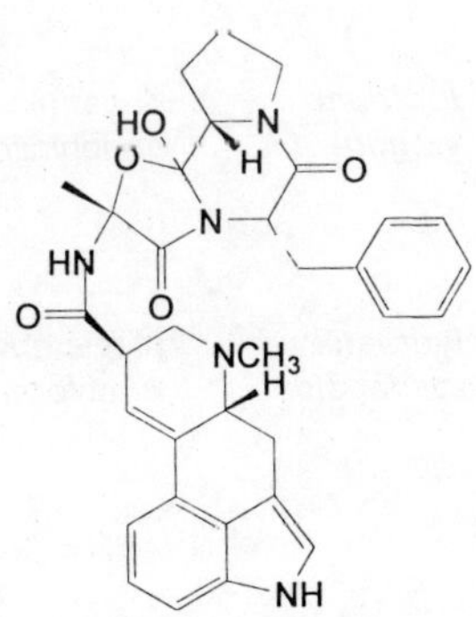	*Claviceps purpurea*	Poisoning in alimentary upsets circulatory disorder, neurological syndrome	Kren *et al.*, 1994

Contd...

Table 4.2–Contd...

Sl.No.	*Bioactive Molecules*	*Chemical Structures*	*Example Sources*	*Biopotentials*	*References*
46.	Galantamine	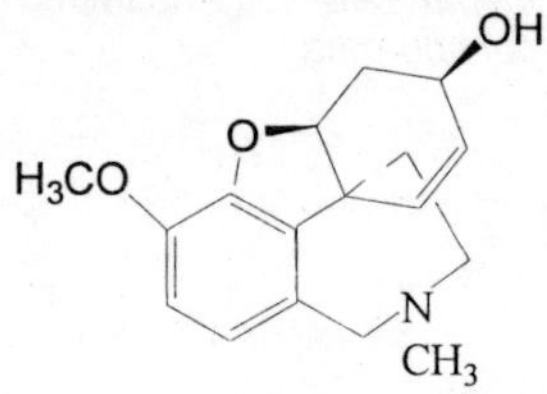	*Galanthus* sps.	In the treatment of Alzheimer's disease	Scott and Goa, 2000
47.	Gentiopicroside	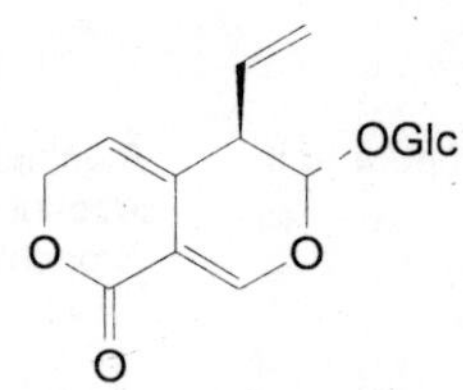	*Gentiana lutea*	In treatment of indigestion, hepatitis, rheumatism	Dewick, 2002
48.	Gramine	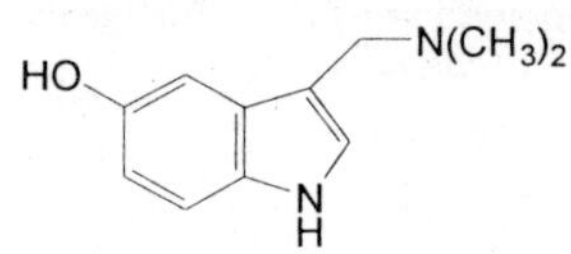	*Hordeum vulgare*	A vasorelaxant acting on 5 HT(2A) receptors	Corcuera, 1993
49.	Harman	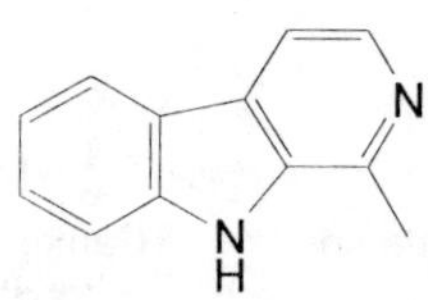	*Peganum harmala*	Psychoactive properties	Dewick, 2002
50.	Holaphyl-lamine	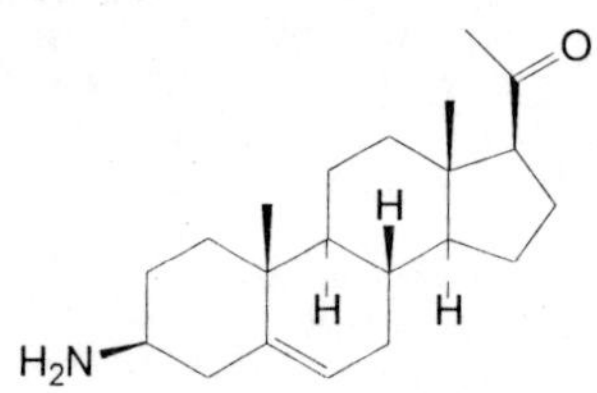	*Holarrhena floribunda*	Hypertrophic activity	Dewick, 2002
51.	Hordenine	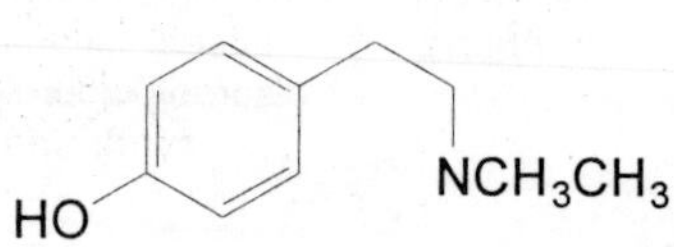	*Hordeum vulgare*	A germination inhibitor	Bhat *et al.*, 2005
52.	Hydrastine	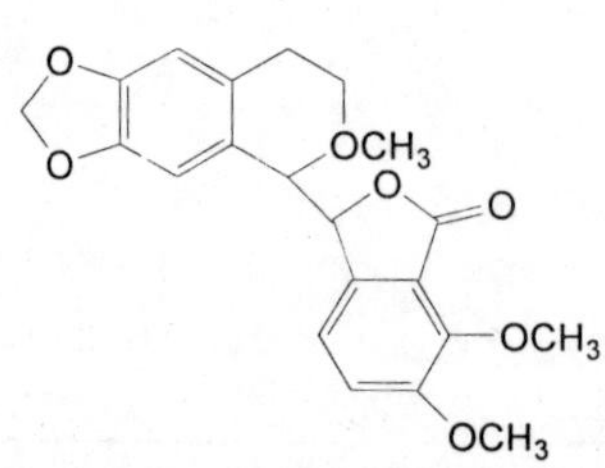	*Hydrastis canadensis*	Antimicrobial and chloretic	Dewick, 2002

Contd...

Table 4.2–Contd...

Sl.No.	Bioactive Molecules	Chemical Structures	Example Sources	Biopotentials	References
53.	Hygrine	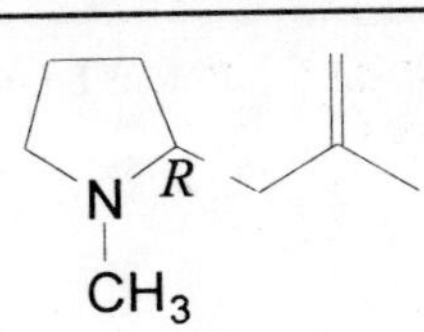	*Erythroxylum coca*	In uterine bleeding	Bhat *et al.*, 2005
54.	Hyoscine	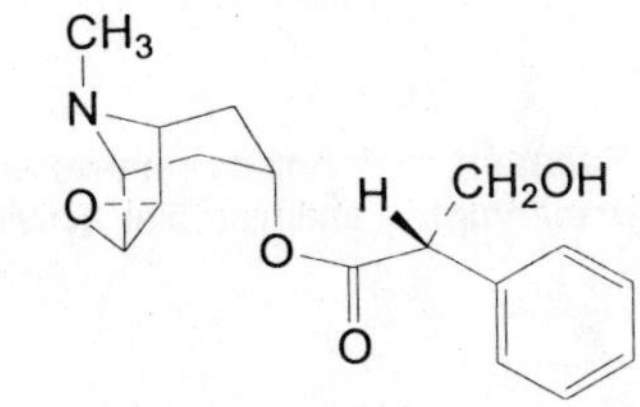	*Hyoscyamus niger*	In treatment of nausea, motion sickness and intestinal cramping	Evans, 1990
55.	Hyoscine butylbromide	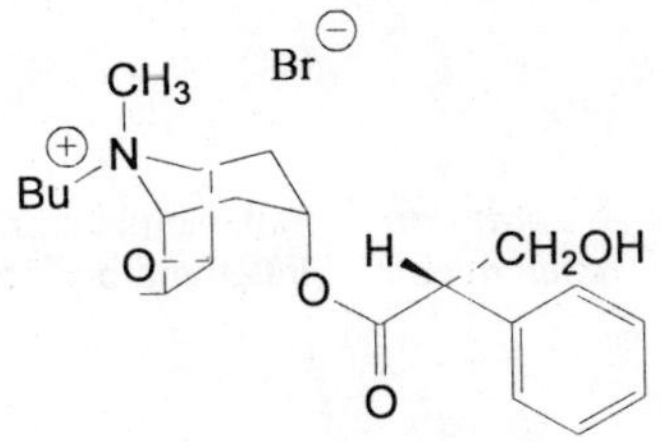	*Tribulus terresstris*	Gastrointestinal dlsorders, antispasmodic	Dewick, 2002
56.	Hyoscyamine	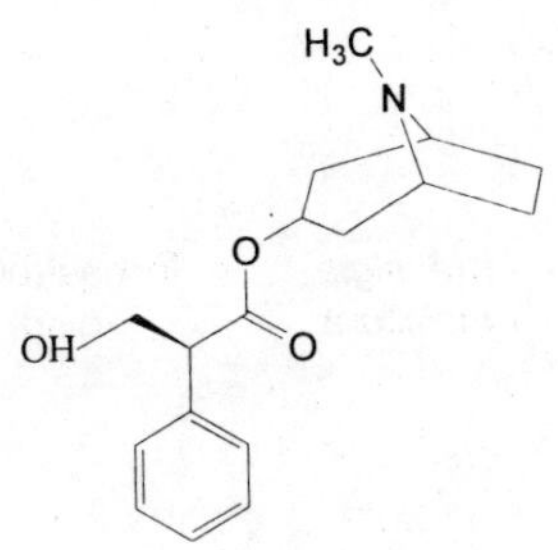	*Datura stramonium*	In gastrointestinal disorders, heart problem, Parkinson's disease	Bhat *et al.*, 2005
57.	Ibogaine	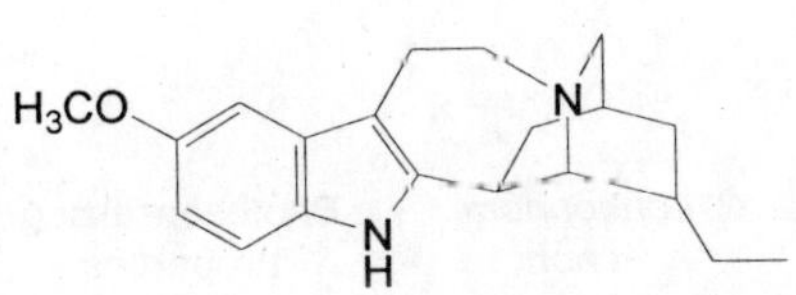	*Tabernanthe iboga*	Antiaddictive activity	Popik and Skolnick, 1999
58.	Indicine-N-oxide	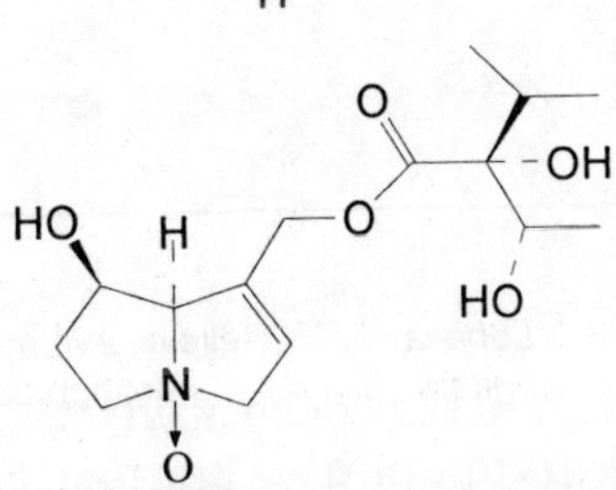	*Heliotropium indicum*	Antileukaemic activity	Dewick, 2002

Contd...

Table 4.2–Contd...

Sl.No.	Bioactive Molecules	Chemical Structures	Example Sources	Biopotentials	References
59.	Ipratropium bromide	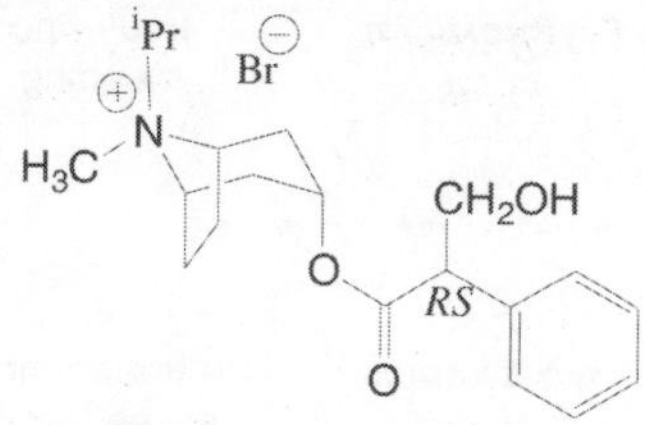	*Adhatoda vasica*	Potent bronchodilator	Dewick, 2002
60.	Isoboldine	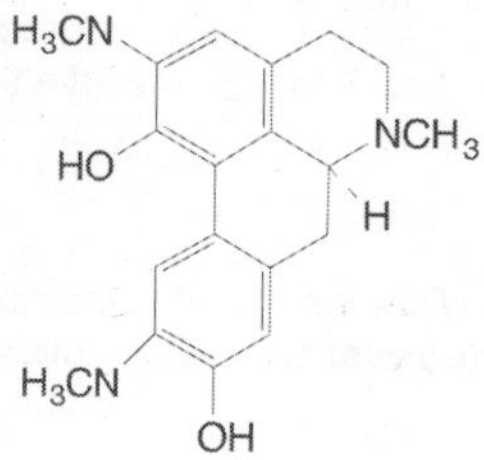	*Papaver sominiferum*	Antileishmanial and antimicrobial activities	Dewick, 2002
61.	Jervine	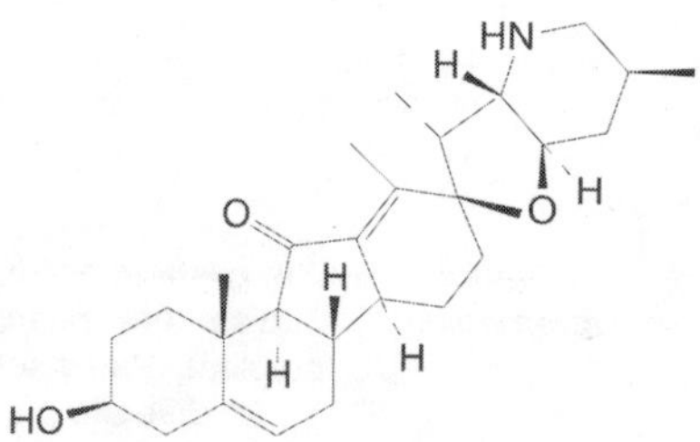	*Veratrum californicum*	Antimicrobial and anti-inflammatory activities	Bhat *et al.*, 2005
62.	Kreysigine	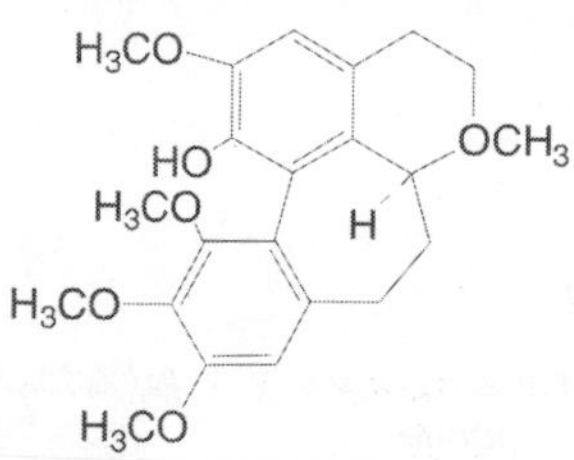	*Kreysigia multiflora*	In gastrointestinal disorders	Dewick, 2002
63.	Lophocerine	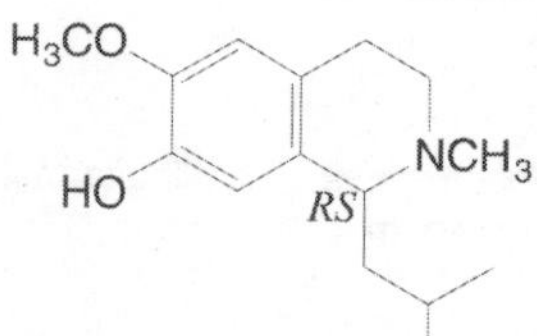	*Lophophora schotti*	Photosensitizing properties	Dewick, 2002
64.	Lobeline	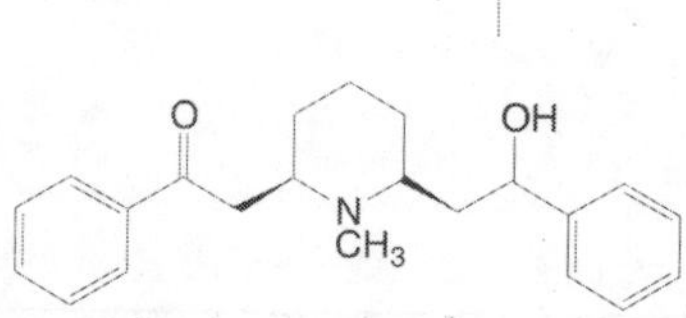	*Lobelia inflata*	Relieve asthma and bronchitis	Dewick, 2002

Contd...

Table 4.2–Contd...

Sl.No.	*Bioactive Molecules*	*Chemical Structures*	*Example Sources*	*Biopotentials*	*References*
65.	Lobelanine	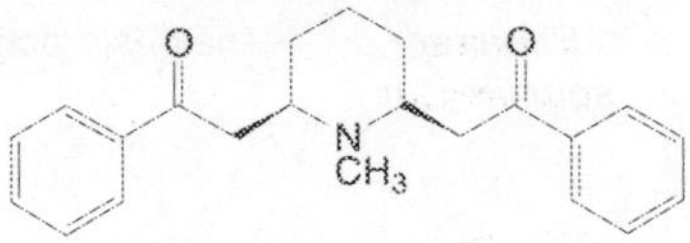	*Lobelia inflata*	A potential pharmaco-therapy for drug addiction	Dewick, 2002
66.	Lupanine	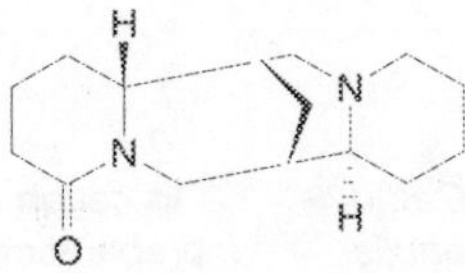	*Lupinus luteus*	Hypoglycemic and human toxic	Dewick, 2002
67.	Lupinine	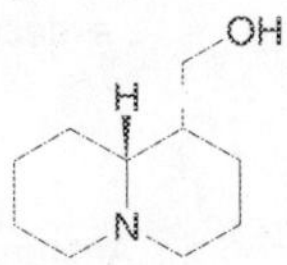	*Lupinus luteus*	Bitter	Dewick, 2002
68.	Lycorine	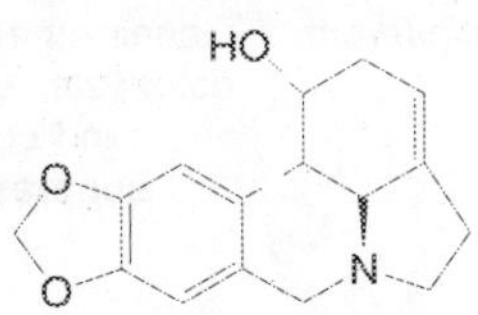	*Lycorus radiata*	Toxic	Dewick, 2002
69.	Melicopicine	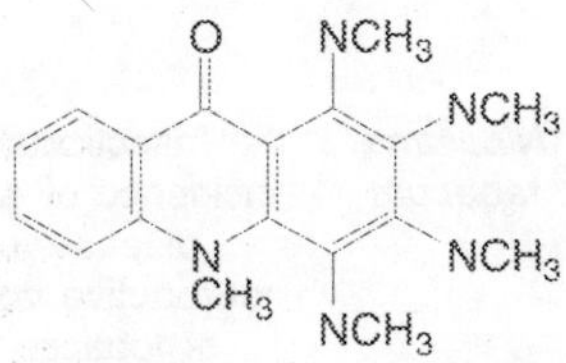	*Melicope fareana*	Antitumor activity	Dewick, 2002
70.	Mescaline	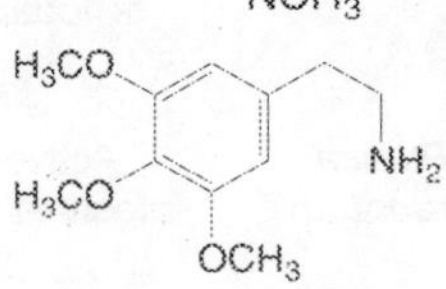	*Lophophora wiliamsii*	Psychoactive, hallucinogenic properties	Bhat *et al.*, 2005
71.	Meteloidino	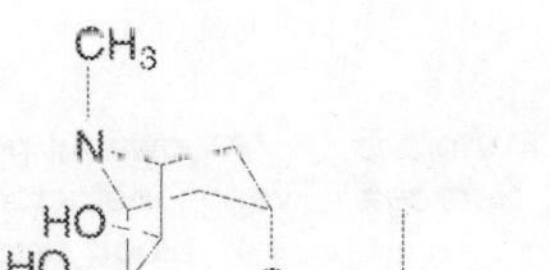	*Datura meteloides*	Hallucinogenic property	Dewick, 2002
72.	Morphine	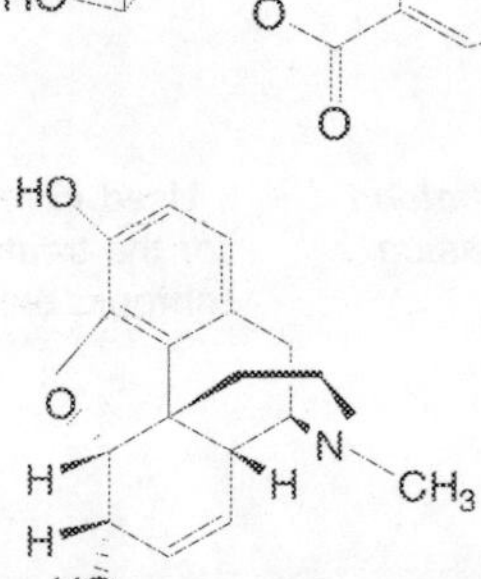	*Papaver sominiferum*	Analgesic, narcotic valuable for relief of severe pain	White *et al.*, 1993

Contd...

Table 4.2–Contd...

Sl.No.	Bioactive Molecules	Chemical Structures	Example Sources	Biopotentials	References
73.	Narceine	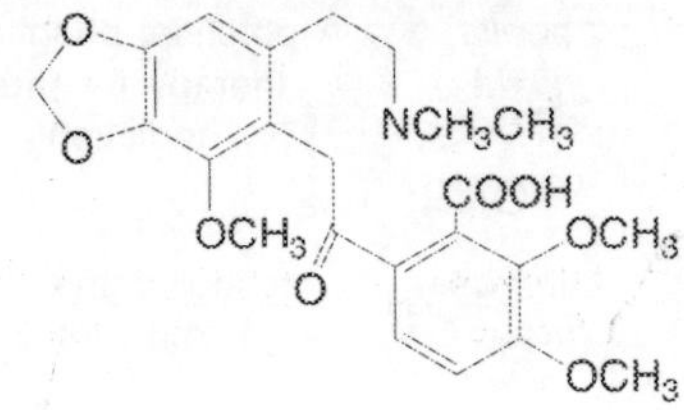	*Papaver somniferum*	Analgesic activity	Dewick, 2002
74.	Norpseudo-ephedrine	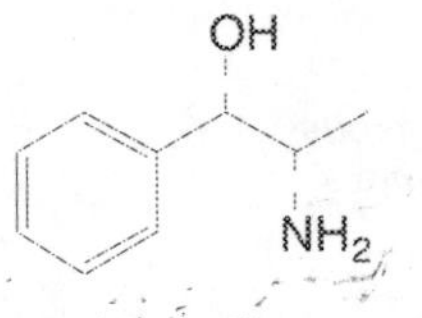	*Catha edulis*	In cough and cold preparations and as a decongestant	Dewick, 2002
75.	Noscapine	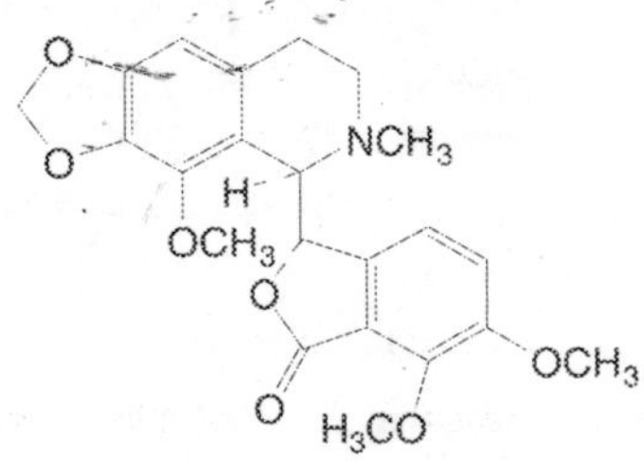	*Papaver sominiferum*	Antitumor activity, chemotherapeutic potentials, antitussive and cough suppressant	Kamei, 1996
76.	Nicotine	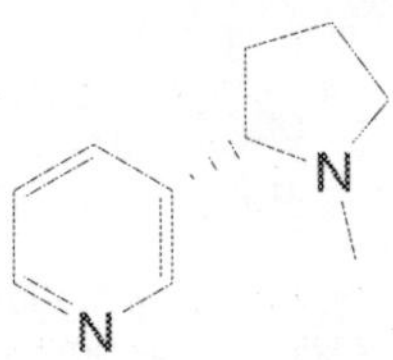	*Nicotiana tabacum*	Insecticidal, low incidence of Alzheimer disease, major neuroactive component of tobacco smog	Dewick, 2002
77.	N-methyl-pelletierine	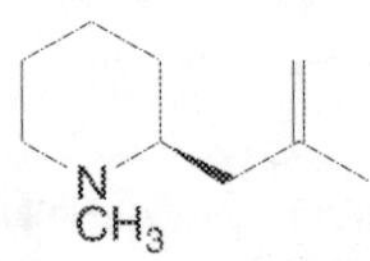	*Punica granatum*	Active against intestinal tapeworms	Dewick, 2002
78.	Noradrenaline	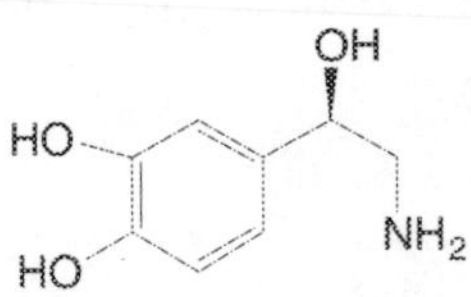	*Portulaca oleracea*	A powerful peripheral vasoconstrictor restoring blood pressure	Dewick, 2002
79.	Oxitropium bromide	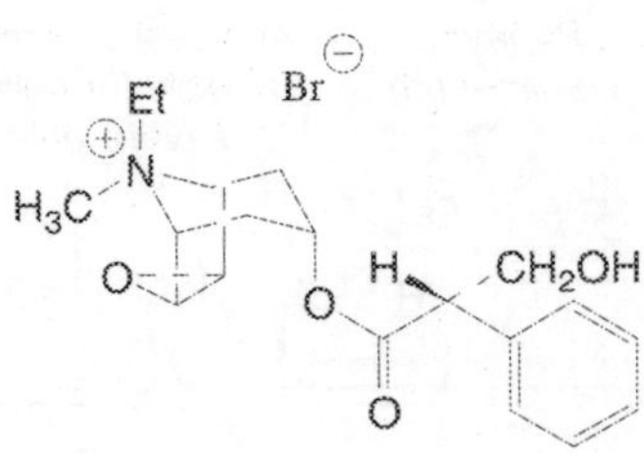	*Adhatoda vasica*	Used in inhalers for the treatment of chronic bronchitis	Dewick, 2002

Contd...

Table 4.2–Contd...

Sl.No.	Bioactive Molecules	Chemical Structures	Example Sources	Biopotentials	References
80.	Papaverine	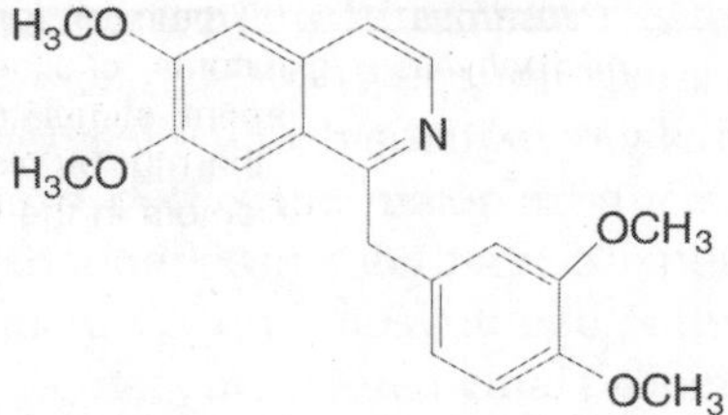	*Papaver sominiferum*	Spasmolytic and vasodilator activity	Gearien and Mede, 1981
81.	Peganine	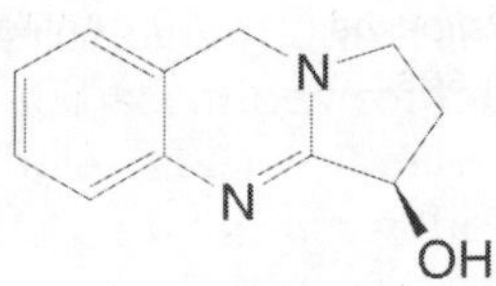	*Peganum harmala*	Bronchodilator activity	Johne *et al.*, 1968
82.	Pelletierine	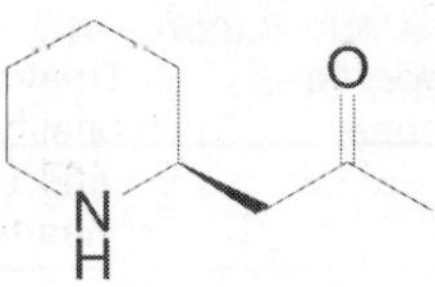	*Punica granatum*	To cure intestinal tapeworms	Bhat *et al.*, 2005
83.	Pilocarpine	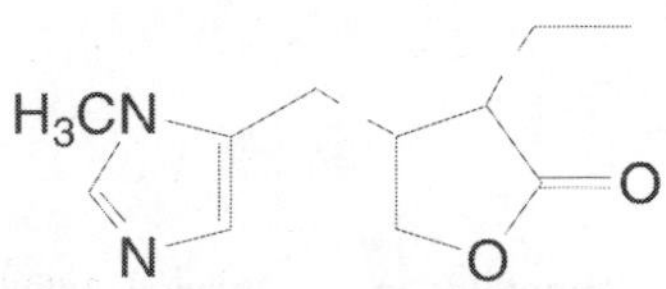	*Pilocarpus microphylus*	In treatment for glaucoma	Brenner, 2000
84.	Pinidine	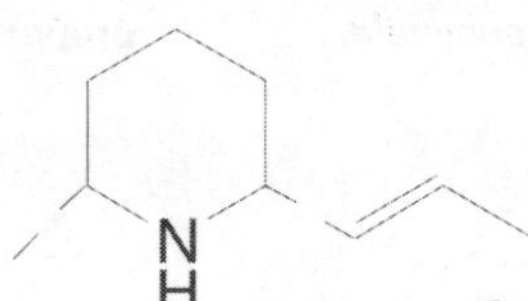	*Pinus* sps.	Antitumor and calcemic activity	Tawara *et al.*, 1995
85.	Piperine	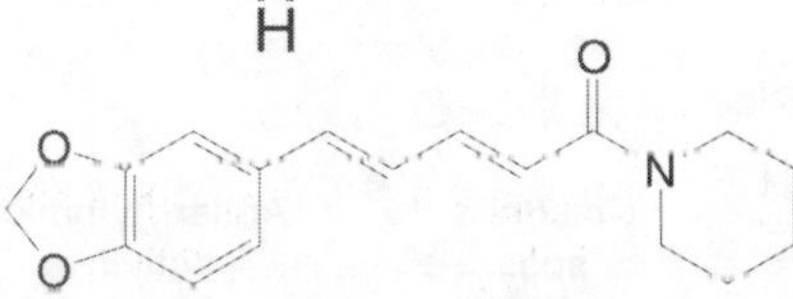	*Piper nigrum*	Pungency, bioavailability enhancer	Bhat *et al.*, 2005
86.	Physostigmine	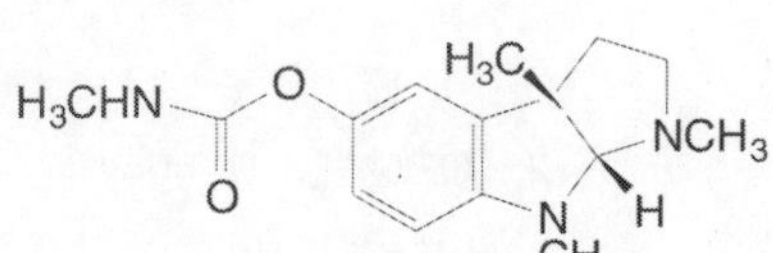	*Physostigma venenosum*	Enhance cholinergic activity, anticholinesterase activity	Brossi *et al.*, 1996
87.	Protopine	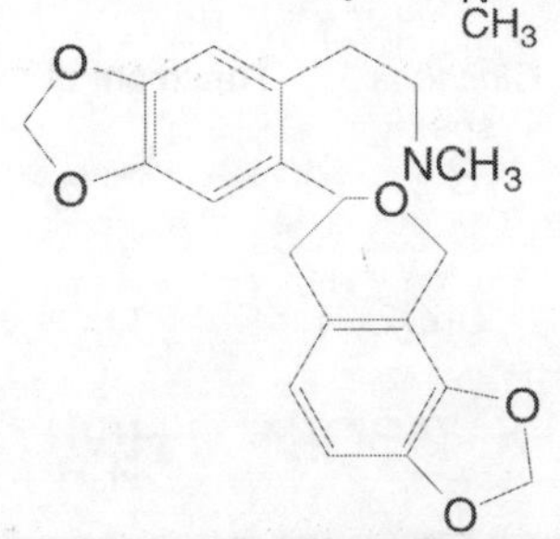	*Chelidonium majus*	Smooth-muscle relaxant, hypotensive, antimicrobial activity	Bhat *et al.*, 2005

Contd...

Table 4.2–Contd...

Sl.No.	*Bioactive Molecules*	*Chemical Structures*	*Example Sources*	*Biopotentials*	*References*
88.	Pilosine	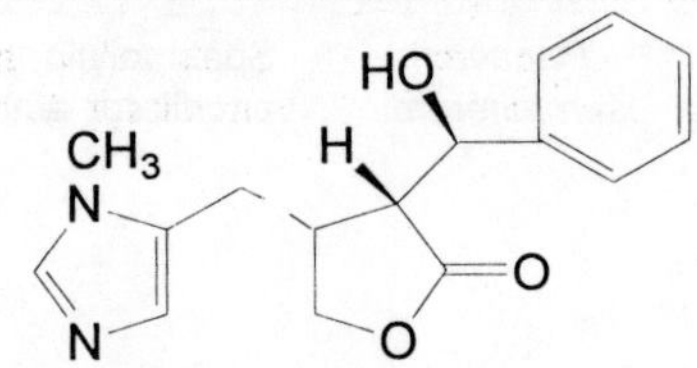	*Pilocarpus microphyllus*	Treatment for glaucoma, cholinergic agent, stimulates the muscarinie receptors in the eye	Dewick, 2002
89.	Psilocin	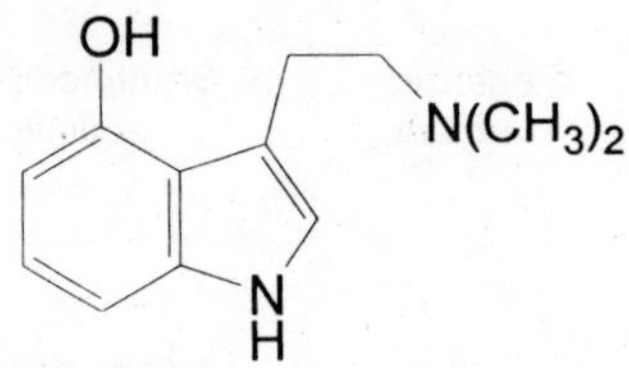	*Psilocybe* sps.	Antitoxic	Dewick, 2002
90.	Psilocybin	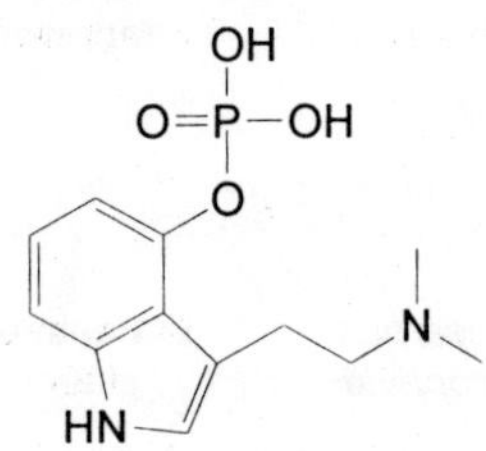	*Psilocybe* sps.	Treatment of personality disorders and cluster headaches	Dewick, 2002
91.	Pumiloside	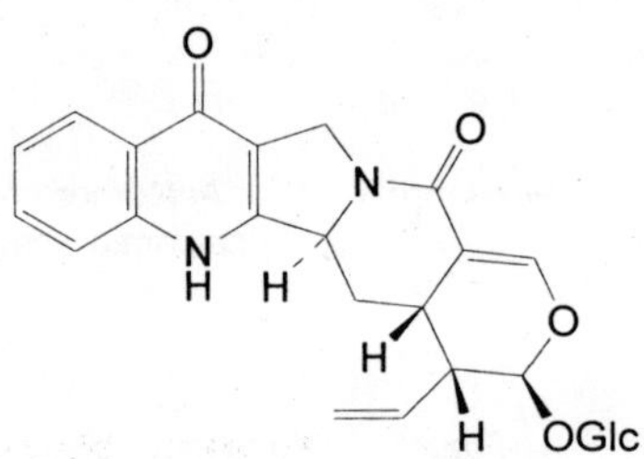	*Camptotheca acuminata*	Antiviral, antibiotic property	Dewick, 2002
92.	Quinidine	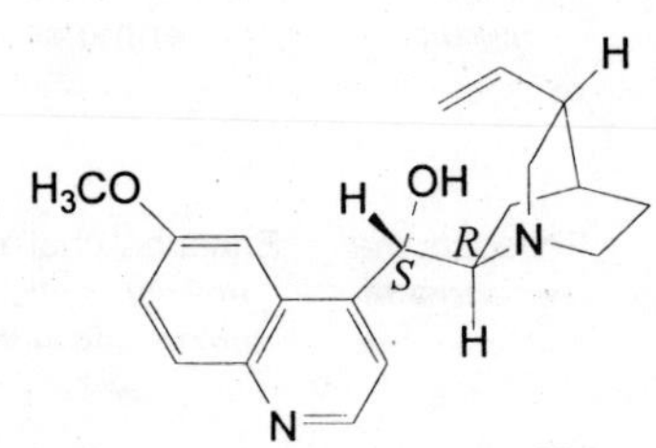	*Cinchona* sps.	Antiarrhythmic activity	Dewick, 2002
93.	Quinine	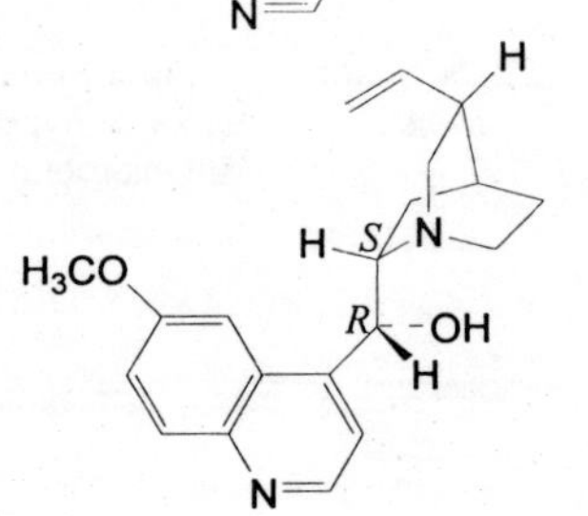	*Cinchona* sps.	Treatment of malaria	Cook and Ikeuchi, 1989

Contd...

Table 4.2–Contd...

Sl.No.	*Bioactive Molecules*	*Chemical Structures*	*Example Sources*	*Biopotentials*	*References*
94.	Rescinnamine	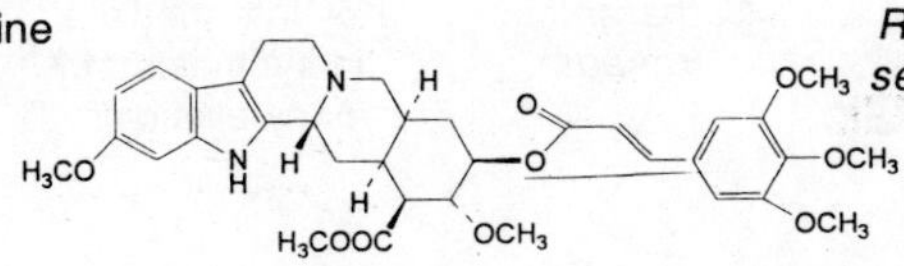	*Rauwolfia serpentina*	Antihypertensive agent	Dewick, 2002
95.	Reserpine	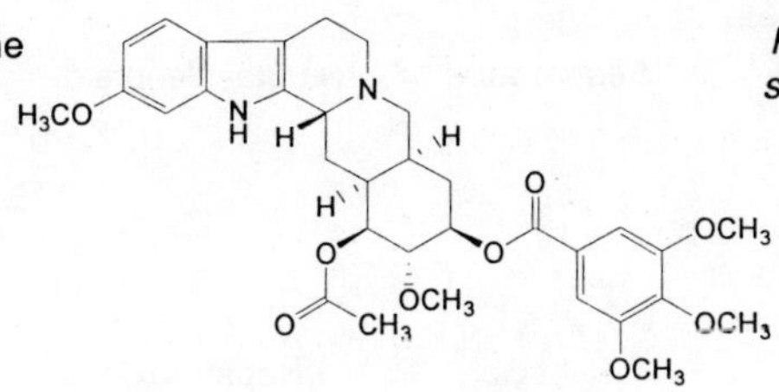	*Rauwolfia serpentina*	Antihypertensive, mild tranquillizer	Ricci and Ricordati, 1955
96.	Retronecine	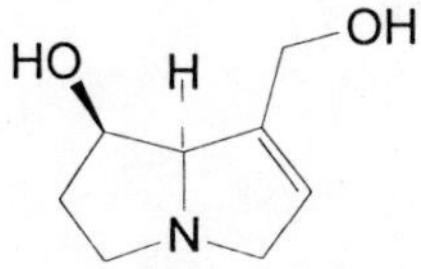	*Senecio tulgaris*	Hepatotoxic	Dewick, 2002
97.	Ricinine	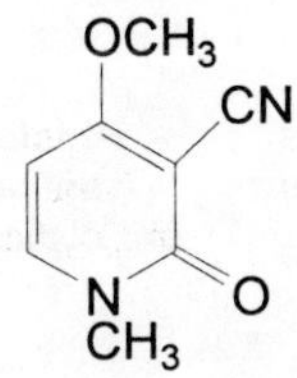	*Ricinus communis*	Toxicity from polypeptide ricin	Robinson and Fowell, 1959
98.	Rutacridone	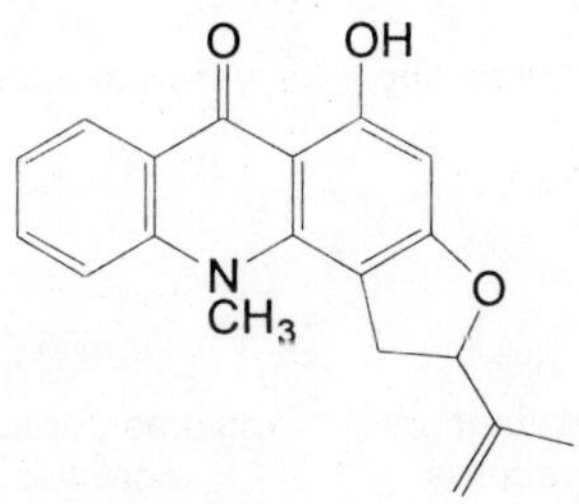	*Ruta graveolens*	Mutagenic property	Roshchina, 2002
99.	Salsolinol	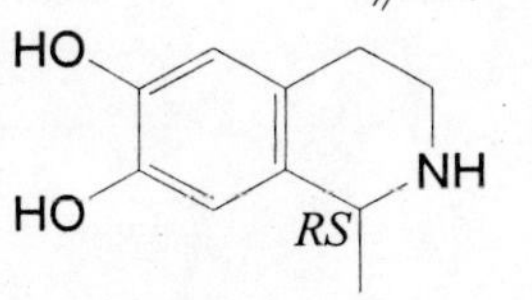	*Corydalis* sps.	Endogenous neurotoxin pathogenesis of Parkinson's disease	Dewick, 2002
100.	Saxitoxin	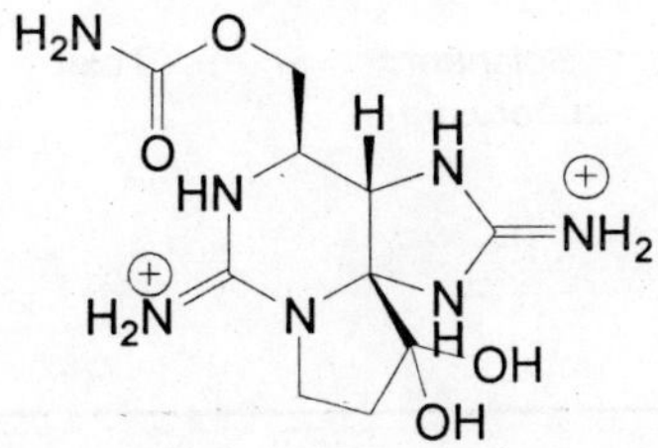	*Saxidomus giganteus*	Neurotoxin	Shimizu, 1993

Table 4.2–Contd...

Sl.No.	*Bioactive Molecules*	*Chemical Structures*	*Example Sources*	*Biopotentials*	*References*
101.	Secologanin	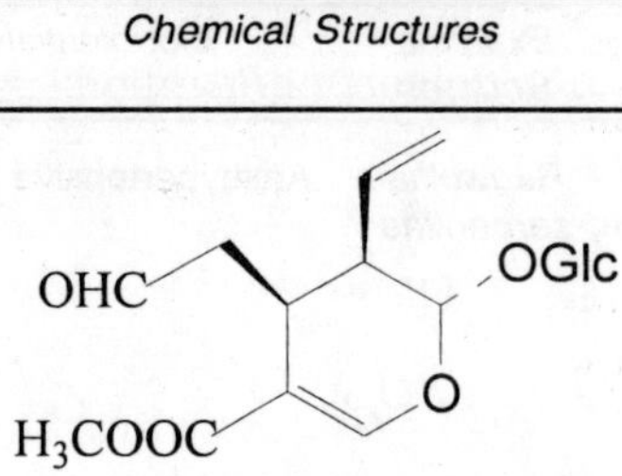	*Catharanthus roseus*	Key intermediate in synthesis of many alkaloids	Leonard, 1999
102.	Sedamine	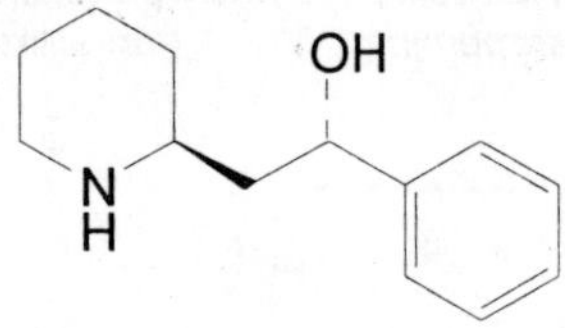	*Sedum acre*	Natural sleep aid	Dewick, 2002
103.	Senecionine	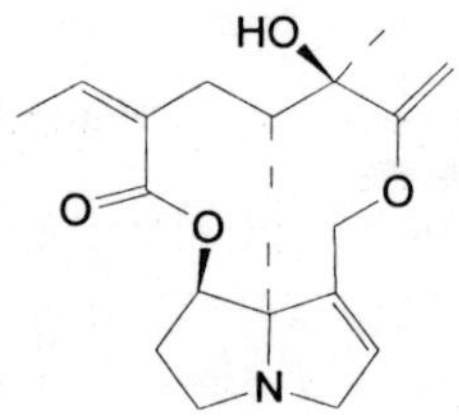	*Senecio* sps.	Hepatotoxic	Dewick, 2002
104.	Serotonin	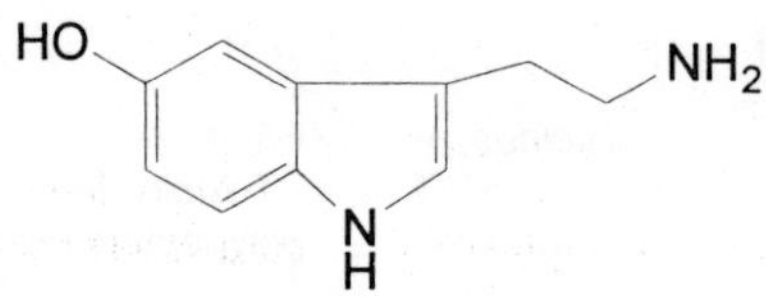	*Agaricus bisporus*	Antidepressant, antipsychotic, anxiolytics, antiemetic	McGowan *et al.,* 1985
105.	Skimmianine	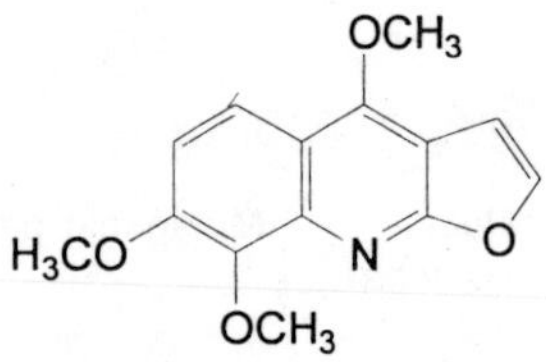	*Skimmia* sps.	Antiviral activity	Dewick, 2002
106.	β-Skytanthine	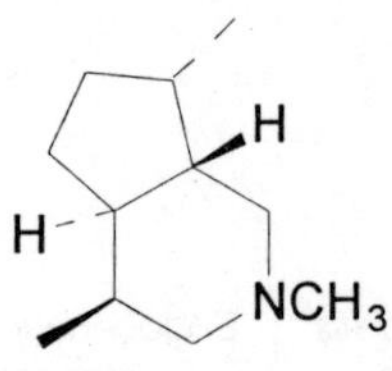	*Skytanthus acutus*	Antitumor, antioxidnt activities	Dewick, 2002
107.	Solanidine	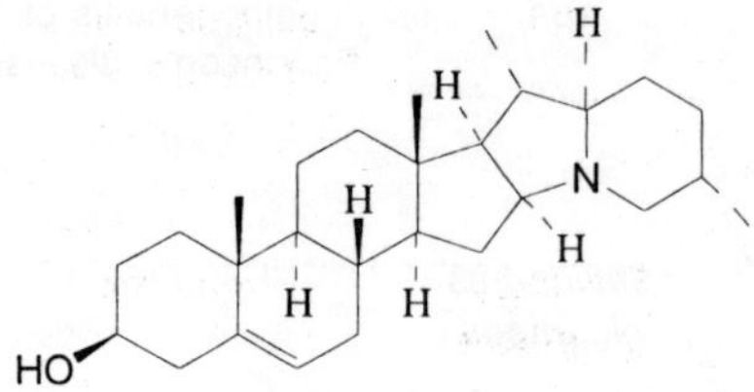	*Solanum tuberosum*	Toxic	Briner, 1969

Contd...

Table 4.2–Contd...

Sl.No.	Bioactive Molecules	Chemical Structures	Example Sources	Biopotentials	References
108.	Sparteine	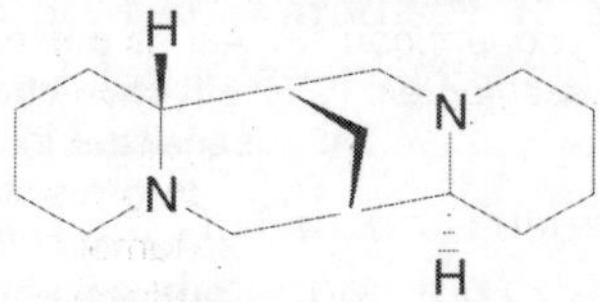	*Baptisis cytisus*	Hypoglycaemic activity	Dewick, 2002
109.	Stephanine	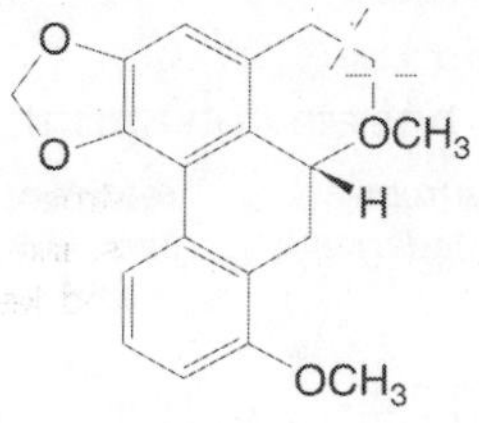	*Stephania* sps.	Analgesic, narcotic valuable analgesic for relief of severe pain	Dewick, 2002
110.	Strychnine	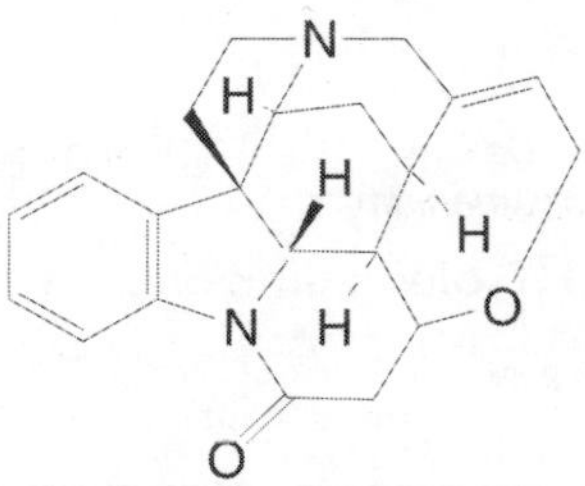	*Strychnos nux-vomica*	Poisonous	Bosch *et al.*, 1996
111.	Swainsonine	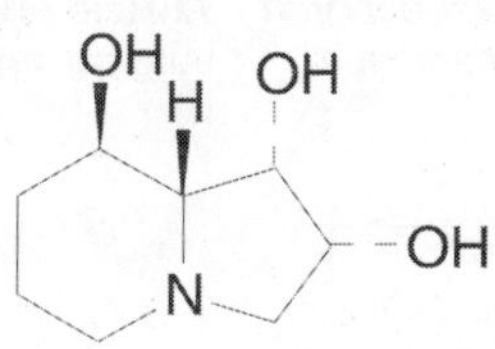	*Swainsona cancescens*	A toxin with potent α–mannosidase inhibitory activity	Dewick, 2002
112.	Tetrandrine	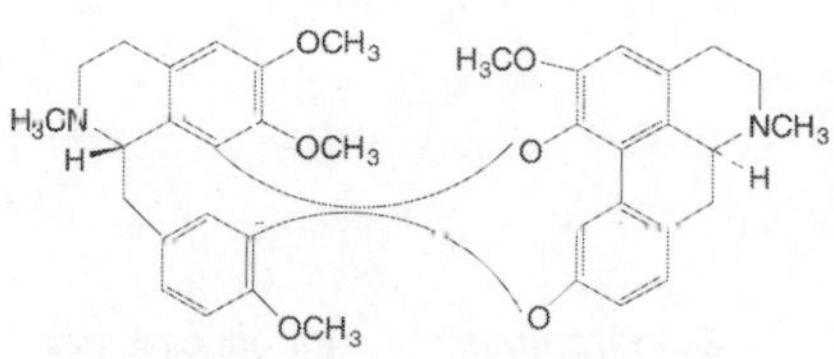	*Stephania tetrandra*	Blocks calcium channels and in treatment of cardio-vascular dlseases	Seow *et al.*, 1986
113.	Thebaine	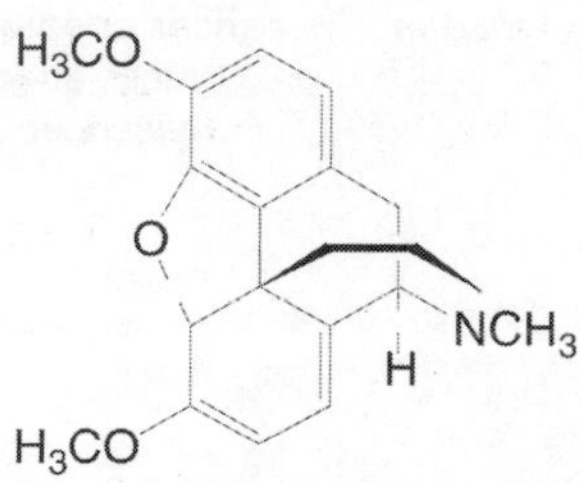	*Papaver sominiferum*	Analgesic, substrate for semi-synthesis of other drugs	Aceto *et al.*, 1999

Contd...

Table 4.2–Contd...

Sl.No.	*Bioactive Molecules*	*Chemical Structures*	*Example Sources*	*Biopotentials*	*References*
114.	Tomatidine	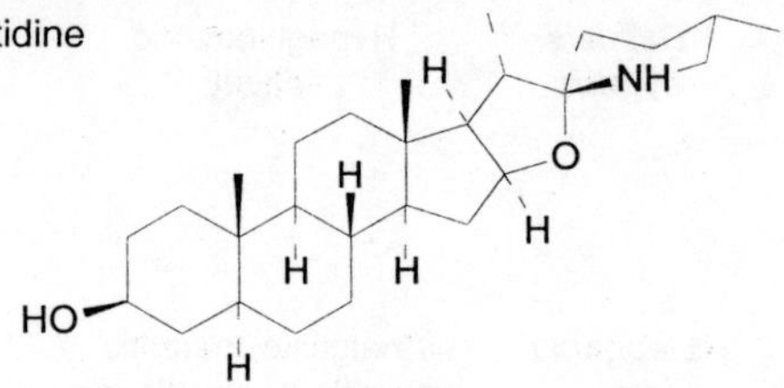	*Lycopersicon esculentem*	Act as potent and effective chemo-sensitizer in multi-drug resistant tumor cells, antiviral activity	Bushway *et al.*, 1994
115.	Tropicamide	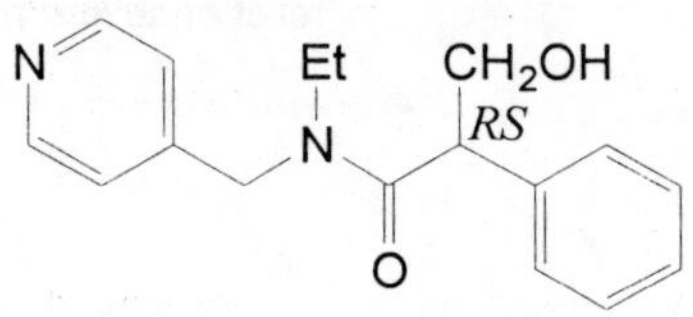	*Atropa belladonna*	Treatment of acute iritis, iridocyclitis, and keratitis	Dewick, 2002
116.	Tropine	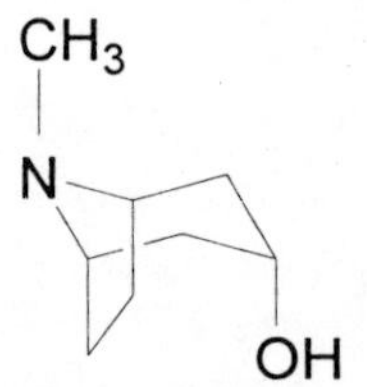	*Datura stramonium*	Poisonous	Dewick, 2002
117.	Tubocurarine	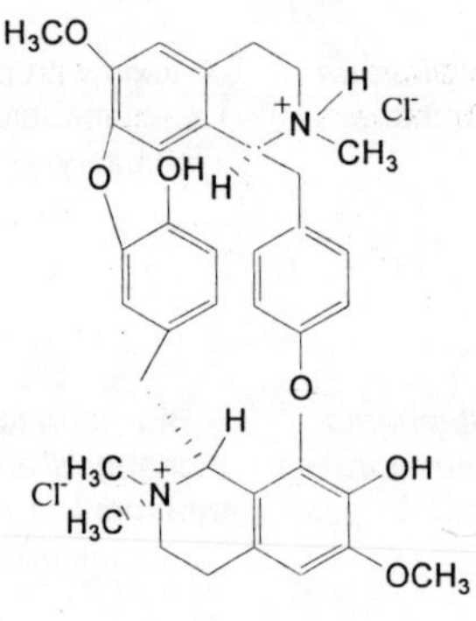	*Chondrodendron tomentosum*	Muscle relaxant in surgical operations	Dewick, 2002
118.	Vincristine	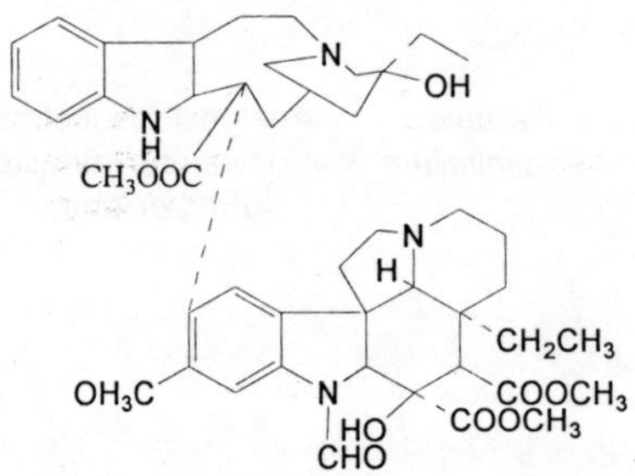	*Catharanthus roseus*	Introduced into cancer chemotherapy, most effective anticancer agent	Noble, 1990

Contd...

Table 4.2–Contd...

Sl.No.	Bioactive Molecules	Chemical Structures	Example Sources	Biopotentials	References
119.	Vincamine	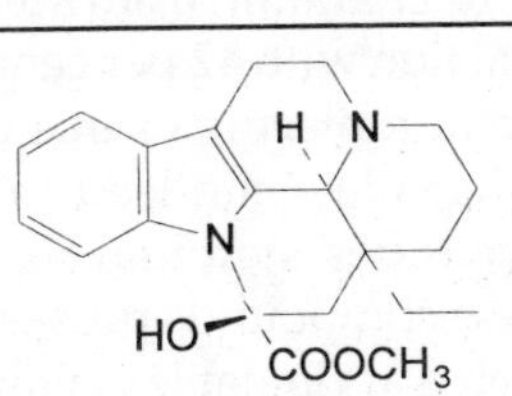	*Vinca minor*	Anticancer activity	Noble, 1990
120.	Vindoline	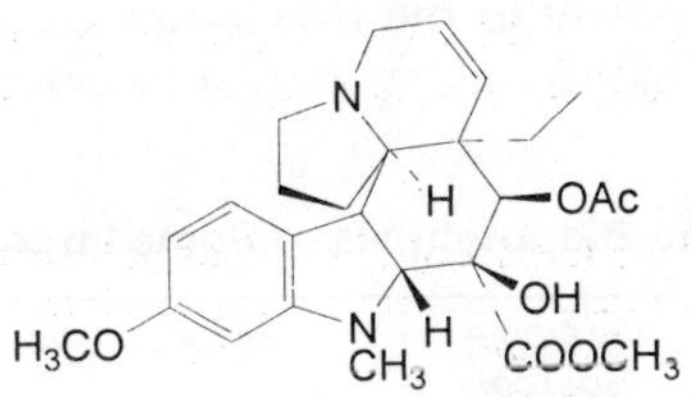	*Aspidosperma* sps.	High value anti-cancer chemotherapy and neoplastic bulk drug	Dewick, 2002
121.	Yohimbine	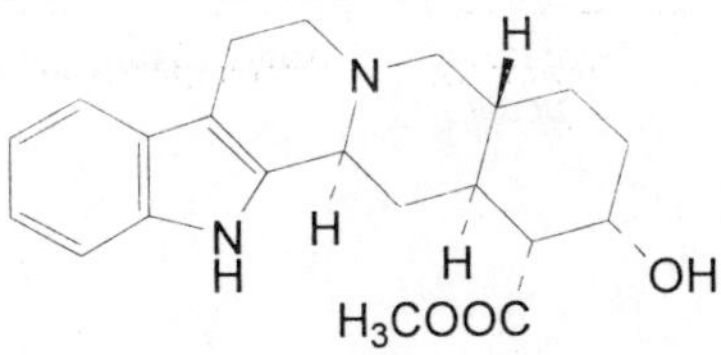	*Pausinystalia yohimbe*	As aphrodisiac–pharmacologically active, known to dilate blood vessels	Shah and Goyal, 1994

Terpenoids

It is a diverse class of secondary metabolites that may be formally considered to be constructed from 'isoprene units'. Isoprene itself had been characterized as a decomposition product from various natural cyclic hydrocarbons, and was suggested as the fundamental building block for these compounds, also referred to as 'isoprenoids'. Several thousand terpenes occur in many genera of higher plants and microorganisms. The isoprenoids in general are very widely distributed through out the whole of the plant kingdom. The terpenoids form a large and structurally diverse family of natural products derived from C_5 isoprene units joined in a head-to-tail fashion. Typical structures contain carbon skeletons represented by $(C_5)n$, and are classified as hemiterpenes (C_5), monoterpenes (C_{10}), sesquiterpenes (C_{15}), diterpenes (C_{20}), sesterterpenes (C_{25}), triterpenes (C_{30}) and tetraterpenes (C_{40}). Higher polymers are encountered in materials such as rubber. Terpenoids find wide application in medicines, industries and other fields, *e.g.*, linalool along with phenyl-ethyl alcohol is used in perfumery, citral as mosquito repellant, farnesol and juvabione as insect juvenile hormones, ecdysones as insect anti-moulting hormones, taxol and cucurbitacins as antitumor compounds and artemisinin as antimalarial agent, etc. Insects use many terpenoids-derived molecules for their communications. Some important terpenoids with their biopotentials are presented in Table 4.3.

Steroids

These are triterpenes which are based on the cyclopentane–perhydrophenanthrene ring system. The 3-hydroxy derivatives which are crystalline solids at room temperature and termed as sterols have been isolated from a large number of species and probably occur in all angiosperms and gymnosperms. Less often studied are the sterols in liverworts, mosses, horsetail and ferns. Because of the profound biological activities encountered, many natural steroids together with a considerable number of synthetic and semisynthetic steroidal compounds are routinely employed in medicine. Steroids are comparable to sulfonylurea-like medicines, *e.g.*, charantin from *Momordica charantia* given orally exhibited pancreatic as well as an extrapancreatic action with 42 per cent lowering blood sugar effect (Lotlikar and Rajaramarao, 1996). The fundamental molecule of this class of compounds is cholesterol, but different modifications in the ring or the side chain lead to a variety of bioactive molecules such as sterols, steroidal saponins, cardiac glycosides, steroidal alkaloids, corticosteroids, sex hormones, bile acids, and ecdysteroids. Although these compounds possess a common structural skeleton but they have markedly different bioefficacies which is attributable mainly to the stereochemistry of the ring fusions, responsible for its shape and partly to the functional groups attached to the nucleus. Some of the compounds of different groups of this class with their biopotentials are presented in Table 4.4.

Table 4.3: Chemical Structure, Example Source and Biopotentials of Some Important Terpenoids

Sl.No.	*Bioactive Molecules*	*Chemical Structures*	*Example Sources*	*Biopotentials*	*References*
1.	β–Amyrin	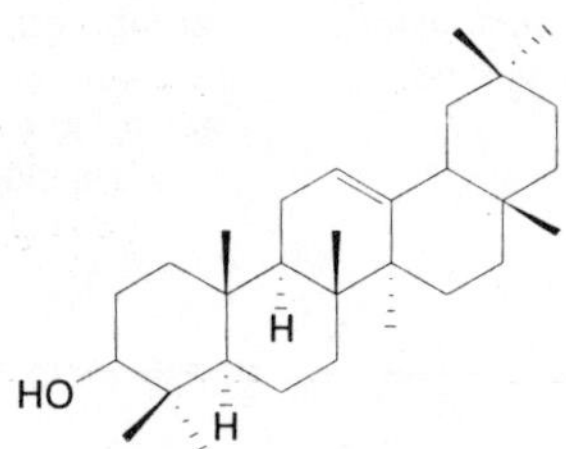	*Euphorbia tirucalli*	Antibacterial activity	Dewick, 2002
2.	Artemisinin	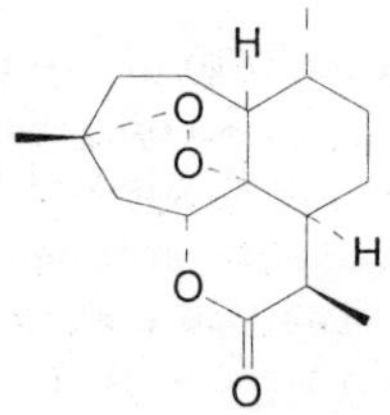	*Artemisia annua*	Antimalarial	Bhattacharya and Sharma, 1999
3.	Azadirachtin	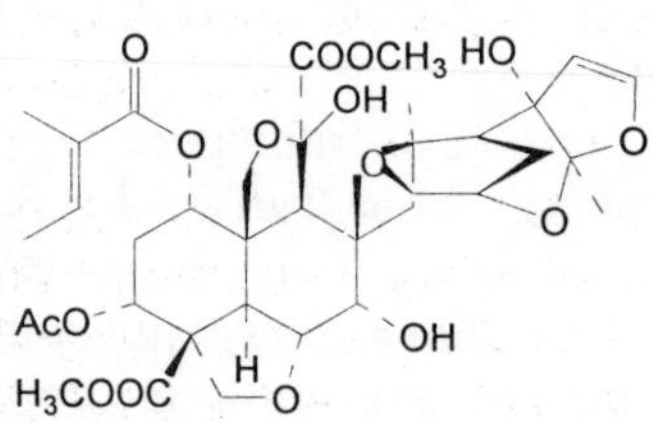	*Azadirachta indica*	Insecticidal activity	Dixit *et al.*, 1992
5.	δ–Cadinene	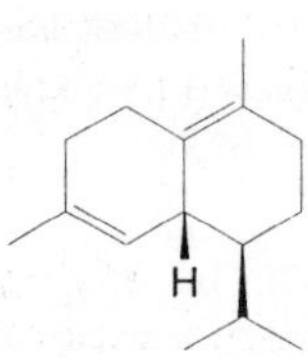	*Juniperus oxycedrus*	Anticarcinogenic, antibacterial, antiacne activities	Chung *et al.*, 1993

Contd...

Table 4.3–Contd...

Sl.No.	Bioactive Molecules	Chemical Structures	Example Sources	Biopotentials	References
6.	Camphor	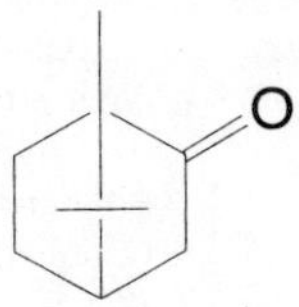	*Salvia officinalis*	Relieves arthritic and rheumatic pains, neuralgia, cold sores, bronchitis	Mann *et al.*, 1994
7.	Camptothecin	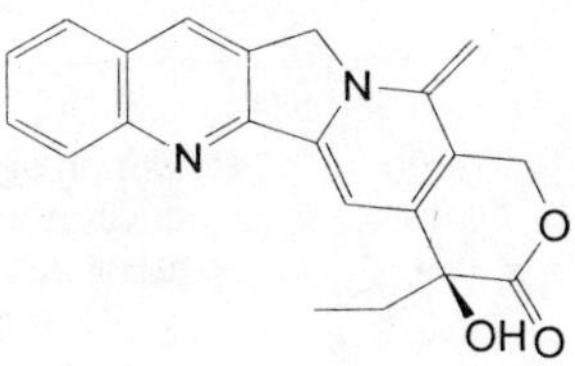	*Camptotheca acuminata*	Active against a series of human tumor cell lines, bioavailability enhancer	Slichenmyer *et al.*, 1993
8.	Capsanthin	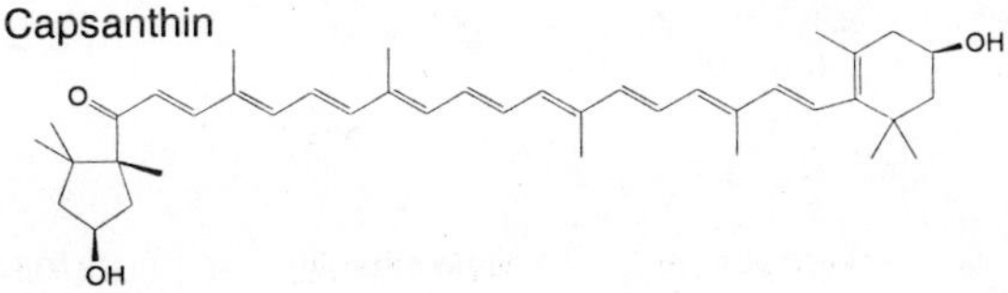	*Capsicum annuum*	Antineoplastic, antioxidant activities	Matsufuji, 1998
9.	β–Carotene	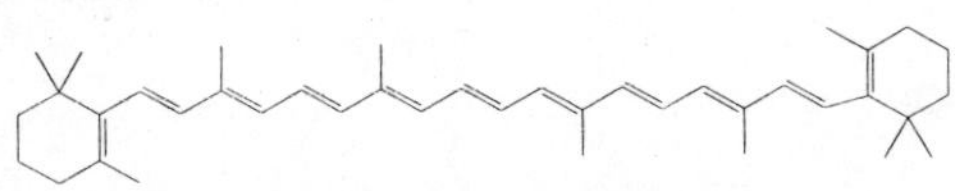	*Docus carota*	Yellow colouring agent–for food, drinks, confectionery and drugs	Lakshmanan and Cama, 1966
10.	Casbene	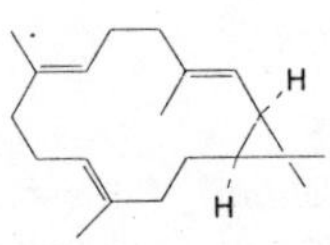	*Ricinus communis*	Antifungal activity	Stekoll and West, 1978
11.	Cinerins	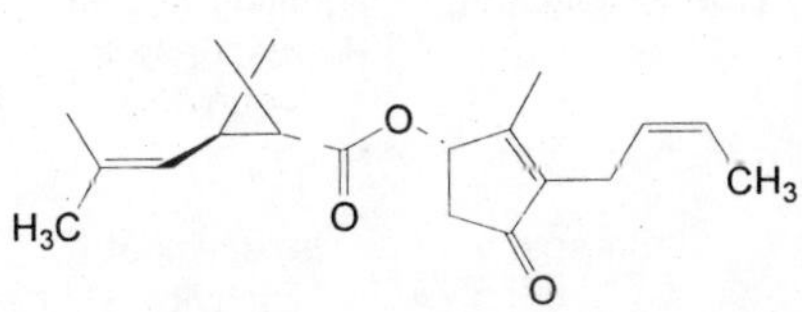	*Chrysanthenum cinerariaefolium*	Insecticidal activity	Casida, 1980
12.	Citronella	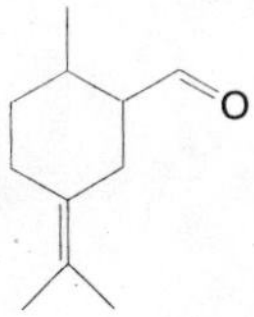	*Cymbopogon nardus*	Insecticidal, repellent, antifeeding	Patinaik *et al.*, 2006
13.	Cucurbitacin E	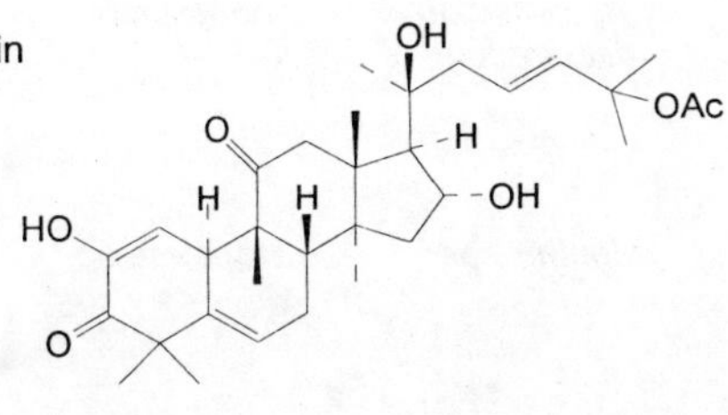	*Cucumber/ melon*	Bitter taste, purgative, extremely cytotoxic	Tallamy *et al.*, 1997

Contd...

Table 4.3–Contd...

Sl.No.	*Bioactive Molecules*	*Chemical Structures*	*Example Sources*	*Biopotentials*	*References*
14.	Forskolin	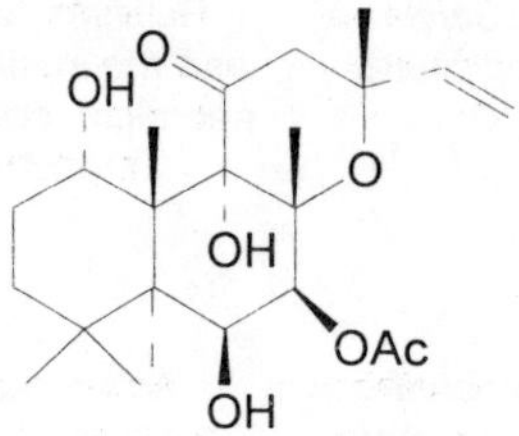	*Coleus forskohii*	Used in Indian system of Medicine, hypotensive, antispasmodic activity	Bhat, 1993
15.	Ginkgolide	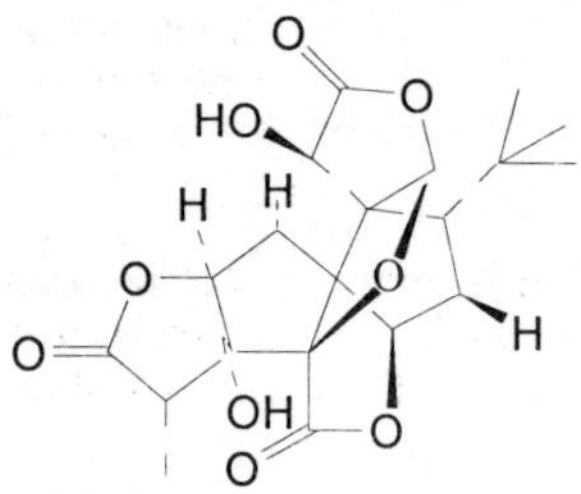	*Ginkgo biloba*	Potent antagonistic activity towards platelet activating factor	Braquet *et al.*, 1991
16.	Gossypol	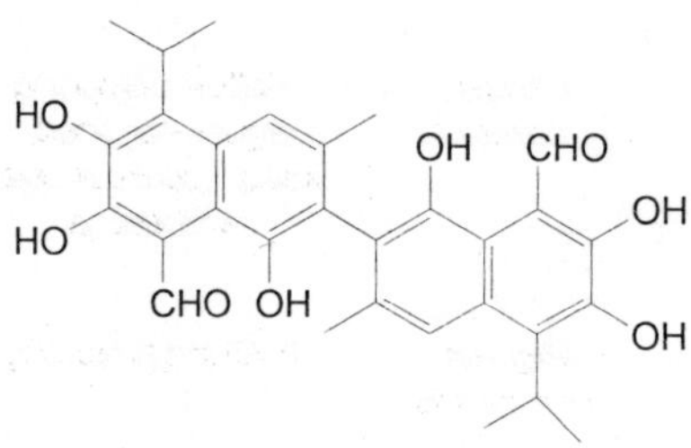	*Gossypium* sps.	Male infertility agent	Jaroszewski *et al.*, 1992
17.	Jasmolin I	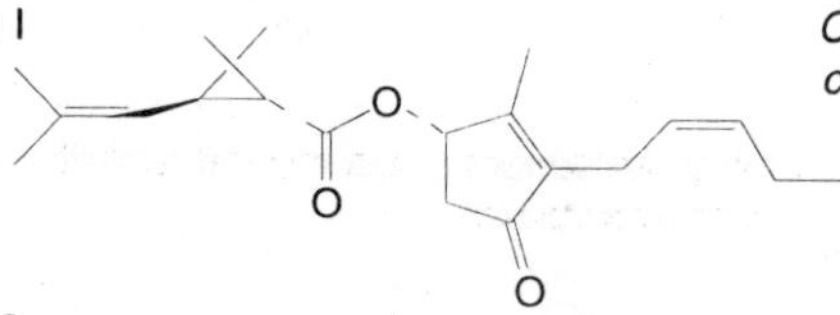	*Chrysanthenum cinerariaefolium*	Insecticidal, as signaling system in response to wounding	Casida, 1980
18.	Limonene	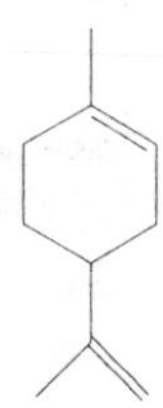	*Citrus* sps.	Insecticidal activity	Mann *et al.*, 1994
19.	Lycopene	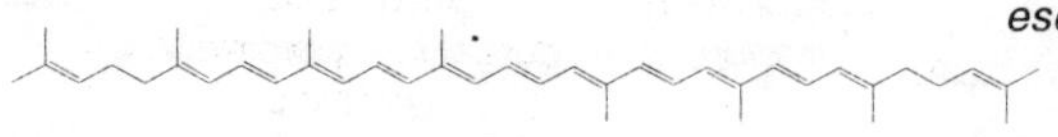	*Lycopersicon esculentum*	Antioxidant	Sies and Stahl, 1998
20.	Menthofuran	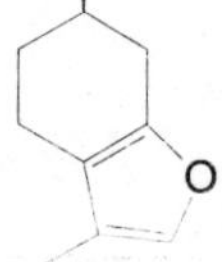	*Mentha* sps.	Hepatotoxic	Wise and Croteau, 1999

Contd...

Table 4.3–Contd...

Sl.No.	Bioactive Molecules	Chemical Structures	Example Sources	Biopotentials	References
21.	Quassin	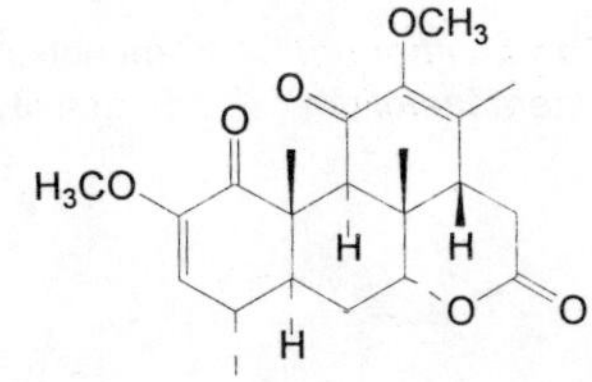	*Quassia amara*	Cytotoxic, antimalarial, amoebicidal activities	Evans and Raj, 1991
22.	Paclitaxel (taxol)	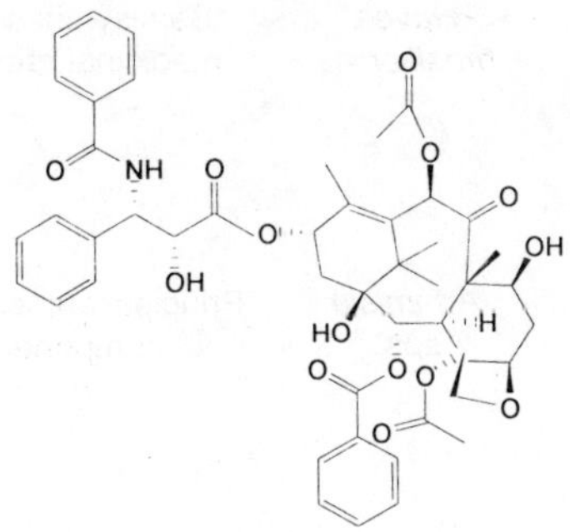	*Taxus brevifolia*	Active against a series of human tumor cell lines, bioavailability enhancer	Heinstein and Chang, 1994
23.	Parthenolide	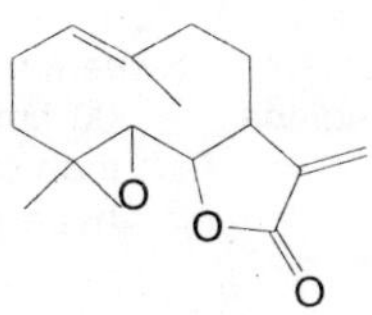	*Tanacetum parthenium*	Antimigraine agent in feverfew	Tiuman *et al.*, 2005
24.	Phellandrene	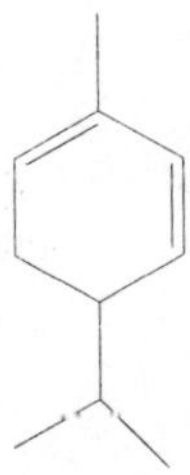	*Myristica fragrans*	Antimicrobial and antioxidant activities	Dewick, 2002
25.	Phorbol	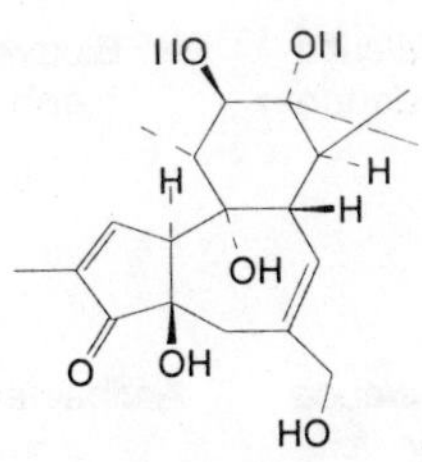	*Euphorbia* sps.	Activates protein kinase–leads to uncontrolled cancerous growth, tumor promoter	Hecker *et al.*,1967
26.	Pulegone	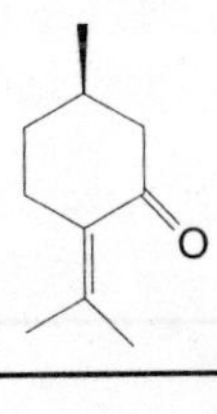	*Mentha pulegium*	Folk history of abortifacient	Grundschober, 1979

Contd...

Table 4.3–Contd...

Sl.No.	*Bioactive Molecules*	*Chemical Structures*	*Example Sources*	*Biopotentials*	*References*
27.	Pyrethrin I	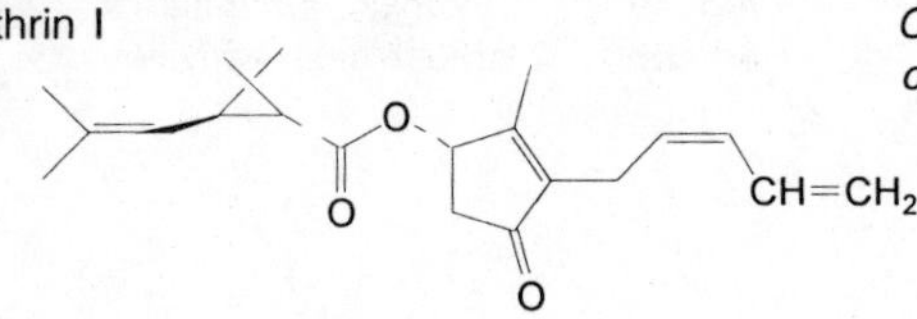	*Chrysanthenum cinerariaefolium*	Insecticidal activity	Casida, 1980
28.	Rubber	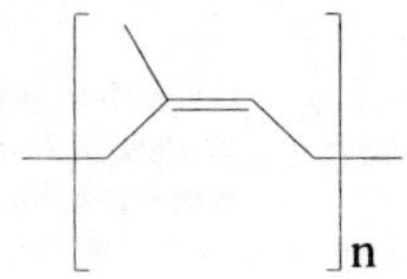	*Hevea brasiliensis*	Semisynthesis of medicinal steroids	Dewick, 2002
29.	Santonin	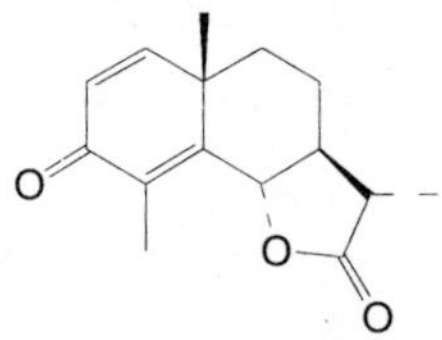	*Artemisia* sps.	Principal anthelmintic component	Dewick, 2002
30.	Stevioside	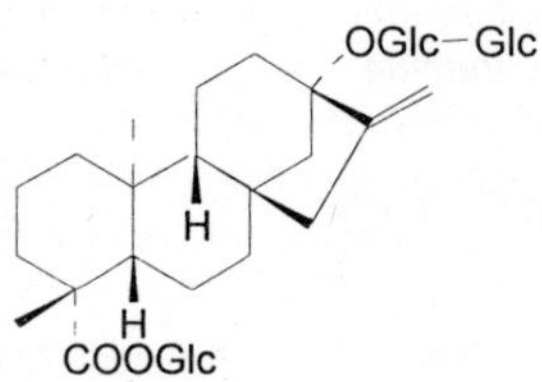	*Stevia reboundiana*	Sweetener component/ 300 times sweeter than sugar, anti-hyperglycaemic	Hanson and Oliveira, 19931
31.	Terpinene	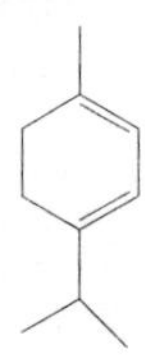	*Myristica fragrans*	Antimicrobial and antioxidant activities	Bhat *et al.*, 2005
32.	Terpineol	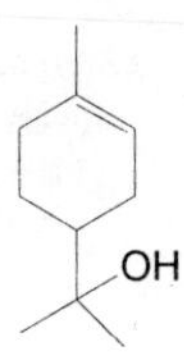	*Melaleuca leucadendron*	Bioavailability enhancer	Bhat *et al.*, 2005
33.	Terpinen-4-ol	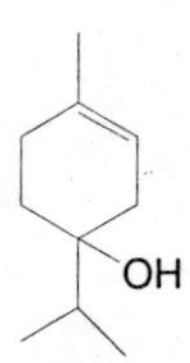	*Melaleuca alternifolia*	Antibacterial activity	Surburg and Panten, 2006

Contd...

Table 4.3–Contd...

Sl.No.	Bioactive Molecules	Chemical Structures	Example Sources	Biopotentials	References
34.	Tetrahydro-cannabinol	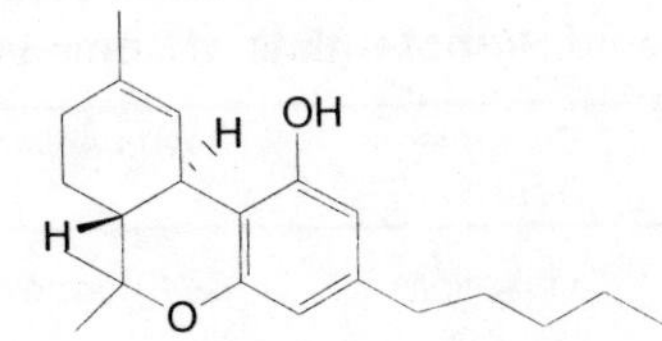	*Cannabis sativa*	Antagonist	Munson *et al.*, 1975
35.	Thapsigargin	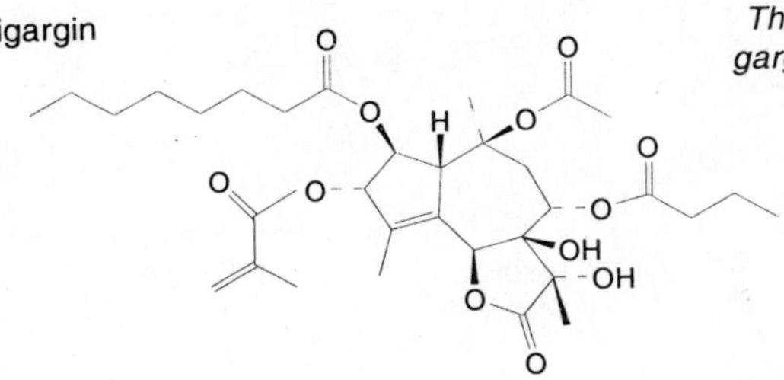	*Thapsia garganica*	As a tumor promoter, potent activator of cells involved in the inflammatory response	Rogers *et al.*, 1995
36.	Thujone	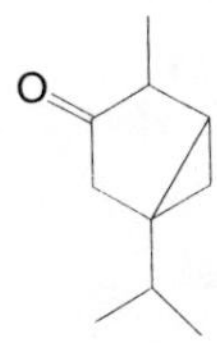	*Artemisia obsinithium*	Neurotoxic agents, used in oral drinks	Naser *et al.*, 1995
37.	Valtrate	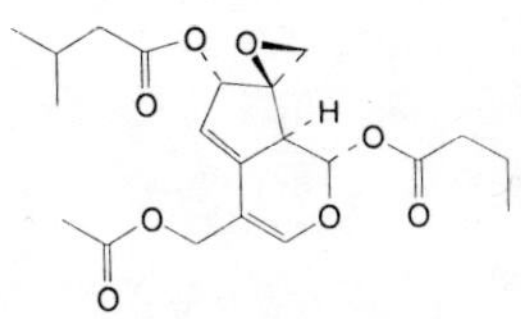	*Valeriana officinalis*	Sedative activity	Dewick, 2002
38.	Vitamin A_1 (Retinol)	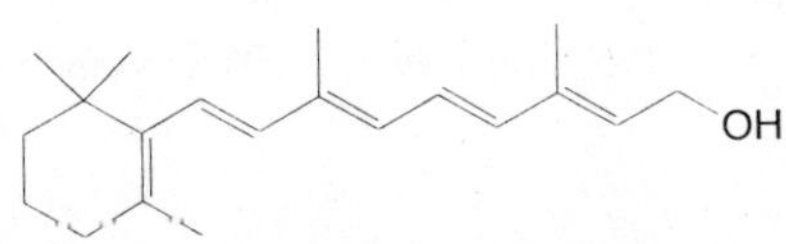	*Daucus carota*	Animal product, essential dletary components/human nutrient	Van Arnum, 1998
39.	Vitamin A_2 (Dehydroretinol)	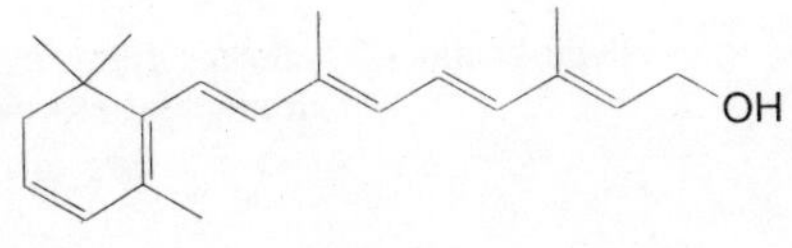	*Daucus carota*	Animal product, essential dietary components/essential human nutrient	Van Arnum, 1998

Saponins

These are glycosides which, even at low concentrations, produce a frothing in aqueous solution, because they have surfactant and soap-like properties. The name comes from the Latin *Sapo*, soap, and plant materials containing saponins were originally used for cleaning clothes, *e.g.*, soapwort (*Saponaria officinalis*) and quillaia or soapbark (*Quillaja saponaria*). These materials also cause haemolysis, lysing red blood cells by increasing the permeability of the plasma membrane, and thus, they are highly toxic when injected into the blood stream. Some saponins containing plant extracts have been used as arrow poison. These are relatively harmless when taken orally and some are valuable food materials, *e.g.*, beans, lentils, soybean, spinach and oats.

Table 4.4: Chemical Structure, Example Source and Biopotentials of Some Important Steroids

Sl.No.	*Bioactive Molecules*	*Chemical Structures*	*Example Sources*	*Biopotentials*	*References*
1.	Andosterone	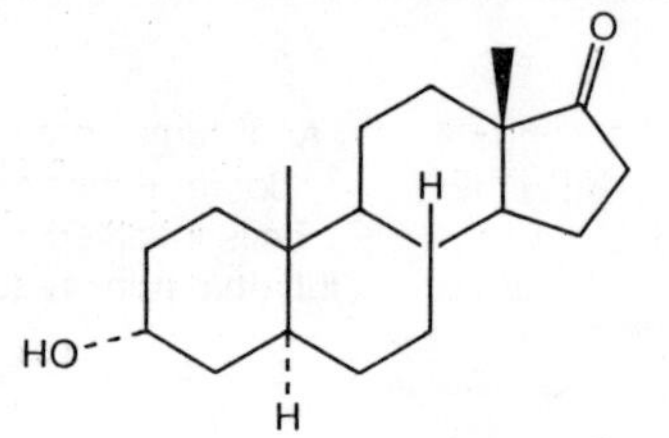	*Pinus nigra*	Sex hormone	Dewick, 2002
2.	17β-Estradiol	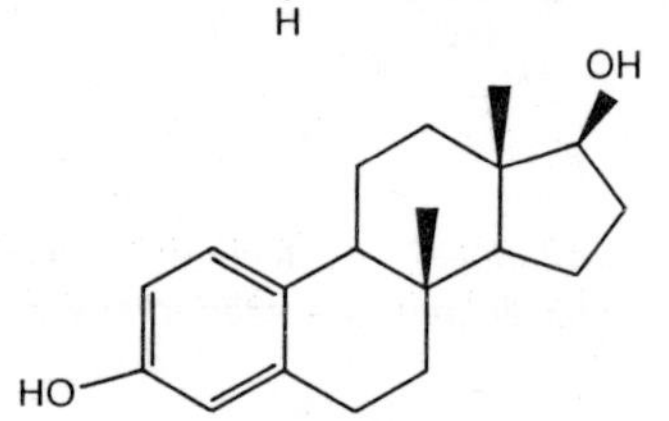	*Phaseolus vulgaris*	Sex hormone	Carani *et al.*, 1997
3.	Fucosterol	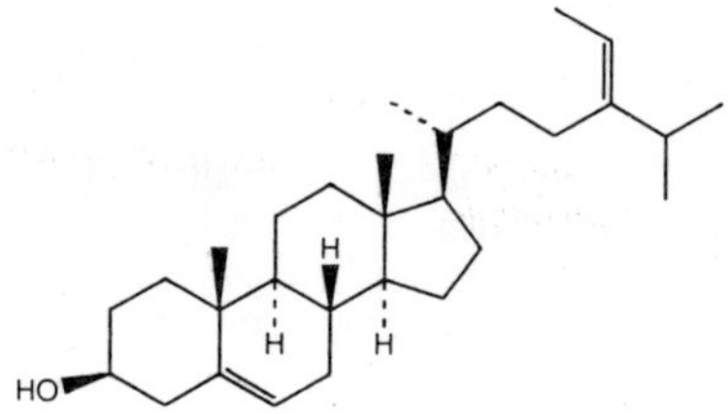	*Fucus* sps.	Antioxidant, antidiabetic	Morisaki *et al.*, 1981
4.	Progesterone	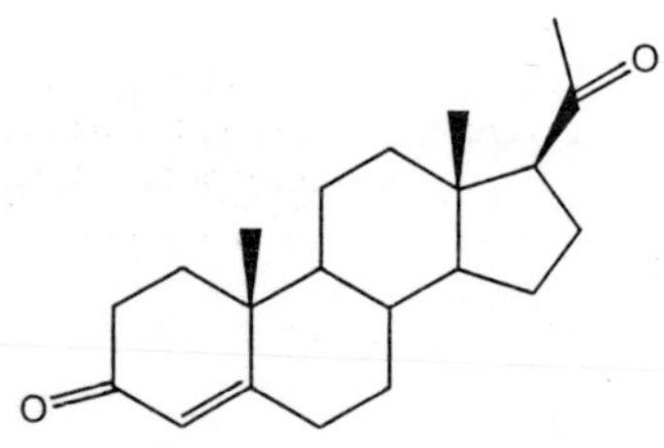	*Digitalis lanata*	Sex hormone	Allen, 1970
5.	Stigmasterol	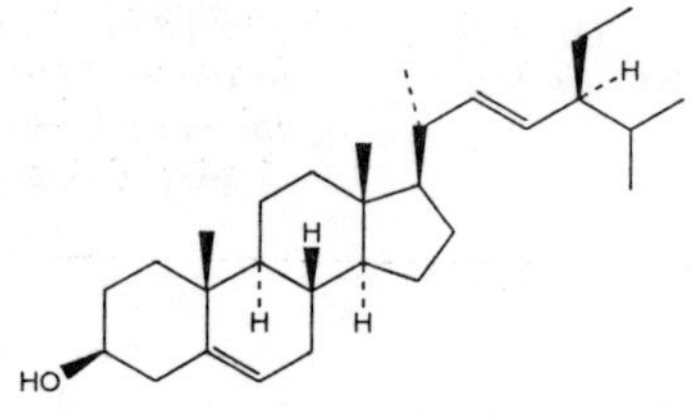	*Glycine max*	Semisynthesis of medicinal steroids	Dewick, 2002
6.	Testosterone	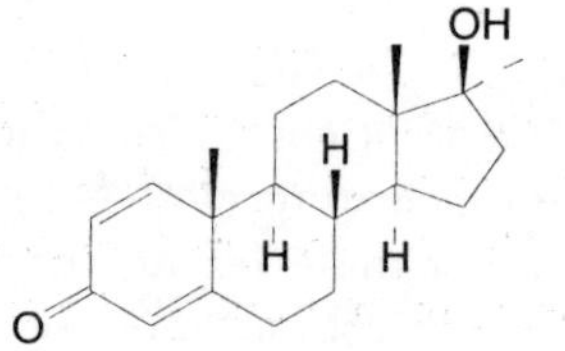	*Pinus sylvestris*	Sex hormone	Freeman *et al.*, 2001

There are two types of saponins: (*i*) triterpenoid saponins which are rare in monocotyledons, but abundant in many dicotyledons families; and ii) steroidal saponins having similar biological properties to the triterpenoid saponins but are less widely distributed in nature. They are found in many monocotyledons families, especially the Dioscoreaceae (*e.g., Discorea*), the Agavaceae (*e.g., Agave, Yucca*) and the Liliaceae (*e.g., Smilax, Trillium*). All the steroidal saponins have the same configuration at the *spiro* centre C-22, but stereoisomers at C-25 exist, *e.g.,* yamogenin and often mixtures of the C-25 stereoisomers co-occur in plant. Some important saponins with their biopotentials are presented in Table 4.5.

Table 4.5: Chemical Structure, Example Source and Biopotentials of Some Important Saponins and Sapogenins

Sl.No.	*Bioactive Molecules*	*Chemical Structures*	*Example Sources*	*Biopotentials*	*References*
1.	Barringtogenol	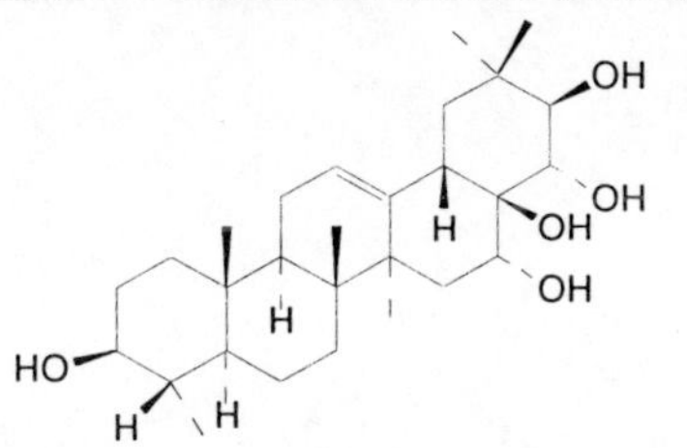	*Aesculus hippocastrum*	Antiinflammatory and antibruising remedy	Khong and Lewis, 1977
2.	Dioscin	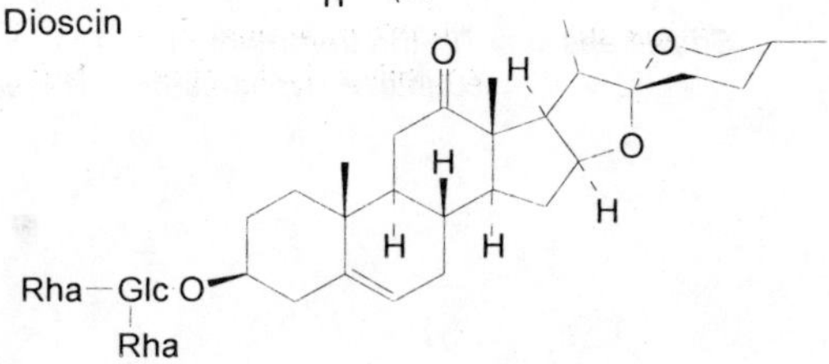	*Dioscorea* sps.	As contraceptive and in the treatment of various disorders of the genitary organs	Zou *et al.*, 2003
3.	Diosgenin	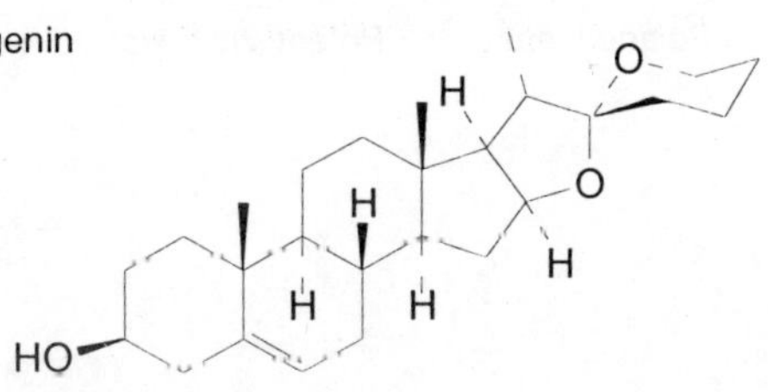	*Dioscorea* sps.	Contraceptive activity	Cayen and Dvornik, 1979
4.	Glycyrrhizic acid	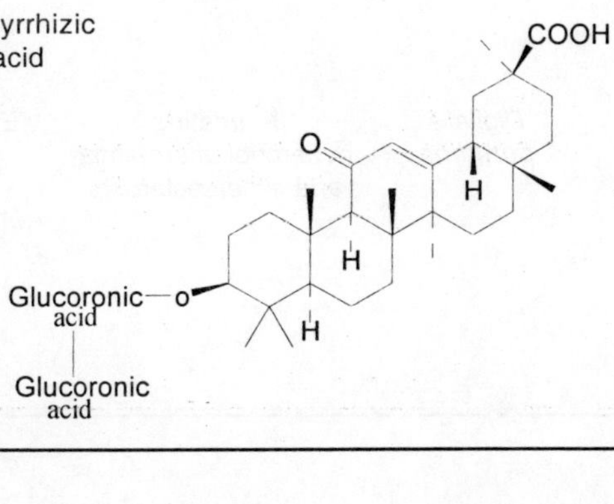	*Glycyrrhiza glabra*	As a sweetener in food products and chewing tobacco	Ploeger *et al.*, 2001

Contd...

Table 4.5–Contd...

Sl.No.	*Bioactive Molecules*	*Chemical Structures*	*Example Sources*	*Biopotentials*	*References*
5.	Hecogenin	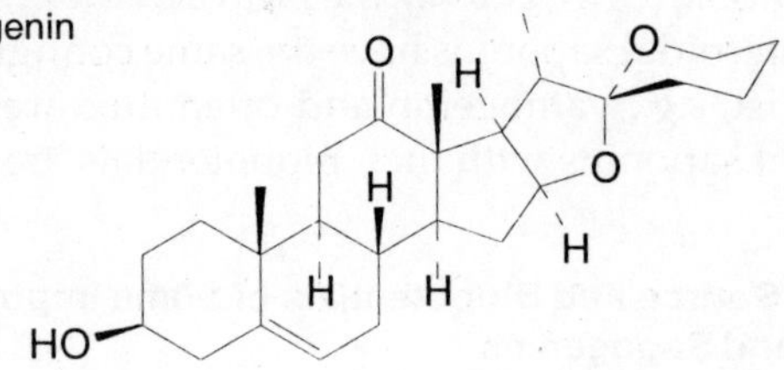	*Agave sisalana*	Antileukemic activity	Pkheidze *et al.*,1991
6.	Protoaescigenin	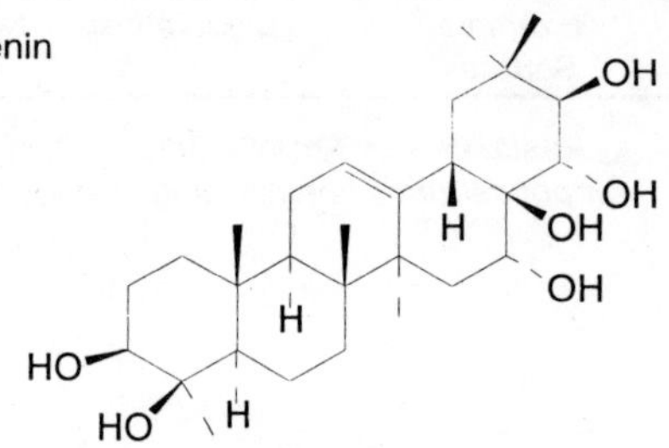	*Aesculus hippocastrum*	Antiinflammatory and antibruising remedy	Zhao *et al.*, 2000
7.	Smilagenin	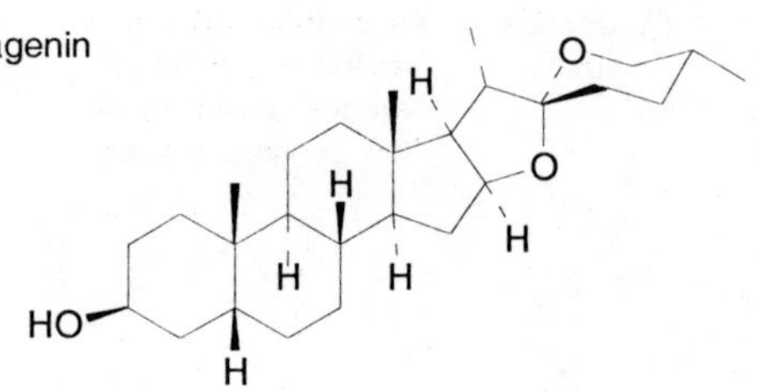	*Smilax* sps.	In the treatment of cognitive dysfunction	Yu and Nasudari, 1971
8.	Solasonine	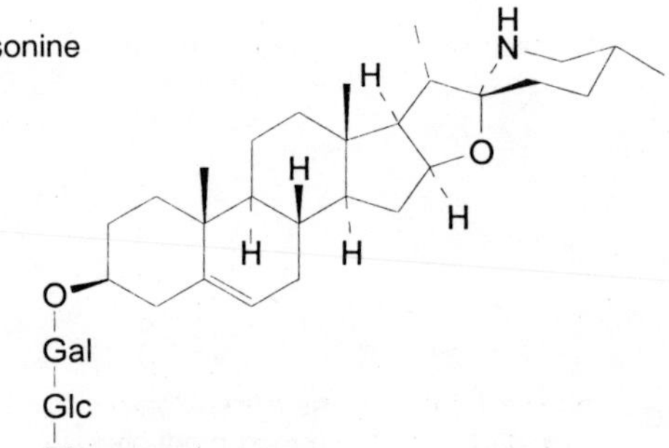	*Solanum* sps.	Potentially toxic	Millward *et al.*, 2005
9.	Tigogenin	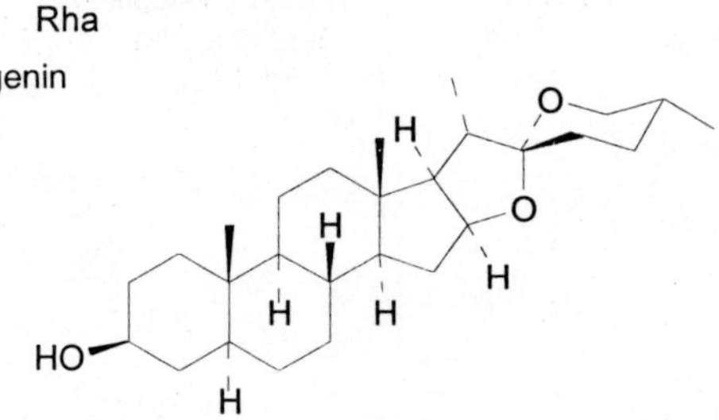	*Digitalis purpurea*	In treating hypercholesterolemia and atherosclerosis	Evans, 1989

Glucosinolates

These are a uniform class of naturally occurring anions which have so far, been found exclusively in the plant kingdom, and only in a limited number of dicotyledonous families. Although all are derivatives of a common general structure, there is a great variation in the chemistry of their aglycones. Glucosinolates are characterized by their ability to be hydrolysed by the enzyme myrosinase to yield glucose and a labile aglycone which spontaneously rearranges with the loss of sulphate to give an isothiocyanate (mustard oil) as the major products. They are glycosides which are enzymically hydrolysed in damaged plant tissues giving rise to potentially toxic material, and they share the early stages of the cynogenic glycoside biosynthetic pathway for their formation in plants (Bones and Rossiter, 1996). Many of them are of medicinal properties *viz.* sulphoraphane from broccoli (*Brassica oleracea italica*) induces carcinogen-detoxifying enzyme systems and accelerates the removal of xenobiotics. Young sprouted seedlings contain some 10-100 times as much glucoraphanin as the mature plant, but, nevertheless, broccoli may be regarded as a valuable dietary vegetable (Nestle, 1997). Some important glucosinolates with their biopotentialities are presented in Table 4.6.

Table 4.6: Chemical Structure, Example Source and Biopotentials of Some Important Glucosinolates

Sl.No.	*Bioactive Molecules*	*Chemical Structures*	*Example Sources*	*Biopotentials*	*References*
1.	Glucoraphanin	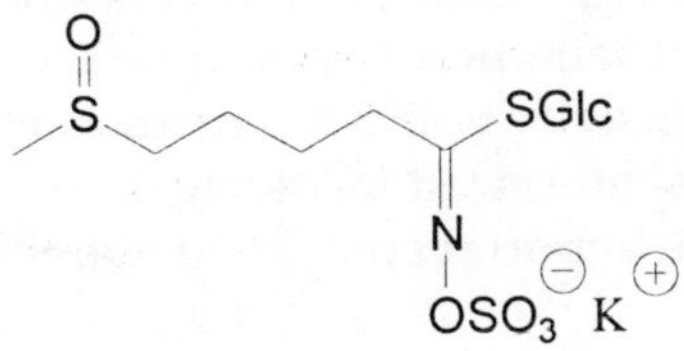	*Brassica oleracea*	Induces carcinogen-detoxifying	Nestle, 1997
2.	Glucobrassicin	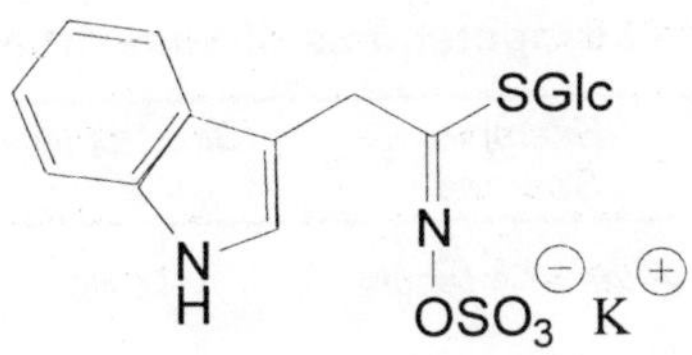	*Armoracia rusticana*	Anticancer	Stefania *et al.*, 2006
3.	Gluconasturtiin	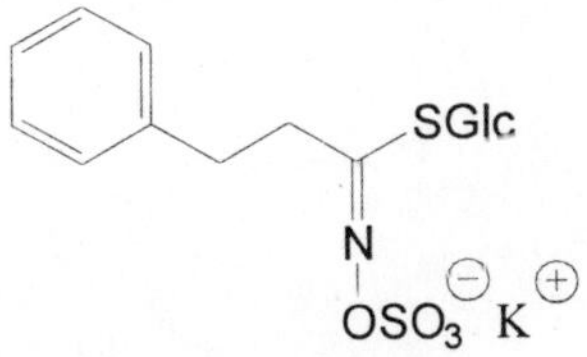	*Brassica napus*	Pungent	Xian and Kushad, 2004
4.	Goitrin	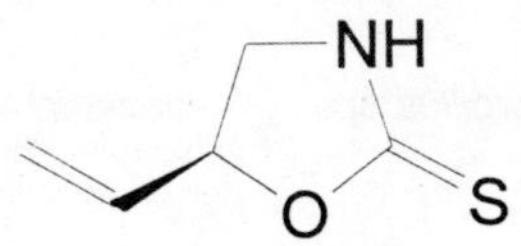	*Brassica napus*	Potent goitrogen, inhibits iodine incorporation and thyroxine formation	Bones and Rossiter, 1996
5.	Progoitrin	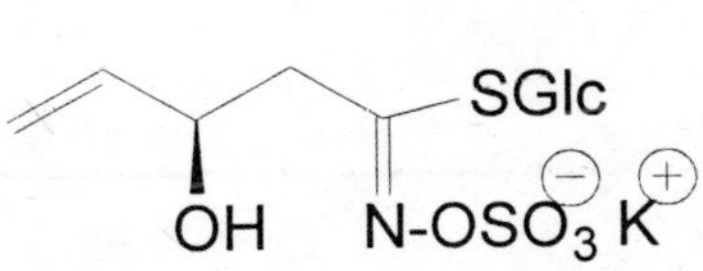	*Brassica napus*	Antithyroid agent	Van Doorne *et al.*, 1998

Contd...

Table 4.6–Contd...

Sl.No.	Bioactive Molecules	Chemical Structures	Example Sources	Biopotentials	References
6.	Sinalbin	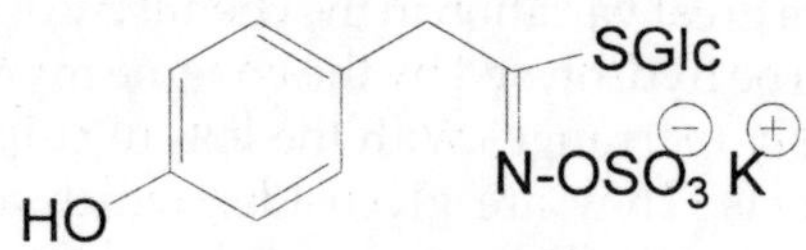	*Sinapis alba*	Pungent	Xian and Kushad, 2004
7.	Sinigrin	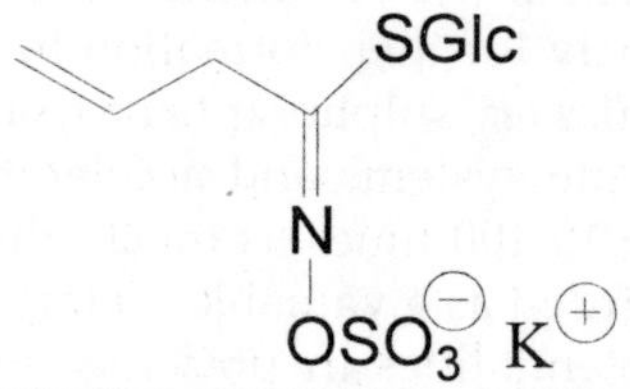	*Brassica nigra*	Pungent	Xian and Kushad, 2004

Polyketides

It forms an enormous class of secondary metabolites synthesized by the bacteria, fungi and plants. These compounds vary in structure can be cyclic, acyclic, small, large, simple or complex molecules. These may also be linked to different sugars and amino sugars since polyketides vary in structure, may be having many different biological activities. About ~10,000 polyketides are known, out of which 1 per cent have demonstrated drug activity which is 5 times as many as the average in natural products. These polyketides are typically synthesized following the onset of stationary phase in the life cycle of different organisms. Some of the important polyketides are listed below with their biopotentials in Table 4.7.

Table 4.7: Chemical Structure, Example Source and Biopotentials of Some Important Polyketides

Sl.No.	Bioactive Molecules	Chemical Structures	Example Sources	Biopotentials	References
1.	Alternariol	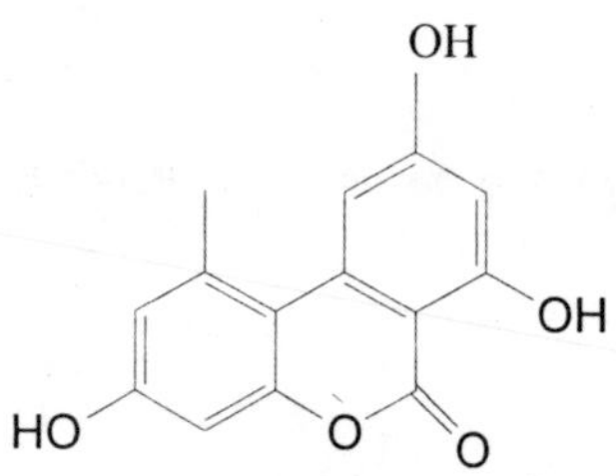	*Alternaria tenuis*	Toxic	Davis and Stack, 1994
2.	Endocrocin	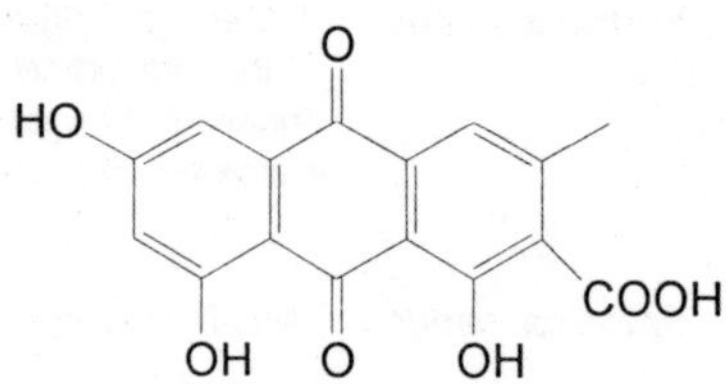	*Aspergillus* sps.	Antioxidant activity	Wolfgang and Wolfgang, 1978

Contd...

Table 4.7–Contd...

Sl.No.	*Bioactive Molecules*	*Chemical Structures*	*Example Sources*	*Biopotentials*	*References*
3.	Griseofulvin	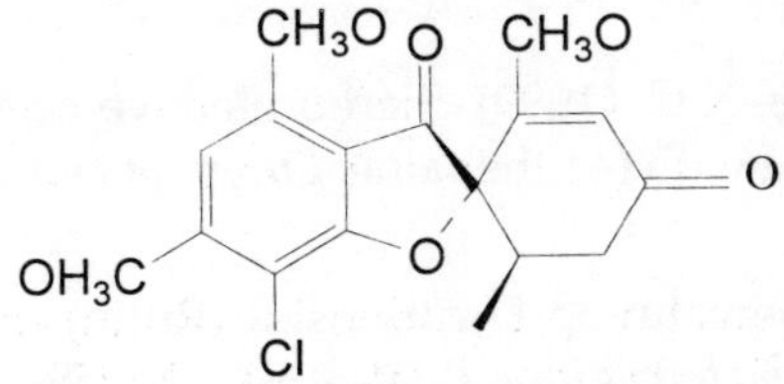	*Penicillium griseofulvin*	Antifungal agent, to treat ringworm infections of the skin and nails	Shah, 1980
4.	Hypericin	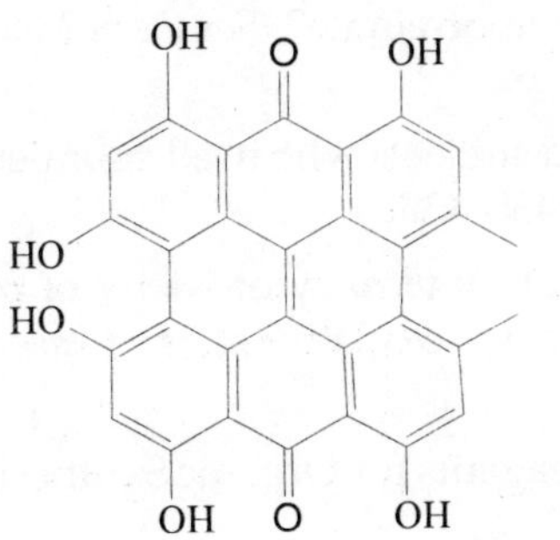	*Hypericum perforatum*	In depression treatment, antiviral, in particularly potential against HIV	Grieve, 1992
5.	6-Methyl-salicylic acid	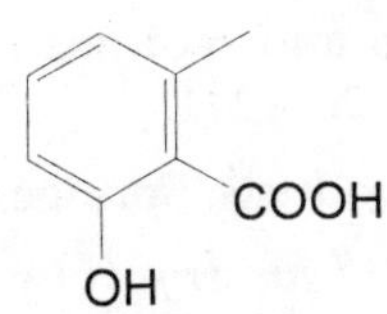	*Penicillium patulum*	Intimately involved in establishing the polyketide biosynthetic pathway	Spencer and Jordan, 1992
6.	Patulin	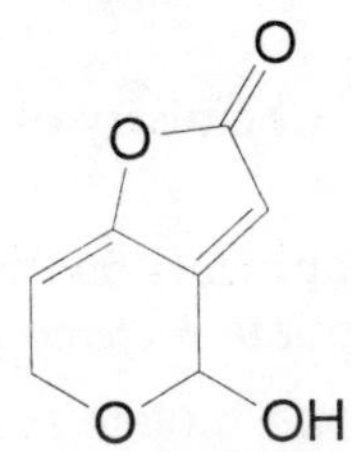	*Penicillium patulum*	Potent carcinogen	D'Arcy, 1999
7.	Penicillic acid	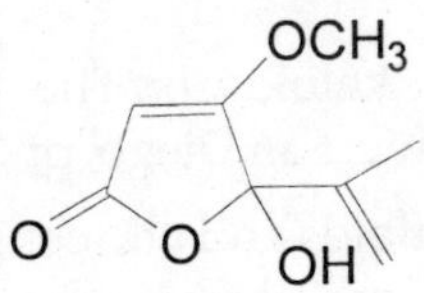	*Penicillium cyclopium*	Potent carcinogen	Lindenfelser and Ciegler, 1977
8.	Urushiols	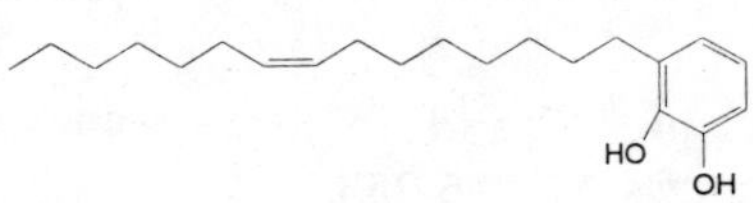	*Rhus toxicodendron*	Allergenic, Poisonous	Schötz, 2004
9.	Visnagin	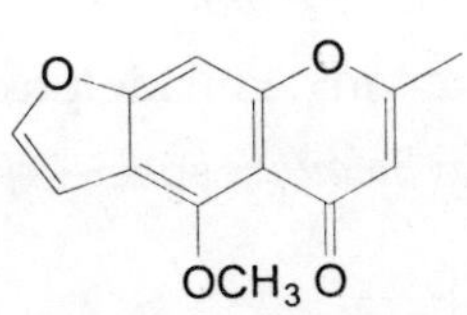	*Ammi visnaga*	Antiasthmatic agent, coronary vasodialator, spasmolytic	Abeysekera *et al.*, 1983

References

Abeysekera, B.R, Abramowski, Z. and Towers, G.H.N. (1983). Genotoxicity of the natural furochromones, khellin and visnagin and the identification of a khellin-thymine photoadduct. *Photochemistry and Photobiology*, 38: 311-315.

Aceto, M.D., Harris, L.S., Abood, M.E. and Rice, K.C. (1999). Stereoselective mu–and delta-opioid receptor-related antinociception and binding with (+)-thebaine. *European Journal of Pharmacology*, 365: 143-147.

Addae-Mensah, I. and Munenge, R.W. (1989). Quercetin-3β-D-rutinoside (Rutin) and other flavonoids as the active hypoglycaemic agents of *Bridelia ferruginea*. *Fitoterapia*, LX: 359-362.

Allen, W.M. (1970). Progesterone: how did the name originate?. *Southern Medical Journal*, 63: 1151-1155.

Autier, P., Dore, J.F. and Cesarini, J.P. (1997). Should subjects who used psoralen suntan activators be screened for melanoma?. *Annals of oncology*, 8: 435-437.

Babich, H., Sedletcaia, A. and Kenigsberg, B. (2002). *In vitro* cytotoxicity of protocatechuic acid to cultured human cells from oral tissue: involvement in oxidative stress. *Pharmacology and Toxicology*, 91: 245–253.

Barner, B.A. (2004). Catechol. *In:* Encyclopedia of Reagents for Organic Synthesis. Ed. By Paquette, L., John Wiley and Sons, New York.

Bayer,T., Colnot, T. and Dekant, W. (2001). Disposition and biotransformation of the estrogenic isoflavone daidzein in rats. *Toxicological Sciences*, 62: 205–211.

Bell, E.A. and Charlwood, B.A. (1980). Secondary Plant Products. Springer-Verlag, Berlin.

Bhat, S.V. (1993). Forskolin and congeners. *Progress in the Chemistry of Organic Natural Products*, 62: 1-74.

Bhat, S.V., Nagasampagi, B.A. and Sivakumar, M. (2005). Chemistry of Natural Products. Narosa Publishing House, New Delhi.

Bhattacharya, A.K. and Sharma, R.P. (1999). Recent developments on the chemistry and biological activity of artemisinin and related antimalarials–an update. *Heterocycles*, 51: 1681-1745.

Bones, A.M. and Rossiter, J.T. (1996). The myrosinase glucosinolate system, its organisation and biochemistry. *Plant Physiology*, 97: 194-208.

Bosch, J., Bonjoch, J. and Amat, M. (1996). The *Strychnos* alkaloids. *In:* The Alkaloids, Chemistry and Pharmacology, Ed. By Cordell, G.A., Vol. 48, Academic, San Diego, pp. 75-189.

Boye, O. and Brossi, A. (1992). Tropolonic Colchicum alkaloids and allo congeners. *In:* The Alkaloids, Chemistry and Pharmacology, Ed. By Brossi, A. and Cordell, G.A., Vol. 41, Academic, San Diego, pp. 125-176.

Braquet, P., Esanu, A., Buisine, E., Hosford, D., Broquet, C. and Koltai, M. (1999). Recent progress in ginkgolide research. *Medical Care Research Reviews*, 11: 295-355.

Brenner, G.M. (2000). Pharmacology, W.B. Saunders Company, Philadelphia, PA.

Briner, J. (1969). Determination of total steroidal bases in *Solanum* species. *Journal of Pharmacological Sciences*, 58: 258-259.

Brossi, A., Pei, X.F. and Greig, N.H. (1996). Phenserine, a novel anticholinesterase related to physostigmine: total synthesis and biological properties. *Australian Journal of Chemistry,* 49: 171-181.

Bushway, R.J., Perkins, L.B., Paradis, L.R. and Vanderpan, S. (1994). High-performance liquid chromatographic determination of the tomato glycoalkaloid, tomatine, in green and red tomatoes. *Journal of Agricultural and Food Chemistry,* 42: 2824-2829.

Carani, C., Qin, K., Simoni, M., Faustini-Fustini, M., Serpente, S., Boyd, J., Korach, K.S. and Simpson, E.R. (1997). Effect of testosterone and estradiol in a man with aromatase deficiency. *New England Journal of Medicine,* 337: 91-95.

Casida, J.E. (1980). Pyrethrum flowers and pyrethroid insecticides. *Environmental Health Perspectives,* 34: 189-202.

Cayen, M.N. and Dvornik, D. (1979). Effect of diosgenin on lipid metabolism in rats. *Journal of Lipid Research,* 20: 162–174.

Cherian, S. and Augusti, K.T. (1993). Antidiabetic effects of a glycoside of leucopelargonidin isolated from *Ficus bengalensis* Linn. *Indian Journal of Experimental Biology,* 31: 26-29.

Christie, J.E., Shering, A. and Ferguson, J. (1981). Physostigmine and arecoline: effects of intravenous infusions in Alzheimer's presenile dementia. *British Journal of Psychiatry,* 138: 46–50.

Chung, T.Y., Eiserich, J.P. and Shibamoto, T. (1993). Volatile compounds isolated from edible Korean chamchwi (Aster scaber Thunb). *Journal of Agricultural and Food Chemistry,* 41: 1693-1697.

Cook, D.I. and Ikeuchi, M. (1989). Tolbutamide as mimic of glucose on β-cells electrical activity. ATP-sensitive K+ channels as common pathway for both stimuli. *Diabetes,* 38: 416-421.

Corcuera, L.J. (1993). Biochemical basis of the resistance of the barley to aphids. *Phytochemistry,* 33: 741-747.

Daly, J.W., Garaffo, H.M., Spande, T.F., Decker, M.W., Sullivan, J.P. and Williams, M. (2000). Alkaloids from frog skin: the discovery of epibatidine and the potential for developing novel non-opioid analgesics. *Natural Product Reports,* 17: 131-135.

D'Arcy H.P. (1999). A change in scientific approach: from alternation to randomized allocation in clinical trials in the 1940s. *British Medical Journal,* 319: 572–573.

Davis, V.M. and Stack, M.E. (1994). Evaluation of alternariol and alternariol methyl ether for mutagenic activity in *Salmonella typhimurium. Applied and Environmental Microbioogy,* 60: 3901–3902.

Debska, W. (1958). Separation and determination of the dissociation constants of chelidonine and protopine by paper chromatography. *Nature,* 182: 666–667.

Dewick, P.M. (2002). Medicinal Natural Products: A Biosynthetic Approach. 2nd ed., John Wiley and Sons Inc., New York.

Dixit, V.P., Jain, P. and Purohit, A.K. (1992) *In:* Recent Advances in Medicinal, Aromatic and Spice Crops, Ed. By Raychaudhuri, S.P., Vol. 2, Today and Tomorrow's Printers and Publishers, New Delhi, pp. 463–471.

Edwards, D.J. and Bernier, S.M. (1996). Inhibitory effect of grapefruit juice and its bitter principal, naringenin, on CYP1A2 dependent metabolism of caffeine in man. *Life Sciences,* 59: 1025–1030.

Etter, J.F. (2006). Cytisine for smoking cessation; a literature review and a meta-analysis. *Archives of Internal Medicine*,166:1553-1559.

Evans, D.A. and Raj, R.K. (1991). Larvicidal efficacy of quassin against *Culex quinquefasciatus. Indian Journal of. Medical Research*, 93: 324–327.

Evans, W.C. (1989). Trease and Evans' Pharmacognosy. 13th ed., Balliere Tindall, London

Evans, W.C. (1990). Datura, a commercial source of hyoscine. *Pharmaceutical Journal*, 244: 651-653.

Farina, A., Ferranti, C. and Marra, C. (2006). An improved synthesis of resveratrol. *Natural Products Research*, 20: 247-252.

Fereidoon, S. and Marian, N. (2004). Phenolics in food and nutraceuticals. CRC Press LLC, Florida, USA, pp. 4.

Ferland, G. and Sadowski, J. (1992). Vitamin K_1 (Phylloquinone) content of green vegetables: Effects of plant maturation and geographical growth location. *Journal of Agricultural and Food Chemistry*, 40: 1874–1877.

Fischer, F.G. (1948). Newer Methods of Preparative Organic Chemistry, Interscience Publishers, New York, pp. 174.

Freeman, E.R., Bloom, D.A. and McGuire, E.J. (2001). A brief history of testosterone. *Journal of Urology*, 165: 371–373.

Garcia, R.M.A., Oliveira, L.O.de., Moreira, M.A. and Barros, W.S. (2005). Variation in emetine and cephaeline contents in roots of wild Ipecac (*Psychotria ipecacuanha*). *Biochemical Systematics and Ecology*, 33: 233-243.

Geahlen, R.L., Koonchanok, N. M., McLaughlin, J.L. and Pratt, D.E. (1989). Inhibition of protein-tyrosine kinase activity by flavonoids and related compounds. *Journal of Natural Products*, 52: 982-986.

Gearien, J.E. and Mede, K. A. (1981). Cholinergics anticholinesterases, antispasmodics. *In:* Principles of Medicinal Chemistry, 2nd ed., Ed. By Foye, W. O., Lea and Febiger, Philadelphia, pp. 353-376.

Grant, I.J., Hamor, T.A., Monteath R. J. and Sim, G.A. (1965). The structure of chimonanthine: X-ray analysis of chimonanthine dihydrobromide. *Journal of Chemical Society*, 5678–5696.

Grieve, M. (1992). Modern Herbal: Medicinal,Culinary and Cosmetic Properties, Tiger Book International, London, pp.707–708.

Grundschober, F. (1979). Literature review of pulegone. *Perfume and Flavorist*, 4: 15–17.

Hargreaves, J.A., Mansfield, J.W. and Coxon, H. (1976). Identification of medicarpin as a phytoalexin in the broad bean plant (*Vicia faba* L.). *Nature*, 262: 318–319.

Hartmann, T. (1999). Chemical ecology of pyrrolizidine alkaloids. *Planta*, 207: 483-495.

Hartwell, J.L. and Schrecker, A.W. (1951). Components of Podophyllin. V. The Constitution of Podophyllotoxin. *Journal of the American Chemical Society*, 73: 2909–2916.

Hasegawa, K. and Hashimoto, T. (1973). Quantitative changes of batatasins and abscisic acid in relation to the development of dormancy in yam bulbils. *Plant and Cell Physiology*, 14: 369-377.

Hanson, J.R. and de Oliveira, B.H. (1993). Stevioside and related sweet diterpenoid glycosides. *Natural Product Reports*, 10: 301-309.

Hecker, E., Bartsch, H., Bresch, H., Gschwendt, M., Härle, B., Kreibich, G., Kubinyi, H., Schairer, H.U., Szczepanski, C.V. and Thielmann, H.W. (1967). Structure and stereochemistry of the tetracyclic diterpene phorbol from *Croton tiglium* L. *Tetrahedron Letters*, 8: 3165–3170.

Heinstein, P.F. and Chang, C-j. (1994). Taxol. *Annual Reviews of Plant Physiology and Plant Molecular Biology*, 45: 663-674.

Hock, B.H. and Elstner, E.F. (2004). Plant Toxicology, CRC Press LLC, Florida, USA, pp. 630.

Huebner, C.F., MacPhillamy, H.B., Schlittler, E. and St. André, A.F. (1955). *Rauwolfia* alkaloids XXI. The stereochemistry of reserpine and deserpidine. *Cellular and Molecular Life Sciences*, 11: 8.

Ignatushchenko, M.V., Winter, R.W., Bächinger, H. P., Hinrichs, D. J. and Riscoe, M.K. (1997). Xanthones as antimalarial agents: studies of a possible mode of action. *FEBS Letters*, 409: 67–73.

Iwu, M. M. (1993). Handbook of African Medicinal Plants. CRC Press LLC, Florida, USA, pp. 130.

Jacob, P. 3rd., Yu, L., Shulgin, A. T. and Benowitz, N. L. (1999). Minor tobacco alkaloids as biomarkers for tobacco use: comparison of users of cigarettes, smokeless tobacco, cigars, and pipes. *American Journal of Public Health*, 89: 731-736.

Jafri,W., Yakoob, J., Hussain, S., Jafri, N. and Islam, M. (2006). Phloroglucinol in irritable bowel syndrome. *Journal of Pakistan Medical Association*, 56: 5-8.

Janot, M.M., Guilhem, J., Contz, O., Venera, G. and Cionga, E. (1979). Contribution to the study of valerian alkaloids (*Valeriana officinalis*, L.): actinidine and naphthyridylmethylketone, a new alkaloid. *Annales Pharmaceutiques Francaises*, 37: 413-420.

Jaroszewki, J.W., Strom-Hansen, T., Hansen, S.H., Thastrup, O. and Kofod, H. (1992). On the botanical distribution of chiral forms of gossypol. *Planta Medica*, 58: 454-458.

Jogia, M.K., Vakamoce, V. and Weavers, R.T. (1985). Synthesis of Some furfural and syringic acid derivatives. *Australian Journal of Chemistry*, 38: 1009–1016.

Johne, S., Gröger, D. and Richter, G. (1968). On the biosynthesis of peganine in *Adhatoda vasica* Nees. *Arch Pharm Ber Dtsch Pharm Ges.*, 301: 721-727.

Johnson, E.L. and Emcho, S.D. (1994). Variation in alkaloid content in *Erythroxylum coca* leaves from leaf bud to leaf drop. *Annals of Botany*, 73: 645-650.

Kamei, J. (1996). Role of opioidergic and serotonergic mechanisms in cough and antitussives. *Pulmonary pharmacology*, 9: 349-356.

Kanazawa, M., Satomi, Y., Mizutani, Y., Ukimura, O., Kawauchi, A., Sakai, T., Baba, M., Okuyama, T., Nishino, H. and Miki, T. (2003). Isoliquiritigenin inhibits the growth of prostate cancer. *European Urology*, 43: 580-586.

Kang, D.G., Yin, M.H., Hyuncheol, O.H., LEE, D.H., Sub, H.O., and Lee, U.B. (2004). Vasorelaxation by amentoflavone isolated from *Selaginella tamariscina*. *Planta Medica*, 70: 718-722.

Kerimov, Yu. B. and Nasudari, A. A. (1971). Smilagenin from *Polygonatum polyanthemum*. *Chemistry of Natural Compounds*, 7: 124-125.

Khanna, S., Sen, C.K., Roy, S., Christen, M.O. and Packer, L. (1998). Protective effects of anethole dithiolethione against oxidative stress-induced cytotoxicity in human Jurkat T cells. *Biochemical Pharmacology*, 56: 61-69.

Khawaled, R., Bruening-Wrightm, A., Adelman, J.P. and Maylie, J. (1999). Bicuculline block of small-conductance calcium-activated potassium channels. *Pflügers Archiv*, 438: 314-321.

Khong, P.W. and Lewis, K.G. (1977). New chemical constituents of *Planchonia careya. Australian Journal of Chemistry*, 30: 1311–1322.

Klaschka, F. (1964). Allergic contact dermatitis from hydroxylbenzoic acid. *Z Haut Geschlechtsk*, 37: 312-314.

Kren, V., Harazim, P. and Malinka, Z. (1994). *Claviceps purpurea* (ergot): Culture and bioproduction of ergot alkaloids. *In:* Biotechnology in Agriculture and Forestry, Vol. 58, Medicinal and Aromatic Plants VII, Ed. By Bajaj, Y.P.S., Springer, Heidelberg, pp. 139-156.

Kumar, L.N. and Rangaswamy, S.N. (1985). Effect of some flavonoids and phenolic acids on seed germination and rooting. *Journal of Experimental Botany*, 36: 1313-1319.

Kumi-Diaka, J., Rodriguez, R. and Goudaze, G. (1998). Influence of genistein (4',5,7-trihydroxyisoflavone) on the growth and proliferation of testicular cell lines. *Journal of Cell Biology*, 90: 349-354.

Kurobane, I., Vining, L.C. and Mcinnes, G.A. (1979). Biosynthetic relationships among the secalonic acids. *Journal of Antibiotics*, 32: 1256-1266.

Kutney, J.P., Brown, R.T. and Pies, A. (1965). Some aspects of the chemistry of catharanthine and cleavamine. *Canadian Journal of Chemistry*, 13: 1545-1552.

Lakshmanan, M.R. and Cama, H.R. (1996). Studies on the visual pigment and the indicator yellow analogues formed from 5,6-monoepoxyretinal. *Biochemical Journal*, 99: 87–92.

Lee, J.H. and Talcott, S.T. (2002). Ellagic acid and ellagitannins affect on sedimentation in muscadine juice and wine. *Journal of Agricultural and Food Chemistry*, 50: 3971-3976.

Lee, W.J. and Zhu, B.T. (2006). Inhibition of DNA methylation by caffeic acid and chlorogenic acid, two common catechol-containing coffee polyphenols. *Carcinogenesis*, 27: 269-277.

Leonard, J. (1999).Recent progress in the chemistry of monoterpenoid alkaloids derived from secologanin. *Natural Product Reports*, 16: 319-338.

Lidell, J.R. (2000). Pyrrolizidine alkaloids. *Natural Product Reports*, 17: 455-462.

Lindenfelser, L.A. and Ciegler, A. (1977). Penicillic acid production in submerged culture. *Applied and Environmental Microbiology*, 34: 553–556.

Lotlikar, M.M. and Rajaramarao, M.R. (1966). Pharmacology of a hypoglycemic principle from *Momordica charantia* L. *Indian Journal of Pharmacology*, 28: 129-133.

Mann, J. (1992). Secondary Metabolism, 2nd ed., Oxford University Press, Oxford, UK, pp. 279-280.

Mann, J., Davidson, R.S., Hobbs, J.B., Banthorpe, D.V. and Harborne, J.B. (1994). Natural Products, Addison Wesley Longman Ltd., Harlow, UK, pp. 309-311.

Matsufuji, H. (1998). Antioxidant activity of capsanthin and the fatty acid esters in paprika (*Capsicum annum*). *Journal of Agricultural and Food Chemistry*, 46: 3468-3472.

McGowan, K., Guerina, V., Wicks, J. and Donowitz, M. (1985). Secretory hormones of *Entamoeba histolytica. Ciba Foundation Symposium*, 112: 139-54.

Mikaberidze, K.G. and Moniava, I.I. (1975). Umbelliferone from tea leaves. *Chemistry of Natural Compounds*, 10: 81.

Millward, M., Powell, A., Tyson, S., Daly, P., Ferguson, R. and Carter, S. (2005). Phase I trial of coramsine (SBP002) in patients with advanced solid tumors. *Journal of Clinical Oncology*, 23: 3105.

Misra, N., Luthra, R., Singh, K.L. and Kumar, S. (1999). Recent advances in biosynthesis of alkaloids. *In:* Comprehensive Natural Products Chemistry, Vol. 4, Elsevier, Amsterdam, pp. 25-59.

Mitsubichi Chemic Industries COLTD (1982). Lathyrines as hypoglycaemic, Japan Kokai, Tokyo, 82: 514.

Molyneux, R.J., Nash, R.J and Asano, N. (1996). Chemistry and biological activity of the calystegines and related nortropane alkaloids. *In:* Alkaloids, Chemical and Biological Perspectives, Vol. 11, Ed. By Pelletier, S.W., Elsevier, Amsterdam, pp 303-343.

Morisaki, M., Ying, B. and Ikekawa, N. (1981). Identification of both fucosterol and isofucosterol in the siklworm, *Bombyx mori. Cellular and Molecular Life Sciences*, 37: 4.

Munson, A.E., Harris, L.S., Friedman, M.A., Dewey, W.L. and Carchman, R.A. (1975). Anticancer activity of cannabinoids. *Journal of the National Cancer Institute*, 55: 597-602.

Naser, B., Bodinet, C., Tegtmeier, M. and Lindequist, U. (2005). *Thuja occidentalis* (Arbor vitae): A review of its pharmaceutical, pharmacological and clinical properties. *Evidence Based Complementary and Alternative Medicine*, 2: 69-78.

Nestle, M. (1997). Broccoli sprouts as inducers of carcinogen-detoxifying enzyme systems: Clinical, dietary, and policy implications. *Proceedings of the National Academy of Sciences*, 94: 11149-11151.

Noble, R.L. (1990). The discovery of the Vinca alkaloids–Chemotherapeutic agents against cancer. *Biochemistry and Cell Biology*, 68: 1344-1351.

O'Donoghue, J.L. (2006). Hydroquinone and its analogues in dermatology–a risk-benefit viewpoint. *Journal of Cosmetic Dermatology*, 5: 196-203.

Park, J.S., Rho, H.S., Kim, D.H. and Chang, I.S. (2006). Enzymatic preparation of kaempferol from green tea seed and its antioxidant activity. *Journal of Agricultural and Food Chemistry*, 54: 2951–2956.

Patinaik, S., Subramanyam, V.R. and Kole, E.C. (2006). Antibacterial and antifungal activity of ten essential oils *in vitro. Microbios*, 86: 237-246.

Pkheidze, T. A., Gvazava, L.N. and Kemertelidze, E.P. (1991). Luvigenin and hecogenin from the leaves of *Yucca gloriosa. Chemistry of Natural Compounds*, 27: 376.

Ploeger, B., Mensinga, T., Sips, A., Seinen, W., Meulenbelt, J. and DeJongh, J. (2001). The pharmacokinetics of glycyrrhizic acid evaluated by physiologically based pharmacokinetic modeling. *Drug Metabolism Reviews*, 33: 25-47.

Popik, P. and Skolnick, P. (1999). Pharmacology of ibogaine and ibogaine-related alkaloids. *In:* The Alkaloids, Chemistry and Biology, Vol. 52, Ed. By Cordell, G.A., Academic, San Diego, pp.197-231.

Prokopenko, A.P., Zhukov, G.A. and Zaitsev, V.G. (1968). Quantitative determination of khellin by thin layer chromatography. *Pharmaceutical Chemistry Journal*, 2: 517-518.

Pryce, R.J. (1971). Lunularic acid, a common endogenous growth inhibitor of liverworts. *Planta*, 97: 4.

Pugsley, T.A. (1994). Epinephrine and norepinephrine. *In:* Kirk-Othmer Encyclopedia of Chemical Technology, Vol. 9, John Wiley, New York, pp 715-730.

Qiming, C. and Mingzhi, X. (1987). Effects of berberine on blood glucose regulation in normal mice. *Yaoxue Xuebao*, 22: 161-165.

Ricci, G.C. and Ricordati, M. (1955). Physiopathological and clinical therapeutic effects of an alkaloid from *Rauwolfia serpentina* and of its total extracts. 1. Glycemic changes caused in normal-and hypoglycemic subjects by reserpine, total extracts plus glucose insulin and adrenaline. *Archivio e Maragliano di Patologia e Clinica*, 11: 359-401.

Robinson, T. and Fowell, E. (1959). A chromatographic analysis for ricinine. *Nature*, 183: 833–834.

Rogers, T.B., Inesi, G., Wade, R. and Lederer, W.J, (1995). Use of thapsigargin to study Ca^{2+} homeostasis in cardiac cells. *Bioscence Reports*, 15: 341-349.

Roshchina, V.V. (2002). Rutacridone as a fluorescent dye for the study of pollen. *Journal of Fluorescence*, 12: 241-243.

Ruidavets, J.B., Teissedre, P.L., Ferrieres, J., Carando, S., Bougard, G. and Cabanis, J.C. (2000). Catechin in the Mediterranean diet : vegetable, fruit or wine? *Atherosclerosis*, 153: 101-117.

Schötz, K. (2004). Quantification of allergenic urushiols in extracts of *Ginkgo biloba* leaves, in simple one-step extracts and refined manufactured material. *Phytochemical Analysis*, 15: 1-8.

Scott, L.J. and Goa, K.L. (2000). Adis Review: Galantamine: a review of its use in Alzheimer's disease. *Drugs*, 60: 1095-122.

Scott, T.A. and Mercer, E.I. (1997). Concise Encyclopedia Biochemistry and Molecular Biology. Walter de Gruyter, Berlin, pp. 24.

Seow, W.K., Li, S.Y. and Thong, Y.H. (1986). Inhibitory effects of tetrandrine on human neutrophil and monocyte adherence. *Immunology Letters*. 13: 83–88.

Shah,G.B. and Goyal, R.K. (1994). Effect of yohimbine in congestive cardiac failure. *Indian Journal of Pharmacology*, 26: 41-43.

Shah, V.P. (1980). Griseofuivin absorption per OS and percutaneous Preusser (eds) Med. Mycology, Zbl, Bakt, Suppl.-8, Gustav Fischer Verlag, Stuttgart, pp. 223-239.

Shimizu, Y. (1993). Microalgal metabolite. *Chemical Reviews*, 93: 1685-1698.

Sies, H., and Stahl, W. (1998). Lycopene: antioxidant and biological effects and its bioavailability in the human. *Proceedings of the Society for Experimental Biology and Medicine*, 218: 121-124.

Slichenmyer, W.J., Rowunsky, E. K., Dohehower, R.C. and Kaufmann, S. H. (1993). The current status of camptothecin analogues as antitumor agents. *Journal of the National Cancer Institute*, 85: 271-291.

Smith, S. and Timmis, G.M. (1932). The Alkaloids of Ergot. Part III. Ergine, a new base obtained by the degradation of ergotoxine and ergotinine. *Journal of Chemical Society*, 1932: 763-766.

Spencer, J.B. and Jordan, P. M. (1992). Purification and properties of 6-methylsalicylic acid synthase from *Penicillium patulum*. *The Biochemical Journal*, 15: 839–846.

Stefania, G., Barillari, J., Iori, R., and Venturi, G. (2006). Glucobrassicin enhancement in wood (*Isatis tinctoria*) leaves by chemical and physical treatments. *Journal of the Science of Food and Agriculture*, 86: 1833-1838.

Stekoll, M. and West, C.A. (1978). Purification and properties of an elicitor of castor bean phytoalexin from culture filtrates of the fungus *Rhizopus stolonifer*. *Plant Physiology*, 61: 38–45.

Surburg, H. and Panten, J. (2006). Common Fragrance and Flavor Materials: Preparation, Properties, and Uses. 5th ed., Ed. By Surburg, H. and Panten, J.,Wiley-VCH, Weinheim, Germany.

Tallamy, D.W., Stull, J., Ehresman, N.P., Gorski, P.M. and Mason, C.E. (1997). Cucurbitacins as feeding and oviposition deterrents to insects. *Environmental Entomology*, 26: 678-688.

Tawara, J.N., Stermitz, R., and Blokhin, A.V. (1995). Alkaloids of young ponderosa pine seedlings and late steps in the biosynthesis of pinidine. *Phytochemistry*, 39: 705-708.

Thomas, T.J., Pauze, D. and Love, J.N. (2008). Are one or two dangerous? Diphenoxylate-atropine exposure in toddlers. *Journal of Emergency Medicine*, 34: 71-75.

Tillequin, F.M.S. and Skaltsounis, A.L. (1998). Acronycine-type alkaloids: Chemistry and biology. *In:* Alkaloids, Chemical and Biological Perspectives, Vol. 12, Ed. By Pelletier, S.W., Elsevier, Amsterdam.

Tiuman, T.S., Ueda-Nakamura, T., Garcia, C.D.A., Dias, F.B.P., Morgado-Diaz, J.A., De Souza, W. and Nakamura, C.V. (2005). Antileishmanial activity of parthenolide, a sesquiterpene lactone isolated from *Tanacetum parthenium*. *Antimicrobial Agents and Chemotherapy*, 49: 176–82.

Truitt, E.B., Duritz, G. and Ebersberger, E.M. (1963). Evidence of monoamine oxidase inhibition by myristicin and nutmeg. *Proceedings of the Society for Experimental Biology and Medicine*, 112: 647-50.

Van Arnum, S.D. (1998). Vitamins (Vitamin A). Kirk-Othmer Encyclopedia of Chemical Technology, 4th Edn. Vol.25, Wiley-Interscience, New York, pp. 1272-192.

Van Doorne, H.E., Van Der Kruk, G.C., Van Holst, G.J., Raaijmakers-Ruijs, N.C.M.E., Postma, E., Groeneweg, B. and Jongen, H.F. (1998). The glucosinolates sinigrin and progoitrin are important determinants for taste preference and bitterness of Brussels sprouts. *Journal of the Science of Food and Agriculture*, 78: 30-38.

Wagner, H., Geyer, B., Fiebig, M., Kiso, Y. and Hikino, H. (2006). Isobutrin and butrin, the antihepatotoxic principles of *Butea monosperma* flowers. *Planta Medica*, 2: 77-79.

Wall, M.E. and Wani, M.C. (1998). History and future prospects of camptothecin and taxol. *In:* The Alkaloids. Chemistry and Pharmacology, Vol. 50, Ed. By Cordell, G.A., Academic, San Diego, pp. 509-536.

Wang, W.J.R., Rebhun, L.I. and Morris, S. (1977). Kupchan· Antimitotic and antitubulin activity of the tumor inhibitor steganacin· *Cancer Research*, 37: 3071-3079.

White, C.W., Ward, C.R., Dombrowski, D.S., Dunlow, L.D., Brase, D.A. and Dewey, W. L. (1993). Effect of intrathecal morphine on the fate of glucose. Comparison with effects of insulin and xanthan gum in mice. *Biochemical Pharmacology*, 45: 459-464.

Wills, S. (1994). Drugs and substance misuse: tobacco and alcohol. *Pharmaceutical Journal*, 253: 158-160.

Wise, M.L. and Croteau, R. (1999). *In:* Comprehensive Natural Products Chemistry: Isoprenoids Including Carotenoids and Steroids, Ed. By Cane, D.E., Vol. 2, Elsevier Science, London, pp. 97-153.

Wolfgang, S. and Wolfgang, R. (1970). A synthesis of endocrocin, endocrocin-9-anthrone, and related compounds. *Journal of Chemical Society*, 33: 178.

Wood, S.A., Rasmussen, J.P., Holland, P. T., Campbell, R. and Crowe, A.L.M. (2007). First report of the cyanotoxin anatoxin-A from *Aphanizomenon issatschenkoi* (cyanobacteria). *Journal of Phycology*, 43: 356-365.

Wu, C.M., Koehler, P.E. and Ayres, J.C. (1972). Isolation and identification of xanthotoxin (8-Methoxypsoralen) and bergapten (5-Methoxypsoralen) from celery Infected with *Sclerotinia sclerotiorum*. *Journal of Applied Microbiology*, 23: 852–856.

Xian, L.I. and Kushad, M.M. (2004). Correlation of glucosinolate content to myrosinase activity in horseradish (*Armoracia rusticana*). *Journal of Agricultural and Food Chemistry*, 52: 6950-6955.

Young. W.K., Sung, H.K., Jong, R.L., Song, J.L., Choon, W.K., Sang, C.K. and Sang, G.K. (2006). Liquiritigenin, an aglycone of liquiritin in *Glycyrrhizae radix*, prevents acute liver injuries in rats induced by acetaminophen with or without buthionine sulfoximine. *Chemico-biological Interactions*, 161: 125-138.

Yu, B.K. and Nasudari, A.A. (1971). Smilagenin from *Polygonatum polyanthemum*. *Chemistry of Natural Compounds*, 7: 119.

Zhao J., Yang X.W., Hattori, M. (2000). Chinese Traditional and Herbal Drugs, 31, 648–651 (2000).

Zou, C.C., Hou, S.J., Shi, Y., Lei, P.S. and Liang, X.T. (2003). The synthesis of gracillin and dioscin: two typical representatives of spirostanol glycosides. *Carbohydrate Research*, 338: 721-727.

Utilisation and Management of Medicinal Plants (2010) *Pages 107–123*
Editors: V.K. Gupta, Anil K. Verma and Sushma Koul
Published by: DAYA PUBLISHING HOUSE, NEW DELHI

Chapter 5

Bioactive Compounds from Fungi: A Review

Nilanjana Das* and Lazar Mathew
School of Biotechnology, Chemical and Biomedical Engineering, VIT University, Vellore – 632 014, Tamil Nadu, India

ABSTRACT

'Bioactive compounds' from natural products have attracted the attention of biologists and chemists throughout the world. Numerous bioactive natural products have been discovered from plants and microorganisms. Fungi are a group of organisms having a great biodiversity. They are important sources of bioactive metabolites. Notable examples from fungal sources are multi-billion dollar classes of antibiotics that include penicillins and cephalosporins, the important and widely used cholesterol–lowering agents lovastatin, compactin, and pravastatin, and the immunosuppresant cyclosporine A. In addition, many other bioactive compounds have also been isolated from fungi and these compounds vary widely in their chemical structure and function. Some of these are now considered as good candidates in the group mostly known as nutraceuticals. The present review documents the information on intensive search for newer and more effective agents isolated from various fungal organisms especially endophytic fungi and macrofungi or mushrooms as a novel source of potentially useful bioactive compounds.

Keywords: *Bioactive compounds, Endophytic fungi, Macrofungi/mushrooms, Natural products, Nutraceuticals.*

---

* Corresponding Author: E-mail: nilanjana00@lycos.com.

Introduction

Biologically active compounds have been searched from the natural products which are traditionally a rich source of chemical diversity. Over the last few decades microorganisms have been seriously exploited as a source of antibiotics and pharmaceuticals though plants have been used for many years for therapeutic applications by numerous civilizations. Fungi are the important sources of bioactive compounds. In order to exploit the full extent of chemical diversity of fungal secondary metabolites, various groups of fungal organisms have been screened. Specialized laboratories have been established in many countries to investigate the potential of bioactive compounds from fungi. Fungal endophytes have been recognized as a repository of novel secondary metabolites, some of which have beneficial biological activities (Bills and Polishook, 1991; Strobel and Daisy, 2003). A recent comprehensive study has indicated that 51 per cent of bioactive substances isolated from endophytic fungi were previously unknown (Schutz, 2001). Hence, the endophytic fungi are expected to be a potential source for new natural bioactive products.

Applying fungi as medicines dates back to 3000 BC when macrofungi or mushrooms were used to cure diseases by mankind especially in the traditional oriental therapies. Macrofungi such as *Ganoderma lucidium, Lentinus edodes, Fomes fomentarius, Fomitopsis officinalis* and many others have been used to cure different diseases for hundred of years in China, Japan, Korea and many other countries. Macrofungi contain several bioactive compounds that belong to polysaccharides, glycoprotein, proteoglycons, terpenoids, fatty acids, proteins, lectins etc. possessing certain medicinal properties. They can be added to the diet and used orally and considered as a safe and useful approach for disease treatment. Several major substances with immunomodulating and/antitumor activity have also been isolated from them. This article reports the potential bioactive compounds derived from various fungal sources throughout the world.

Endophytic Fungi as Source of Bioactive Compounds

In the past few decades plant scientists have begun to realize that plants may serve as a reservoir of untold number of organisms known as endophytes (Bacon, 2000). Endophytic fungi which live inside the living plants are special biotope and account for some biological activity of their host (Schulz *et al.*,2002).Some of these fungi are potential sources of diverse bioactive metabolites which may have potential for therapeutic purposes and could be used as research tools (Tan and Zou, 2001; Tan *et al.*, 2000). Endophytic fungal communities have been explored throughout the world and following endophytes have been reported as potential sources of bioactive metabolites.

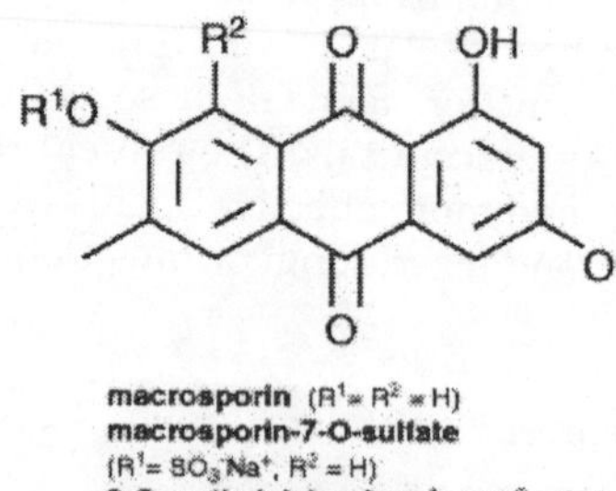

macrosporin ($R^1 = R^2 = H$)
macrosporin-7-O-sulfate ($R^1 = SO_3^-Na^+$, $R^2 = H$)
3-O-methylalaternin ($R^1 = H$, $R^2 = OH$)
3-O-methylalaternin-7-O-sulfate ($R^1 = SO_3^-Na^+$, $R^2 = OH$)

Ampelomyces sp.

The fungal endophyte *Ampelomyces* sp. isolated from the medicinal plant *Urospermum picroides* yielded 14 natural products out of which six (macrosporin-7-*O*-sulfate, 3-*O*-methylalaternin-7-*O*-sulfate, ampelopyrone, desmethyldiaportinol, desmethyldichlorodiaportin, and ampelanol) were bioactive compounds. The known macrosporin and 3-*O*-methylalaternin were also identified in the host plant *Urospermum picroides*, indicating that they are also produced by the endophytes in plants (Aly *et al.*, 2008).

Hypocrea sp.

An endophytic fungus, *Hypocrea* spp.NSF-08 associated with tropical tree species *Dillenia indica* Linn, has a broad spectrum antimicrobial property against human and plant pathogenic microorganisms (Gogoi *et al.*, 2008). The fungus was identified as a teleomorphic genus of *Trichoderma*, based on morphological, sporulation and molecular characteristics. The antimicrobial agent produced by *Hypocrea* sp. was extracted with ethyl acetate as solvent and purified by TLC. The purified active compound with UV λ-max 242 nm got the lowest minimum inhibitory concentration (MIC) against *Staphylococcus aureus* and *Fusarium oxysporum*, whereas no activity recorded against *Pseudomonas aeruginosa*.

Edenia gomezpompae

The newly discovered endophytic fungus, *Edenia gomezpompae* isolated from the leaves of *Callicarpa acuminata* (Verbenaceae) resulted in the isolation of napthoquinone spiroketals, including three new compounds and palmarumycin CP_2 (4). The trivial names proposed for these compounds are preussomerin EG_1 (1), preussomerin EG_2 (2) and preussomerin EG_3 (3) (Macías-Rubalcava *et al.*, 2008).

The bioactivity of the mycelial organic extracts and the pure compounds were tested against three endophytic fungi (*Collectotrichum* sp., *Phomopsis* sp. and *Guignardia mangifera*) isolated from the same plant species (*Callicarpa acuminata*, Verbenaceae) and four economically important phytopathogenic microorganisms (*viz.* two fungoid oomycetes, *Phythophtora capsici* and *Phythophtora parasitia* and the fungi *Fusarium oxysporum* and *Alternaria solani*). All compounds caused significant inhibition of the diameter growth of four phytopathogenic microorganisms. Compound 1 showed the strongest bioactivity. This is the first report of allelochemicals with antifungal activity from the newly discovered endophytic fungus, *Edenia gomezpompae*.

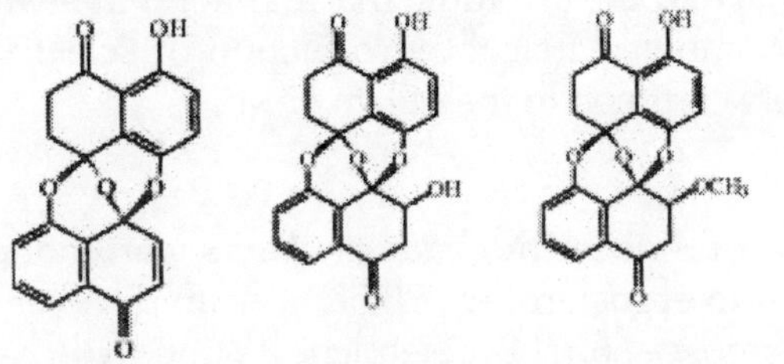

Bioactive Compounds Preussomerin EG_1 (1), Preussomerin EG_2 (2) and Preussomerin EG_3 (3)

Muscodor albus

It is a novel endophytic fungus that produces bioactive volatile organic compounds (VOCs) reported by Strobel (2006). It has enormous potential for uses in Agriculture, industry and medicine. *Muscodor albus* produces a mixture of VOCs that act synergistically to kill a wide variety of plant and human pathogenic fungi and bacteria. This mixture of gases consists of various alcohols, acids, esters, ketones and lipids. Artificial mixtures of the VOCs mimic the biological effects of the fungal VOCs when tested against a wide range of fungal and bacterial pathogens. Many practical applications for 'mycofumigation' by *M. albus* have been investigated and the fungus is now in the market place.

Aspergillus fumigatus

The endophytic fungus, *Aspergillus fumigatus* CY018 was recognized as an versatile producer of new and bioactive metabolites for the first time in the leaf of *Cynodon dactylon* (Liu *et al.*, 2004). The two new metabolites *viz.*, asperfumoid (1) and asperfumin (2), together with six known bioactive compounds including monomethylsulochrin, fumigaclavine C, fumitremorgin C, physcion, helvolic acid and 5α,8α-epidioxy-ergosta-6,22-diene-3β-ol as well as other four known compounds ergosta-4,22-diene-3β-ol, ergosterol, *cyclo*(Ala-Leu) and *cyclo*(Ala-Ile) were isolated from the fungus. All of the 12 isolates were subjected to *in vitro* bioactive assays against three human pathogenic fungi *Candida albicans, Tricophyton rubrum* and *Aspergillus niger*. As a result, asperfumoid, fumigaclavine C, fumitremorgin C, physcion and helvolic acid were shown to inhibit *C. albicans* with MICs of 75.0, 31.5, 62.5, 125.0 and 31.5 μg/mL, respectively.

Gliocladium sp.

An endophytic isolate of *Gliocladium* sp. was obtained from the Patagonian Eucryphiacean tree–*Eucryphia cordifolia*, known locally as "ulmo". The fungus was identified on the basis of its morphology and aspects of its molecular biology. This fungus produces a mixture of volatile organic compounds (VOCs) lethal to such plant pathogenic fungi as *Pythium ultimum* and *Verticillum dahliae*, while other pathogens were only inhibited by its volatiles (Stinson *et al.*,2003). Some of the same volatile bioactive compounds exuded by *Gliocladium* sp. such as 1-butanol, 3-methyl-, phenylethyl alcohol and acetic acid, 2-phenylethyl ester, as well as various propanoic acid esters, are also produced by *Muscodor albus*, a well known volatile antimicrobial producer. In fact, *M. albus* was used as a selection tool to effectively isolate *Gliocladium* sp. since it is resistant to VOC's produced by *M. albus.* However, the primary volatile compound produced by *Gliocladium* sp. is 1,3,5,7-cyclooctatetraene or annulene, which by itself, was an effective inhibitor of fungal growth. The authenticated VOC's of *Gliocladium* sp. were inhibitory to all, and lethal to some test fungi in a manner that nearly mimicked the gases of *Gliocladium* sp. itself. This report showed that the production of selective volatile antibiotics by endophytic fungi is not exclusively confined to the *Muscodor* sp.

Collectotrichum sp.

New bioactive metabolites were produced by *Collectotrichum sp.*, an endophytic fungus in *Artemisia annua* (Lu *et.al.*,2000). In addition to ergosterol (I), 3β,5α,6β-trihydroxyergosta-7,22-diene (II), 3β-hydroxy-ergosta-5-ene (III), 3-oxo-ergosta-4,6,8(14),22-tetraene (IV), 3β-hydroxy-5α,8α-epidioxy-ergosta-6,22-diene(V),3β-hydroxy-5α,8α-epidioxy-ergosta6,9(11),22-triene (VI) and 3-oxo-ergosta-4-ene (VII), a plant hormone indole-3-acetic acid (IAA) and three new antimicrobial metabolites were characterized from the culture of *Colletotrichum* sp. The structures of the new metabolites were elucidated by a combination of spectroscopic methods (IR, MS, ^{1}H and ^{13}C NMR) as 6-isoprenylindole-3-carboxylic acid (1),3β,5α-dihydroxy-6β-acetoxy-ergosta-7,22-diene(2)and3β,5α-dihydroxy-6β-phenylacetyloxy–ergosta-7,22-diene (3), respectively. The compounds 1–3 and III–V inhibited the growth of all the tested bacteria (*Bacillus subtilis, Staphylococcus aureus, Sarcina lutea* and *Pseudomonas* sp.) with minimal inhibitory concentrations (MICs) ranging from 25 to 75 μg/ml. Moreover, metabolites 2 and 3, together with the known sterols III and V, were inhibitory against the fungi *Candida albicans* and *Aspergillus niger* with MICs between together with the known sterols III and V, were inhibitory against the fungi *Candida albicans* and *Aspergillus niger* with MICs between 50 and 100 μg/ml. At 200 μg/ml,compounds 1–3, III and IV were shown to be fungistatic to the crop pathogenic fungi *Gaeumannomyces graminis* var. *tritici, Rhizoctonia cerealis, Helminthosporium sativum* and *Phytophthora capsici*. This was the first report on the endophytic fungus from *A. annua* and the bioactive metabolites thereof.

Artemisia annua (*A. annua*) L. (Asteraceae), a traditional Chinese medicinal herb well recognized for its synthesis of artemisinin (an antimalarial drug), was found to be a widespread species that can thrive in many geographically different areas. In addition to the remarkable ecological adaptability, this plant is strongly resistant to insects and pathogens. The study was thus undertaken in order to ascertain the presence of endophytes inside the plant, and if any the potential for synthesizing bioactive compounds. Therefore it was conceived that *Colletotrichum* sp., an endophyte in *A. annua* can produce in vitro metabolites that were shown to be antimicrobial. Others are known to be plant growth regulatory.

Taxol Producing Endophytes

Taxol, a highly functionalized diterpenoid, is found in each of the world's yew (*Taxus*) species (Suffness, 1995). This compound is the world's first billion dollar anticancer drug, and it is used to treat a number of other human tissue proliferating diseases as well. Its cost makes it unavailable to many people worldwide. Therefore alternative sources were needed, since organic synthesis, is not economically feasible. Some endophytic fungi have been found to be the potential sources for taxol.

Taxomyces andreanae

By the early 1990s, however, no endophytic fungi had been isolated or even known from any of the world's representative yew species. After several years, a novel taxol producing endophytic fungus, *Taxomyces andreanae* was discovered in *Taxus brevifolia* (Strobel *et al.*, 1993).

Pestalotiopsis microspora

One of the most commonly found endophytes of World's yews is *Pestalotiopsis* sp (Strobel *et al.*, 1996). It was reported that *Pestalotiopsis microspora* is one of the most common endophyte isolated from *Taxus wallichiana* which may produce taxol. Furthermore, several other *P. microspora* isolates were obtained from bald cypress in South Carolina and were shown to produce taxol (Li *et al.*,1996). This was the first indication that endophytes residing in plants other than *Taxus* spp. were producing taxol.

Pestalotiopsis guepini

A specific search was conducted for taxol producing endophytes exists in South America and Australia. The endophyytic fungus *Pestalotiopsis guepini* isolated from rare Wollemia pine, *Wollemia nobilis* was shown to produce taxol. (Strobel *et al.*,1997).

Periconia sp.

The endophytic fungus–*Periconia* sp isolated from *Torreya grandifolia* was noted to produce taxol. It was stated that fungi more commonly produce taxol than higher plants and the distribution of those fungi making taxol is worldwide and not confined to endophytes of yew (Li *et al.*,1998). In addition, several fungal endophytes of *Torreya grandifolia* produce taxol in culture (Hoffman *et al.*, 1998).

Seimatoantlerium tepuiense

A rubiaceous plant–*Manguireothamnus speciosus* yielded a noble fungus *Seimatoantlerium tepuiense* that produces taxol. This endemic plant grows on the top of the tequis in the Venzuelan–Guyana in southwestern Venezuela (Strobel *et al.*,1999).

Tubercularia sp.

There are reports on taxol production by *Tubercularia* sp. isolated from Southern Chinese yew (*Taxus mairei*) in Southeastern China.(Wang *et al.*, 2000). In addition, other endophytes of *T. wallichiana* produce taxol including *Sporormia minima* and *Trichothecium* sp. has also been reported (Shrestha, 2001).

It can be stated that taxol is made by a number of higher plants in the world as well as their associated endophytes. Uses for taxol in medical applications have been proved. Some oomycetes group of pathogenic fungi like *Phytopthora*, *Pythium* and *Aphanomyces* are extremely sensitive to taxol. In fact, these fungi are killed in identical manner by taxol as certain sensitive human cells, such as those originating from breast and ovarian cancer cell lines (Schiff and Horowitz, 1980; Young *et al.*, 1992). The mode of action of taxol is to preclude tubulin molecules from depolymarizing during the process of cell division (Schiff and Horowitz, 1980). Tubulin molecules in taxol–sensitive fungi such as oomycetes are affected in the same manner as human cancer cells (Young *et al.*, 1992). The tubulin gene in *Pythium* sp. is virtually identical to the tubulin gene in humans. Therefore, it seems reasonable to think that taxol is serving as fungicide in nature and *Taxus* spp. shows no infection caused by oomycetes. A search for taxol compound using oomycetes as a screening tool seems to be a reasonable approach.

Anti-Candida Metabolism from Endopytic Fungi

Five species of endophytic fungi were screened against *Candida albicans* and six bioactive compounds were isolated and identified, *viz.* cerulenin (1), arundifungin (2), sphaeropsidin A (3), 5-(1,3-butadiene-1-yl)-3-(propene-1-yl)-2-(5H)-furanone (4), ascosteroside A (formerly called ascosteroside; 5) and a derivative of 5, ascosteroside B (6). Considerably more Ascomycota (11–16 per cent) than Basidiomycota (3.5 per cent) produced metabolites with activity against *C. albicans.* (Weber *et al.*, 2007).

Immunosupressive Compounds from *Fusarium subglotinans*: An Endophytic Fungus

Immunosuppressive drugs are used toady to prevent allograft rejection in transplant patients, and in future they could be used to treat autoimmune diseases such as rheumatic arthritis and insulin dependent diabetes. Screening have revealed that fungi are potential sources of immunosuppressive agents such as cyclosporine A, FK506 and rapamycin, but these agents also showed some undesirable side effects such as nephrotoxicity (Allison,2000).Two novel immunosuppressive compounds *viz.* Subglutinols A and B which are noncytotoxic diterpene pyrones have been discovered by Lee *et al.* (1995) from the endophytic fungus *Fusarium subglutinans* isolated from perennial twinning vine *Tripterygium wilfordii.*

Non-Endophytic Fungi Producing Bioactive Compounds

Chaetomium brasiliense

Chaetochalasin A (1), a new fungal metabolite with a novel ring system, was isolated from *Chaetomium brasiliense* (Oh *et al.*,1998). The compound showed potent insecticidal properties and also known as Chaetoglobosins. The structure of (1) was determined by NMR experiments and single-crystal X-ray diffraction analysis.

Malbranchea filamentosa

The fungus was isolated from an Argentine soil sample (Hosoe *et al.*,2005). Screening of *Malbranchea filamentosa* IFM 41300 for bioactive compounds led to the discovery of furanone derivative–benzyl-3-

phenyl-5*H*-furan-2-one (1) as a vasodialator and the isolation of erythroglaucin (2) which was previously reported (Braün,1981; Chandrasenan, 1960; Siliva *et al.*, 1979).

The structure of (1) was established on the basis of spectroscopic and chemical investigations.

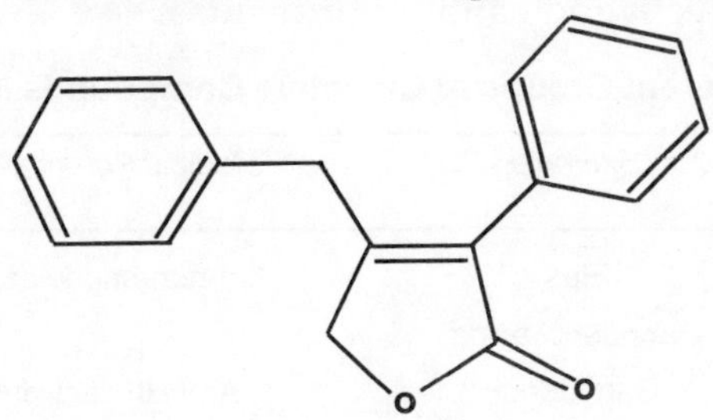

II

Chemical Structure of Compound 1

Penicillium simplicissimum

A soil isolate *Penicillium simplicissimum* ATCC 90288 produced novel insecticidal indole alkaloids designated as okaramines (Hayashi, 2005). Random screening was carried out using okara (an insoluble residue of the whole soybean homogenate) as a culture medium in order to get fungal isolates). Okaramines were also found to be produced by other strains of *Penicillium simplicissimum*. Three kinds of activities *viz.* insecticidal activity, convulsive activity and paralytic activity were observed against silkworms.

Macrofungi as Source of Bioactive Compounds

Macrofungi or mushrooms have an established history of use in traditional oriental therapies. Medicinal effects have been demonstrated for many traditionally used mushrooms, including extracts of *Favolus alveolarious* (Chang *et al.*, 1988), *Phellinus linteus* (Chung *et al.*, 1993; Kim *at al.*, 2001), *Agaricus campestris* (Gray and Flatt, 1998) *Pestalotiopsis* sp. (Kiho *et al.*, 1997)), *Lentinus edodes* (Kim and Park, 1979; Sugano *et al.*, 1985; Song *et.al.*, 1998), *Pleurotus ostreatus* (Kim and Park, 1979), *Tricholoma* sp. (Wang *et al.*, 1995; Wang *et al.*, 1996a; Liu *et al.*, 1996), and *Coriolus versicolor* (Kim and Park, 1979; Mayer and Drews, 1980; Fujita *et al.*, 1988; Li *et al.*, 1990; Yang *et al.*, 1992a; Han *et al.*, 1996, Ng 1998; Chu *et al.*, 2002).

Bioactive molecules of macrofungi belong to Polysaccharides, glycoproteins, proteoglycans, terpenoids, fatty acids, proteins, lectins etc. that possess certain medicinal properties (Table 5.1). They can be added to the diet and used orally and considered as a safe and useful for disease treatment. These compounds are found in the fruiting bodies, mycelia, spores and culture broth of macrofungi. Several major substances with immunomodulating and/or anticancer activity have been isolated from them.

Immunomodulating and Anticancer Agents from Macrofungi

Compounds that are capable of interacting with the immune system to upregulate or downregulate specific aspects of the host response can be classified as immunomodulators or biologic response modifiers. Whether certain compounds enhance or suppress immune responses can depend on a number of factors, including dose, route of administration, and timing of administration of the compound in question. The type of activity can also depend on their mechanism of action or the site of activity (Tzianabos,2000). Many compounds isolated from macrofungi that are known as immonumodulators that almost related to polysaccharides and their peptide or protein derivates and Fips. Also in some cases triterpenoids have closed to immunomodulating activity. These compounds are also worthwhile anti-infective and antitumor agents.

Table 5.1: The Different Groups of Bioactive Compounds Isolated from Macrofungi

Major Bioactive Compound Group	*Example*	*Medical Potentiality*	*Reference*
Proteins	Fips	Immunomodulator	Lin *et al.* (1997)
	Ganoderic acids		El-Mekkawy *et al.* (1998)
	Ganoderiol	Anti-HIV activity	Chairul *et al.* (1991)
	Ganoderinic acids	Antitumor	Toth *et al.* (1983)
	Lucidinic acids	Cytotoxic	Toth *et al.* (1983)
Polysaccharides	Grifolan	Immunomodulator	Bohn and BeMiller (1995)
	Lentinan	Antitumor	Yap and Ng (2003)
	Schizophyllan	Antiviral	Sarkar *et al.* (1993)
Polysaccharopeptide	PSP	Antitumor	Maeda and Chihara (1999)
	PSK	Antiviral	Oh *et al.* (2000)
		Cytotoxic	Ooi (2001)
Terpenoids	Ganolucidic acids	Histamin release inhibition	Kohda *et al.* (1985)
	Lucidimols	Antihypertension	Morigiwa (1986)
Steroids	Polyoxygenated derivatives	Cytotoxic	Lin and Tome (1991)
	of ergosterol	Antitumor	Bok *et al.* (1999)
		Antibacterial	Keller *et al.* (1996)
	Linolenic acid	Antimutagenic	Menoli *et al.* (2001)
Fatty acids	Palmitic acid	Antibacterial	Moradali *et al.* (2004)
Nucleotides	Adenosine	Platelet aggregate inhibition	Shimizu *et al.* (1995)
Polyacetylenic compounds	Biformyne, agrocybin, Nemotinic acid, marasmin, quadrifidins	As antibiotic	Gottlieb and Shaw (1967)

Now a days macrofungi are distinguished as important natural resources of immunomodulating and anticancer agents and with regard to the increase in diseases involving immune dysfunction, cancer, autoimmune conditions in recent years, applying such immunomodulator agents especially with the natural original is vital (Moradali *et al.*, 2007). These compounds belong mainly to polysaccharides especially β-d-glucan derivates, glycopeptide/protein complexes(polysaccharide-peptide/proteincomplexes),proteoglycons,proteins and triterpenoids.

Major Immunomodulating and Antitumor Agents

Polysaccharides and Glyco-conjugates

Numerous bioactive polysaccharides, glycoproteins, glycopeptides, and proteoglycans from macrofungi are considered as immunomodulators affecting on proliferation and differentiation of immune cells and cytokines, interleukins and receptors production due to recognition these compounds by the certain receptors located on the leukocytes and other immune cells that lead to enhance the innate and cell-mediate immune responses. In virtue of these activities also induction of different types of antitumor effector cells such as cytotoxic T cells, NK cells and macrophages occur. In addition to these activities some of them possess antiviral, antibacterial, antifungal and antiprotosoal activities (Wasser and Weis, 1999). Macrofungi are rich in such components in their cell wall structures.

Polysaccharides are carbohydrate polymers that can be found abundantly in higher fungi cell wall. They involve different chemical compositions including β-glucans, hetero-β-glucans, heteroglycans, ∗-manno-β-glucan complexes that are found in macrofungi and all have showed immunomodulating and antitumor properties (Table 5.2). Among them β-glucans are most important polysaccharides with immunomodulating and antitumor activity. β-glucans are glucose polymers that can exist as a non-branched (1→3)-β-linked backbone or as a (1→3)-β-linked backbone with (1→6)-β-branches and they occur as a primary component in the cell walls of higher fungi in the great deals. Heteroglucans side chains contain glucuronic acid, xylose, galactose, mannose, arabinose and ribose that may combined with other components. Glycans are other polysaccharides that have been found in macrofungi. These polysaccharides, in general, contain units other than glucose in their backbone. They are classified as galactans, fucans, xylans, and mannans by individual sugar components in the backbone.

Table 5.2: Some Immunomodulating and Antitumor Polysaccharides Isolated from Macrofungi

Macrofungi	*Bioactive Compound*	*Reference*
Lentinus edodes	Galactoglucomannan	Fujii *et al.*,1979
Inonotus obliquus	Xylogalactoglucan	Mizuno,1999
Polyporus confluens	Xyloglucan	Mizuno,1999
Flammulina velutipes	Galactomannoglucan	Ikekawa *et al.*,1982
Ganoderma tsugae	Glucogalactan, Arabinoglucan	Zhuang *et al.*,1994
Ganoderma lucidum	β-(1→3)-glucuronoglucan, Mannogalactoglucan	Cho *et al.*,1999
Hericium erinaceum	Galactoxyloglucan, Mannoglucoxylan, Glucoxylan, Xylan	Mizuno,1999
Grifola frondosa	Mannoxyloglucan, Xylogluoan, β-(1→6); β-(1→3)-glucan, Mannogalactofucan	Zhuang *et al.*,1994
Agaricus blazei	Mannogalactoglucan, β-(1 ›6); ∗-(1→3)-glucan, ∗-(1→4); β-(1→6)-glucan, ∗-(1→6); ∗-(1→4)-glucan,	Mizuno,1999

PSK and PSP from *Coriolus versicolor*

The best known commercial polysaccharopeptide obtained from *C. versicolor* are polysaccharopeptide Krestin (PSK) and polysaccharopeptide PSP which are taken orally for gastric and other cancers and commercially the best established. Both the products are obtained from the extraction of *C. versicolor* mycelia. PSK and PSP are Japanese and Chinese products, respectively. Both products have similar physiological activities but are structurally different. PSK was commercialized by Kureha Chemicals, Japan. After extensive clinical trials, PSK was approved for use in Japan in 1977, and by 1985, it ranked 19th on the list of the world's most commercially successful drugs (Yang *et al.*, 1992a). Annual Japanese sales of PSK in 1987 were worth US$357 million (Yang *et al.*, 1992a). PSP appeared on the market about 10 years after PSK. In addition to clinically tested PSK and PSP, numerous other extract preparations of *C. versicolor* are on the market as nutraceuticals and traditional medicines. Neutraceutical polysaccharopeptide preparations are sold worldwide in the form of capsules, ground biomass tablets, syrups, food additives,and teas. Traditional usage, pharmacological activities, and clinical effects of *C. versicolor* preparations have been reported by Chu *et al.* (2002).

Polysaccharide-polypeptide Complexes from *Ganoderma lucidum*

The fungus *G. lucidum* (fruit body and spore) contains kinds of glycopeptide complexes with antitumor and immunostimulating activities. Some of them stimulate the expression of cytokines, especially IL-1, IL-2 and INF-γ (Wang *et al.*, 2002; Won *et al.*, 1989)

Antioxidant Compounds from the Fruiting Body of Edible Mushroom, *Agrocybe aegerita*

The search for bioactive natural products from edible mushroom *Agrocybe aegerita* was carried out by Zhang *et al.* (2003). The methanol extract of the mushroom yielded a fatty acid fraction (FAF) along with palmitic acid (1), ergosterol (2), 5,8-epidioxy-ergosta-6,22-dien-3β-ol (3), mannitol (4) and trehalose (5). The composition of FAF was confirmed by GC-MS and by comparison to the retention values of authentic samples of palmitic, stearic, oleic and linoleic acids. The structures of 1–5 were established using spectroscopic methods. FAF and compounds 1–3 showed cyclooxygenase (COX) enzyme inhibitory and antioxidant activities. Compounds 1, 3 and fatty acids were isolated here for the first time from the fruiting body of *A. aegerita*.

Anti-tumour and Immunomodulating Effects of *Pleurotus ostreatus*

Pleurotus ostreatus is one of the widely cultivated edible mushrooms. Water-soluble proteoglycan fractions from *P. ostreatus* mycelia were purified by alcohol-precipitation, ion exchange and followed by gel permeation (Sephadex G-100) chromatography. Three neutral fractions were found which had polysaccharide to protein ratios 14.2, 26.4 and 18.3, respectively. These fractions were tested for *in vitro* and *in vivo* immunomodulatory and anticancer effects on Sarcoma-180-bearing mouse model (Sarangi *et al.*, 2006). The three neutral proteoglycans derived from the mushroom mycelia could be used as immunomodulators and anti cancer agents.

Eritadenine from *Lentinus edodes*

Eritadenine is an hypocholesterolemic agent which has been found to be present in the edible Shitake fungus, *Lentinus edodes.* The study was conducted by Enman *et al.* (2007) to quantify the amount of cholesterol reducing agent eritadenine to be used in natural medicine against blood cholesterol. The results indicated the potential for delivery of therapeutic amounts of eritadenine extracted from selected strains of *Lentinus edodes.*

Grifolin, Anticancer Agents from *Albatrellus confluens*

Grifolin, a potential antitumour natural product has been obtained from the mushroom *Albatrellus confluen* (Ye *et al.*, 2007).

Nutraceuticals from Macrofungi

In recent days human beings are constantly searching for new products which can improve biological functions and make people fitter and healthier. These products have been called as vitamins, dietary supplements, functional foods, phyto-chemicals, nutraceuticals (Brower, 1998; Zeisel, 1999) and nutriceuticals (Chang and Buswell, 1996).They are designed to supplement the human diet, not to be used as a regular food, by increasing the intake of bioactive compounds for the enhancement of health and fitness. The industries involved in providing these substances are expanding in the United States.

Macrofungi or edible mushrooms can be taken as a source of functional foods. The extractable products or nutriceuticals from mushrooms are likely to be of increasing interest throughout the world. The use of standardised extracts of the mycelium or fruiting bodies of the mushroom is what distinguishes nutriceuticals (Mushroom medicines) from both the use of whole mushrooms (as food) and of single chemical (as a drug). Whole mushrooms, like all other natural materials, vary considerably in their quality, and their beneficial action may be unreliable. Single chemical often provide such intense responses that they are accompanied by very unpleasant side effects. Nutriceuticals, which are extracted products, occupy a middle ground between these extremes and have proven to be very useful. However, to obtain a good quality and trustworthy product is of paramount importance. Differing from most pharmaceuticals, the biologically active compounds that are extracted from mushrooms (nutriceuticals) have extraordinarily low toxicity, even at high doses. Long viewed as tonics, it is now known that they can profoundly improve the quality of human health.

Medicinal mushrooms have been used as a dietary supplement or medicinal food in China for over 2,000 years. In the late 1980s, their extractable ingredients received great attention as products for improving biological function, thus making people fitter and healthier. In some cases, these dietary supplements were used in the prevention and treatment of various human diseases. Francia *et al.* (1999) listed six groups, (1) six species which reduce the total cholesterol level, *Auricularia auriculajudae, Cordyceps sinensis, Ganoderma lucidum, Grifola frondosa, Pleurotus ostreatus,* and *Tremella fuciformis;* (2) two species which reduce the "bad cholesterol–the low-density lipoprotein (LDL) level", *Auricularia auriculajudae and Tremella fuciformis;* (3) three species which reduce the triglyceride level, *Cordyceps sinensis, Grifola frondosa,* and *Lentinua edodes;* (4) six species which reduce platelet binding (in vitro), *Auricularia auriculajudae, Calyptella* sp., *Ganoderma lucidum, Kuehneromyces* sp., *Neolentinus adhaerens* and *Panus* sp.; (5) three species which may reduce the arterial pressure, *Ganoderma lucidum, Grifola frondosa* and *Tricholoma mongolicum* and (6) six species which may decrease glycemia, *Agaricus bisporus, Agrocybe aegerita, Cordyceps sinensis, Tremella aurantia, Grifola frondosa* and *Coprinus comatus*. There is intense industrial interest currently in a novel class of compounds extractable either from the mycelium or fruiting body of mushrooms. The compounds called "mushroom nutriceuticals" (Chang and Buswell, 1996), exhibit either medicinal and/or tonic qualities and have immense potential as dietary supplements for use in the prevention and treatment of various human diseases.

In conclusion, numerous bioactive compounds appear to have beneficial health effects. Much scientific research needs to be conducted before we begin to make science based dietary recommendations. Despite this, there is sufficient evidence to recommend consuming food sources rich in bioactive compounds.

References

Allison, A.C. (2000). Immunosuppressive drugs : the first 50 years and a glance. *Immunopharmacology,* 47: 63-85.

Aly, A.H., Ebel, R.E., Wray, V., Werner, E., Müller, G., Kozytska, S., Hentschel, U., Proksch, P., and Ebel, R.(2008). Bioactive compounds from the endophytic fungus *Ampelomyces* sp.isolated from the medicinal plant *Urospermum picroides. Phytochmistry,* (in Press).

Bacon, C.W., and White, J.F (2000). Microbial Endophytes, Marcel Deker Inc., New York.

Bills, G.F., and Polishook, J.D.(1991). Microfungi from *Carpinus caroliniana, Canadian J. of Botany*, 69: 1477-1482.

Bohn J.A., and. BeMiller, J.N (1995). (1-3)-β-d-glucans as biological response modifiers: a review of structure-functional activity relationships, *Carbohydr Polym.*, 28 : 3–14.

Bok, J.W., Lermer, L., Chilton, J., .Klingeman H.G., and Towers, G.H.(1999).Antitumor sterols from the mycelia of *Cordyceps sinensis*. *Phytochemistry*, 51: 891–898.

Braun, M.(1981). Regioselektive Synthese der nuturlich vorkommenden anthrachinone digitopurpon, islandicin, catenarin und erythroglaucin, *Liebigs. Ann. Chem.*, 12: 2247–2257.

Brower, V. (1988). Nutraceuticals : Poised for a healthy slice of the healthcare market ? *Nature Biotechnology*, 16: 728–731.

Chairul *et al.*, (1991). Applanoxidic acids A, B, C and D, biologically active tetracyclic triterpenes from *Ganoderma applanatum*, *Phytochemistry*, 30 : 4105–4109.

Chandrasenan, K., Neelakantan, S., and Seshadri, T.R. (1960).A new synthesis of catenarin and erythroglaucin, *Proc. Ind. Acad. Sci., Sect. A*, 51: 298–300.

Chang, S. T., and J. A. Buswell.(1996). Mushroom Nutriceuticals. *World J. Microb Biotech.*, 12: 473–476.

Chang, J.B., Park, W.H., Choi, E.C., and Kim, B.K. (1988). Studies on constituents of the higher fungi of Korea (LIV). Anticancer components of *Favolus alveolarius*. *Arch. Pharmacol. Res.*, 11: 203–212.

Cho, S.M., . Park, J.S., . Kim, K.P D.Y. Cha, H.M. Kim., and. Yoo, I.D.(1999). Chemical features and purification of immunostimulating polysaccharides from the fruit bodies of *Agaricus blazei*, *Korean J Mycol.*, 27 :170–174.

Chu, K.K.W., Ho, S.S.S. and Chow, A.H.L. (2002) *Coriolus versicolor*: a medicinal mushroom with promising immunotherapeutic values. *J. Clin. Pharmacol.*, 42 : 976–984.

Chung, K.S., Kim, S.S., Kim, H.S., Kim, K.Y., Han, M.W., and Kim, K.H. (1993.).Effect of Kp, an antitumor protein polysaccharide from mycelial culture of *Phellinus linteus* on the humoral immune response of tumor bearing ICR mice to sheep red blood cells. *Arch. Pharmacol. Res.*, 16 : 336–338.

El-Mekkawy., S *et al.* (1998), Anti-HIV-1 and anti-HIV-1-protease substances from *Ganoderma lucidum*, *Phytochemistry*, 49: 1651–1657.

Enman, J., Rova, U., and Berglund K.A.(2007). Quantification of the bioactive compound eritadenine in selected strain *(Lentinus edodes)*. *Agric. Food Chem.*, 55 (4) : 1177-1180.

Francia, C., Rapior, S., Courtecuisse, R., and Siroux, Y.(1999).Current Research findings on the effects of selected mushrooms on cardiovascular diseases. *International Journal of Medicinal Mushrooms*, 1 : 169-172.

Fujii T, Ishida N, Maeda H, Mizutani I, Suzuki F, KS-2-A. US Patent 4163780, 1979.

Fujita, H., Ogawa, K., Ikuzawa, M., Muto, S., Matsuki, M., Nakajima, S. *et al.* (1988). Effect of PSK, a protein-bound polysaccharide from *Coriolus versicolor*, on drug- metabolizing enzymes in sarcoma-180 bearing and normal mice. *Int. J. Immunopharmacol.*, 10: 445–450.

Gogoi, D.K., Mazumder, S., Saikia, R., and Bora, T.C. (2008).Impact of submerged culture conditions on growth and bioactive metabolites produced by endophyte *Hypocrea* spp. NSF-08 isolated from *Dillenia indica* Linn. in North East India. *Journal of Medical Mycology*, 18 (1): 1-9.

Gottlieb, D and Shaw, P.D (1967) Antibiotics, Springer-Verlag Press, Berlin.

Gray, A.M., and Flatt, P.R., (1998) Insulin-releasing and insulin-like activity of *Agaricus campestris* (mushroom). *J. Endocrinol.*, 157 a : 259–266.

Hayashi, H (2005) Bioactive alkaloids of fungal origin. *Studies in Natural Products Chemistry*, 32 (12) : 549-609.

Han, S.N., Wu, D., Leka, L.S. and Meydani, S.N. (1996.) Effect of mushroom (*Coriolus* polysaccharides of *Flammulina velutipes* 2. The structure of EA-3 and further purification of EA-5, *J Pharmacobio-Dyn.*, 5 : 576–581

Hoffman, A., Khan, W., Worapong, J., Strobel, G., Griffin, DArbigast, B., Borofosky, D., R.B., Boone, R.B., Ning, L., Zheng, P., and Daley, L.(1998). Bioprospecting for taxol in angiosperms plant extracts. *Spectroscopy*, 13: 22-32.

Hosoe, T., Iizuka, T., Komai, S., Wakana, D., Itabashi, T., Nozawa, K., Kazutaka Fukushima, K., and Kawai, K (2005). 4–Benzyl 3–phenyl–5H furan–2-one, a vasodilator isolated from *Malbranchea filamentosa* IEM300. *Phytochemistry*, 66, (23) : 2776-2779.

Ikekawa, T.., Ikeda, Y, . Yoshioka, Y., Nakanishi, Y., Yokoyama, E., and Yamazaki, E.(1982). Antitumor polysaccharides of *Flammulina velutipes* 2. The structure of EA-3 and further purification of EA-5, *J Pharmacobio-Dyn.*, 5 : 576–581.

Keller, A.C., Maillard M.P., and. Hostettmann, K.(1996).Antimicrobial steroids from the fungus *Fomitopsis pinicola*, *Phytochemistry*, 41 : 1041–1046.

Kim, B.K., and Park, E.K.(1979). Studies on the constituents of the higher fungi of Korea 1. Anti-neoplastic components of *Coriolus versicolor* Fr, *Pleurotus ostreatus* (Fr)

Kummer and *Lentinus edodes* (BERK) Singer. *J. Nat. Prod.*, 42: 684.

Kim, D.H., Yang, B.K., Jeong, S.C., Park, J.B., Cho, S.P., Das, S. *et al*. (2001). Production of a hypoglycemic, extracellular polysaccharide from the submerged culture of the mushroom, *Phellinus linteus*. *Biotechnol. Lett.*, 23: 513–517.

Kiho, T., Itahashi, S., Sakushima, M., Matsunaga, T., Usui, S., Ukai, S. *et al*. (1997). Polysaccharide in fungi, XXXVIII. Anti-diabetic activity and structural features of galatomannan elaborated by *Pestalotiopsis* species. *Biol. Pharm. Bull.*, 20: 118–121.

Kohda, H., Tokumoto, W. and Sakamoto K *et al*. (1985).The biologically active constituents of *Ganoderma lucidum* (Fr.) Karst, Histamine release-inhibitory triterpenes, *Chem Pharm Bull.*, 33: 1367–1374.

Lee, J.C., Lobkovsky, E., Pliam, N.B., Strobel, G., and Clardy, J. (1995). Subglutinols A and B : Immunosuppressive compounds from endophytic fungus *Fusarium subglutinans*. *J.Org. Chem.*, 60: 7076-7077.

Li, X.Y., Wang, J.F., Zhu, P.P., Liu, L., Ge, J.B. and Yang, S.X. (1990). Immune enhancement of a polysaccharides peptides isolated from *Coriolus versicolor*. *Acta Pharmacol. Sinica*, 11, pp. 542–545

Li, J.Y., Strobel, G.A., Sidhu, R., Hess, W.M., and Ford, E. (1996). Endophytic taxol producing fungi from Bald Cypress *Taxodium distichum*. *Microbiol.*, 142 : 2223–2226.

Li, J.Y., Sidhu, R.S., Ford, E., Hess, W.M.andStrobel, G.A.(1998). The induction of Taxol production in the endophytic fungus–*Periconia* sp. from *Torreya grandifolia*. *J. Ind. Microbiol.*, 20: 259-264.

Lin C.N., and Tome, W.P.(1991). Novel cytotoxic principle of formosan *Ganoderma lucidum*, *J Nat Prod.*, 54 : 998–1002.

Lin, W.H., . Hung, C.H., Hsu, C.I. and. Lin, J.Y. (1997.Dimerzation of the N-terminal amphipathic alpha-helix domain of the fungal immunomodulatory protein from *Ganoderma tsugae* (Fip-gts) defined by a yeast two-hybrid system and site- directed mutagenesis, *J Biol Chem.*, 272 : 20044–20048.

Liu, F., Ooi, V.E.C., Liu, W.K. and Chang, S.T., (1996). Immunomodulation and antitumor activity of polysaccharide–protein complex from the culture filtrates of a local edible mushroom, *Tricholoma lobayense*. *Gen. Pharmacol*, ., 27: 621–624.

Liu.J.Y., Song, Z., Zhang, Z Wang, Z *et al.* (2004).*Aspergillus fumigatus* CY108, an endophytic fungus in Cynodon as a versatile producer of new and bioactive metabolites. *Journal of Biotechnology*, 114 (3): 279-287.

Lu, H., Zou, W.X., Meng, J.C., Hu, J., and Tan R.X. (2000).New bioactive metabolites produced by *Collectotrichum* sp, an endophytic fungus in *Artemisia annua*.*Plant Science*, 151(1) : 67-73.

Macías-Rubalcava M.L., Hernández-Bautista, B.E., Jiménez-Estrada, M., *et al.*, (2008). Napthoquinone spiroketal with allelochemical activity from the newly discovered endophytic fungus *Edenia gomezpompae*. *Phytochemistry*, 69 (5): 1185-1196.

Maeda Y.Y. and Chihara, G (1999). Immunomodulator agents from plants. In: H. Wagner, Editor.

Mayer, P. and Drews, J. (1980).Effect of a protein-bound polysaccharide from *Coriolus versicolor* on immunological parameters and experimental infections in mice. *Infection*, 8 : 13–21.

Menoli, RC., . Mantovani, R M.S., Ribeiro, L.R., Speit, G and Jordão, Q(2001)Antimutagenic effects of the mushroom *Agaricus blazei* Murrill extracts on V79 cells, *Mutnat Res.*, 496 : 5–13.

Moradali, M. F., Mostafavi, H., Ghods, S and Hedjarou, G.A.(2007). Immunomodulating and anticancer agents in the realm of macromycetes fungi (macrofungi). *International Immunopharmacology*, 7 (6) : 701-724.

Moradali, M.F., Mostafavi, H., Abbasi, M., Ghods, S., and Salahi, A.(2004).Investigation of antibacterial potentiality of methanol extraction from fungus *Ganoderma applanatum*, *World Conference on Magic Bullets Celebrating Paul Ehrlich 150th Birthday, Nürnberg, Germany*.

Morigiwa, A., Kitabatake, K., . Fujimoto Y and. Ikekawa, N.(1986). Angiotensin converting enzyme–inhibitory triterpenes from *Ganoderma lucidum*, *Chem Pharm Bull.*, 34: 3025–3028.

Mizuno, T.(1999). The extraction and development of antitumor-active polysaccharides from medicinal mushrooms in Japan [Review], *Int J Med Mushroom*, 1 : 9–30.

Ng, T.B.(1998.) A review of research on the protein-bound polysaccharide (polysaccharopeptide, PSP) from the mushroom *Coriolus versicolor* (Basidiomycetes: Polyporaceae). *Gen. Pharmacol.*, 30: 1–4.

Oh, H., Swenson, D.C., Gloer, J.B., Wicklow, D.T., and Dowd, P.F. (1998). Chaetochalasin A : A new bioactive metabolite from *Chaetomium brasiliense*. *Tetrahedron Letters*, 39(42) : 7633-7636.

Oh, K.W., Lee, C.K., Kim, Y.S., . Eo, S.K., and Han, S.S. (2000).Antiherpetic activities of acidic protein bound polysaccharide isolated from *Ganoderma lucidum* alone and in combinations with acyclovir and vidarabine, *J Ethnopharmacol*, 72: 221–227.

Ooi, V. E.C (2001) Pharmacological studies on certain mushroom from China, *Int J Med Mushroom*, 3.

Sarangi, I., Ghosh, D., Bhutia, S.K., Mallick, S.K. and Maiti, T.K (2006) Anti-tumour and immunomodulating effects of Pleurotus ostreatus mycelia derived proteoglycans. *International Immunopharmacology*, 6 (8) : 1287-1297.

Sarkar, S., Koga, J., Whitley, R.J., and Chatterjee, S.(1993). Antiviral effect of the extract of culture medium of *Lentinus edodes* mycelia on the replication of herpes simplex virus 1, *Antivir Res.*, 20 : 293–303.

Schiff, P. B and Horowitz, S.B(1980) Taxol stabilizes microtubules in mouse fibroblast cells. *Proc. Natl. Acad. Sci.* USA, 77 : 1561-1565.

Schutz, B. (2001).Endophytic fungi : a source of novel biologically active secondary metabolites, British Mycological Society, International Symposium Proceedings. Bioactive fungal Metabolites–Impact and Exploitation. University of Wales, Swansea.

Schulz, B., Boyle, C., Draeger, S., Rommert, A.K., and Krohn, K. (2002). Endophytic fungi : a source of novel biologically active secondary metabolites, *Mycological Research*, 106 : 996–1004.

Shimizu, A., Yano, T., Saito, Y and Inada, Y.(1985).Isolation of an inhibitor of platelet aggregation from a fungus, *Ganoderma lucidum*, *Chem Pharm Bull.*, 33 : 3012–3015.

Shrestha, K., Strobel, G.A., Prakash, S., and Gewali, S.M. (2001). Evidence for paclitaxel from three new endophytic fungi of Himalayan yew of Nepal, *Planta Medica*, 67 : 374–376.

Siliva, S.O., M. Watanabe, M., and V. Snieckus (1979). General route to anthraquinone natural products via directed metalation of *N*, *N*-diethylbenzamides, *J. Org. Chem.*, 44 : 4802–4808.

Song, C.H., Jeon, Y.J., Yang, B.K., Ra, K.S. and Kim, H.I., (1998). Anti-complementary activity of endo-polymers produced from submerged mycelial culture of higher fungi with particular reference to *Lentinus edodes*. *Biotechnol. Lett.*, 20: 741–744.

Stinson, M., Ezra, D., Hess, W.M., Sears, J., and Strobel, G. (2003). An endophytic *Gliocladium* sp. of *Eucryphia cordifolia* producing selective volatile antimicrobial compounds *Plant Science*, 165 (4): 913-922

Strobel, G.A., Stierle, A., Stierle D., and Hess, W.M. (1993).*Taxomyces andreanae* a proposed new taxon for a bulbilliferous hyphomycete associated with pacific yew. *Mycotaxon*, 47: 71-78.

Strobel G, Yang X., Sears J, Kramer R., Sidhu, S., and Hess, W.M.(1996). Taxol from *Pestalotiopsis microspora*, an endophytic fungus of *Taxus wallichiana*. *Microbiol.*, 142: 435-440.

Strobel, G.A., Hess, W.M., Li, J.Y., Ford, E., Sears, J., Sidhu, R.S., and Summerell, B. (1997). *Pestalotiopsis guepini*, a taxol producing endophyte of the Wollemi Pine, *Wollemia nobilis*. *Aust.J. Bot.*, 45: 1073-1082.

Strobel, G.A., Ford, , ., Li, J.Y, Sears, J., Sidhu, R.S., and Hess, W.M.(1999).*Seimatoantlerium tepuiense* gen.nov. A unique epiphyte fungus producing taxol from the Venezuelan- Guayana System. *Appl. Microbiol.*, 22: 426-433.

Strobel, G., and Daisy, B (2003). Bioprospecting for microbial endophytes and their natural products. *Microbiology and Molecular Biology Reviews*, 67: 491-502.

Strobel., G. (2006) Harnessing endophytes for industrial microbiology.*Current opinion* in *Microbiology*, 9 (3) : 240-244.

Sugano, N., Choji, Y., Hibino, Y., Yasumura, S. and Maeda, H., (1985). Anti-carcinogenic action of an alcohol-insoluble fraction (LAP1) from culture medium of *Lentinus edodes* mycelia. *Cancer Lett.*, 27: 1–6.

Suffness, M.(1995). Taxol Science and Applications, CRC Press, Boca Raton, Florida. Tan, R.X., and Zou, W.X (2001). Endophytes : a rich source of functional metabolites, *Natural Products Reports*, 18: 448-459.

Tan, R.X., Meng, J.C., , and Hostettmann, K (2000). Phytochemical investigation of some traditional Chinese medicines and endophyte cultures. *Pharmaceutical Biology*, 38: 22-32.

Toth, J.O., Luu, B., and Ourisson, G. (1983). Ganoderic acid T and Z: cytotoxic triterpenes from *Ganoderma lucidum* (Polyporaceae), *Tetrahedron Lett.*, 24 : 1081–1084.

Tzianabos, A.O. (2000). Polysaccharide immunomodulators as therapeutic agents: structural aspects and biologic function, *Clin Microbiol Rev.*, 13: 523–533.

Tsukagoshi, S. Krestin (PSK), (1984) *Cancer Treat Rev.*, 11): 131–155.

Wang, H.X., Liu, W.K., Ng, T.B., Ooi, V.E.C. and Chang, S.T(1995.). Immunomodulatory and antitumor activities of a polysaccharide-peptide complex from a mycelial culture of *Tricholoma* sp., a local edible mushroom. *Life Sci.*, 57: 269–281.

Wang, H.X., Ng, T.B., Ooi, V.E.C., Liu, W.K. and Chang, S.T. (1996a).A polysaccharide– peptide complex from cultured mycelia of the mushroom *Tricholoma mongolicum* with immunoenhancing and antitumor activities. *Biochem. Cell. Biol.*, 74: 95–100.

Wang J., Li, G., Lu, H., Zheng, Z., Huang, Y., and Su, W. (2000). Taxol from *Tubercularia* sp strainTF5, an endophytic fungus of Taxus mairei, FEMS *Microbiol. Lett.*, 193: 249-253.

Wang, Y., Khoo, K.H., Chen, S.T., Lin, C.C., Wong C.H., and Lin C.H.(2002). Studies on the immunomodulating and antitumor activities of *Ganoderma lucidum* (Reishi) polysaccharides: functional and proteomic analyses of a fucose-containing glycoprotein fraction responsible for the activities, *Bioorg Med Chem.*, 10: 1057–1062.

Wasser, S.P and. Weis, A.L (1999). Therapeutic effects of substances occurring in higher basidiomycetes mushrooms: a modern perspective, *Crit Rev Immunol.*, 19 : 65–96.

Weber W.S. R., Kappe, R., Paululat, T., Mösker, E., and Anke, H. (2007). Anti-*Candida* metabolites from endophytic fungi. *Phytochemistry*, 68, (6): 886-892.

Won, S.J., Lee, S.S., Ke, Y.H., and. Lin, M.T. (1989). Enhancement of splenic NK cytotoxic activity by extracts of *Ganoderma lucidum* mycelium in mice, *J Biomed Lab Sci.*, 55: 201–213.

Young, D.H., Michelotti., E.J. Sivendell., C.S., and Krauss., N.E (1992).Antifungal properties of taxol and various anlogues. *Experientia*, 48: 882-885.

Yap, A.T., and Ng, M.L (2003). Immunopotentiating properties of Lentinan (1→3)-β-d-glucan extracted from culinary-medicinal mushroom *Lentinus edodes* (Berk.) Singer (Agaricomycetideae), *Int J Med Mushroom*, 5.

Yang, Q.Y., Jong, S.C., Li, X.Y., Zhou, J.X., Chen, R.T. and Xu, L.Z., (1992.a). Antitumor and immunomodulating activities of the polysaccharide–peptide (PSP) of *Coriolus versicolor*. *J. Immunol. Immunopharmacol.*, 12 :29–34.

Ye, M., Luo, X., Li, L., Shi, Y., Tan, M., Weng, X., Li, W., Liu, J and Cao, Y.(2007). Grifolin, a potential antitumour natural product from the mushroom *Albatrellus confluens*, induces cell-cycle arrest in GI phase via the ERK1/2 pathway. *Cancer Letters*, 258 (2): 199-207.

Zeisel, S.H. (1999). Regulation of ' Neutraceuticals'. *Science*, 285: 1853-1855.

Zhang, Y., Mills, G.L., and Nair, M.G. (2003). Cyclooxygenase inhibitory and antioxidant compounds from the fruiting body of an edible mushroom, *Agrocybe aegerita*. *Phytomedicine*, 10 (5): 386-390.

Zhuang, C., Mizuno, T., Ito, H. Shimura, K and Sumiya, T (1994). Chemical modification and antitumor activity of polysaccharides from the mycelium of liquid-cultured *Grifola frondosa*, *Nippon Shokuhin Kogyo Gakkaishi*, 41 : 733–740.

Utilisation and Management of Medicinal Plants (2010) *Pages 124–135*
Editors: **V.K. Gupta, Anil K. Verma and Sushma Koul**
Published by: **DAYA PUBLISHING HOUSE, NEW DELHI**

Chapter 6

Elevated Carbon Dioxide Levels Enhance Rosmarinic Acid Production in Spearmint Plantlets

Brent Tisserat*, Mark Berhow and Steven F. Vaughn
New Crops Processing and Technology Research,
National Center of Agricultural Utilization Research, USDA-ARS,
1815 N. University St., Peoria, IL 61604

ABSTRACT

The phenolic rosmarinic acid (RA) is synthesized in the phenylpropanoid pathway and is constitutively expressed in spearmint (*Mentha spicata* L.) plantlets grown *in vitro*. RA levels within plantlet leaves were found to be readily manipulated by the nutritional and physical environments. Higher RA levels, about a 100 per cent increase, occurred from plantlets cultured on a Murashige and Skoog medium with 3 per cent sucrose (BM) compared to plantlets on BM without sucrose. Plantlets were grown on BM under either 350 or 10,000 μmol mol^{-1} CO_2 and subjected to various Photosynthetic photon flux density (PPFD) levels (34, 80, 120 and 180 $\mu mole{\cdot}m^{-2}{\cdot}s^{-1}$) to determine the optimum light level to conduct experiments. The best light level was determined to be 120 $\mu mole{\cdot}m^{-2}{\cdot}s^{-1}$ because it allowed for high growth and RA production. Spearmint shoots on BM were grown under 350, 1,500, 3,000, 10,000 or 30,000 μmol mol^{-1} CO_2 for 8 wks. Generally, increasing levels of CO_2 produced increased growth, morphogenesis and

* Corresponding Author: Tel: +011-309-681-6289; Fax: +011-309-681-6524; E-mail: brent.tisserat@ars.usda.gov.

RA concentrations. Mint cv. '557789' plantlets produced about a 5-fold increase in RA concentration over the control. High positive correlations occur between CO_2 levels and spearmint plantlet growth (fresh weight), morphogenetic responses (leaves, roots and shoots) and secondary metabolism (RA).

Keywords: *Mentha spicata, Secondary metabolism, Shoots, Phytochemicals, Lamiaceae, Phenolics.*

Introduction

Rosmarinic acid (RA), is an ester of caffeic acid and 3-4-dihydroxyphenyllacetic acid and common among species of the Boraginaceae and Lamiaceae families (Petersen 1991; Shetty, 2001). RA has been shown to have health promotive effects and may be employed for gastrointestinal disorders and urinary anti-inflammation, and also has anti-HIV activity (Arda *et al.*, 1997; Yang and Shetty, 1998; Kang *et al.*, 2003; Takano *et al.*, 2004). RA is constitutively expressed in certain cell suspensions and callus cultures (Zenk *et al.*, 1977; De-Eknamkul and Ellis, 1984; Whitaker *et al.*, 1984; Elis, 1985; Kim *et al.*, 2001; Petersen, 1991; Hippolyte *et al.*, 1992), micro-shoots (Shetty, 1997; 2001) and cultured roots (Karam *et al.*, 2003; Li *et al.*, 2005). RA is an attractive metabolic candidate to be produced commercially *in vitro* because it is readily expressed in a wide variety of cultured tissue types, and has a high economic dollar value. Although cell suspensions and callus have been employed in most past RA studies, no commercialization using these cell types to manufacture RA has materialized. Certain disadvantages are associated when employing undifferentiated cell suspensions, such as genetic instability and the high bioreactor production system costs (Shetty, 2001). Plantlets and micro-shoots should be considered as a viable source of secondary metabolites because they are composed of the same tissues and organs found in plants grown in the field (Tisserat and Vaughn, 2001; Tisserat *et al.*, 2002). In addition, microshoots and plantlets readily express the same secondary metabolites as found in plants grown in the soil (Mitra *et al.*, 1997; Yang and Shetty, 1998; Tisserat and Vaughn, 2001; Nogueira and Romano, 2002; Tisserat *et al.*, 2002). Mint microshoots transition readily into plantlets with distinct root and shoot systems on medium without growth regulators (Shetty, 1997; Tisserat and Silman, 2000; Shetty, 2001; Nogueira and Romano, 2002). Tissue culture plantlets are capable of expressing high photosynthetic activity in either heterotrophic or autotrophic environments in the presence of ultra-high CO_2 environments (Tisserat and Silman, 2000; Tisserat *et al.*, 2001). The outward physical expression of high photosynthetic activity and enhanced primary metabolism is increased biomass (fresh weight) and morphogenesis (leaf, root and shoot production) (Tisserat and Silman, 2000; Tisserat *et al.*, 2001). Recently, it has been shown that microshoots of C-3 plant species exposed to elevated CO_2 environments exhibit the simultaneous occurrence of high production rates of secondary metabolism as well as enhanced growth and morphogenesis responses (Mitra *et al.*, 1997; Tisserat and Vaughn, 2001; Nogueira and Romano, 2002; Tisserat *et al.*, 2002). These observations suggest a strong correlation between the photosynthesis assimilates, plant growth, morphogenetic responses, and secondary metabolism that occurs within cultured plantlets. To date, the influence of CO_2 concentrations on RA production *in vitro* has not been studied.

The basic strategy of this research effort was to develop a plantlet system which produces secondary metabolites of commercial and research interest that can be manipulated by the nutritional and physical environments. We sought to determine how various levels of CO_2 affect plantlet growth, morphogenesis and RA metabolism. Our goal was to optimize the atmospheric environment in order to obtain high plantlet biomass responses coupled with high secondary metabolite (*i.e.*, RA) production. Initially, we compared the ability of spearmint plantlets and callus to produce RA to verify that cultured plantlets had merit to study RA production *in vitro*. The influence of various photosynthetic photon flux density (PPFD) levels on growth and RA production in the presence of ambient or elevated CO_2 (*i.e.*, 10,000 µmol mol^{-1} CO_2) was determined. Then, finally, we tested various concentrations of CO_2 on mint plantlets of various cvs. to maximize growth, morphogenesis and RA production.

Materials and Methods

Medium and Plant Culture

The basal medium (BM) consisted of Murashige and Skoog (1962) salts plus ($mg \cdot l^{-1}$): 0.5 thiamine.HCl, 100 myo-inositol, 30,000 sucrose, and 8,000 agar (Difco Laboratories, Detroit, MI). Medium pH was adjusted to 5.7±0.1 with 0.1 N HCl or NaOH before the addition of agar, then melted and dispensed in 25-mL aliquots into 25 × 150 mm borosilicate glass culture tubes. Tubes were capped with translucent polypropylene closures (Sigma Chemical Co., St. Louis, MO). Medium was autoclaved for 15 min at 1.05 $kg \cdot cm^{-2}$ at 121 °C. Stocks of shoots of spearmint (*Mentha spicata* L.) were maintained on BM under ambient air prior to testing. For experiments, a single 3-cm long shoot was cultured per vessel. Callus was developed from 1-cm long internodal shoot sections on BM with 0.1 $mg \cdot l^{-1}$ 2,4-dichlorophenoxyacetic acid (2,4-D) and 1.0 $mg \cdot l^{-1}$ benzyl adenine (BA) for 24 weeks. Cultures were transferred to fresh medium every eight weeks. Mint cultivars (cvs.) employed in this study were originally obtained from the U. S. Department of Agriculture, Agricultural Research Service, National Germplasm Repository, Corvallis, Oregon.

CO_2 Flow Systems

The CO_2 flow-through testing chamber consisted of a transparent polycarbonate box and lid (Consolidated Plastics, Twinsburg, OH) (32.5 cm width × 30 cm length × 26.3 cm depth; 17.6-l capacity). A silicone tape gasket (Furon, New Haven, CT) was attached to the lid. The box was modified by mounting three polypropylene spigots (Ark-Plas Products, Flippin, AR) attached to 0.45 µm air vents (Gelman Science, Ann Arbor, MI). The box and lid were clamped with 10 equally spaced stationery binding clips (50 mm length). CO_2 was provided by a gas cylinder (BOC Gases, Edison, NJ) rated 99.8 per cent pure and was mixed with an ambient air (*i.e.*, 350 µmol mol^{-1} CO_2) flow produced by an aquarium air pump (Whisper 2000, Carolina Biological Supply Company, Burlington, NC) via a flow meter (Cole Parmer Instrument Co., Niles, IL) to provide 350, 1,500, 3,000, 10,000, and 30,000 µmol mol^{-1} CO_2. CO_2 ranges ≥ 10,000 µmol mol^{-1} CO_2 were adjusted using a LIRA infrared gas analyzer, (model #3000, Mine Safety Appliances Company, Pittsburgh, PA) and CO_2 ranges ≤ 3,000 µmol mol^{-1} CO_2 were adjusted with a Li-Cor CO_2/H_20 infrared gas analyzer (model LI-6262, Li-Cor, Inc., Lincoln, NE). The CO_2 and air streams were added at 2,000 ml min^{-1} during the photoperiod. Control cultures were given a stream of ambient air generated by the aquarium pump only. No CO_2 or air control was applied during the dark. Culture tubes were measured to have 1.4 h^{-1} air exchanges (Tisserat and Silman, 2000). The time to achieve the given CO_2 concentration employed in this experiment, within the culture tube, required 45 min of gas application and was constantly obtained for the duration of the photoperiod.

Plant Tissue Culture Experiments

Mint callus and shoot cultures from three mint cvs., '294099', '557789' and '557793', were analyzed for their RA content. To determine the influence of exogenous carbohydrate additions on growth and RA production, mint shoots of cvs.'557704' and '557823' were grown on BM with and without 3 per cent sucrose. To determine the influence of PPFD and CO_2 on growth and RA production, shoots of cvs.'557804' were grown on BM with 3 per cent sucrose under either 350 or 10,000 μmol mol^{-1} CO_2 and given 40, 80, 120, or 180 μmol·m^{-2}·s^{-1}. To study the influence of CO_2 on spearmint shoot growth, morphogenesis and secondary metabolism, mint microshoots from cvs. '557807', '557789' and '557793' were cultured on BM with 3 per cent sucrose and given 350, 1,500, 3,000, 10,000, or 30,000 μmol mol^{-1} CO_2. A single 3-cm long shoot was cultured per culture tube. Cultures were grown in a culture room maintained at 25±1 °C and employed at a photoperiod of 16 hr light/8 hr dark. Light was supplied by a combination of Cool white fluorescent tubes at a total PPFD of 120 μmol·m^{-2}·s^{-1} at the vessel periphery, unless otherwise stated.

Statistical Analysis

All experiments were conducted for eight weeks, except for the callus production experiments which were conducted for 24 weeks. Experiments were repeated twice with 20 replications per treatment. Data on fresh weight, leaf number, root number, and shoot number were recorded from five cultures and the remaining cultures were employed in essential oil analysis (*i.e.*, RA). As appropriate, data were analyzed using the REG procedure of the statistical analysis system (SAS Institute, Cary, NC). To calculate the significance of predicted values of experimental parameter and growth, morphogenesis and essential oil responses, 95 per cent confidence intervals were used. For each equation, statistical comparisons of mean predicted × levels were conducted with significant differences attributed to non-overlap of the 95 per cent confidence limits. Secondary metabolic data of shoots and callus from various mint cvs were analyzed by t-test ($P < 0.05$).

Sample Preparation and Extraction

Plants from the culture systems were dried in an oven at 45 °C for 48 hours (Fletcher *et al.*, 2005). Samples were ground to fine powder with mortar and pestle, strained through a number 30 mesh sieves to remove un-ground stem elements. For single step extraction analysis, samples (typically 0.25 g) were placed in a 15 x 45 mm vial (5 cc capacity) and 2 ml of methanol was added. The vials were capped and wrapped with sealing tape, sonicated in a sonic waterbath (Model 2510, Branson, Danbury, CT) at 42 KHz±6 per cent for 15 min at room temperature and allowed to stand at room temperature overnight. An aliquot was removed from the vial and filtered through a 0.45 μm nylon 66 filter for HPLC analysis.

Analytical Methodology

Samples were run on a stand-alone Shimadzu 10A HPLC system (SCL-10A system controller, two LC-10A pumps, CTO-10A column oven, and SIL-10A auto injector). Peaks were monitored using a Hewlett-Packard 1040A photodiode array detector running under the HP Chemstation software version A.02.05. The column used was an Inertsil ODS-3 reverse phase C-18 column (5 μm, 250 x 4.6 mm, with a Metaguard column, from Varian). The initial conditions were 20 per cent methanol and 80 per cent 0.01 M phosphoric acid at a flow rate of 1 ml min^{-1}. The effluent was monitored at 285 nanometer (nm). After injection (15 μl), the column was held at the initial conditions for two minutes, then developed to 100 per cent methanol in a linear gradient over 55 min. A standard curve was prepared from pure RA (Chromadex, Santa Ana, CA) based on absorbance (peak area) versus nM concentration.

LC-ESI-MS Analysis

The presence of RA was confirmed by LC-MS by comparison of retention time and mass spectra. Samples were run on a ThermoFinnigan LCQ DECA XP Plus LC-MS system with a Surveyor HPLC system (autoinjector, pump, degasser, and PDA detector) and a nitrogen generator all running under the Xcaliber 1.3 software system. The MS was run with the ESI probe in the positive mode. The column was a 3 mm x 150 mm Inertsil reverse phase C-18, ODS 3, 3μ column (Varian, Torrance, CA) with a Metaguard guard column. The source inlet temperature was set at 250 °C, the sheath gas rate was set at 70 arbitrary units and the sweep (auxiliary) gas rate was set at 20 arbitrary units. The MS was optimized for the detection of RA by using the autotune feature of the software while infusing a solution of RA standard in with the effluent of the column and tuning on m/z 361 $[M+H]^+$. The initial HPLC conditions were 20 per cent methanol and 0.25 per cent acetic acid in water, at a flow rate of 0.3 ml min^{-1}. The column was then developed to 100 per cent methanol and 0.25 per cent acetic acid over 50 min. The effluent was also monitored at 285 nm on the PDA. The spectra and retention time of the RA in the mint extracts was identical to that of the standard.

Results and Discussion

Influence of Culture Morphology on Secondary Metabolism

Callus cultures had significantly different RA levels than that occurring in foliage from cultured plantlets for each of the three cvs. tested (Table 6.1). RA concentrations in leaves were higher in two cvs. ('294099' and '557789') and lower in one cv. ('557793') compared to that occurring in the callus. These results show that cultured shoots readily express RA secondary metabolism *in vitro*. Both high-yielding and low-yielding RA suspension cultures of rosemary have been described to be derived from a single cv. (Whitaker *et al.*, 1984). Low yielding clones may produce minuscule to no RA while high yielding clones have been shown to produce up to 6.5 per cent RA (Whitaker *et al.*, 1984). In our spearmint studies, we evaluated callus for RA production which exhibited rapid and vigorous growth. Callus and cell suspension from Lamiaceae species require auxin and cytokinin additions to promote cell proliferations and also benefit from inclusion of elicitors to stimulate high RA production (Shetty, 1997; Kim *et al.*, 2001). In contrast, plantlets grown on simple BM without any additives or growth regulators readily expressed high levels of RA. Clearly, it would be difficult to compare RA studies dealing with cell suspension and callus cultures with mint plantlet cultures, since media composition, culture morphology and tested parameters are so dissimilar (De-Eknamkul *et al.*, 1984; Sumaryono *et al.*, 1991; Hippolyte *et al.*, 1992; Shetty, 1997; 2001; Li *et al.*, 2005).

Table 6.1: Comparing RA Production for Three Different Spearmint cvs. Grown in Culture Tubes Containing 25-ml agar BM (shoots) or BM with 0.1 mg·l^{-1} 2,4-D and 1.0 mg·l^{-1} BA (callus) After 24 Weeks, Respectively. RA production data were averaged for 5 replications per treatment. Mean separation for each cultivar and secondary metabolites (rosmarinic acid) by t-test ($P< 0.05$) were conducted. Cultivar RA concentrations with the same letter in the same row are not significantly different.

Cvs.	*Shoot RA (mg/g dwt)*	*Callus RA (mg/g dwt)*
'294099'	5.66±1.04 a	0.47±0.05 b
'557789'	8.81±0.97 a	0.91±0.03 b
'557793'	14.83±0.11 a	18.56±0.13 b

Influence of Sucrose and PFFD Levels

Mint microshoots can survive on BM without sucrose, but grow slowly, and resultant plantlets are more stunted compared to microshoots obtained in BM containing 3 per cent sucrose. For example, mint cv '557804' microshoots cultured on BM without sucrose produced 0.38±0.01 g fresh weight and 0.68±0.09 mg RA/g dwt while shoots on BM with 3 per cent sucrose produced 0.85±0.02 g fresh weight and 1.24±0.07 mg RA/g dwt. Therefore, in later experiments, BM with sucrose was employed in order to obtain the optimum growth and RA production. Similarly, the benefit of increasing sucrose levels on fresh weight and RA production has been shown in cell suspension cultures of *Coleus blumei* (Zenk *et al.*, 1977). The beneficial effect of exogenous sugar in mint plantlets could act through carbon nutrition, genetic signaling or osmotic media modifier.

PPFD levels influences both fresh weights and RA levels (Table 6.2). Microshoots grown under ambient CO_2 levels (*i.e.*, 350 μmol mol^{-1} CO_2) were relatively unaffected in terms of fresh weight and RA content by varying PPFD concentrations, except for the 180 μmol·m^{-2}·s^{-1} level which slightly depressed fresh weight without effecting RA content. When microshoots were cultured under elevated CO_2, (*i.e.*, 10,000 μmol mol^{-1} CO_2) increasing PPFD values caused fresh weight to increase up to 120 μmol·m^{-2}·s^{-1}, and higher PPFD levels caused a decline in fresh weight. Apparently, the elevated CO_2 levels are utilized more efficiently as the PPFD values increase. Although the highest RA values were obtained from plantlets grown under 180 μmol·m^{-2}·s^{-1} with elevated CO_2, fresh weights were only half as much as obtained from plantlets grown under 120 μmol·m^{-2}·s^{-1}. From these results, it was determined that 120 PPFD would be employed in further CO_2 experiments.

Table 6.2: Comparing Growth and RA Production for Spearmint Plants cv. '557704' Grown in Culture Tubes Containing 25-mL agar BM Under Various PFFD Levels with Either 350 or 10,000 μmol mol^{-1} CO_2 After 8 Weeks Incubation. RA data were averaged for 5 replications per treatment. Mean separation for each PPFD level and growth rate or RA by t-test ($P< 0.05$) were conducted. Cultivar fresh weights and RA values with the same letter in the same column are not significantly different.

PPFD	*Fwt. (g)*		*RA (mg/g dwt)*	
	350	*10,000*	*350*	*10,000*
40	0.39±0.03 a	0.98±0.08 a	1.08±0.01 a	3.85±0.03 a
80	0.58±0.08 a	2.06±0.11 b	1.18±0.02 a	4.34±0,05 a
120	0.46±0.03 a	2.78±0.30 b	1.17±0.05 a	6.75±0.18 b
180	0.33±0.03 a	1.30±0.14 a	0.91±0.04 a	8.08±0.09 b

Influence of Carbon Dioxide on Growth, Morphogenesis and Secondary Metabolism

Eight-week exposures to various CO_2 levels significantly affected growth and morphogenesis for all three mint cvs. (Figures 6.1–6.3). Generally, increasing CO_2 concentrations up to 10,000 μmol mol^{-1} CO_2 increased fresh weight, leaf number, root number and shoots. No significant increases for growth and morphogenesis responses of mint plantlets occurred for plants grown under 350 or 1500 μmol mol^{-1} CO_2 compared to that obtained employing 10,000 μmol mol^{-1} CO_2. For example, fresh weights of plantlets, leaf number, root number, and shoots number in mint cv '557793' increased 627 per cent, 369 per cent, 784 per cent, and 31 per cent, respectively, after 8-week exposure to 10,000 μmol mol^{-1} CO_2 over those obtained from plantlets grown under ambient CO_2 (Figure 1). Associated with increasing growth and morphogenesis caused by increasing CO_2 levels was the simultaneous

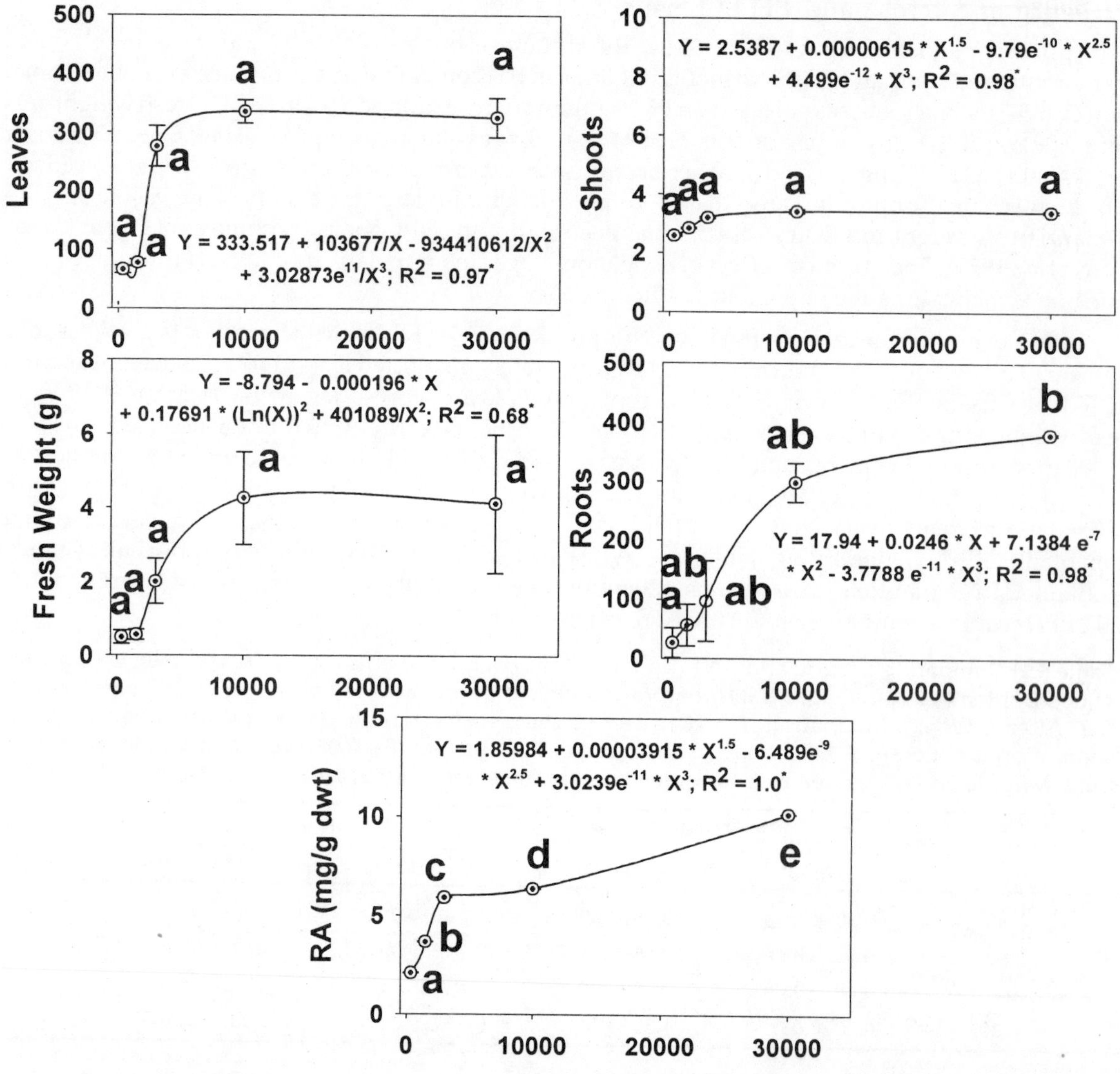

Figure 6.1: Influence of the Carbon Dioxide Concentrations on the Growth, Morphogenesis and RA Concentrations in Spearmint cv. '557793' Plants Cultured in Tubes Containing BM After 8-Weeks. Regression coefficients (R^2) between carbon dioxide concentrations and leaves, shoots, fresh weight, roots, and rosmarinic acid concentrations are given. All regressions were significant at P = 0.05 if denoted by asterisk. Letters represent statistical comparisons of mean predicted carbon dioxide concentrations. Different letters represent non-overlap of the 95 per cent confidence limits.

occurrence of enhanced RA production (Table 6.3; Figures 6.1–6.3). These observations contribute towards our original goal of obtaining high secondary metabolism, coupled with high biomass production, which may be advantageous for potential commercialization. We speculate that when mint plantlets are grown under ultra-high CO_2 levels, enhanced photosynthesis occurs, resulting in

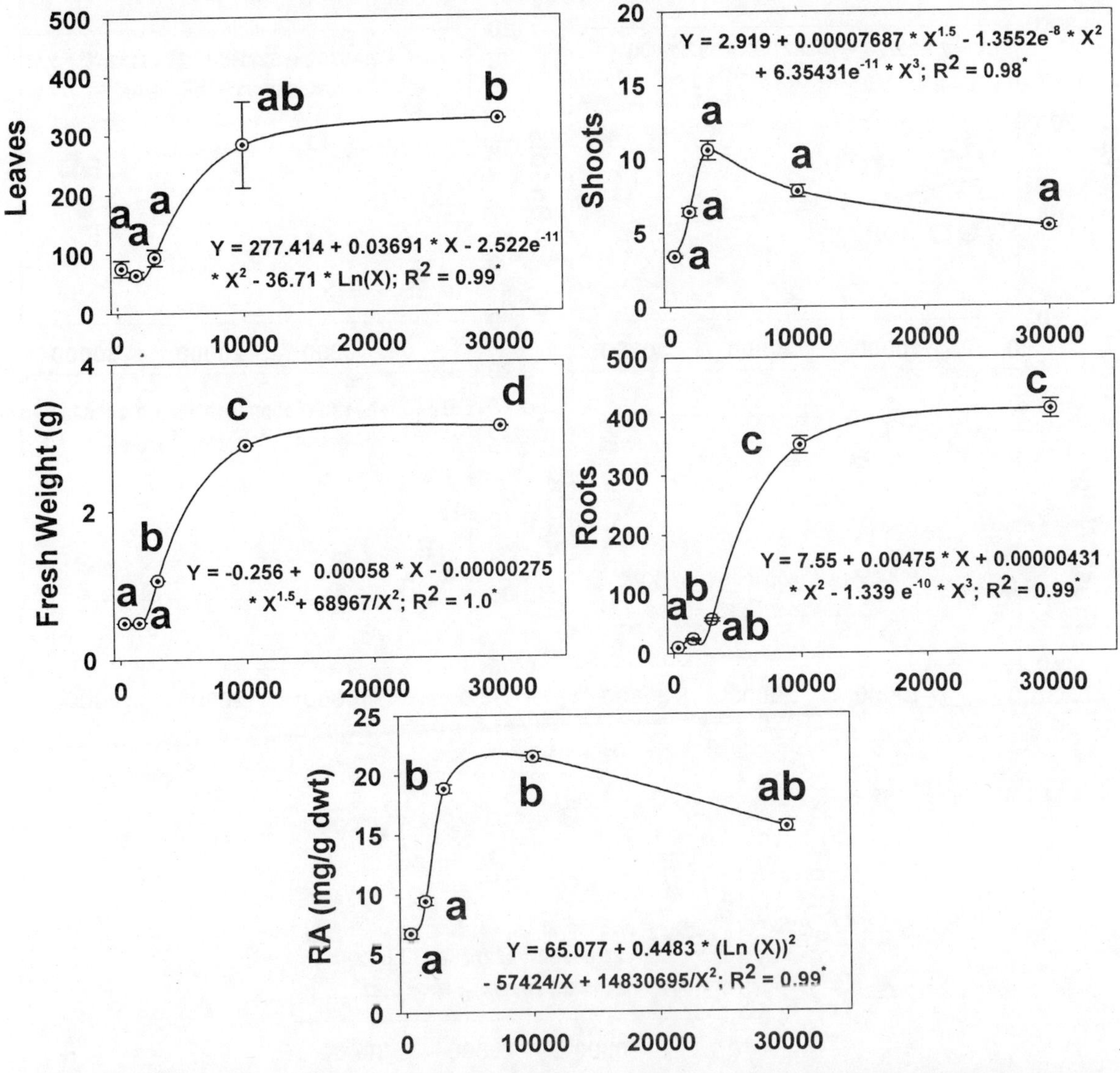

Figure 6.2: Influence of the Carbon Dioxide Concentrations on the Growth, Morphogenesis and RA Concentrations in Spearmint cv. '557789' Plants Cultured in Tubes Containing BM After 8-Weeks. Regression coefficients (R^2) between carbon dioxide concentrations and leaves, shoots, fresh weight, roots, and rosmarinic acid concentrations are given. All regressions were significant at P = 0.05 if denoted by asterisk. Letters represent statistical comparisons of mean predicted carbon dioxide concentrations. Different letters represent non-overlap of the 95 per cent confidence limits.

enhanced primary metabolism, which is physically expressed in higher growth rates and morphogenesis response. In addition, more photosynthetic assimilates are also being channeled at higher levels into various secondary metabolic pathways, such as the shikimic acid and phenylpropanoid pathways, which produce RA. The culture system employed in these experiments

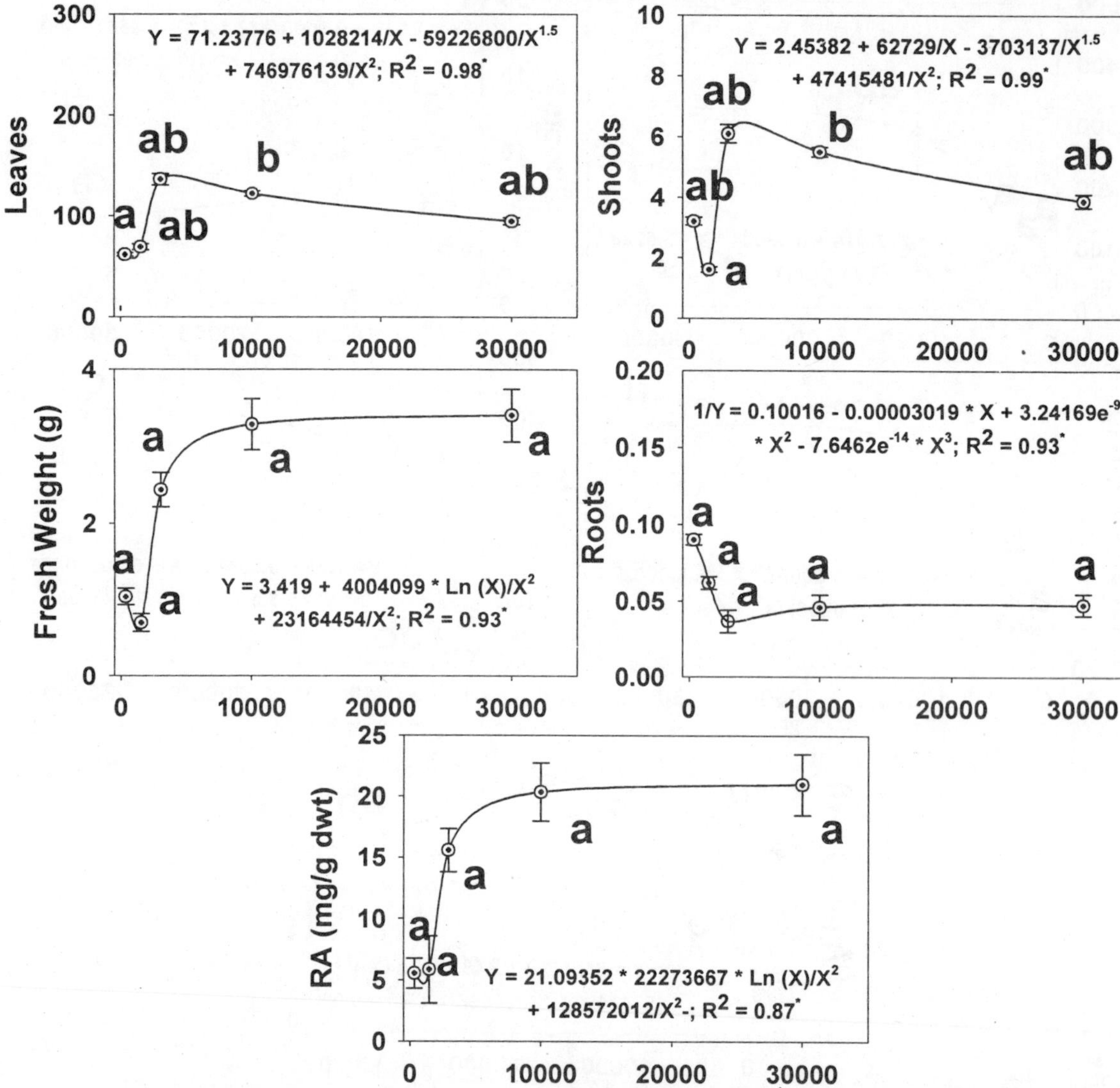

Figure 6.3: Influence of the Carbon Dioxide Concentrations on the Growth, Morphogenesis and RA Concentrations in Spearmint cv. '557807' Plants Cultured in Tubes Containing BM After 8-Weeks. Regression coefficients (R^2) between carbon dioxide concentrations and leaves, shoots, fresh weight, roots, and rosmarinic acid concentrations are given. All regressions were significant at P = 0.05 if denoted by asterisk. Letters represent statistical comparisons of mean predicted carbon dioxide concentrations. Different letters represent non-overlap of the 95 per cent confidence limits.

is relatively simplistic (*i.e.*, culture tubes containing 25 ml BM), yet they are useful for the study of the influence of various chemical and physical environments on plantlets. The addition of growth regulators and complex additives were not needed for either growth or RA expression as in suspension and callus cultures (De-Eknamkul and Ellis, 1984; Sumaryono *et al.*, 1991; Hippolyte *et al.*, 1992; Kim *et al.*, 2001; Karam *et al.*, 2003). It is interesting that plantlets grown on BM containing sucrose grow significantly better and produce higher RA values when supplemented with ultra-high levels of CO_2. This observation follows our work (Tisserat and Vaughn, 2001), where we have shown that CO_2 enhanced the concentrations of volatile monoterpenes produced by the mevalonate pathway. Apparently, in the plantlet culture system, exogenous carbohydrates and enhanced photosynthesis provided by the ultra-high CO_2 applications has a synergistic effect on both primary and secondary metabolism. We have been able to obtain 20 to 25 mg RA/g dwt in mint plantlet on BM under ultra-high CO_2 levels (Figures 6.1–6.3).

Table 6.3: Pearson Correlation Coefficients Values for Growth, Morphogenesis, RA, and Carbon Dioxide Concentrations for Various Mint cvs.[a]

Cvs. and Parameters	*Carbon Dioxide*	*Shoots*	*Leaves*	*Roots*	*Fwt. (g)*
		cv. '557789'			
Carbon dioxide	---	0.083	0.733*	0.858*	0.811*
Shoots	0.083	---	0.022	0.059	0.079
Leaves	0.733*	0.022*	---	0.819*	0.843*
Roots	0.858*	0.059	0.819*	---	0.949*
Fwt. (g)	0.811*	0.079	0.843*	0.949*	---
RA (mg/g dwt)	0.557*	0.649*	0.504	0.598*	0.648*
		cv. '557793'			
Carbon dioxide	---	0.363	0.679*	0.725*	0.729*
Shoots	0.363	---	0.561*	0.509*	0.546*
Leaves	0.679*	0.561*	---	0.946*	0.945*
Roots	0.725*	0.509*	0.946*	---	0.907*
Fwt. (g)	0.729*	0.546*	0.945*	0.907*	---
RA (mg/g dwt)	0.856*	0.555*	0.805*	0.834*	0.854*
		cv. '557807'			
Carbon dioxide	---	0.099	0.126	0.104	0.535*
Shoots	0.099	---	0.664*	0.701*	0.679*
Leaves	0.126	0.664*	---	0.744*	0.764*
Roots	0.104	0.701*	0.744*	---	0.685*
Fwt. (g)	0.535*	0.679*	0.764*	0.685*	---
RA (mg/g dwt)	0.577*	0.599*	0.814*	0.689*	0.825*

a: Values with asterisks were significant at P = 0.05. Observations: Carbon dioxide parameters, 25; Leaves, 25; Shoots, 25; Fwt. (g), 25; Roots, 25; RA, 15.

In this study we employed several different mint cultivars to test the parameters associated with ultra-high CO_2 on primary and secondary metabolism; our philosophy in doing this was to demonstrate that the response obtained were universal in various mint cultivars. Research needs to be continued in order to develop a viable commercial plantlet culture system. Obviously, single plantlets grown in single containers are not commercially viable due to their spatial requirements; but they have been useful bioassay study systems to explore important parameters that would enhance secondary metabolism. Continued effort should be addressed to understand how plantlet systems may express high secondary metabolism coupled with high biomass production. Once these parameters are understood, efforts should then be directed to the establishment of mass proliferating plantlet clumps or batches which are capable of manifesting the basic morphology and biochemistry of the plant. These systems could then employ ultra-high CO_2 levels with exogenous carbohydrates to obtain concentrations of high secondary metabolites.

Acknowledgements

The authors wish to thank R. Holloway, S. Tisserat and T. Tisserat for technical assistance in RA analysis. Names are necessary to report factually on available data; however, the USDA neither guarantees nor warrants the standard of the product, and the use of the name by USDA implies no approval of the product to the exclusion of others that may also be suitable.

References

Arda N., Goren N., Kuru A., Pengsuparp T., Pezzuto J.M., Qiu S.X., and Cordell G.A. (1997). Saniculoside N from *Sanicula europaea* L. *Journal of Natural Products*, 60:1170-1173.

De-Eknamkul W. and Ellis B.E. (1984). Rosmarinic acid production and growth characteristics of *Anchusa officinalis* cell suspension cultures. *Planta Medica*, 51:346-350.

Ellis, B.I. (1985). Characterization of clonal cultures of *Anchusa officinalis* derived from single cells of known productivity. *Journal of Plant Physiology*, 19:149-158.

Fletcher, R.S., Slimmon T., McAuley Y., and Kott L.S. (2005). Heast stress reduces the accumulation of rosmarinic acid and total antioxidant capacity in spearmint (*Mentha spicata* L.). *Journal of Science and Food Agriculture*, 85:2429-2436.

Hippolyte I., Marin B., Baccou J.C., and Jonard R. (1992). Growth and rosmarinic acid production in cell suspension cultures of *Salvia officinalis* L. *Plant Cell Reports*, 11:109-112.

Kang M.-A., Yun S.-Y., and Won J. (2003) Rosmarinic acid inhibits Ca^{2+}-dependent pathways of T-cell antigen receptor-mediated signaling by inhibiting the PLC-γ1 and Itk activity. *Blood*, 101:3534-3542.

Karam N.S., Jawad F.M., Arikat N.A., and Shibli R.A. (2003). Growth and rosmarinic acid accumulation in callus, cell suspension, and root cultures of wild *Salvia fruticosa*. *Plant Cell, Tissue and Organ Culture*, 73:117-121.

Kim H.K., Oh S.–R., Lee H.–K., and Huh, H. (2001). Benzothiadiazole enhances the elicitation of rosmarinic acid production in a suspension culture of *Agastache rugosa* O. Kuntze. *Biotechnology Letters*, 23:55-60.

Li W., Koike K., Asada Y., Yoshikawa T., and Nikaido T. (2005) Rosmarinic acid production of *Coleus forskohlii* hairy root cultures. *Plant Cell, Tissue and Organ Culture*, 80:151-155.

Mitra A., Khan B.M., and Rawal S.K. (1997) Photoautotrophic shoot culture: an economical alternative for the production of total alkaloid from *Cartharanthus roseus* (L.) G. Don. *Current Science*, 73:608-609.

Murashige T. and Skoog, F. (1962) A revised medium for rapid growth and bioassays with tobacco tissue cultures. *Physiologia Plantarum*, 15:473-497.

Nogueira J.M.F. and Romano A. (2002). Essential oils from micropropagated plants of *Lavandula viridis*. *Photochemistry Analysis*, 13:4-7.

Petersen M.S. (1991). Characterization of rosmarinic acid synthase from cell cultures of *Coleus blumei*. *Phytochemistry*, 30:2877-2881.

Shetty K. (1997). Biotechnology to harness the benefits of dietary phenolics; focus in Lamiaceae. *Asia Pacific Journal of Clinical Nutrition*, 6:162-171.

Shetty K. (2001). Biosynthesis and medical applications of rosmarinic acid. *Journal of Herbs, Spices and Medicinal Plants*, 8:161-192.

Sumaryono W., Proksch, P., Hartmann T., Nimtz M., and Wray V. (1991). Induction of rosmarinic acid accumulation in cell suspension cultures of *Orthosiphon aristatus* after treatment with yeast extract. *Phytochemistry*, 30:3267-3271.

Takano H., Osakabe N., Sanbongi C., Yanagisawa R., Inoue K.-I., Yasuda A., Natsume M., Baba S., Ichishi E.-I., and Yoshidawa T. (2004). Extract of *Perilla frutescens* enriched for rosmarinic acid, a polyphenolic phytochemical, inhibits seasonal allergic rhioconjunctivitis in humans. *Experimental Biological Medicine*, 229:247-254.

Tisserat B. and Silman R. (2000). Interactions of culture vessels, media volume, culture density, and carbon dioxide levels on lettuce and spearmint shoot growth in vitro. *Plant Cell Reports*, 19:464-471.

Tisserat B., Vaughn S., and Silman R. (2002). Influence of modified oxygen and carbon dioxide atmospheres on mint and thyme plant growth, morphogenesis and secondary metabolism in vitro. *Plant Cell Reports*, 20:912-916.

Tisserat B. and Vaughn S.F. (2001). Essential oils enhanced by ultra-high carbon dioxide levels from Lamiaceae species grown in vitro and in vivo. *Plant Cell Reports*, 20:361-368.

Whitaker R.J., Hashimoto T., and Evans D.A. (1984). Production of the secondary metabolite, rosmarinic acid, by plant cell suspension cultures. *Annals of the New York Academy of Science*, 435:364-368.

Yang R., and Shetty K. (1998). Stimulation of rosmarinic acid in shoot cultures of oregano (*Origanum vulgare*) clonal line in response to proline, proline analog and proline precursors. J *Agricultural Food Chemistry*, 46:2888-2893.

Zenk M., El-Shagi H., and Ulbrich B. (1977) Production of rosmarinic acid by cell suspension cultures of *Coleus blumei*. *Naturwissenschaften*, 64:585-586.

Abbreviations

BA: Benzyl adenine; BM: Basal medium, Murashige and Skoog salts with 3 per cent sucrose; CO_2: Carbon dioxide; HPLC: High pressure liquid chromatography; LC-MS: Liquid chromatography-mass spectroscopy; 2,4-D: 2,4-dichlorophenoxyacetic acid.

Utilisation and Management of Medicinal Plants (2010) *Pages 136–156*
Editors: **V.K. Gupta, Anil K. Verma and Sushma Koul**
Published by: **DAYA PUBLISHING HOUSE, NEW DELHI**

Chapter 7

Approaches for Enhancing Yield of Artemisinin: A Novel Antimalarial Compound, in *Artemisia annua* L. Plants

M.Z. Abdin[1]*, Mauji Ram[1], Usha Kiran[2] and M.A. Khan[1]
[1]Centre for Transgenic plant Development, Department of Biotechnology, Faculty of Science, Jamia Hamdard, New Delhi – 110 062, India
[2]Faculty of Interdisciplinary Research Studies, Jamia Hamdard, New Delhi – 110 062, India

ABSTRACT

Malaria is probably as old as mankind and continues to affect millions of people throughout the world. Today some 500 million people in Africa, India, South East Asia and South America are exposed to endemic malaria and it is estimated to cause two and half million deaths annually, one million of which are children. As a consequence, effective therapeutic agents against malaria are continuously being sought, especially against those strains of *P. falciparum*, which have become resistant to nearly all antimalarial drugs, including chloroquine and quinine. In absence of reports of artemisinin resistance in malaria parasite, WHO now recommends the use of Artemisinin based Combination Therapies (ACTs) with formulations containing an artemisinin derivative. Artemisinin, a sesquiterpene endoperoxide lactone, is isolated from the shoots of *Artemisia annua* L. plants. Apart from a novel and potent antimalarial drug, artemisinin and its derivatives are also used in therapies against hepatitis, leismaniasis and schistosomiasis. Artemisinin also possess lethal activities against cancerous cells, fungi and bacteria. It has also shown to be immune-suppressant in mammals and a potent herbicide.

* Corresponding Author: E-mail: mzabdin@rediffmail.com.

Despite of its immense commercial value, the production of artemisinin is not cost effective because of its low concentration (0.01-1.1 per cent) in the plant. Moreover, its *de novo* synthesis is complex, uneconomical and gives low yields. Further, classical breeding and selection techniques have failed to develop high yielding strains of *Artemisia annua* L. plants. Efforts are therefore, needed to elucidate the complex pathway of artemisinin biosynthesis and its biochemical and molecular regulation. Non conventional approaches have to be developed to evolve novel strains of the plant to optimize and scale-up the production of artemisinin in bulk and make it available to ACT manufacturers at a price much lower than their current cost in turn making an important contribution towards attaining the goals of global malaria eradication programs. The details of past and current status of both conventional and non-conventional approaches for enhancing artemisinin content in *Artemisia annua* L. plants and its yield have been discussed in this chapter.

***Keywords**: Malaria, Artemisinin, Artemisia annuna, Non conventional approaches.*

Introduction

Being the world's most severe parasitic infection, malaria caused more than a million deaths and 500 million cases annually. Despite tremendous efforts for the control of malaria, the global morbidity and mortality have not been significantly changed in the 50 years (Reley, 1995). The key problem is the failure to find effective medicines against malaria. Obtained from a Chinese medicinal plant *Artemisia annua* L., artemisinin, a sesquiterpene lactone containing an endoperoxide bridge, has become increasingly popular as an effective and safe alternative therapy against malaria (Luo and Shen, 1987). Artemisinin and its derivative are effective against multi-drug resistant *Plasmodium falciparum* strain mainly in Southeast Asia and more recently in Africa, without any reported cases of resistance (Mohapatra *et al.*, 1996; Krishana *et al.*, 2004).

A. annua is a cosmopolitan species, growing wild in many countries, *e.g.* in China and Vietnam, the Balkan, the former Soviet Union, Argentina and Southern Europe (Van Geldre *et al.*, 1997), and large differences exist in artemisinin content between different varieties of *A. annua* (Delabays *et al.*, 1993; Woerdenbag *et al.*, 1993). A substantial increase in the content of artemisinin would be required to make artemisinin available on a large scale also to the people in the Third World. Selection for high-producing lines and traditional breeding, and research on the effects of environmental conditions and cultural practices could perhaps lead to an improvement of artemisinin content (Delabays *et al.*, 1993; Ferreira *et al.*, 1995; Gupta *et al.*, 1996).

Artemisinin, a sesquiterpene-lactone isolated from the aerial parts of *Artemisia annua* L. plants. Besides being currently the best therapeutic agent against both drug-resistant and cerebral malaria causing strains of *Plasmodium* sp. (Newton and White, 1999). It is also effective against other infectious diseases such as Schistosomiasis, hepatitis B and Leishmaniasis (Borrmann *et al.*, 2001; Utzinger *et al.*, 2001; Romero *et al.*, 2005 and Sen *et al.*, 2007). More recently, it has also been shown to be effective against a variety of cancer cell lines including breast cancer, human leukemia, colon cancer and small cell-lung carcinomas (Efferth *et al.*, 2001; Singh and Lai, 2001). Due to its current use in artemisinin based-combination therapy (ACT), its global demand continuously is increasing. The relatively low yield of artemisinin in *A. annua* L. plant leaves (0.01-0.8 per cent) is however, a serious limitation to the commercialization of the drug (Van Agtmael *et al.*, 1999; Laughlin *et al.*, 1994; Abdin *et al.*, 2003).

Artemisinin (qinghaosu), an unusual sesquiterpene-lactone endoperoxide from *Artemisia annua* L., is an effective antimalarial drug, particularly against chloroquine-resistant *Plasmodium falciparum* infection and cerebral malaria. Artemisinin and its semisynthetic analogues have undergone clinical trials as new life saving antimalarials under the auspices of the World Health Organization and have been intensively studied due to their unique structure, with an endoperoxide (1,2,4-trioxane) linkage, their novel mechanism of action as the first non-nitrogenous antimalarial, and the worldwide resurgence of drug-resistant falciparum infections. The state-of-the-art of production of artemisinin by chemical and biotechnological methods and analytical aspects has recently been reviewed. Five different approaches have been employed to increase artemisinin content in the plant including conventional breeding, biochemical, physiological and molecular approaches, hairy root culture techniques, for the artemisinin biosynthetic pathway in *A. annua* L. (Abdin *et al.*, 2003; Martin *et al.*, 2003; Ro *et al.*, 2006; Liu *et al.*, 1999; Smith *et al.*, 1997; Wang *et al.*, 2002; Zeng *et al.*, 2007; Chang *et al.*, 2000; Newman *et al.*, 2006; Weathers *et al.*, 2005; Picaud *et al.*, 2005; Wallaart *et al.*, 2001). Chemical synthesis has also been attempted (Xu *et al.*, 1986; Avery *et al.*, 1992), but the yield of artemisinin is very low. Thus, it is economically not viable for the large-scale production of artemisinin. Two genes of artemisinin biosynthesis pathway (Fernasyl Diphosphate Synthase and Amorpha-4, 11-diene synthase) were over expressed (Han *et el.*, 2006; Ping *et al.*, 2008) and artemisinin content was increased by 34.4 per cent.

Agrotechnology

Artemisia annua (family Asteraceae), also known as qinghao (Chinese), annual or sweet wormwood, or sweet Annie, is an annual herb native to Asia, most probably China (McVaugh, 1984). *Artemisia annua* occurs naturally as part of the steppe vegetation in the northern parts of Chahar and Suiyuan provinces (408N, 1098E) in Northern China (now incorporated into Inner Mongolia), at 1000–1500m above sea level (Wang, 1961). The plant now grows wild in many countries, such as Argentina, Bulgaria, France, Hungary, Romania (cultivated for its essential oil), Italy, Spain, USA and former Yugoslavia (Klayman *et al.*, 1989, 1993). In addition, it has been introduced into experimental cultivation in India (Singh *et al.*, 1986), Vietnam, Thailand, Myanmar, Madagascar, Malaysia, USA, Brazil, Australia (Tasmania) and in Europe into the Netherlands, Switzerland, France and as far north as Finland (Laughlin *et al.*, 2002).

Artemisia annua is a xeromorphic temperate plant belonging to Asteraceae family that contains promising antimalarial drugs, the sesquiterpene lactone artemisinin and derivatives of this compound. An examination of the growth and flowering behavior of *Artemisia annua* in the subtropical climate region of India demonstrated the plant grew normally and flowered profusely in the winter cropping season, late October to late April, at Lucknow, India. Considerable inter-plant variation was observed, however, in growth habit and flowering time. Plants could be grouped into four classes: early maturing dwarf, early maturing tall, late maturing dwarf, and late maturing tall. Early maturing plants which flowered in February and March, produced fertile achenes, completing the life cycle in 7 to 8 months. Late flowering plants that flowered in May and June, when the maximum day temperature was over 40°C, produced florets without seeds. The high temperature conditions to which the late flowering plants were exposed, appeared to prematurely dry the stigma. Late flowering plants sprouted branches from the vegetative and flowering parts of the plant during the rainy season.

A. annua appears to be the only *Artemisia* species that contain appreciable amounts of artemisinin. Chinese scientists have reported that extracts from 30 other different species of *Artemisia* did not show anti-malarial activity (UNDP/World Bank/WHO special programme for Research and Training in

Tropical Diseases *Artemisia* species, 1981), American Scientist have failed to detect artemisinin in various species endemic to America (Klayman *et al.*, 1984). In India, Balachandran *et al.* (1987) also did not find artemisinin in various *Artemisia* species of Indian origin. Considering the importance of artemisinin which is tedious and difficult to synthesize chemically, an all out programme was undertaken to develop *Artemisia annua* plant varieties with high artemisinin content starting with development of agro technology for increased yield of these compounds, followed by improved extraction procedure. More particularly, the program focused on agro-technology involving method of optimizing the planting time, transplanting scheduling, population density, number of harvests and harvesting schedule leading to enhanced yields of artemisinin and related metabolites which have pharmaceutical value of anti-infectives, particularly as antimalarial drug. In this direction the inventors were successful in developing and releasing a variety named "Jeevan Raksha" from an isolated population containing high artemisinin in the foliage (0.5 to 1.0 per cent) (Kumar *et al.*,1999). This plant "Jeevan Raksha" not only produces high artemisinin but also maintains the synchronized conversion to higher level of artemisinin during May to October. As the content of artemisinin fluctuates from zero level at the time of planting to more than 0.4 to 1.00 per cent during May and June with subsequent functions of increase till October, it was necessary to scientifically develop cultivation methodology for the crop to maximize the vigour of the foliage and biosynthesis of artemisinin by systematic scheduling. For this purpose the inventors carried out planned experiments with variation in planting times, population density and number of harvest from the crop to increase the yield from limited area within optimum span of time. Until now, artemisinin production has depended on extraction from *A. annua* L. plants grown outdoors. There are two methods to enhance artemisinin production in intact *A. annua* plants. One method is to define the appropriate developmental stage at which to harvest the leaves of the plants. At this developmental stage, both the highest artemisinin content and leaves yielding can be obtained. The other method is to breed high artemisinin yielding strains.

Biochemical and Physiological Approach

Although artemisinin is an effective medicine for treating malaria, the application of this medicine is limited by the availability of the source. The artemisinin content in the leaves or florets of *A. annua* is very low, and the chemical method for the synthesis of this compound is difficult. These factors make the medicine expensive and hardly available on a global scale for patients (Geldre *et al.*, 1997; Abdin *et al.*, 2003). Despite the commercial value of artemisinin, exact biosynthetic pathway of artemisinin in *Artemisia annua*, particularly about the early enzymatic steps leading to (dihydro) artemisinic acid. Several authors have demonstrated that *A. annua* converts artemisinic acid and dihydroartemisinic acid to artemisinin (Sangwan *et al.*, 1993a; Wallaart *et al.*, 1999b). Akhila *et al.* (1990) hypothesized a pathway in which the formation from FDP of an unidentified enzyme-bound sesquiterpene-like intermediate represents the first committed step in the biosynthesis of artemisinin. In addition, many authors have analysed extracts of *A. annua* to search for possible intermediates in the biosynthesis of artemisinin. Artemisinic and dihydroartemisinic acid were reported by many authors, as well as many olefinic mono–and sesquiterpenes and putative intermediates *en route* from dihydroartemisinic acid to artemisinin (Brown, 1994; Jung *et al.*, 1990; Ranasinghe *et al.*, 1993; Wallaart *et al.*, 1999b; Woerdenbag *et al.*, 1993). However, none of the reported olefinic sesquiterpenes seemed to fit in the biosynthetic pathway, nor was a possible intermediate between the sesquiterpene olefin and artemisinic acid ever detected, with the exception of artemisinic alcohol, which was tentatively identified in the roots of *A. annua* (Woerdenbag *et al.*, 1993). It has been shown by several groups that the cyclization of the ubiquitous precursors geranyl diphosphate, farnesyl diphosphate (FDP) and geranyl diphosphate to the respective olefinic mono-, sesqui–and diterpene skeletons represents the regulatory step in the biosynthesis of terpenoids (Gershenzon and Croteau, 1990; McGarvey and Croteau 1995). The accumulation of artemisinic acid and dihydroartemisinic acid and the absence of any intermediates en route from FDP to these two compounds support that the first step(s) in the biosynthetic pathway of artemisinin [and again some step(s) from (dihydro) artemisinic acid to artemisinin] are indeed regulatory/rate-limiting. Here we describe the elucidation of the unknown four intermediates and the corresponding five enzymatic steps that constitute the first part of the artemisinin biosynthetic pathway. The implications for strategies to improve artemisinin production are discussed. Chemical synthesis of artemisinin is an expensive multistep process; the plant remains the only commercial source of the drug.

In our biosynthetic studies on artemisinin toward purification of endoperoxidase enzyme from *A. annua*, and determination of the source of the endoperoxide Oxygen Bridge by ^{18}O-isotope labeling in plant cell-free and tissue culture, we required an experimental method suitable for direct detection, quantitation, and isotopomeric analysis since artemisinin is unstable and lacks a chromophore for UV detection in HPLC.

Alternatively, the C11-C13 double-bond reduction may occur in artemisinic alcohol or artemisinic aldehyde, yielding dihydroartemisinic alcohol or dihydroartemisinic aldehyde as intermediates, respectively. To study this unknown part of the pathway, we analysed the presence of putative intermediates and enzymes involved in the conversion of these intermediates in leaves and glandular-trichome extracts of *A. annua*. Hereto first a number of reference compounds such as artemisinic alcohol, dihydroartemisinic alcohol, artemisinic aldehyde and dihydroartemisinic aldehyde were synthesized using artemisinic acid and dihydroartemisinic acid as starting materials or isolated (artemisinic aldehyde). The structures of all isolated or synthesized compounds were confirmed using NMR and MS (Bertea *et al.*, 2005). Subsequently, we looked for these compounds in extracts of *A. annua* leaves as well as in extracts of isolated trichomes. The chromatograms obtained with these two extracts were very similar, indicating that most (if not all) of *A. annua* terpenoids are present in the trichomes. In both cases, artemisinic alcohol, artemisinic aldehyde, artemisinic acid, dihydroartemisinic alcohol, dihydroartemisinic aldehyde, dihydroartemisinic acid and a series of olefinic terpenes were detected (Bertea *et al.*, 2005). Artemisinic acid, dihydroartemisinic acid and the sesquiterpene olefins have been reported before as constituents of *A. annua* (Bouwmeester *et al.*, 1999a; Wallaart *et al.*, 1999b) but this was the first time artemisinic alcohol, artemisinic aldehyde, dihydroartemisinic alcohol and dihydroartemisinic aldehyde have been identified in *A. annua*. In enzyme assays with microsomal pellets of *A. annua* leaf extracts, using amorpha-4, 11-diene as a substrate and in the presence of NADPH, we found a small, but consistent amorpha-4, 11-diene hydroxylase activity which was absent in the soluble protein fraction (150,000*g* supernatant), confirming that a cytochrome-P450 enzyme catalyses the formation of artemisinic alcohol from amorpha-4, 11-diene. The next putative enzymatic step was assayed by incubating a mixture of artemisinic alcohol and dihydroartemisinic alcohol with the 150,000 g young-leaf supernatant in the presence of $NAD^+/NADP^+$ at pH 9.0. In the presence of cofactors, the ratio between artemisinic alcohol and dihydroartemisinic alcohol strongly decreased showing that artemisinic alcohol was converted to artemisinic aldehyde, dihydroartemisinic aldehyde and dihydroartemisinic acid (Bertea *et al.*, 2005). None of these intermediates were formed in the absence of cofactors. Artemisinic acid was not detected in any of these experiments. To test whether the conversion of dihydroartemisinic aldehyde to dihydroartemisinic acid that was observed in leaf extracts also occurred in trichomes, we incubated the 150,000*g* supernatant of the glandular trichomes with dihydroartemisinic aldehyde in the presence of $NAD^+/NADP^+$. Under these conditions we detected conversion of dihydroartemisinic aldehyde into dihydroartemisinic acid, whereas conversion did not occur in the absence of cofactors.

Artemisinin was first isolated from the aerial parts of *A. annua* by the Chinese scientists and later characterized by others. But, the details of isolation procedure were not published for long time (reviewed by Klayman, 1985). The researchers at the Walter Reed Army Institute of Research, USA spotted some *A.annua* growing in the neighbourhood of Washington D.C. and extracted its various air-dried parts with a number of apolar organic solvents. The petroleum ether extraction proved most satisfactory for the isolation of artemisinin and its derivatives (Klayman, 1985).

Artemisinin has been reported to accumulate in leaves, small green stems, buds, flowers and seeds (Acton *et al.*, 1985; Ferreira *et al.*, 1995. Liersch *et al.*, 1986; Martinez and Staba, 1988). Its content was found more in leaves and inflorescence, but neither artemisinin nor its precursors were detected in roots (Trigg, 1990; Charles *et al.*, 1990). Duke *et al.* (1994) showed that artemisinin is sequestered in glandular trichome of *A. annua*. Artemisinin content in full bloomed flowers was 4-5 times higher than in leaves (Ferreria *et al.*, 1995). The artemisinin yield estimated at different steps of development reveals a possible correlation between plant age and artemisinin content. This is assumed to be due to both an increase in leaf yield and artemisinin content with the progressive increase in plant growth (Singh *et al.*, 1988). Our own observations have revealed that the artemisinin content was highest at full vegetative stage. Some researchers reported that artemisinin content is highest just prior to flowering (Acton and Klayman, 1985, ElSholy *et al.*, 1990, Liersch *et al.*, 1986, Woerdenbag *et al.*, 1991, 1993); others found an artemisinin peak at full flowering stage (Morales *et al.*, 1993; Pras *et al.*, 1990; Singh *et al.*, 1986).

Artemisinin yields reported from plants in China range from 0.01 to 0.5 per cent (w/w), varieties growing in Siachuan Province showing the highest content. Klayman *et al.* (1984) reported 0.06 per cent (w/w) yield form *A. annua* growing wild in Washington D.C. Other reports claim the yield to be 0.09-0.17 per cent (Liersch *et al.*, 1986; Singh *et al.*, 1986; UNDP/World bank/WHO special program for research/Training in Tropical Diseases 1986). The yields of the related sesquiterpenes *i.e.* artemisinic acid and arteannuin B also show variation in their contents. In USA, artemisinic acid content is 8-10 times more than the artemisinin (Jung *et al.*, 1990; Roth and Acton, 1987) followed by arteannuin B (Klaymna, 1993). In India the yield of arteannuin B (0.27 per cent) is relatively higher than the other two sesquiterpenes (Singh *et al.*, 1986; Gulati *et al.*, 1996a).

A study on effect of levels of nitrogen (0,50 and 100 kg ha^{-1}) phosphorus (0 and 50 kg ha^{-1}) and potassium (0 and 50 kg ha^{-1}) on growth, oil and artemisinin yield revealed that application of 50 and 100 kgN/ha increased herbage, oil and artemisinin yield by 26.2 and 40.1 per cent, respectively compared with control (no nitrogen) (Singh, 2000). The influence of micro-nutrient imbalance on growth and artemisinin contents shows that *A. annua* was very sensitive to boron (B) deficiency. Boron deficient plants did not show flowering and there was approximately 50 per cent reduction in artemisinin content. Similarly artemisinin content declined by 25-30 per cent in Fe, Mn, Zn and Cu deficient plants (Srivastava, 1990). Effect of plant growth regulators on yield, oil composition and artemisinin content of *A. annua* under temperate condition was studied in 1998 by Yaseen. Foliar application of IAA at 100 ppm produced significantly higher herb and oil yields than the control, due to increase in plant height, leaf/stem ratio and oil content, and delayed leaf senescence. Although the Artemisia ketone in the oil was highest following application of GA_3 and IAA at 150 ppm, the artemisinin content was higher in the plants treated with 6 ppm triacontanol. Effect of bio-regulators, chlormequat and triacontanol, was studied for artemisinin content, growth parameters and leaf yield. Plants treated with chlormequat were found to have more herbage yield, but the effect of higher dose was not statistically significant (Shukla *et al.*, 1992). Level of ABA in chlormequat treated plants was higher than in control plants, whereas treatment with triacontanol lowered the abscisic acid level. On the contrary, application of triacontanol increased the level of endogenous GA_3 like components while chlormequat caused reduction in their concentration. According to Liersch *et al.* (1986) chlormequat was able to increase the artemisinin contents by 30 per cent. Local climatic conditions, season of harvesting as well as the post harvest handling seem to play an important role in the levels of artemisinin content (Chen *et al.*, 1987; Ferrieta *et al.*, 1995; Martinez and Staba, 1988; Singh *et al.*, 1986). The time of planting seem to play an important role on the yield of essential oils and artemisinin in *A. annua*. Plants planted between September and December produced significantly higher herbage yields (on the basis of fresh weight and dry weight) as compared with that of plants planted in February. Plants planted in September produced the highest amount of artemisinin. Plants established during pre-winter (August-September) and allowed to grow through the entire winter synthesized and accumulated more artemisinin than plants established during early (October-November) and late (February) winter periods. It was concluded that the artemisinin content was dependent on the weather conditions (Muni Ram *et al.*, 1997). Environmental stress, such as light, temperature, water and salt significantly alter artemisinin yields (Weathers *et al.*, 1994; Wallaart *et al.*, 2000).

Genetic studies on *A. annua* have confirmed that the diploid plants are 2n= 18 (CIMAP India, 1986-87). The average artemisinin level in tetraploids was 38 per cent higher than that of the wild type (diploid) as measured over the whole vegetation period (Wallaart *et al.*, 1999). A hybrid form of *A. annua* was successfully cultivated in Central Africa. The aerial parts of the plants contained 0.63-0.7 per cent artemisinin on dry weight basis (Mueller *et al.*, 2000).

Biotechnological Production of Artemisinin

The commercial sources of most artemisinin are from field grown leaves and flowering tops of *A. annua*, which are subjected to seasonal and somatic variation and infestation of bacteria, fungi, and insects that can affect the functional medicinal content of this plant (Klayman, 1985; Luo and Shen, 1987). The total organic synthesis is very complicated with low yields, and economically unattractive (Avery *et al.*, 1992; Xu *et al.*, 1986). In view of these problems, artemisinin production from *in vitro* plant tissue culture has been considered as an attractive alternative. The biosynthesis of artemisinin was studied in the calli, suspension cells, shoots, and hairy roots of *A. annua* during their cultivation *in vitro* (He *et al.*, 1983; Tawfiq *et al.*, 1989; Weathers *et al.*, 1994; Paniego and Giulietti, 1996; Liu *et al.*, 1997; Nair *et al.*, 1986; Teo *et al.*, 1995). A certain degree of differentiation of *A. annua* tissue cultures is a prerequisite for the synthesis of artemisinin. Paniego and Giuletti (1994) reported that no artemisinin was found in cell suspension cultures of *A. annua*, whereas trace amounts were found in the multiple shoot cultures. Woerdenbag *et al.* (1993) reported a high percentage of artemisinin content in *A. annua* shoots cultured on 1/2 MS medium supplemented with 0.05 mg/l naphthaleneacetic acid, 0.2 mg/l benzyladenine (BA), and 2 per cent sucrose. The flowering of *A. annua* was observed *in vitro* by supplementing with gibberellic acid (GA_3) where artemisinin content reached 0.1 per cent in *A. annua* plantlets, and the highest artemisinin content in the plantlets was observed in full bloom (Gulati *et al.*, 1996). Most groups did not find artemisinin in root part of *A. annua* plant. However, artemisinin content in the shoot part of cultured plantlet was higher than that in the cultured shoots without roots (Ferreira and Janick, 1996; Martinez and Staba, 1988). Attempts were also made to improve the artemisinin production by optimizing chemical and physical environmental factors. Wang and Tan (2002) reported the influence of the ratio of NO_3/NH_4 and total initial nitrogen concentration on the artemisinin yield in hairy roots. With the ratio of NO_3/NH_4 at 5:1(w/w), the optimum concentration of total nitrogen for artemisinin production was 20 mM. Under this concentration, artemisinin production was 57 per cent higher than that in the standard MS medium. Weathers' research group investigated the effects of media sterilization method and types of sugar on growth and artemisinin accumulation of *A. annua* hairy roots. They found that biomass from filter-sterilized medium was greater than that from autoclaved medium, but artemisinin accumulation from filter-sterilized medium was less than that from autoclaved medium. Growth of hairy roots in the medium with sucrose (3.99 g DW/l) was equivalent to the growth in the medium with fructose (3.75 g DW/l) and significantly better than in the medium with glucose (2.16 g DW/l), while the roots that grew in glucose showed a dramatic stimulation in artemisinin content which is three–and twofold higher than that in medium with sucrose and fructose (Weathers *et al.*, 2004). Casein hydrolysate, a source of amino acids and oligopeptides, at low concentration enhances artemisinin production in *A. annua* shoot cultures (Woerdenbag *et al.*, 1993). A combination of BA and kinetin increased the yields of artemisinin in cultured shoots by 3.6 and 2.6 fold (Whipkey *et al.*, 1992). GA3, a plant hormone that can induce blooming, has been reported to improve growth and artemisinin biosynthesis in shoot cultures, root cultures, and plantlets of *A. annua* (Fulzele *et al.*, 1995; Charles *et al.*, 1990; Smith *et al.*, 1997; Weathers *et al.*, 2005). The effects of light irradiation on growth and production of artemisinin were studied in hairy root cultures of *A. annua* L. by Liu *et al.* (2002). They found that when the hairy roots were cultured under illumination of 3,000 lx for 16 h using several cool-white fluorescent lamps, the dry weight and artemisinin concentration reached 13.8 g/l and 244.5 mg/l, respectively (Liu *et al.*, 2002). Wang *et al.* (2001) investigated the dependence of biomass of hairy roots and artemisinin content on the light spectrum. They found that the highest biomass (5.73 g DW/l) and artemisinin content (31 mg/g) were obtained under red light at 660 nm which were 17 and 67 per cent higher than those obtained under white light, respectively. Temperature in the range of 15–35 °C also affected growth and artemisinin biosynthesis in the cultured *A. annua* hairy roots. The maximum hairy root growth was found at 25 °C. However, the highest artemisinin content in the root cultures was observed at 30 °C (Guo *et al.*, 2004). Enhancing the artemisinin production by precursor feeding was also investigated. Addition of artemisinin precursors to the medium used for tissue cultures of *A. annua* resulted in a fourfold increase of artemisinin in the tissue and an 11-fold increase of artemisinin in the spent medium (Weathers *et al.*, 1994). The feeding of mevalonic acid alone, however, did not induce an enhancement of artemisinin production (Woerdenbag *et al.*, 1993). But the addition of some compounds such as naphtiphine (an inhibitor of the enzyme squalene epoxidase) to the medium improved the artemisinin production. Other additions, such as 5-azacytidine (a gene regulator), colchicine (a gene regulator), miconazole (an inhibitor of sterol demethylase), and terbinaphine (an inhibitor of the enzyme squalene epoxidase), were too toxic for the cultures to induce an enhancement of the artemisinin production (Woerdenbag *et al.*, 1993). Kudakasseril *et al.* (1987), however, reported a concentration-dependent increase in the levels of artemisinin and growth of shoot cultures with miconazole. Other sterol inhibitors, such as chlorocholine chloride, 2-isopropyl-4-(trimethylammonium chloride)-5-methylphenylpiperidinecarboxylate, and 4-chloro-2-(2–diethylaminoethoxyphenyl)-2-(4-methyl-phenyl)-benzeneethanol, increased both the incorporation of 14C-IPP into artemisinin by cell-free extracts and the production of artemisinin in shoot culture of *A. annua*. Sterol inhibitors inhibited the enzyme in the mevalonate pathway, resulting in increased terpenoid production rather than sterol production. To develop more potent antimalarial agents with improved in vivo stability, tremendous efforts have been made toward structure modification of artemisinin and analogue synthesis. Due to the difficulties of structural modification by conventional chemical methods, microbial transformation serves as a valuable tool that comes to play an important role in the modification. To date, a number of oxidating products of artemisinin at different positions of artemisinin structure have been reported.

These transformations include conversion to 3α-hydroxydeoxyartemisinin and deoxyartemisinin, conversion to 9β-Hydroxy-artemisinin and 3α-hydroxy-artemisinin, and conversion to 10-hydroxy-artemisinin and 9β-hydroxy-11α-artemisinin. In addition, microbial transformations on some artemisinin analogue, such as artemether, arteether, artemisitene, and 12-deoxoartemisinin, have been reported to produce oxidative products by different microorganisms (Liu *et al.*, 2006).

Many studies have been performed trying to enhance artemisinin content using bioengineering methods. Because *A. annua* is easily propagated *in vitro*, the production of artemisinin by cultures of cells or tissues (Nair *et al.*, 1986; Kudakasseril *et al.*, 1987; Martinez *et al.*, 1988; Tawfiq *et al.*, 1989; Paniego *et al.*, 1994), transformed hairy root (Qin *et al.*, 1994; Jaziri *et al.*, 1995; Wang *et al.*, 2000; Xie *et al.*, 2000; Kim *et al.*, 2002, 2003; Souret *et al.*, 2003), and shoot cluster (He *et al.*, 1983; Woerdenbag *et al.*, 1993) has been investigated widely. However, the yield of artemisinin remained low and undifferentiated cell or callus cultures, in particular, contained null or trace amounts of artemisinin. The production of artemisinin in shoot clusters and transformed hairy root is still disappointing at present.

A threefold enhancement in production of the putative anti-malarial, anti-cancer agent artemisinin has been reported in transgenic *Artemisia* plants overexpressing farnesyl diphosphate synthase, the enzyme immediately preceding the first committed biosynthetic step Ri-mediated transformation of *Artemisia annua* with a recombinant farnesyl diphosphate synthase gene for artemisinin production and expression of a chimeric farnesyl diphosphate synthase gene in *Artemisia annua* L. transgenic plants via *Agrobacterium tumefaciens*-mediated transformation (Chen *et al.*, 1999 and 2000).

When the bacterial gene *ipt*, which promotes the endogenous production of cytokinin growth hormones, is expressed in *Artemisia* there is a coordinated increase in hormone, chlorophyll and artemisinin levels and effects of *ipt* gene expression on the physiological and chemical characteristics of *Artemisia annua* L (Geng *et al.*, 2001).

Combinatorial Biosynthesis of Artemisinin

Naturally occurring terpenoids are produced in small quantities, and thus, their purification results in low yields. Further, the complex structure of these molecules makes chemical synthesis challenging and often uneconomical due to poor yields. Metabolic engineering of these pathways in a common industrial biological host (*E. coli*) offers an attractive alternative to extractions from plants or chemical syntheses for producing large quantities of these complex molecules. To accomplish this goal may require altering the MVA and the MEP pathways along with addition of very specialized enzymes, *e.g.* ADS. Based on preliminary work by others who described engineering of the MEP pathway to increase isoprenoid precursors for high-level production of carotenoids (Kajiwara *et al.*, 1997; Farmer and Liao, 2001; Kim and Keasling, 2001; Abdin *et al.*, 2003), Keasling's group further developed a base technology for production of amorphadiene in *E. coli* (Martin *et al.*, 2003). Bacteria already contain the MEP pathway for production of IPP/DMAPP, but they lack the MVA pathway. Keasling's group posited that the MEP pathway is likely linked to unknown control elements in bacteria and that direct alteration might impair growth. Instead, they added a truncated MVA pathway from *Saccharomyces cerevisiae* that was coupled to ADS in *E. coli* resulting in good bacterial growth and high-level production of amorphadiene estimated at.100 mg l21 in 12 h. Keasling's work is important because these engineered *E. coli* strains can serve as platform hosts for the production of essentially any terpenoid for which the biosynthetic genes are available because IPP and DMAPP produced by either arm of the terpenoid pathway are universal precursors to all terpenoids. More recently, Teoh *et al.* (2006) have isolated the next enzyme in the artemisinin pathway, a cytochrome P450 enzyme

(CYP71AV1); this enzyme appears to catalyze the next three steps in artemisinin biosynthesis, an enzymatic function also confirmed by Keasling's group (J. Keasling, personal communication). Once cloned into a bacterial host and after optimization of the culture conditions, it should be possible to produce very large quantities of a close precursor to artemisinin in *E. coli*, thus making this important drug readily available in much larger quantities than previously thought possible. The concept of *E. coli* as a host cell producing sesquiterpenoids out of the endogenous pool of farnesyl diphosphate (FDP) has been investigated (Martin *et al.*, 2001). This work resulted in the production of 10.3 µg of (+)-δ-cadinene, 0.24 µg of 5-epi-aristolochene, or 6.4 µg vetispiradiene per liter of bacterial culture. Furthermore the authors concluded that the poor expression of the plant terpene cyclases was limiting for the synthesis of sesquiterpenes and not the endogenous supply of FDP. This has been confirmed in their further work by coexpressing the *E. coli dxs* gene, which did not result in an increase of sesquiterpenoids produced where it did result in an increase of lycopene production in *E. coli* (Harker and Bramley, 1999; Kim and Keasling, 2001). To overcome the low enzyme levels, the expression of amorphadiene synthase has been optimized by constructing a synthetic amorphadiene synthase gene completely optimized for the expression in the bacterial host. This strategy has been combined with engineering of genes from the mevalonate dependent isoprenoid pathway (Figure 7.1), which resulted in an *E. coli* strain producing 24 µg/ml amorpha-4,11-diene (calculated as caryophyllene equivalent) from acetyl-CoA after supplementation of 0.8 per cent glycerol (Martin *et al.*, 2003). Recently, attempts to use *S. cerevisiae* for the production of artemisinin precursors have been described. The expression of the amorphadiene synthase gene in yeast using plasmids and chromosomal integration led to the production of respectively 600 and 100 µg/amorpha-4, 11-diene after 16 days batch cultivation (Lindahl *et al.*, 2006). Using a *S. cerevisiae* strain containing an engineered MVA pathway coupled with the genes encoding amorphadiene synthase and CYP71AV1 the production of artemisinic acid up to 100 mg/l has been reported (Ro *et al.*, 2006). This strain transported the artemisinin precursor outside the yeast cell, which makes purification of the product less complex. Artemisininc acid can be used for the semi-synthesis of artemisinin, but to lower the costs for production of the drug bioprocessing must be optimized (Liu *et al.*, 1998).

Breeding and Marker Assisted Breeding

Because the *A. annua* is a hybrid species, these transformed strains can only be preserved in flasks in the laboratory and the characteristic of high artemisinin content will be lost through sexual propagation. Although the transgenic strains can be multiplied on a large scale using micropropagation methods, the cost is high.

By bringing herbs into cultivation, traditional and biotechnological plant-breeding techniques can be applied at the genetic level to improve yield and uniformity, and to modify potency or toxicity. The high heritability and useful range of variation for artemisinin suggests that the development of molecular tags for the trait and their exploitation in a marker-assisted breeding programme are feasible (Delabays *et al.*, 2001). Although the impact to date has been minimal, it is certain that the '-omics' revolution, as it spreads out from model species to those with more complex genomes (so-called 'muddle' species) will influence research and exploitation of medicinal species as it will plants in general.

Increasing the production of active phytochemical constituents is a well-established target for genetic manipulation but presents some severe challenges. In particular, the metabolic pathways by which active compounds are biosynthesized are mostly poorly understood, and relatively few genes for key enzymatic or regulatory steps have been isolated. Nevertheless, there are examples of pathway

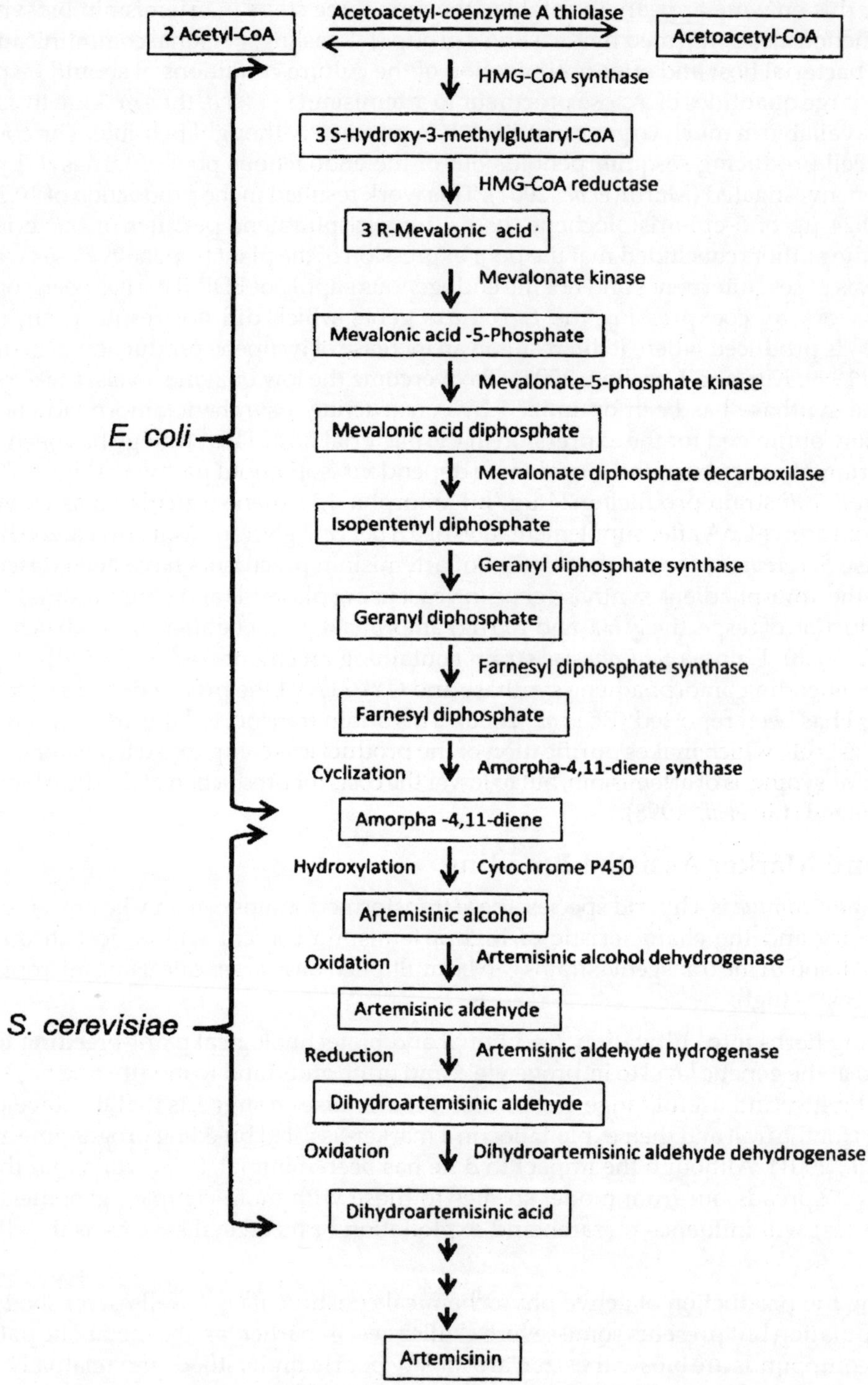

Figure 7.1: Proposed Biosynthetic Pathway for the Biosynthesis of Artemisinin Starting from Acetyl Coenzyme A. Adapted from Martin *et al.* (2003) and Ro *et al.* (2006).

engineering leading to improvements of potential value in the breeding of medicinal plants (Ferreira and Duke, 1997; Charlwood and Pletsch, 2002).

The artemisinin content is distinctly different in *A. annua* of diverse origins. Although the artemisinin content in leaves is influenced by environmental factors and the developmental situation of the herb, the primary factor contributing to variations in the artemisinin content is genetic (Delabays *et al.*, 2001). So, it is important to analyze genetic variations of different strains of *annua* that have different artemisinin contents. To evaluate the availability of the genetic variability of strains of *A. annua*, Zhang *et al*. (2006) performed RAPD analysis of selected chemotypes. The data clearly supported the conclusion of distinct variation of heredity among these chemotypes (Sangwan *et al.*, 1999). Studying the variation of heredity between high–and low-yielding strains by RAPD techniques is more accessible for the selection and breeding of high-yielding strains of *A. annu*a. In the present study, the OPA151000 band could be used as a marker to predict the strains with high artemisinin content.

A recent project in our department includes the study of the production of an antimalarial compound, artemisinin in *Artemisia annua*. Artemisinin is currently still extracted from the plant itself, but due to the low amount of artemisinin in the plant there is a shortage in the production (Cyranoski, 2004). In the case of *Artemisia annua*, it has been shown that the genetic variability linked to artemisinin content can be used to generate improved high-yielding varieties (Delabays *et al.*, 2001); thus, it is likely that genetic factors will be identified that are involved in the low or high artemisinin trait. A biosynthetic pathway of artemisinin has been proposed, but most of the genes underlying the synthesis and the control of it, are not yet identified (Bertea *et al.*, 2005; Bouwmeester *et al.*, in press). In our department the biosynthesis of artemisinin will be studied using cDNA–AFLP gene profiling. The knowledge of genes activated upon artemisinin biosynthesis, combined with metabolome data from the same time points as used for the transcript profiling, will allow us to identify key genes, encoding enzymes and/or transcription factors involved in the biosysthesis of artemisinin and the regulation of this pathway. This information will be the basis for a more detailed study, which will ideally give the information needed to engineer a high artemisinin producing plant through metabolic engineering.

Current Status and Future Prospective

Knowledge of the exact biosynthesis of artemisinin should enable us to influence its formation in a direct way, for example by metabolic engineering. As an alternative to targeting an individual rate-limiting enzyme reaction, exploiting transcription factors that turn whole secondary pathways on or off shows great promise as a metabolic engineering strategy (Figure 7.2). New genomic approaches and efficient gene isolation methods applied to difficult secondary pathways in medicinal plant metabolism will undoubtedly expand the range and precision of manipulations via transgenesis, providing potentially superior material for the breeder. Plant natural products have been a very productive source in drug development. The study of plant secondary metabolism is a fully expanding and challenging field in molecular biology and biotechnology, with many opportunities ahead. New tools of functional genomics combined with metabolomics and proteomics will revolutionize our knowledge on the pathways and enzymes involved in the synthesis of natural products, and thus allow a more focused approach for their production. With the increasing need for novel drugs for newly identified molecular targets, this field will likely become increasingly relevant. The appealing economic aspects of large-scale production of pharmaceuticals in plants could attract increasing investments and create new opportunities in this promising research field. It would be interesting to develop transgenic plants of *A. annua* to ensure a constant high production of artemisinin after the introduction of genes encoding enzyme(s) regulating the biosynthesis pathway of artemisinin.

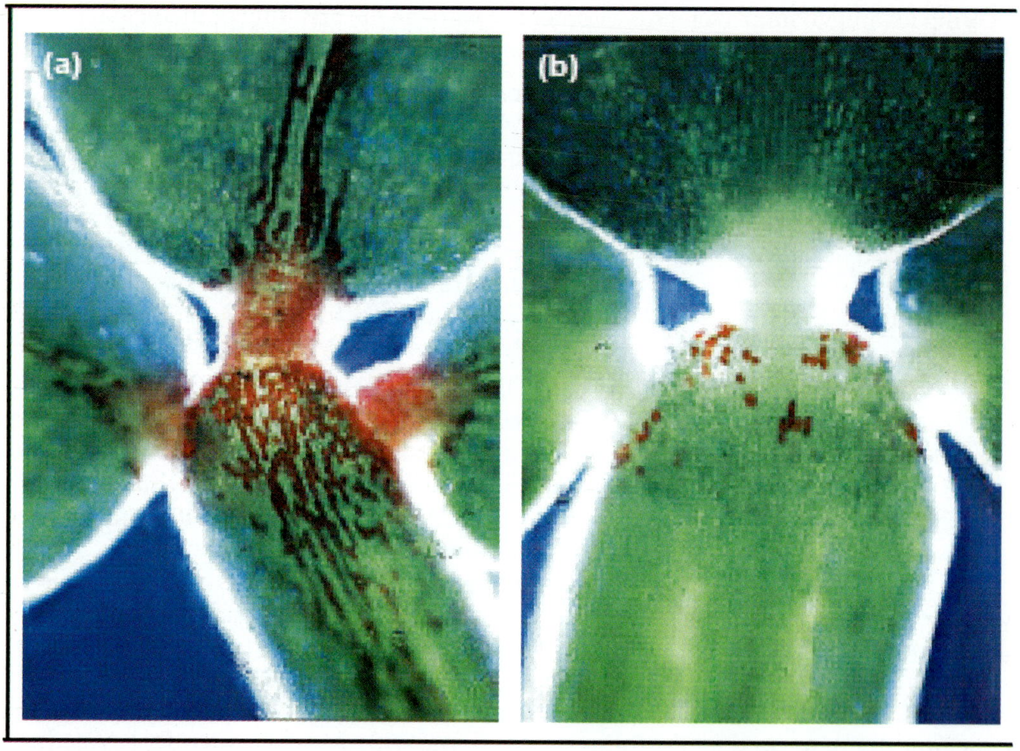

Figure 7.1: Manipulation of the Levels and Sites of Expression of an Entire Pathway of Secondary Metabolism in *Lotus comiculatus* by Transformation with a Transposition Bactor.

Introduction of Sn (a maize myo-class gene) resultes in subepidermal phenolic metabolism, visible as accumulation of red anthocyanins in subepidermal cell layers of the leaf base and petiole. It also induces differentiation of cells that biosynthesize condensed tannins in lineages leading to spongy and pallisade mesophyll in the leaves. (a) Transgenic line (b) untransformed control. Reproduced with permission from Oxford university Press.

Conclusion and Summary

Artemisia annua is the main source of artemisinin, the potent and efficacious antimalarial after quinine. Recently, artemisinin has also been proved to be a selective anti-cancer drug (Moore *et al.*, 1995; Efferth *et al.*, 2001). Currently, the limited availability of artemisinin and the lack of real competition among producers of raw material seem to be major barriers to scaling-up production and are partially responsible for its high price (World Bank, 2003). Also, the lack of affordable certified seeds hampers the extension of *A. annua* cultivation around the world. Breeding high-yielding, late flowering cultivars of *A. annual* adapted to the tropics, where malaria is endemic, is a desirable approach that needs to be pursued. Scientists are trying to understand the intricate and self-regulated biosynthetic pathway of artemisinin, its potential increase by the manipulation of terpene cyclase genes, although commercially feasible results are still to be seen. Currently, the hope to curb malaria rests on hampering the spread of the disease by mosquito vectors, on the availability of an effective and affordable vaccine, on the widespread use of insecticide-treated nets, on new antimalarial drugs effective against multidrug-resistant Plasmodium, and on meeting the world demand for artemisinin-combination treatments. Of course this last factor depends on a steady production of artemisinin, at affordable prices, to meet global demand. Although field production of *A. annua* is presently the most commercially feasible approach to produce artemisinin and related compounds, farmers must have access to good-quality seed generated from high-artemisinin parents. Although these seeds do not constitute 'true hybrids' because the parents are not homozygous, artemisinin content found currently in seeds available for research is approximately twice as high as it was 10 years ago (1.0 per cent compared to less than 0.5 per cent). Also, the agricultural aspects of artemisinin production such as soil fertility and pH, plant density, water availability, latitude and altitude, hormones, harvesting and drying protocols must be fine-tuned for each geographic area where artemisinin is to be produced as a raw material.

In addition, factors that affect temporal (when artemisinin reaches its maximum) or spatial (tissue localization) accumulation must not be ignored when evaluating the commercial potential of *Artemisia annua* as a new crop for tropical or temperate regions. Artemisinin based combination therapies (ACTs) have been long considered more effective than the existing drugs. ACTs are much more expensive than other drugs because of the relatively low yields of artemisinin in *A. annua*. Therefore, there have been many efforts to enhance the production of artemisinin *in vivo* and *in vitro* by biotechnology. Even though viable methods of increasing artemisinin content, *e.g.*, *A. annua* organ culture, hormone medium, and metabolic manipulation, have been investigated, and show potential for future development, the improvements delivered by these methods have not yet met the demand. To increase the yield of artemisinin by biotechnology, it is necessary to study the enzymatic pathway. Enzymes and precursors involved in the artemisinin biosynthesis have to be isolated and characterized. In recent years, many researchers have focused their efforts on investigating the molecular regulation of artemisinin biosynthesis and the genes coding for the key enzymes involved in the artemisinin biosynthesis. The high efficiency of genetic transformation and regeneration procedure developed by Han *et al.* (2006) allows the manipulation of artemisinin biosynthesis by genetic methods. By genetic engineering, we can overexpress the key enzymes involved in biosynthesis of artemisinin, or inhibit the enzymes involved in other pathways competing for its precursors to obtain transgenic high-yield *A. annua*. Although greatly improved yields were obtained by combining the expression of a synthetic sesquiterpene synthase with a recombinant mevalonate pathway, the data suggest that a maximum yield was not attained. Furthermore, *in vitro* evolution and combinatorial biosynthesis of sesquiterpene biochemical pathways in microbes may lead to artemisinin derivatives or even new sesquiterpene compounds. Efforts, therefore, are being made to enhance the production of artemisinin both *in vivo* and *in vitro*. Chemical synthesis of artemisinin is very complex and uneconomical. Breeding of high artemisinin yielding plants as well as the manipulation of culture conditions, growth media, and hormone levels to increase the yield of artemisinin in tissue and cell culture have not been successful. It is, therefore, essential to look for non-conventional, alternate strategies, which are economically viable for commercial production of artemisinin. Two approaches can be used to achieve this goal. The first approach could be the use of a semi synthetic route for the synthesis of artemisinin from its simple precursors such as artemisinic acid and arteannuin-B. The second approach could involve the use of genetic engineering to overexpress enzyme(s) catalyzing the rate limiting steps of artemisinin biosynthesis or by using anti-sense RNA technology to inhibit the enzyme(s) of other pathway competing for its precursors.

References

Abdin MZ, Israr M, Rehman RU, Jain SK (2003). Artemisinin, a novel antimalarial drug: Biochemical and molecular approaches for enhanced production. *Planta Med.*, 69: 289-299.

Acton N, Roth RS (1985). On the conversion of dihydorartemisinic acid into artemisinin. *J Org Chem.*, 57: 3610-3614.

Akhila A, Kumkum R, Thakur RS (1990). Biosynthesis of artemisinin in *Artemisia annua*. *Phytochemistry*, 29: 2129-2132.

Avery MA, Chong WKM, Jennings-White C (1992). Stereoselective total synthesis of (+)-artemisinin the antimalarial constituent of *Artemisia annua* L. *J. Am. Chem. Soc.*, 114: 974-979.

Ranasinghe A, Sweatlock JD and Cooks RG (1993). A rapid screening method for artemisinin and its congeners using MS/MS: search for new analogues in *Artemisia annua*. *Journal of Natural Products*, 56: 552-563

Bertea CM, Freije JR, van der Woude H, Verstappen FW, Perk L, Marquez V, de Kraker JW, Posthumus MA, Jansen BJ, de Groot A, Franssen MC, Bouwmeester HJ (2005). Identification of intermediates and enzymes involved in the early steps of artemisinin biosynthesis in *Artemisia annua*. *Planta Med.*,71:40–47

Borrmann S, Szlezak N, Faucher JF, Matsiegui PB, Neubauer R, Biner RK, Lell B and Kremsner PG (2001). Artesunate and praziquantel for the treatment of Shistosoma haematobium infections: a doubleblind, randomized, placebo-controlled study. *J Infect Dis.*, 184: 1363-1366

Boumeester HJ, Wallaart TE, Janssen MH, van Loo B, Jansen BJ, Post-humus MA, Schmidt CO, de Kraker JW, Knig WA, Franssen MC (1999). Amorpha-4,11-diene synthase catalyze the first probable step in artemisinin biosynthesis. *Phytochemistry*, 52:843–854

Brown GD (1994) Secondary metabolism in tissue culture of *Artemisia annua*. *J Nat Prod.*,57(7):975-977

Chang YJ, Song SH, Park SH, Kim SU (2000). Amorpha-4, 11-diene synthase of *Artemisia annua*: cDNA isolation and bacterial expression of a terpene synthase involved in artemisinin biosynthesis. *Arch Biochem Biophys.*, 383:178–184

Charles DJ, Simon JE, Wood KV, Heinsten P (1990). Germplasm variation in artemisinin content of *Artemisinin annua* using an alternative method of artemisinin analysis from crude plant extracts. *J Nat Prod.*, 53:157–160

Charlwood BV and Pletsch M (2002). Manipulation of natural product accumulation in plants through genetic engineering. *J. Herbs Spices Med Plants.*, 9: 139–151

Chen D, Ye H, Li G (2000). Expression of a chimeric farnesyl diphosphate synthase gene in *Artemisia annua* L. transgenic plants via *Agrobacterium tumefaciens*-mediated transformation. *Plant Science*, 155: 179-185

Chen D, Liu C, Ye H, L I G, Liu B, Meng Y and Chen X (1999). Ri-mediated transformation of *Artemisia annua* with a recombinant farnesyl diphosphate synthase gene for artemisinin production. *Plant Cell Tissue Organ Cult.*, 57: 157–162

Cyranoski D (2004). Campaign to fight malaria hit by surge in demand for medicine. *Nature*, 432 (7015): 259

Delabays N, Benakis A, and Collet G (1993). Selection and breeding for high artemisinin (qinghaosu) yielding strains of *Artemsia annua*. *Acta Hort.*, 330:203-206.

Delabays N, Simonnet X, Gaudin M (2001). The genetics of artemisinin content in *Artemisia annua* and the breeding of high yielding cultivars. *Curr Med Chem.*, 8:1795?1801

Duke MV, Paul RN (1994) Localization of artemisinin and artemisitene in foliar tissue of glanded and glandless biotypes of *Artemisia annua. Int J Plant Sci.*, 155:365–372

Efferth T, Dunstan H, Sauerbrey A, Miyachi H and Chitambar CR (2001). The anti-malarial artesunate is also active against cancer. *International Journal of Oncology*, 18: 767–773.

ElSohly HN (1990). A large-scale extraction technique of artemisinin from *Artemisia annua. Journal of Natural Products*, 53: 1560–1564.

Ferreira, J.F.S., J.E. Simon, and J. Janick. (1995a). Developmental studies of *Artemisia annua*: Flowering and artemisinin production under greenhouse and field conditions. *Planta Med.*, 61:167-170.

Ferreira JFS and Janick J (1996). Distribution of artemisinin in *Artemisia annua*. In: Progress in New Crops. Janick, J. ed. ASHS Press, Arlington, VA. pp 579-584

Ferreira JFS and Duke SO (1997). Approaches for maximizing biosynthesis of medicinal plant secondary metabolites. *Ag. Biotech News and Information*, 9: 309N-316N

Fulzele DP, Heble MR, Rao PS (1995). Production of terpenoid from *Artemisia annua* L. plantlet cultures in bioreactor. *J Biotechnol.*, 40:139–143

Geldre EV, Vergauwe A, Eecdkhout EVD (1997). State of the art of the production of the antimalarial compound artemisinin in plants. *Plant Mol Biol.*, 33: 199?209

Geng S, Ye HC, Li GF (2001). Effects of ipt gene expression on the physiological and chemical characteristics of *Artemisia annua* L. *Plant Sci.*, 160: 691-698

Gershenzon and Croteau (1990). Regulation of monoterpene biosynthesis in higher plants. *Recent Advance in phytochemistry*, 24:99-160

Gulati A, Bharel S, Jain SK, Abdin MZ, Srivastava PS (1996). *In vitro* micropropagation and flowering in *Artemisia annua. J. Plant Biochem. Biotechnol.*, 5:31-35

Guo C, Liu CZ, Ye HC, Li GF (2004). Effect of temperature on growth and artemisinin biosynthesis in hairy root cultures of *Artemisia annua. Acta Bot Boreal-Occident Sin.*, 24:1828–1831

Gupta MM, Jain DC, Mathur AK, Singh AK and Verma RK (1996). *Planta Med.*, 62: 280

Han JL, Liu BY, Ye HC, Wang H, Li ZQ and Li GF (2006). Effects of overexpression of the edogenous farnesyl diphosphate synthesis on the artemisinin content in *Artemisia annua* L. *J Integr Palnt Biol.*, 48 (4): 482-487

He XC, Zeng MY, Li GF, Liang Z (1983). Callus induction and regeneration of plantlets from *Artemisia annua* and changes of qinghaosu contents. *Acta Bot Sin.*, 25:87–90

Jung M, ElSohly HN, Mc Chesney JD. (1990). Artemisinic acid: a versatile chiral synthon and bioprecursor to natural products. *Planta Med.*, 56: 624

Luo XD and Shen CC (1987). The chemistry, pharmacology and clinical application of (qinghaosu) artemisinin and its derivatives. *Med Res Rev.*, 7: 29-52

Kim YJ, Wyslouzil BE, Weathers PJ (2002). Secondary metabolism of hairy root cultures in bioreactors. *In Vitro Cell Dev Biol Plant*, 38:1–10

Kim YJ, Weathers PJ, Wyslouzil BE (2003). Growth dynamics of *Artemisia annua* hairy roots in three culture systems. *Biotechnol Bioeng.*, 83:428–443

Klayman DL (1989). Weeding out malaria. *Natural History October*: 18–26

Klayman DL (1993). *Artemisia annua*: from weed to respectable antimalarial plant. In: Kinghorn AD and Balandri MF (eds) Human Medicinal Agents from Plants. Washington, DC: *American Chemical Society*, pp. 242–255.

Klayman, DL (1985). Qinghaosu (Artemisinin): an antimalarial drug from China. *Science*, 228:1049-1055

Klayman DL, Lin AJ, Acton N, Scovill JP, Hock JM, Milhous WK and Theoharides AD (1984). Isolation of artemisinin (qinghaosu) from *Artemisia annua* growing in the United States. *J Nat Prod.*, 47:715-717

Krishna S, Uhlemann AC, Haynes RK (2004). Artemisinins: mechanisms of action and potential for resistance. *Drug Resist Updat.*, 7:233–244

Kumar S, Khanuja SPS, Shasany AK, Darokar MP (1999). "Jeevan Raksha" from an isolated population containing high artemisinin in foliage (0.5-1.0 per cent). *J Med Arom Plant Sicences*, 21:47-48

Laughlin JC (2002). Post-harvest drying treatment effects on antimalarial constituents of *Artemisia annua* L. *Acta hortic.*, 576:315–320

Laughlin JC (l994). Agricultural production of artemisinin: A review. *Trans Royal Soc Trop Med Hyg.*, 88 (Suppl.1):21-22

Liersch R, Soicke H, Stehr C (1986). Formation of artemisinin in *Artemisia annua* during one vegetation period. *Planta Med.*, 52: 387?388

Liu C, Zhao Y, Wang Y (2006). Artemisinin: current state and perspectives for biotechnological production of an antimalarial drug. *Appl. Microbiol. Biotechnol.*, 72: 11-20

Liu CZ, Guo C, Wang YC, Ouyang F (2002). Effect of light irradiation on hairy root growth and artemisinin biosynthesis of *Artemisia annua* L.*Process Biochem.*, 38: 581-585

Liu CZ, Wang YC, Ouyang F, Ye HC, Li GF (1999). Improvement of artemisinin accumulation in hairy root culture of *Artemisia annua* L. by fungal elicitor. *Bioprocess Engineering*, 20:161-164

Liu CZ, Wang YC, Ouyang F, Ye HC, Li GF (1997). Production of artemisinin by hairy root culture of *Artemisia annua* L. *Biotechnology Letters*, 19:927-929

Mc garry and Croteau (1995). Terpenoid Metabolism. *Plant Cell*, 7(7):1015-1026

McVaugh R (1984). A descriptive account of the vascular plants of Western Mexico. In: Andersohn WR (ed.) Flora Novo-Galiciana Vol. 12. Compositae. Ann Arbor: University of Michigan Press

Martinez BC, Staba EJ (1988). The production of artemisinin in *Artemisia annua* L. tissue cultures. *Adv Cell Cult.*, 6:69–87

Martin VJJ, Pitera DJ, Withers ST, Newman JD, Keasling JD (2003). Engineering a mevalonate pathway in Escherichia coli for production of terpenoids. *Nat Biotechnol.*, 21:796–802

Mohapatra, PK, Khan AM, Prakash A, Mahanta J and Srivastava VK (1996). Effect of arteether alpha/beta on uncomplicated falciparum malaria cases in Upper Assam. *Ind J Med Res.*, 104: 284–287

Moore JC, Lai H, Li J-R, Ren R-L, McDougall JA, Singh NP and Chou C-K (1995). Oral administration of dihydroartemisinin and ferrous sulfate retarded implanted fibrosarcoma growth in the rat. *Cancer Letters*, 98: 83–87

Morales MR, Charles DJ, Simon JE (1993). Seasonal accumulation of artemisinin in *Artemisia annua* L. *Acta Hort.*, 344: 416-420

Mueller MS, Karhagombc IB, Hirt HM, Wemakor E, (2000). The potential of *Artemisia annua* L. as locally produced remedy for malaria in the tropics: agricultural, chemical and clinical aspects. *Ethanopharmacol.*, 73: 487-493

Nair MS, Acton N, Klayman DL, Kendrick K, Basile DV, Mante S. (1986). Production of artemisinin in tissue cultures of *Artemisia annua. J Nat Prod.*, 49 (3):504–507

Newman JD, Marshall J, Chang MCY, Nowroozi F, Paradise E, Pitera D, Newman KL, Keasling JD (2006). High-level production of amorpha-4,11-diene in a two phase partitioning bioreactor of metabolically engineered Escherichia coli. *Biotechnol Bioeng.*, 95:684–691

Newton P, White N (1999). Malaria: new development in treatment and prevention. *Ann Rev Med.*, 50:179–192

Paniego NB, Giulietti AM (1996). Artemisinin production by *Artemisia annua* L.-transformed organ cultures. *Enzyme Microb.Technol.*, 18: 526–530

Paniego NB, and AM Giuliette (1994). *Artemisia annua* L.: dedifferentiated and differentiated cultures. *Plant Cell Tiss Organ Cult.*, 36:163-168

Picaud S, Olifsson L, Brodelius PE (2005). Expression, purification and characterization of recombinant amorpha-4,11-diene synthase from *Artemisia annua* L. *Arch Biochem Biophys.*, 436:215–226

Ping ZQ, Chang Z, Lulu Y, Yi YR, Mei ZX, Ying H, ling FL and Qiu YX (2008). Cloning of artemisinin biosynthetic cDNA and novel gene overexpression. *Sci China Ser C-Life Sci.*, 51:232-244

Pras N, Visser JF, Batterman S, Woerdenbag HJ, Maligre TM, Lugt CB (1991). Laboratory selection of *Artemisia annua* L. for high artemisinin yielding types. *Phytochem Anal.*, 2: 80-83

Qin MB, Li GZ, Yun Y, Ye HC, Li GF (1994). Induction of hairy root from Artemisia annua with *Agrobacterium rhizogenes* and its culture *in vitro*. *Acta Bot Sin.*, 36:165–170 (Suppl)

Ram M, Gupta MM, Dwivedi S and Kumar S (1997). Effect of plant density on the yields of artemisinin and essential oil in *Artemisia annua* cropped under low input cost management in north-central India. *Planta Medica*, 63:372–374

Riley EM (1995). The London School of Tropical Medicine: a new century of malarial research. *Mem Inst Oswaldo Cruz.*, 95:25–32

Ro DK, Paradise EM, Ouellet M, Fisher KJ, Newman KL, Ndungu JM, Ho KA, Eachus RA, Ham TS, Kirby J, Chang MC, Withers ST, Shiba Y, Sarpong R, Keasling JD (2006). Production of the antimalarial drug precursor artemisinic acid in engineered yeast. *Nature*, 440:940–943

Romero MR, Effeth T, Serrano MA, Castano B, Macias RI, Briz O, Martin JJ (2005). Effect of artemisinin/artesunate as inhibitors of hepatitis B virus production in an *'in vitro'* system. *Antiviral Res.*, 68:75-83

Roth RJ, Acton N (1987). A simple conversion of artemisinic acid into artemisinin. *Planta Med.*, 53: 501

Sangwan RS, Agarwal K, Luthra R, Thakur RS, Sangwan NS (1993). Biotransformation of arteannuic acid into arteannuin B and artemisinin in *Artemisia annua*. *Phytochemistry*, 34:1301–1302

Sangwan RS, Sangwan NS, Jain DC, Kumar S, Ranade SA (1999). RAPD profile based genetic characterization of chemotypic variants of *Artemisia annua* L. *Biochem Mol Biol Int.*, 47(6): 935-44

Sen R, Bandyopadhyay S, Dutta A, Mandal G, Ganguly S and Saha P (2007). Artemisinin triggers induction of cell-cycle arrest and apoptosis in Leishmania dovani promastigotes. *J Med Microbiol.*, 56: 1213-1218

Singh A, Kaul VK, Mahajan VP, Sing A, Misra LN, Thakur RS, Husain A (1986). Introduction of *Artemisia annua* in India and isolation of artemisinin, a promising antimalarial drug. *Indian J Pharmaceut Sci.*, 48: 137-138

Singh A, Vishwakarma RA, Husain A (1988). Evaluation of *Artemisia annua* strain for higher artemisinin production. *Planta Med.*, 54: 475?477

Singh M (2000) Effect of nitrogen, phosphorus and potassium nutrition on herb, oil and artemisinin yield of *Artemsia annua* undersemi-arid tropical condition. *J Med Aro Plant Sci.*, 22:368-9

Singh NP and Lai H (2001). Selective toxicity of dehydroartemisinin and holotransferrin on human breast cancer cells. *Life Sciences*, 70:49-56

Smith TC, Weathers PJ, Cheetham RC (1997). Effect of gibberellic acid on hair root cultures of *Artemisia annua* growth and artemisinin production. *In vitro Cell Dev Biol Plant*, 33:75–79

Srivastava NK and Sharma S (1990). Influence of micronutrient imbalance on growth and artemisinin content in *Artemisia annua*. *Ind J Pharm Sci.*, 52: 225

Shukla A, Abad Farooqi AH, Shukla YN, Sharma S(1992). Effect of tricontanol and chlormequat on growth, plant hormones and artemisinin yield in *Artemisia annua* L. *Plant growth regul.*, 11: 165-171

Souret FF, Kim Y, Wyslouzil BE, Wobbe KK, Weathers PJ (2003). Scale-up of *Artemisia annua* L. hairy root cultures producescomplex patterns of terpenoid gene expression. *Biotechnol Bioeng.*, 83:653–667

Tawfiq NK, Anderson LA, Roberts MF, Phillipson JD, Bray DH, Warhurst DC (1989). Antiplasmodial activity of *Artemisia annua* plant cell cultures. *Plant Cell Rep.*, 8:425–428

Teo CKH, Yap AW, Chan KL, Gan EK, Tanaka M (1995). Artemisinin production from callus of *Artemisia annua* cultured in fluorocarbon polymer film culture bag. *Asia-Pac J Mol Biol Biotechnol.*, 3:317–321

Trigg PL (1990). Qinghaosu as an antimalarial drug. *Econ Med Plant Res.*, 3:20-25

Utzinger J, Xiao S, N'Goran EK,Berquist R and Tanner M (2001). The potential of artemether for the control of shistosomiasis. *Int J Parasitol.*, 31: 1549-1562

Van Agtmael MA, Eggetle TA and Van Boxtel CJ (1999). Artemisinin drugs in the treatment of malaria: from medicinal herb to registered medication. *Trends pharmacol. Sci.*, 20 199-204

Wallaart TE, Van Uden W, Lubberink HG, Woerdenbag HJ, Pras N, Quax WJ (1999a). Isolation and identification of dihydroartemisinic acid from *Artemisia annua* and its possible role in the biosynthesis of artemisinin. *J Nat Prod.*, 62:430–433

Wallaart TE, Van Uden W, Lubberink HG, Woerdenbag HJ, Pras N, Quax WJ (1999b). Isolation and identification of dihydroartemisinic acid from *Artemisia annua*: a novel biosynthetic precursor of artemisinin. *J Nat Prod.*, 62:1160-1162

Wallaart TE, Pras N, Beekman AC, Quax WJ (2000). Seasonal variation of artemisinin and its biosynthetic precursors in plants of *Artemisia annua* of different geographical origin: proof for the existence of chemotypes. *Plant Med.*, 66: 57–62

Wallaart TE, Boumeester HJ, Hille J, Poppinga L, Maijers NCA (2001). Amorpha-4,11-diene synthase: cloning and functional expression of a key enzyme in the biosynthetic pathway of the novel antimalarial drug artemisinin. *Planta*, 212:460–465

Wang CW (1961). The forests of China, with a survey of grassland and desert vegetations. In Harvard University Maria Moors Cabot Foundation No. 5. Cambridge, MA: Harvard University Press, pp. 171–187

Wang JW, and Tan RX (2002). Artemisinin production in *Artemisia annua* hairy root cultures with improved growth by altering the nitrogen source of the medium. *Biotechnol Lett.*, 24:1153-1156

Wang JW, Zhang Z, and Tan X (2001). Stimulation of artemisinin production in *Artemisia annua* hairy roots by the elicitor from the endophytic Colletotrichum sp. *Biotechnol Lett.*, 23: 857-860

Wang H, Ye HC, Li GF, Liu BY, Chong K (2000). Effects of fungal elicitors on cell growth and artemisinin accumulation in hairy root cultures of *Artemisia annua*. *Acta Botanica Sinica.*, 42: 905-909

Weathers PJ, Cheetham RD, Follansbee E, and Tesh K (1994). Artemisinin production by transformed roots of *Artemisia annua*. *Biotech Lett.*, 16:1281-1286

Weathers PJ, Bunk G, Mccoy MC (2005). The effect of phytohormones on growth and artemisinin production in *Artemisia annua* hairy roots. *In Vitro Cell Dev Biol Plant*, 41:47–53

Weathers PJ, DeJesus-Gonzalez L and Kim YJ (2004). Alteration of biomass and artemisinin production in Artemisia annua hairy roots by media sterilization method and sugars. *Plant Cell Rep.*, 23:414–418

WHO (2001). Antimalarial drug combination therapy: report of a WHO technical consultation. WHO/CDS/RBM/2001/35, reiterated in 2003

Whipkey A, Simon JE, Charles DJ, Janick J (1992). *In vitro* production of artemisinin from *Artemisia annua* L. *Phytother Res.*, 1:15–25

Woerdenbag HJ, Lüers JFJ, van Uden W, Pras N, Malingré TM, Alfermann AW (1993). Production of the new antimalarial drug artemisinin in shoot cultures of *Artemisia annua* L. *Plant Cell, Tiss. Org. Cult.*, 32:247-257

World Bank (2003). Expert Consultation on the Procurement and Financing of Antimalarial Drugs. Meeting Report, Draft 3, 7 November 2003. Washington, DC: World Bank

Boumeester HJ, Wallaart TE, Janssen MH, van Loo B, Jansen BJ, Posthumus MA, Schmidt CO, de Kraker JW, Knig WA, Franssen MC (1999). Amorpha-4,11-diene synthase catalyze the first probable step in artemisinin biosynthesis. *Phytochemistry*, 52:843–854

Xie DY, Wang LH, Ye HC, Li GF (2000). Isolation and production of artemisinin and stigmasterol in hairy root cultures of *Artemisia annua*. *Plant Cell Tiss Org Cult.*, 63: 161?166

Xu XX, Zhu J, Huang DZ, Zhou WS (1986). Total synthesis of arteannuin and deoxyarteannuin. *Tetrahedron*, 42: 819-828

Yaseen M, Tajuddin (1998). Effect of Plant growth regulators on yield, oil composition and artemisinin from *Artemisia annua* under temperate condition. *Journal of Medicinal and Aromatic plant sciences*, 20: 1038-1041

Zeng QP, Qiu F and Yuan L (2007). Production of artemisinin by genetically modified microbes. Biotechnology letters: DOI 10.1007/s10529-007-9596-y

Zhang L, Ye H and Li G (2006). Effect of development satge on the artemisinin content and the sequence characterized amplified region (SCAR) markers of high-artemisinin yielding strains of *Artemisia annua* L. *J Intg Plant Biol.*, 48:1054-1062

Utilisation and Management of Medicinal Plants (2010) *Pages 157–173*
Editors: **V.K. Gupta, Anil K. Verma and Sushma Koul**
Published by: **DAYA PUBLISHING HOUSE, NEW DELHI**

Chapter 8

Pieris brassicae as Laboratory of Synthesis of New Compounds with Biological Potential: Interaction with *Brassica oleracea* var. *costata* and *Brassica rapa* var. *rapa*.

David M. Pereira[1], Patrícia Valentão[1], Federico Ferreres[2], Rosa Seabra[1] and Paula B. Andrade[1]*

[1]REQUIMTE/Serviço de Farmacognosia, Faculdade de Farmácia, Universidade do Porto, R. Aníbal Cunha, 164, 4050-047 Porto, Portugal

[2]Research Group on Quality, Safety and Bioactivity of Plant Foods, Department of Food Science and Technology, CEBAS (CSIC), P.O. Box 164, 30100 Campus University Espinardo, Murcia, Spain

ABSTRACT

Interactions between insects and plants have been studied for a long time, showing beneficial and deleterious effects for both organisms. A general overview about the relationship between glucosinolates, flavonoids and insects will be presented. Several aspects of the complex interactions established by cabbage white butterfly (*Pieris brassicae* L.; Lepidoptera: Pieridae) are also considered. The larvae of this species constitute a frequent pest of some *Brassica* species, which are an important way of subsistence in several countries. As insects are unable to synthesize

* Corresponding Author: E-mail: pandrade@ff.up.pt.

phenolic compounds or their precursors, their presence in the different stages of *P. brassicae* life cycle can only arise from the food it has ingested. Deacylation, deglycosylation and sulphating steps are known to be involved in the metabolic process. Thus, with this study we intend to demonstrate the possible use of *P. brassicae* as a source of compounds with interest for the health, unusual in nature and hard to be synthesized in the laboratory. Two examples will be presented: the sequestration of phenolics by *P. brassicae* larvae fed with tronchuda cabbage leaves (*Brassica oleracea* L. var. *costata* DC) and kept without food for one hour, and the phenolic profiles of *P. brassicae* at different development stages (larvae, exuviae and butterfly), its excrements and its host plant *Brassica rapa* var. *rapa* L.

Keywords: *Brassica oleracea var. costata, Brassica oleracea var. rapa, Flavonoids, Glucosinolates, Insect-plant interactions, Pieris brassicae.*

Introduction

The role of plant chemistry in shaping plant-insect relationships is well recognized, with a close association of certain oligophagous insects with specific chemicals of their host plants (Renwick, 2002).

Large white butterfly *Pieris brassicae* L. (Lepidoptera: Pieridae), an insect whose larvae constitutes a frequent pest of some *Brassica* species, has a life cycle that lasts about 45 days from egg to adult. The larvae feed exclusively on crucifers (namely, cauliflower, cabbage, turnip, nasturtium and, more rarely, on red cabbage and radish), while adults feed on the nectar of several plants (Renwick, 2002; Muriel and Grez, 2002).

Herein, it will be presented a general overview about the relationship between glucosinolates, flavonoids and insects, with special emphasis on *P. brassicae*. Additionally, two examples of the interaction between this insect with two different host plants (*Brassica oleraceae* L. var. *costata* DC and *Brassica rapa* var. *rapa* L.) will be presented. These examples reveal that those interactions produced interesting bioactive compounds.

Interactions Insect-Plant

Glucosinolates

Glucosinolates (Figure 8.1) are β-thioglucoside N-hydroxysulfates [also known as (Z)-(or *cis*)-N-hydroximinosulfate esters or S-glucopyranosyl thiohydroximates], with a side chain (R) and a sulfur-linked β-d-glucopyranose moiety. The side chain (R) is characterized by a wide variety of chemical structures, which depends on the aminoacid precursor. So, they are subdivided into three classes: aliphatic, indolic and aromatic (Fahey *et al.*, 2001).

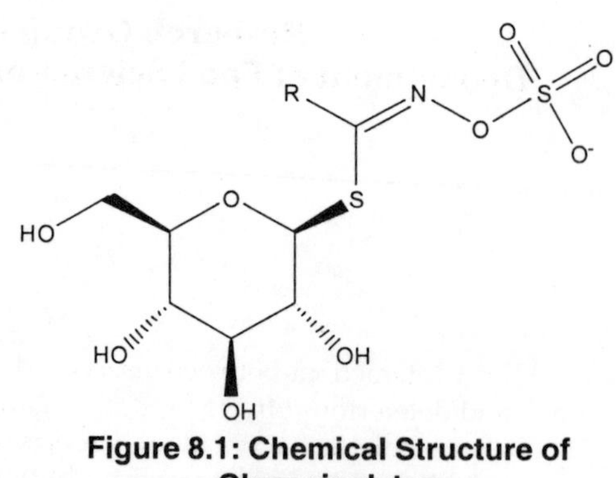

Figure 8.1: Chemical Structure of Glucosinolates

Glucosinolates have frequently been quoted as both a defense against generalist herbivores and an agent for host choice by specialist herbivores (Moyes *et al.*, 2000).

In what concerns to plant-insect interactions, the most important reaction of glucosinolates is their hydrolysis by the enzyme myrosinase, with the production of compounds, including isothiocyanates, referred as the mustard oils. Glucosinolates and these volatile compounds are largely responsible for the close association between crucifers and their specialist insect invaders. Isothiocyanates may serve to attract specialist insects to their hosts, whereas glucosinolates often trigger oviposition or feeding after an insect lands on the plant (Renwick, 2002). Once glucosinolates, or their hydrolysis products, are generally toxic to non-adapted insects, specialists have ways to prevent the potential toxicity of these compounds. This may occur by rapid excretion, glucosides hydrolysis, inhibition of hydrolysis, the action of protective enzymes, or by sequestering the glucosinolates (Schoonhoven *et al.*, 1998). This association was already demonstrated in the specific case of *Pieris* sp. larvae (Renwick, 2002).

In a general way, sequestration of plant toxic compounds in herbivores is correlated with aposematic coloration and gregarious behaviour. Once larvae of *P. brassicae* present these characteristics, it was suggested that it sequester glucosinolates of their host plants. In opposition, *Pieris rapae* L. (Lepidoptera: Pieridae) are camouflaged and solitary, so there's no expectation of occurrence of that sequestration. To test this hypothesis and to check the repeatability of a study that did report the presence of the glucosinolate sinigrin (Figure 8.2A) in *P. brassicae*, Müller *et al.* (2003) analysed the glucosinolate composition of larvae reared on three species of Brassicaceae (*Sinapis alba*, *Brassica nigra* and *Barbarea stricta*). Host plant glucosinolates were found only in traces or not at all in the larvae of *P. rapae* and of *P. brassicae* reared on *S. alba*, *B. nigra* or *B. stricta*. Thus, the larvae of both species do not sequester these secondary metabolites from their host plants. The results obtained by Aplin *et al.* (1975) indicating the accumulation of sinigrin in *P. brassicae* pupae wasn't confirmed. Also, the authors didn't find a correlation between glucosinolate sequestration and aposematism or gregariousness in the two *Pieris* spp.

The explanation for the presence of glucosinolates only in vestigial traces in larvae and faeces of both *Pieris* species, was their hydrolysis by myrosinase present in the ingested leaf tissue and/or metabolisation by the insect. Larvae feeding on *S. alba* excreted a progenitor of 4-hydroxybenzylcyanide (HBC) in the faeces. One possible justification for the detection of HBC after sulfatase treatment of

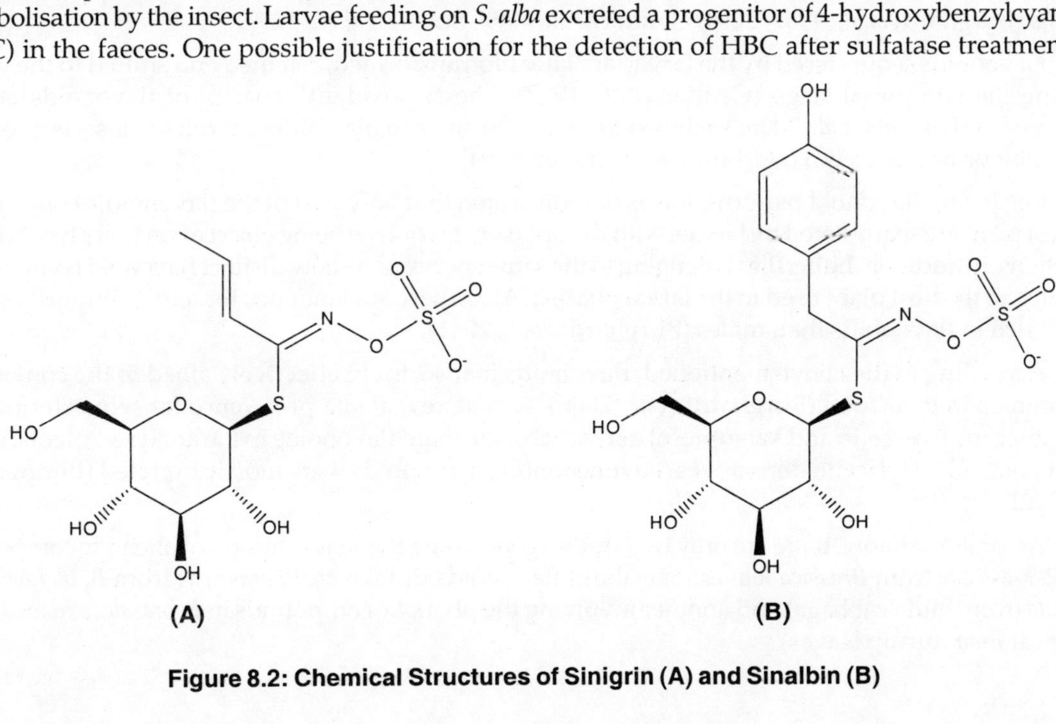

Figure 8.2: Chemical Structures of Sinigrin (A) and Sinalbin (B)

faecal extracts is that sinalbin, in the *Pieris* digestive tract or body, is hydrolysed into HBC and that enzymatic conversion of HBC into HBC-sulfate occurs subsequently. As Müller *et al.* (2003) referred, conjugation of phenols (case of sinalbin, Figure 8.2A) with sulfate is a detoxification path, increasing water solubility, which allows the excretion of a dietary compound, an example of the so called 'Phase 2 Metabolism' (Brattsten 1992).

Later, it was demonstrate by Agerbirk *et al.* (2006) that caterpillars of *P. rapae* convert 4-hydroxybenzylglucosinolate (sinalbin, Figure 8.2B) of brassicaceous plants into 4-hydroxybenzylcyanide sulfate (HBC sulfate), having 4-hydroxybenzylcyanide (HBC) as intermediate. This apparently serves as a detoxification process, as alternative formation of a mustard oil is avoided.

It would be interesting to assess the biological activity of these products of detoxification of glucosinolates by insects, namely by *P. brassicae.*

Flavonoids

Like glucosinolates, flavonoids can influence the feeding behaviour of larvae and oviposition of adult insects (van Loon *et al.*, 2002).

Flavonoids uptake is relatively diffused in the Lepidoptera, namely in butterfly families as Papilionidae, Nymphalidae and Lycaenidae, in which they participate in wing pigmentation (Burghardt *et al.*, 1997, 2001; Schittko *et al.*, 1999). Actually, although most pigments are likely to be synthesised *de novo* during scale development in the pupa, others are secondary plant metabolites obtained from the larval diet once insects are incapable to synthesise flavonoids or their precursors (Knüttel and Fiedler, 2001). Several studies confirmed that flavonoids in insects arise from the diet (Harborne and Grayer, 1994; Burghardt *et al.*, 1997; Schittko *et al.*, 1999; Knüttel and Fiedler, 2001). So, flavonoid uptake and metabolization is effectively depending on the specific flavonoid pattern of host plants (Burghardt *et al.*, 1997, 2001; Geuder *et al.*, 1997; Schittko *et al.*, 1999).

Flavonoids sequestered by the larvae are later biotransformed, retained and shifted to the wings during the late pupal stage (Geuder *et al.*, 1997). The antioxidant capacity of flavonoids is well recognized (Ferreres *et al.*, 2006; Vrchovská *et al.*, 2006) and can play different roles in insects, working as antibiotic and antiviral (Harborne and Grayer, 1994).

Regarding flavonoid patterns, it was demonstrated that only part of the flavonoidic compounds of host plant are sequestered by larvae, with the uptaken flavonoids being object of several glycosylation reactions. In addition, butterflies belonging to the same species can show distinct flavonoid composition (related to the host plant used in the larval phases). Also, there is a tendency for female butterflies to be more rich in flavonoids than males (Burghardt *et al.*, 2001).

According to the above mentioned, flavonoids in insects are effectively allied to the contents of flavonoids in their food (Burghardt *et al.*, 2000). Larvae revealed a preference for sequestering and metabolising quercetin and kaempferol derivatives, the main flavonoids in the analysed plants. Other flavonoids like myricetin derivatives, flavones and isoflavonoids were mostly excreted (Burghardt *et al.*, 2001).

As far as we know, there are only two studies concerning the sequestration of phenolic compounds by *P. brassicae* from *Brassica* leaves: one about flavonoids uptake by *P. brassicae* from *B. oleracea* var. *costata* (tronchuda cabbage) and another involving the phenolic compounds in *P. brassicae* reared on *B. rapa* var *rapa* (turnip leaves).

These studies can be important, attending to the fact that the larvae may accumulate and/or metabolize host plant constituents, namely complex flavonol glycosides (Ferreres *et al.*, 2005, 2006), constituting a source of potential bioactive compounds not available in nature.

Flavonoid Pattern of Larvae of *Pieris brassicae* Reared on *Brassica oleraceae* var. *costata*

The flavonoid pattern of larvae of cabbage white butterfly (*P. brassicae*) (Figure 8.3) reared on the leaves of tronchuda cabbage was analyzed by HPLC-DAD-MS/MS-ESI, a highly advanced and valuable technique for the characterization of complex phenolic molecules (Ferreres *et al.*, 2007a).

Wild *P. brassicae* larvae (fourth instar) and respective tronchuda cabbage external leaves (from three individuals with 45 days-old) host plants were collected on fields located in Samil, Bragança, northeastern Portugal.

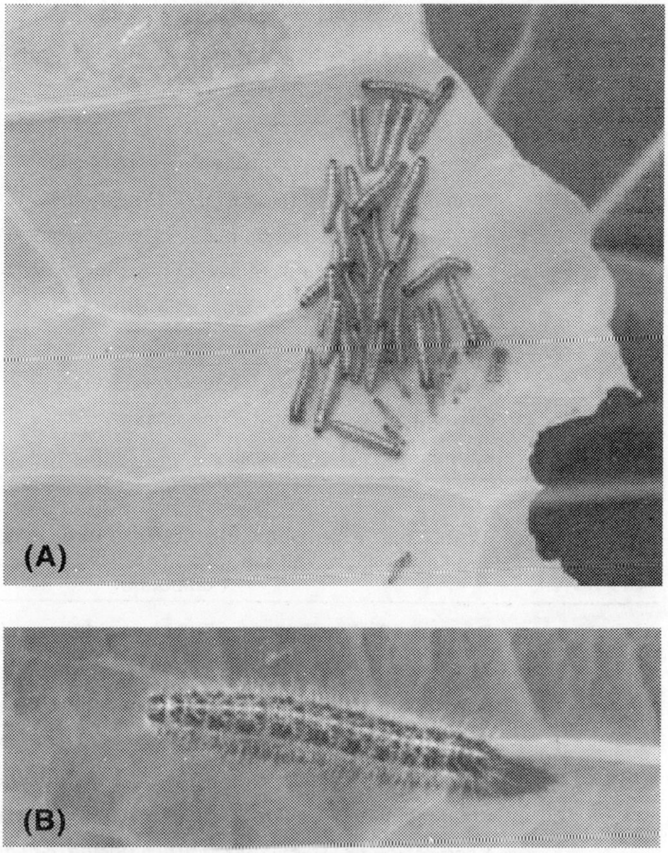

Figure 8.3: *Brassica oleraceae* var. *costata* Plant Material (A), Infested with *Picris brassicae* Larvae (B), *Pieris brassicae* Larvae

The phenolic composition of the tronchuda cabbage external leaves had already been studied in a previous work (Ferreres *et al.*, 2005). The composition of the host leaves, from which the larvae feed, revealed to be similar to that described before, being detected thirteen kaempferol derivatives (Table 8.1). The flavonoid profile obtained with *P. brassicae* (Figures 8.4 and 8.5) was then compared with that of the cabbage. Kaempferol-3-*O*-sophoroside-7-*O*-glucoside, kaempferol-3-*O*-sophoroside-7-*O*-sophoroside and kaempferol-3-*O*-sophoroside were the only compounds that the larvae and cabbage had in common.

Although the glycosylation pattern of the flavonols was the same in both extracts, it was observed that the flavonol 3-*O*-glycosides represented more than ca. 50 per cent in the larvae extract (Table 8.2), while they corresponded to ca.12 per cent of their food plant (Table 8.1). This was ascribed to the metabolism of the flavonols glycosylated at 3 and 7 positions present on tronchuda cabbage, or to a higher efficiency of sequestration of flavonol-3-*O*-glycosides (Ferreres *et al.*, 2007a).

Kaempferol-3-*O*-sophoroside was the most abundant flavonol glycoside derivative without acylation, corresponding to ca. 16 per cent of the total amount of phenolic compounds of the larvae (Table 8.2), while in tronchuda cabbage leaves it only represented ca. 5 per cent (Table 8.1). This difference can result from the metabolism of kaempferol-3-*O*-sophoroside-7-*O*-glucoside and its acylated derivatives, which are the most abundant compounds of tronchuda cabbage external leaves.

Table 8.1: Phenolic Composition of *Brassica oleracea* var. *costata* External Leaves (Ferreres *et al.*, 2007a)

	Compound	*Per cent*
21 +	Kaempferol-3-*O*-sophorotrioside-7-*O*-glucoside	7.6
22	Kaempferol-3-*O*-(methoxycaffeoyl/caffeoyl)-sophoroside-7-*O*-glucoside	
2	Kaempferol-3-*O*-sophoroside-7-*O*-glucoside	22.9
23	Kaempferol-3-*O*-sophorotrioside-7-*O*-sophoroside	1.4
3 +	Kaempferol-3-*O*-sophoroside-7-*O*-sophoroside	11.4
24	Kaempferol-3-*O*-tetraglucoside-7-*O*-sophoroside	
25	Kaempferol-3-*O*-(sinapoyl/caffeoyl)-sophoroside-7-*O*-glucoside	17.1
26	Kaempferol-3-*O*–(feruloyl/caffeoyl)-sophoroside-7-*O*-glucoside	27.8
27 +	Kaempferol-3-*O*-sophorotrioside	5.1
28	Kaempferol-3-*O*-(sinapoyl)-sophoroside	
29	Kaempferol-3-*O*-(feruloyl)-sophorotrioside	0.4
30	Kaempferol-3-*O*-(feruloyl)-sophoroside	1.1
15	Kaempferol-3-*O*-sophoroside	5.2

Table 8.2: Phenolic Composition of *P. brassicae* (Ferreres *et al.*, 2007a)

	Compound	*Per cent*
1	Quercetin-3-*O*-sophoroside-7-*O*-glucoside	8.7
2	Kaempferol-3-*O*-sophoroside-7-*O*-glucoside	10.0
3	Kaempferol-3-*O*-sophoroside-7-*O*-sophoroside	6.6
4	Quercetin-3-*O*-(feruloyl)-triglucoside-7-O-glucoside	4.5
5	Kaempferol-3-*O*-(sinapoyl)-triglucoside-7-O-glucoside	5.0
6	Kaempferol-3-*O*-(feruloyl)-triglucoside-7-*O*-glucoside	5.6
7	Kaempferol-3-*O*-(*p*-coumaroyl)-triglucoside-7-*O*-glucoside	2.6
8	Kaempferol-3-*O*-(methoxycaffeoyl)-sophoroside-7-O-glucoside	0.5
9	Kaempferol-3-*O*-(caffeoyl)-sophoroside-7-O-glucoside	1.8
10	Quercetin-3-*O*-(*p*-coumaroyl)-sophoroside	3.4
11	Kaempferol-3-*O*-(*p*-coumaroyl)–triglucoside	3.3
12	Kaempferol-3-*O*-(*p*-coumaroyl)-sophoroside	13.4
13 +	Kaempferol-3-*O*-(methoxycaffeoyl)-sophoroside	9.2
14	Quercetin-3-*O*-sophoroside	
15	Kaempferol-3-*O*-sophoroside	15.8
16	Kaempferol-3-*O*-(*p*-coumaroyl)-sophoroside (isomer)	2.4
17	Kaempferol-3-*O*-(disinapoyl)-triglucoside-7-O-glucoside	2.1
18	Kaempferol-3-*O*-(feruloyl/sinapoyl)-triglucoside-7-O-glucoside	1.3
19	Quercetin-3-*O*-(feruloyl)-triglucoside	1.9
20	Kaempferol-3-*O*-glucoside	1.9

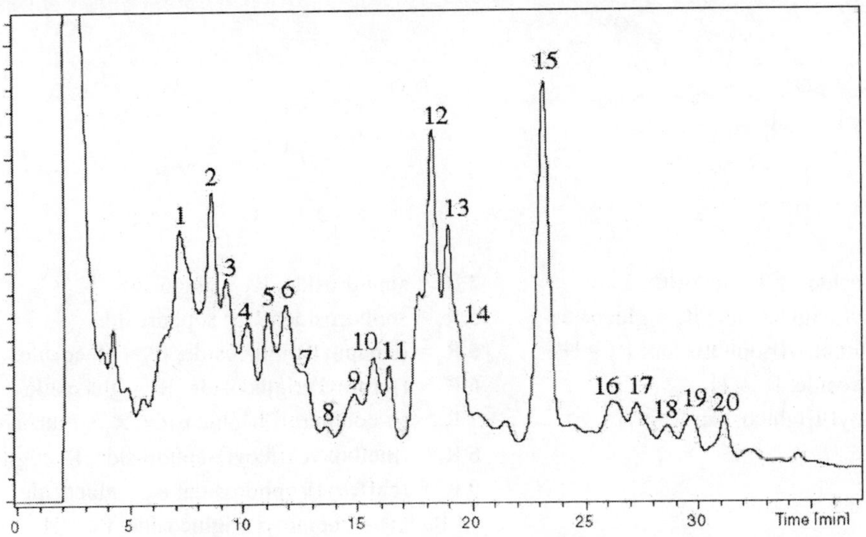

Figure 8.4: HPLC-DAD Phenolic Profile of *Pieris brassicae* Larvae Hydromethanolic Extract, Reared with *B. oleracea* var. *costata*.

Detection at 330 nm. Peaks: (1) quercetin-3-*O*-sophoroside-7-*O*-glucoside; (2) kaempferol-3-*O*-sophoroside-7-*O*-glucoside; (3) kaempferol-3-*O*-sophoroside-7-*O*-sophoroside; (4) quercetin-3-*O*-(feruloyl)-triglucoside-7-*O*-glucoside; (5) kaempferol-3-*O*-(sinapoyl)-triglucoside-7-*O*-glucoside; (6) kaempferol-3-*O*-(feruloyl)-triglucoside-7-*O*-glucoside; (7) kaempferol-3-*O*-(*p*-coumaroyl)-triglucoside-7-*O*-glucoside; (8) kaempferol-3-*O*-(methoxycaffeoyl)-sophoroside-7-*O*-glucoside; (9) kaempferol-3-*O*-(caffeoyl)-sophoroside-7-O-glucoside; (10) quercetin-3-*O*-(*p*-coumaroyl)-sophoroside; (11) kaempferol-3-*O*-(*p*-coumaroyl)–triglucoside; (12) kaempferol-3-*O*-(*p*-coumaroyl)-sophoroside; (13) kaempferol-3-*O*-(methoxycaffeoyl)-sophoroside; (14) quercetin-3-*O*-sophoroside; (15) kaempferol-3-*O*-sophoroside; (16) kaempferol-3-*O*-(*p*-coumaroyl)-sophoroside (isomer); (17) kaempferol-3-*O*-(disinapoyl)-triglucoside-7-*O*-glucoside; (18) kaempferol-3-*O*-(feruloyl/sinapoyl)-triglucoside-7-*O*-glucoside; (19) quercetin-3-*O*-(feruloyl)-triglucoside; (20) kaempferol-3-*O*-glucoside (Ferreres *et al.*, 2007a).

In what concerns the presence of quercetin derivatives, the authors mention that they have re-analysed the composition of the external leaves of tronchuda cabbage (Ferreres *et al.*, 2005) and they had detected these compounds in vestigial amounts, which also happened with the tronchuda cabbage external leaves eaten by *P. brassicae*. The larvae contained high amounts of quercetin derivatives (ca. 18 per cent of the total amount of phenolic compounds) (Table 8.2), while in tronchuda cabbage these compounds were present only in trace amounts, which suggests that *P. brassicae* selectively sequesters these flavonoids or that the kaempferol glycosides are metabolised into quercetin glycosides by the larvae.

The presence of *p*-coumaroyl derivatives (kaempferol-3-*O*-(*p*-coumaroyl)-triglucoside-7-*O*-glucoside, quercetin-3-*O*-(*p*-coumaroyl)-sophoroside, kaempferol-3-*O*-(*p*-coumaroyl)–triglucoside, kaempferol-3-*O*-(*p*-coumaroyl)-sophoroside and respective isomer) in larvae aqueous extract (Figure 8.2), which had not been found on either the internal or external leaves of tronchuda cabbage (Ferreres *et al.*, 2005; Sousa *et al.*, 2005) were explained by the demethoxylation of the sinapoyl and/or feruloyl

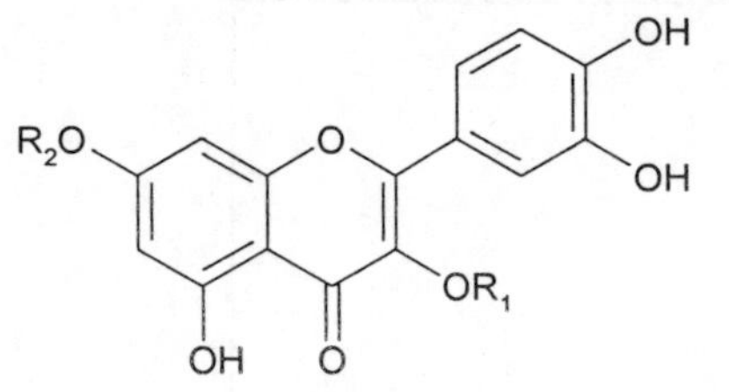

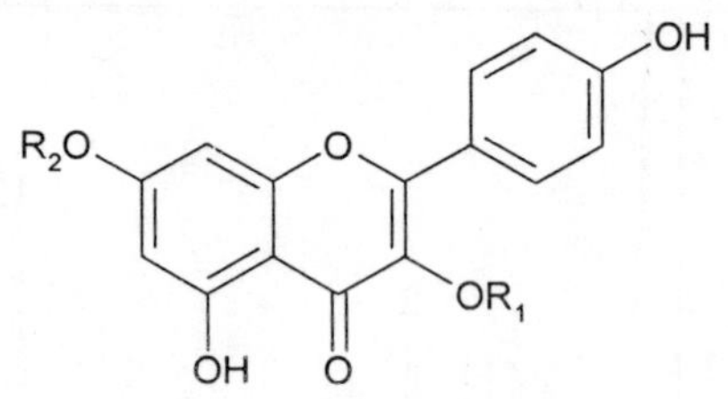

1 R_1 = sophoroside; R_2 = glucoside
4 R_1 = (feruloyl)triglucoside; R_2 = glucoside
10 R_1 = (*p*-coumaroyl)sophorosido; R_2 = H
14 R_1 = sophoroside; R_2 = H
19 R_1 = (feruloyl)triglucoside; R_2 = H

2 R_1 = sophoroside; R_2 = glucoside
3 R_1 = sophoroside; R_2 = sophoroside
5 R_1 = (sinapoyl)triglucoside; R_2 = glucoside
6 R_1 = (feruloyl)triglucoside; R_2 = glucoside
7 R_1 = (*p*-coumaroil)triglucoside; R_2 = glucoside
8 R_1 = (methoxycaffeoyl)sophoroside; R_2 = glucoside
9 R_1 = (caffeoyl)sophoroside; R_2 = glucoside
11 R_1 = (*p*-coumaroyl)triglucoside; R_2 = H
12, 16 R_1 = (*p*-coumaroyl)sophoroside; R_2 = H
13 R_1 = (methoxycaffeoyl)sophoroside; R_2 = H
15 R_1 = sophoroside; R_2 = H
17 R_1 = (disinapoyl)triglucoside; R_2 = glucoside
18 R_1 = (feruloyl/sinapoyl)triglucoside; R_2 = glucoside
20 R_1 = glucoside; R_2 = H
21 R_1 = sophorotrioside; R_2 = glucoside
22 R_1 = (methoxycaffeoyl/caffeoyl)sophoroside; R_2 = glucoside
23 R_1 = sophorotrioside; R_2 = sophoroside
24 R_1 = tetraglucoside; R_2 = sophoroside
25 R_1 = (sinapoyl/caffeoyl)sophoroside; R_2 = glucoside
26 R_1 = (feruloyl/caffeoyl)sophoroside; R_2 = glucoside
27 R_1 = sophorotrioside; R_2 = H
28 R_1 = (sinapoyl)sophoroside; R_2 = H
29 R_1 = (feruloyl)sophorotrioside; R_2 = H
30 R_1 = (feruloyl)sophoroside; R2 = H

Figure 8.5: Structures of the Phenolic Compounds Identified in *Pieris brassicae* and *Brassica oleracea* var. *costata*. Identity of compounds as in Tables 8.1 and 8.2.

derivatives during the metabolism process in the larvae. On the other hand, Ferreres *et al.* (2007) referred that the absorbance of the peaks observed in Figure 4 for acylated flavonoid derivatives, could not be taken as proportional to their abundance, as some of them co-eluted with other unidentified cinnamoyl acids' derivatives, presenting a similar UV spectrum and contributing to the overall absorbance of those peaks. Another advanced explanation was that, despite their existence in tronchuda cabbage leaves in concentrations below the detection limits, *P. brassicae* selective uptakes and accumulates them.

The existence of two methoxylated flavonol derivatives in *P. brassicae* (kaempferol-3-*O*-(methoxycaffeoyl)-sophoroside-7-*O*-glucoside and kaempferol-3-*O*-(methoxycaffeoyl)-sophoroside) (Figure 8.4) were explained as a result from the metabolism of kaempferol-3-*O*-(methoxycaffeoyl/caffeoyl)-sophoroside-7-*O*-glucoside present on the external leaves of the tronchuda cabbage.

Phenolics in *Pieris brassicae* Related on *Brassica rapa* var. *rapa*

The aim of the study of Ferreres *et al.* (2008) was to characterize the phenolic compounds of *B. rapa* var. *rapa* leaves and to establish possible relations with their ingestion, metabolism and accumulation by *P. brassicae* in the different stages of its life cycle (Figure 8.6). For this purpose, turnip leaves, *P. brassicae* larvae reared on this leaves and deprived of food for 12 hours, their excrements, exuviae and butterflies were analysed by HPLC-DAD-MS/MS-ESI.

In *B. rapa* var. *rapa* leaves it were characterized for all the acylated derivatives (methoxycaffeic, caffeic, sinapic, ferulic and *p*-coumaric acids) of quercetin-3-*O*-sophoroside-7-*O*-glucoside, kaempferol-3-*O*-sophoroside-7-*O*-glucoside and kaempferol-3-*O*-sophoroside (Figure 8.7). The kaempferol-3-*O*-sophoroside-7-*O*-glucoside derivatives are the most abundant ones (Figure 8.7B), while those of kaempferol-3-*O*-sophoroside were present in trace amounts. Quercetin-3-*O*-sophoroside-7-*O*-glucoside derivatives are found in considerable contents (Figure 8.7B). However, the deacylated glycosides were detected only in vestigial amounts in the saponificated hydromethanolic extract (Figure 8.7A). This can be due to the alkaline decomposition, during the saponification process, of phenolic compounds with an *o*-dihydroxy group, resulting in the presence of quercetin derivatives in trace amounts while caffeic acid is not observed.

In general, this kind of acylated derivatives (Figures 8.7B and 8.10) are very common in Brassicacea (Llorach *et al.*, 2003, Vallejo *et al.*, 2004, Ferreres *et al.*, 2005, 2006 and 2007b), and particularly in distinct *B. rapa* subspecies (Romani *et al.*, 2006; Rochfort *et al.*, 2006). On the other hand, the presence of flavonol-3,7-di-*O*-glucosides, namely non-acylated isorhamnetin-3,7-di-*O*-glucoside characterizes *B. rapa* (Fernandes *et al*, 2007; Romani *et al.*, 2006; Rochfort *et al.*, 2006) relatively to other *Brassica* species. Despite contributing to the organoleptic characteristics of the plant, these compounds may participate in the defence against external aggressions.

The two main phenolic compounds in excrements' hydromethanolic extract (Figure 8.8) were ferulic and sinapic acids (Figure 8.10). Other compounds present in considerable amounts, and that have been found before in the native hydromethanolic extract of *B. rapa* var. *rapa* leaves, were kaempferol-3-*O*-sophoroside, isorhamnetin-3,7-di-*O*-glucoside and isorhamnetin-3-*O*-glucoside. Some of the acylated derivatives already described were also detected, in low or trace amounts: kaempferol-3-*O*-(caffeoyl)sophoroside-7-*O*-glucoside, quercetin-3-*O*-(sinapoyl)sophoroside-7-*O*-glucoside, quercetin-3-*O*-(feruloyl)sophoroside-7-*O*-glucoside, quercetin-3-*O*-(*p*-coumaroyl)sophoroside-7-*O*-glucoside), kaempferol-3-*O*-(feruloyl)sophoroside-7-*O*-glucoside, kaempferol-3-*O*-(*p*-coumaroyl)sophoroside-7-*O*-glucoside and kaempferol-3-*O*-(*p*-coumaroyl)sophoroside. Other compounds that were not found in the native extract of the leaves were kaempferol-3-*O*-sophoroside-7-*O*-glucoside, described in the saponificated extract, quercetin-3-*O*-sophoroside, kaempferol-3-*O*-sophorotrioside and three isomers of kaempferol-3-*O*-(*p*-coumaroyl)sophoroside. In the first part of the chromatogram (Figure 8.8) several flavonoids derivatives were detected and were identified as sulphate flavonoids: isorhamnetin-3,7-di-*O*-glucoside sulphate and monoglucosides (kaempferol-3-*O*-glucoside sulphate isomers and isorhamnetin-3-*O*-glucoside sulphate isomers). This kind of compounds is very usual in animals' metabolic process. Considering the obtained results it was inferred that during the metabolic process of *P. brassicae* it occurs the deacylation of flavonoids, leading to the disappearance or decrease of

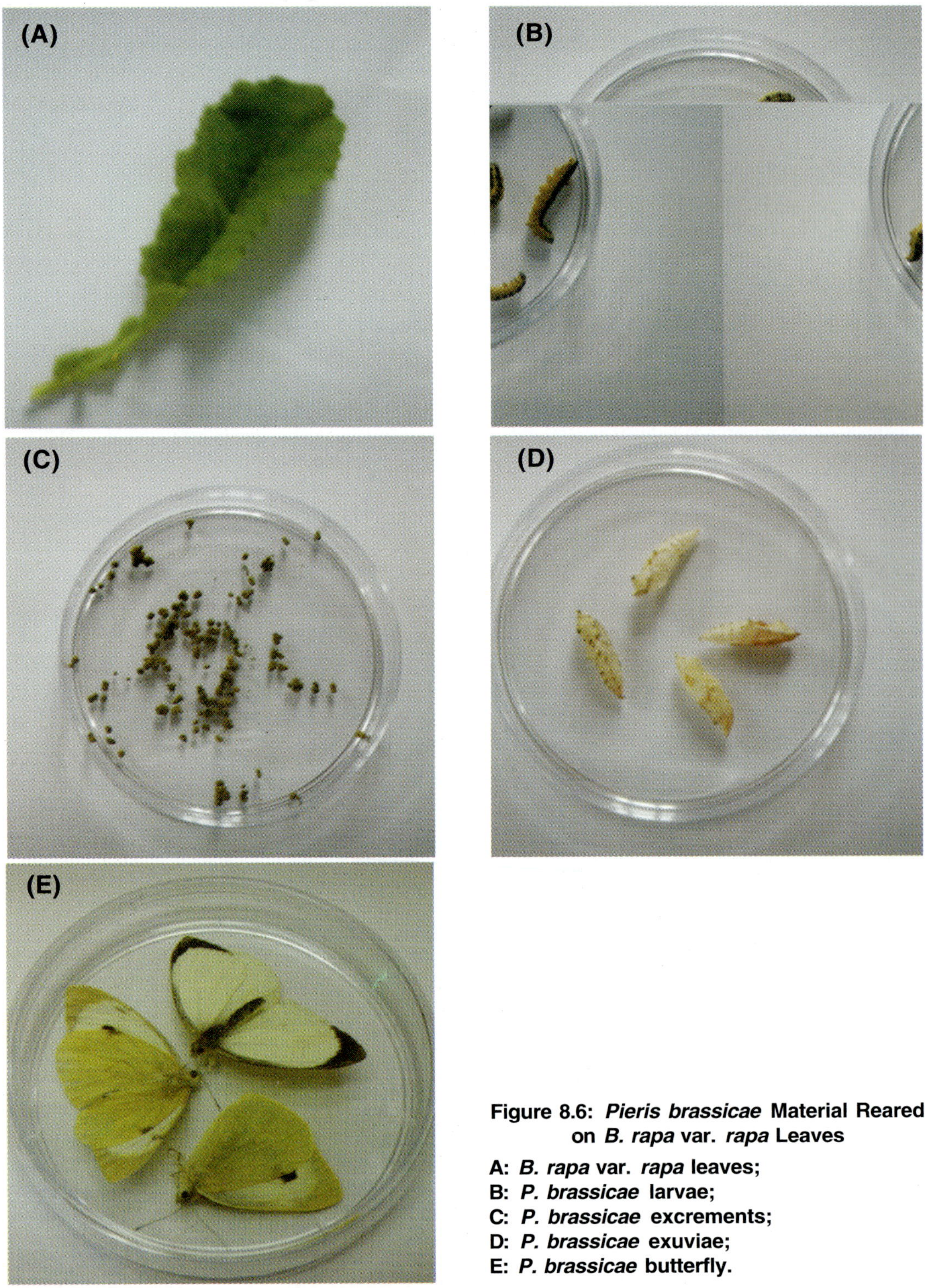

Figure 8.6: *Pieris brassicae* Material Reared on *B. rapa* var. *rapa* Leaves

A: *B. rapa* var. *rapa* leaves;
B: *P. brassicae* larvae;
C: *P. brassicae* excrements;
D: *P. brassicae* exuviae;
E: *P. brassicae* butterfly.

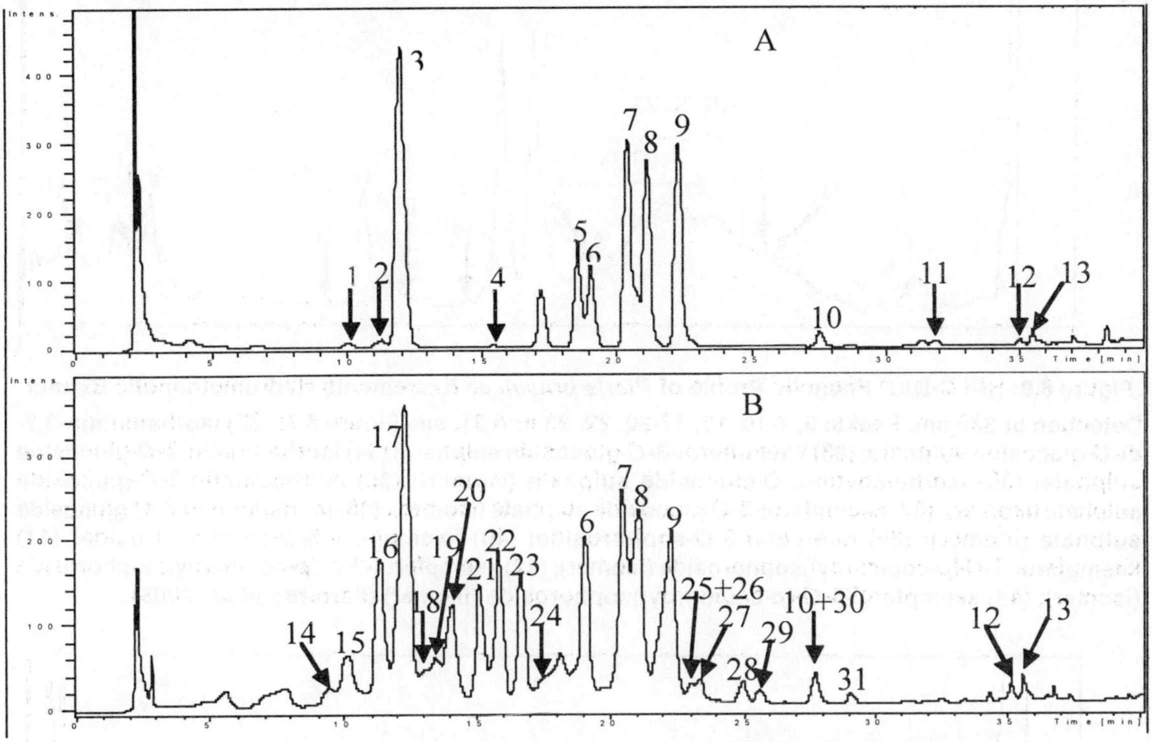

Figure 8.7: HPLC-DAD Phenolic Profile of *Brassica rapa* var. *rapa* Leaves. (A) saponified hydromethanolic extract and (B) native hydromethanolic extract.

Detection at 330 nm. Peaks: (1) quercetin-3-*O*-sophoroside-7-*O*-glucoside; (2) kaempferol-3-*O*-sophorotrioside-7-*O*-glucoside; (3) kaempferol-3-*O*-sophoroside-7-*O*-glucoside; (4) quercetin-3,7-di-*O*-glucoside; (5) *p*-coumaric acid; (6) kaempferol-3,7-di-*O*-glucoside; (7) isorhamnetin-3,7-di-*O*-glucoside; (8) ferulic acid; (9) sinapic acid; (10) kaempferol-3-*O*-sophoroside; (11) kaempferol-7-*O*-glucoside; (12) kaempferol-3-*O*-glucoside; (13) isorhamnetin-3-*O*-glucoside; (14) quercetin-3-*O*-(methoxycaffeoyl)sophoroside-7-*O*-glucoside; (15) quercetin-3-*O*-(caffeoyl)sophoroside-7-*O*-glucoside; (16) kaempferol-3-*O*-(methoxycaffeoyl)sophoroside-7-*O*-glucoside; (17) kaempferol-3-*O*-(caffeoyl)sophoroside-7-*O* glucoside; (18) quercetin-3-*O*-(sinapoyl)sophoroside-7-*O*-glucoside; (19) quercetin-3-*O*-(feruloyl)sophoroside-7-*O*-glucoside; (20) quercetin-3-*O*-(*p*-coumaroyl)sophoroside-7-*O*-glucoside; (21) kaempferol-3-*O*-(sinapoyl)sophoroside-7-*O*-glucoside; (22) kaempferol-3-*O*-(feruloyl)sophoroside-7-*O*-glucoside; (23) kaempferol-3-*O*-(*p*-coumaroyl)sophoroside-7-*O*-glucoside; (24) quercetin-3-*O*-(caffeoyl)sophoroside-7-*O*-glucoside (isomer); (25) kaempferol-3-*O*-(feruloyl)sophoroside-7-*O*-glucoside (isomer); (26) kaempferol-3-*O*-(methoxycaffeoyl)sophoroside; (27) kaempferol-3-*O*-(*p*-coumaroyl)sophoroside-7-*O*-glucoside (isomer); (28) kaempferol-3-*O*-(caffeoyl)sophoroside; (29) kaempferol-3-*O*-(sinapoyl)sophoroside; (30) kaempferol-3-*O*-(feruloyl)sophoroside; (31) kaempferol-3-*O*-(*p*-coumaroyl)sophoroside (Ferreres *et al.*, 2008).

acylated derivatives. Besides this, the absence of glycosilation in the 7 position in the majority of flavonoid sulphates, as well as in the remaining compounds, indicates the loss of the sugar in this position, together with the above mentioned deacylation, in the derivatives of kaempferol-3-*O*-sophoroside-7-*O*-glucoside and of quercetin-3-*O*-sophoroside-7-*O*-glucoside and in kaempferol-3-*O*-

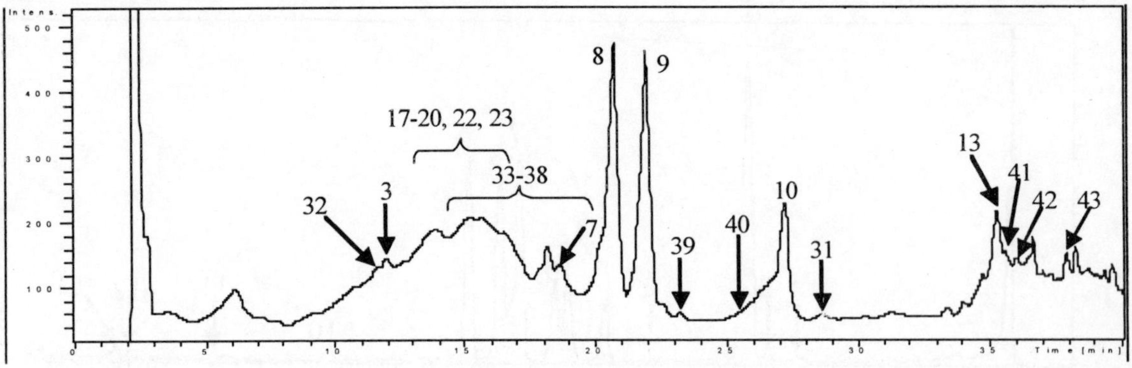

Figure 8.8: HPLC-DAD Phenolic Profile of *Pieris brassicae* Excrements Hydromethanolic Extract Detection at 330 nm. Peaks: 3, 7-10, 13, 17-20, 22, 23 and 31, see Figure 8.7; (32) isorhamnetin-3,7-di-*O*-glucoside sulphate; (33) kaempferol-3-*O*-glucoside sulphate; (34) isorhamnetin-3-*O*-glucoside sulphate; (35) isorhamnetin-3-*O*-glucoside sulphate (isomer); (36) isorhamnetin-3-*O*-glucoside sulphate (isomer); (37) kaempferol-3-*O*-glucoside sulphate (isomer); (38) isorhamnetin-3-*O*-glucoside sulphate (isomer); (39) quercetin-3-*O*-sophoroside; (40) kaempferol-3-*O*-sophorotrioside; (41) kaempferol-3-*O*-(*p*-coumaroyl)sophoroside (isomer); (42) kaempferol-3-*O*-(*p*-coumaroyl)sophoroside (isomer); (43) kaempferol-3-*O*-(*p*-coumaroyl)sophoroside (isomer) (Ferreres *et al.*, 2008).

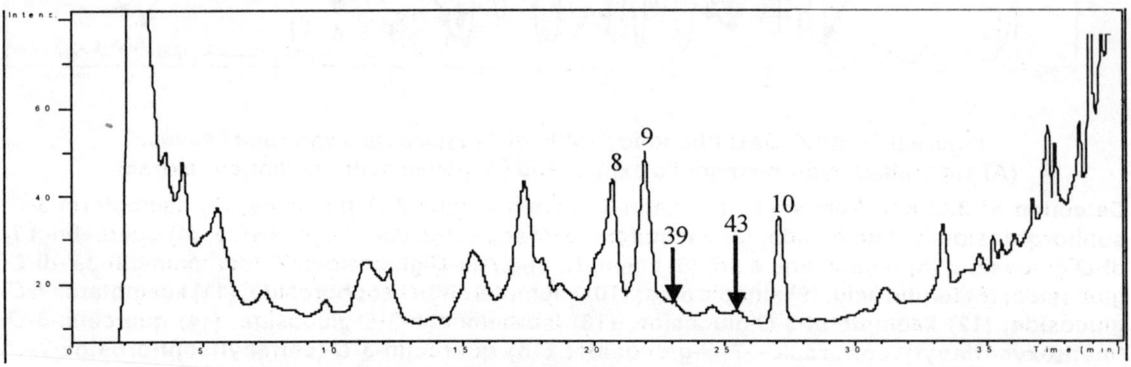

Figure 8.9: HPLC-DAD Phenolic Profile of *Pieris brassicae* Larvae Hydromethanolic Extract Detection at 330 nm. Peaks: 8, 9 and 10 see Figure 8.7; 39 see Figure 8.8; (43) kaempferol-3-*O*-sophorotrioside (Ferreres *et al.*, 2008).

sophorotrioside-7-*O*-glucoside and isorhamnetin-3,7-di-*O*-glucoside, to originate kaempferol-3-*O*-sophoroside, quercetin-3-*O*-sophoroside, kaempferol-3-*O*-sophorotrioside and isorhamnetin-3-O-glucoside, respectively. On the other hand, monoglycosilation of the majoraty of sulphate flavonoids points to a new deglycosilation process.

The hydromethanolic extract of *P. brassicae* larvae presented compounds found in the excrements: ferulic and sinapic acids and kaempferol-3-*O*-sophoroside (Figures 8.9 and 8.10). Vestigial amounts of quercetin-3-*O*-sophoroside and kaempferol-3-*O*-sophorotrioside, detected in the excrements too, were also identified. These compounds may contribute to protect the larvae from external aggressions, like light, undesirable environmental conditions, oxidative phenomena or microbial agents.

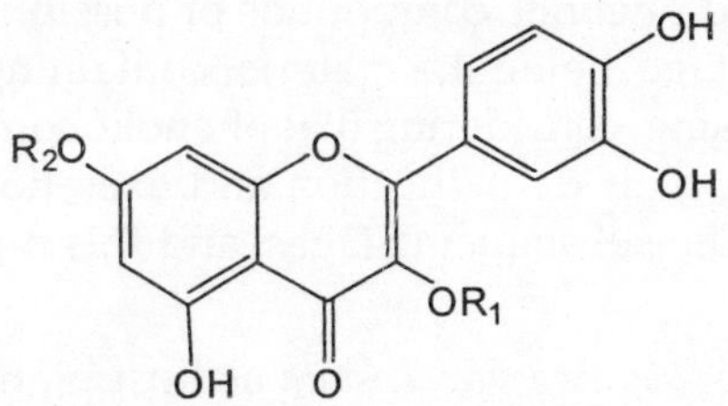

1 R_1 = sophorose; R_2 = glucose
4 $R_1 = R_2$ = glucose
14 R_1 = (methoxycaffeoyl)sophorose; R_2 = glucose
15, 24 R_1 = (caffeoyl)sophorose; R_2 = glucose
18 R_1 = (sinapoyl)sophorose; R_2 = glucose
19 R_1 = (feruloyl)sophorose; R_2 = glucose
20 R_1 = (*p*-coumaroyl)sophorose; R_2 = glucose
39 R_1 = sophorose; R_2 = H

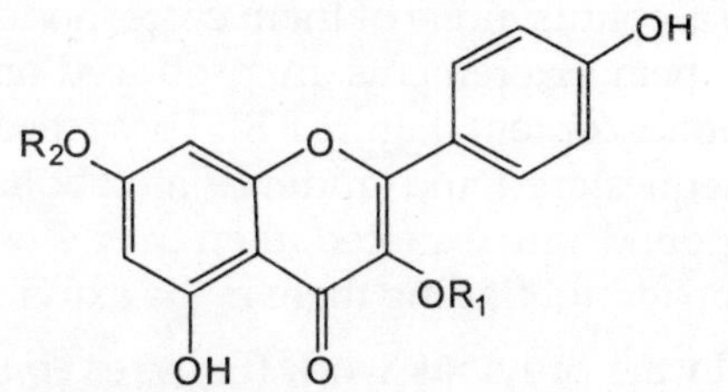

2 R_1 = sophorotriose; R_2 = glucose
3 R_1 = sophorose; R_2 = glucose
6 $R_1 = R_2$ = glucose
10 R_1 = sophorose; R_2 = H
11 R_1 = H; R_2 = glucose
12 R_1 = glucose; R_2 = H
16 R_1 = (methoxycaffeoyl)sophorose; R_2 = glucose
17 R_1 = (caffeoyl)sophorose; R_2 = glucose
21 R_1 = (sinapoyl)sophorose; R_2 = glucose
22, 25 R_1 = (feruloyl)sophorose; R_2 = glucose
23, 27 R_1 = (*p*-coumaroyl)sophorose; R_2 = glucose
26 R_1 = (methoxycaffeoyl)sophorose; R_2 = H
28 R_1 = (caffeoyl)sophorose; R_2 = H
29 R_1 = (sinapoyl)sophorose; R_2 = H
30 R_1 = (feruloyl)sophorose; R_2 = H
31, 41, 42, 43 R_1 = (*p*-coumaroyl)sophorose; R_2 = H
40 R_1 = sophorotriose; R_2 = H

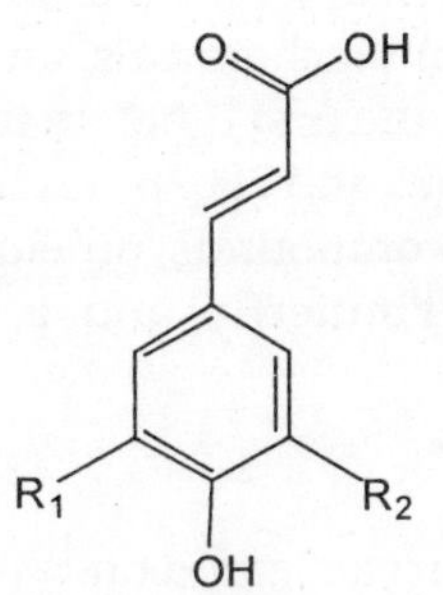

5 $R_1 = R_2$ = H
8 $R_1 = OCH_3$; R_2 = H
9 $R_1 = R_2 = OCH_3$

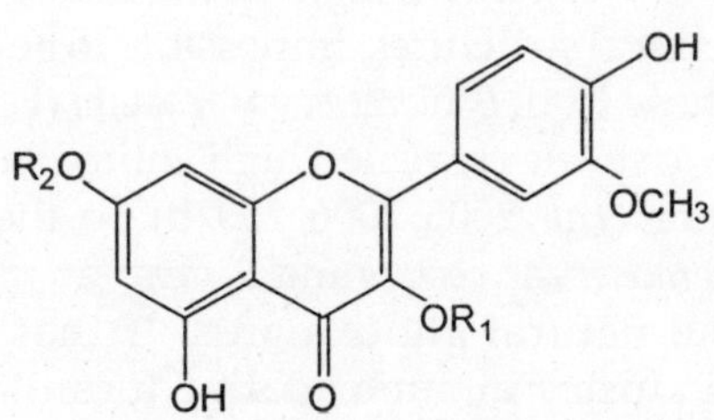

7 $R_1 = R_2$ = glucose
13 R_1 = glucose; R_2 = H

Figure 8.10: Chemical Structures of Several Phenolic Compounds Identified in *Pieris brassicae* Material and in the Host *Brassica rapa* var. *rapa* Leaves. Identity of compounds as in Figures 8.6–8.8

Hydromethanolic extracts of exuviae and butterflies analysed by HPLC-MS revealed peaks in trace amounts, none of them corresponding to the studied phenolic compounds or possibly related with them. Excrements are produced only at the larval stage, being the material containing higher phenolics content (Figure 8.8). These results are not surprising, considering that phenolic compounds are sequestered and undergo metabolization, regarding their detoxification and excretion. If the compounds are excreted, then they won't be present in the subsequent stages, and this maybe the reason for not finding them in the exuviae and butterflies.

In the previous work (Ferreres *et al.*, 2007a) using *B. oleracea* var. *costata* as host plant, it was already possible to see that the larva can sequester and metabolize this type of compounds. The phenolics of these two *Brassica* species are different, so, the phenolic profile found for the larvae is also distinct form that observed before. This fact confirms the strong dependency on the phenolic pattern of the host plant. In addition, the study involving *P. brassicae* excrements, exuviae and butterflies (Ferreres *et al.*, 2008), allowed to accomplish that, besides deacylation and deglycosylation already reported (Ferreres *et al.*, 2007a), sulphating reactions also occur in the metabolic process of the larvae, and that phenolics are mainly excreted and not transferred into the wings.

As insects are unable to synthesize phenolic compounds or their precursors, their presence in the different stages of *P. brassicae* life cycle can only arise from the food it has ingested, that is, from the complex flavonoid derivatives and free phenolic acids of *B. rapa* var. *rapa* leaves. So, the detection of this kind of compounds in the larvae indicates that it has the ability to sequester them. Additionally, the fact that both larvae and excrements exhibit phenolic compounds distinct from those of the host plant evidences that the larvae has the capacity to metabolize these phytochemicals, and to excrete them by the faeces, which included sulphate derivatives, reported for the first time. As these kind of flavonoids are known for their antioxidant potential (Ferreres *et al.*, 2006 and 2007b; Vrchovská *et al.*, *2006*), in what concerns the obtainment of potential health promoting compounds, unusual in nature and of difficult laboratorial synthesis, *P. brassicae* (larvae, exuviae and butterfly) and its excrements may constitute a promising source.

Conclusion

The two examples presented herein showed that the *P. brassicae* larvae reared on *B. oleraceae* var. *costata* and *B. rapa* var. *rapa* leaves their excrements, exuviae and butterflies presented new compounds, with complex chemical structures, impossible to be synthesized in the laboratory. These compounds are related with those from *B. oleracea* var. *costata* (Ferreres *et al.*, 2005) and *B. rapa* var. *rapa* (Ferreres *et al.*, 2008). These two species revealed high antioxidant capacity for which its phenolic compounds are responsible (Ferreres *et al.*, 2005, 2006, 2007b). So, there's a strong possibility that extracts of *P. brassicae* larvae reared *B. oleraceae* var. *costata* and *B. rapa* var. *rapa* leaves, their excrements, exuviae and butterflies provide powerful natural antioxidants. If that happens, those extracts may be used by the pharmaceutical industry in antioxidative formulations for prevention of free radicals-mediated diseases, or even as preservative of other oxidizable formulations. The same can be applied to cosmetic industry, for which it can be further used in anti-ageing formulations. Food industry may employ it to prevent the oxidation of its products, maintaining their quality and safety and extending their shelf-life, or to improve their nutritional value, by incorporating the extract in foodstuffs, thus increasing the dietary supply of antioxidants. In addition, it may constitute an economical advantage for *B. oleracea* var *costata* and *B. rapa* var. *rapa* producers, who have great losses caused by *P. brassicae* infestations.

Acknowledgements

The authors are grateful to Fundação para a Ciência e a Tecnologia (PTDC/AGR-AAM/64150/2006) for financial support of this work.

REFERENCES

Agerbirk, N., Müller, Olse, C.E.,Chew, F.S. (2006). A common pathway for metabolism of 4-hydroxybenzylglucosinolate in *Pieris* and *Anthocaris* (Lepidoptera: Pieridae). *Biochemical Systematics and Ecology*, 34: 189–198.

Aplin, R.T, D'Arcy W.R, and Rothschild, M. (1975). Examination of the large white butterflies and small white butterflies (*Pieris* spp.) for the presence of mustard oils and mustard oil glycosides. *Journal of Entomology A*, 50:73–78.

Brattsten L.B. (1992). Metabolic defences against plant allelochemicals. *In:* Herbivores and their Interactions with Secondary Plant Metabolites, Vol. 2. Ed. By Rosenthal, G.A., and Berenbaum, M.R., Academic Press, USA, pp. 175-242.

Burghardt, F., Fiedler, K., and Proksch, P. (1997). Uptake of flavonoids from *Vicia villosa* (Fabaceae) by the lycaenid butterfly, *Polyommatus icarus* (Lepidoptera: Lycaenidae). *Biochemical Systematics and Ecology*, 25: 527-536.

Burghardt, F., Knüttel, H., Becker, M., and Fiedler, K. (2000). Flavonoid wing pigments increase attractiveness of female common blue (*Polyommatus icarus*) butterflies to mate-searching males. *Naturwissenschaften*, 87: 304-307.

Burghardt, F., Proksch, P., and Fiedler, K. (2001). Flavonoid sequestration by the common blue butterfly *Polyommatus icarus*: quantitative intraspecific variation in relation to larval hostplant, sex and body size. *Biochemical Systematics and Ecology*, 29: 875-889.

Fahey, J.W., Zalcmann, A.T., and Talalay, P. (2001). The chemical diversity and distribution of glucosinolates and isothiocyanates among plants. *Phytochemistry*, 56: 5–51.

Fernandes, F., Valentão, P., Sousa, C., Pereira, J.A., Seabra, R.M., AND Andrade, P.B. (2007). Chemical and antioxidative assessment of dietary turnip (*Brassica rapa* var. *rapa* L.). *Food Chemistry*, 105: 1003-1010.

Ferreres, F., Sousa, C., Valentão, P., Pereira, J.A., Seabra, R.M., and Andrade, P.B. (2007a). Tronchuda cabbage flavonoids uptake by *Pieris brassicae*. *Phytochemistry*, 68: 361-367.

Ferreres, F., Sousa, C., Valentão, P., Seabra, R.M., Pereira, J.A., and Andrade, P.B. (2007b). Tronchuda cabbage (*Brassica oleracea* L. var. *costata* DC) seeds: Phytochemical characterization and antioxidant potential. *Food Chemistry*, 101, 549-558.

Ferreres, F., Sousa, C., Vrchovská, V., Valentão, P., Pereira, J.A., Seabra, R.M., and Andrade, P.B. (2006). Chemical composition and antioxidant activity of tronchuda cabbage internal leaves. *European Food Research and Technology*, 222: 88-98.

Ferreres, F., Valentão, P., Llorach, R., Pinheiro, C., Cardoso, L., Pereira, J.A., Sousa, C., Seabra, R.M., and Andrade, P.B. (2005). Phenolic compounds in external leaves of tronchuda cabbage (*Brassica oleracea* L. var. *costata* DC). *Journal of Agricultural and Food Chemistry*, 53: 2901-2907.

Ferreres, F., Valentão, P., Pereira, J.A., Bento, A., Noites, A., Seabra, R.M., and Andrade, P.B. (2008). HPLC-DAD-MS/MS-ESI Screening of phenolic compounds in *Pieris brassicae* L. reared on *Brassica rapa* var *rapa* L. *Journal of Agricultural and Food Chemistry*, 56: 844-853.

Geuder, M., Wray, V., Fiedler, K., and Proksch, P. (1997). Sequestration and metabolism of host-plant flavonóides by the lycaenid butterfly *Polyommatus bellargus*. *Journal of Chemical Ecology*, 23: 1361-1372.

Harborne, J.B., and Grayer, R.J. (1994). Flavonoids and insects. *In:* The Flavonoids–Advances in Research since 1986, Ed. By Harborne, J.B., Chapman and Hall, London, pp. 589-618.

Knüttel, H., and Fiedler, K. (2001). Host-plant-derived variation in ultraviolet wing patterns influences mate selection by male butterflies. *The Journal of Experimental Biology*, 204: 2447-2459.

Llorach, R., Gil-Izquierdo, A., Ferreres, F., and Tomás-Barberán, F.A. (2003). HPLC-DAD-MS/MS ESI characterization of unusual highly glycosylated acylated flavonoids from cauliflower (*Brassica oleracea* L. *var. botrytis*) agroindustrial byproducts. *Journal of Agricultural and Food Chemistry*, 51: 3895-3899.

Moyes, C.L., Collin, H.A., Britton, G., and Raybould, A. (2000). Glucosinolates and differential herbivory in wild populations of *Brassica oleracea*. *Journal of Chemical Ecology*, 26: 2625-2641.

Müller, C., Agerbirk, Niels, and Olsen, C.E. (2003). Lack of sequestration of host plant glucosinolates in *Pieris rapae* and *P. brassicae*. *Chemoecology*, 13: 47–54.

Muriel, S. B., and Grez, A.A. (2002). Effect of plant patch shape on the distribution and abundance of three lepidopteran species associated with *Brassica oleracea*. *Agricultural and Forest Entomology*, 4: 179-185.

Renwick, J.A.A. (2002). The chemical world of crucivores: lures, treats and traps. *Entomologia Experimentalis et Applicata*, 104: 35-42.

Rochfort, S.J., Imsic, M., Jones, R., Trenerry, V.C., and Tomkins, B. (2006). Characterization of flavonol conjugates in immature leaves of pak choi (*Brassica rapa* L. ssp. *chinensis* L. (Hanelt.)) by HPLC-DAD and LC-MS/MS. *Journal of Agricultural and Food Chemistry*, 54: 4855-4860.

Romani, A., Vignolini, P., Isolani, L., Ieri, F., and Heimler, D. (2006). HPLC-DAD/MS characterization of flavonoids and hydroxycinnamic derivatives in turnip tops (*Brassica rapa* L. Subsp. *sylvestris* L.). *Journal of Agricultural and Food Chemistry*, 54: 1342-1346.

Schittko, U., Burghardt, F., Fiedler, K., Wray, V., and Proksch, P. (1999). Sequestration and distribution of flavonoids in the common blue butterfly *Polyommatus icarus* reared on *Trifolium repens*. *Phytochemistry*, 51: 609-614.

Schoonhoven, L.M., Jermy, T., and van Loon, J.J.A. (1998). Insect-Plant Biology: From Physiology to Evolution. Chapman and Hall, London.

Sousa, C., Valentão, P., Rangel, J., Lopes, G., Pereira, J.A., Ferreres, F., Seabra, R.M., and Andrade, P.B. (2005). Influence of two fertilization regimens on the amounts of organic acids and phenolic compounds of tronchuda cabbage (*Brassica oleracea* L. var. *costata* DC). *Journal of Agricultural and Food Chemistry*, 53: 9128-9132.

Vallejo, F., Tomás-Barberán, F.A., and Ferreres, F. (2004). Characterisation of flavonols in broccoli (*Brassica oleracea* L. var. *italica*) by liquid chromatography–UV diode-array detection–electrospray ionisation mass spectrometry. *Journal of Chromatography A.*, 1054: 181-193.

van Loon, J.J.A., Wang, C.Z., Nielsen, J.K., Gols, R., and Qiu, Y.T. (2002). Flavonoids from cabbage are feeding stimulants for diamondback moth larvae additional to glucosinolates: Chemoreception and behaviour. *Entomologia Experimentalis et Applicata*, 104: 27-34.

Vrchovská, V., Sousa, C., Valentão, P., Ferreres, F., Pereira, J.A., Seabra, R.M., and Andrade, P.B. (2006). Antioxidative properties of tronchuda cabbage (*Brassica oleracea* L. var. *costata* DC) external leaves against DPPH, superoxide radical, hydroxyl radical and hypochlorous acid. *Food Chemistry*, 98: 416-425.

Utilisation and Management of Medicinal Plants (2010) *Pages 174–182*
Editors: **V.K. Gupta, Anil K. Verma and Sushma Koul**
Published by: **DAYA PUBLISHING HOUSE, NEW DELHI**

Chapter 9

Medicinal Properties of Mistletoe: A Review

P.O. Osadebe[1]*, I.C. Uzochukwu[2] and E.O. Omege[1]
[1]Department of Pharmaceutical and Medicinal Chemistry, University of Nigeria, Nsukka, Enugu State, Nigeria
[2]Department of Pharmaceutical and Medicinal Chemistry, Nnamdi Azikiwe University Awka,Anambra State, Nigeria

ABSTRACT

There has been a paradigm shift from sourcing of new drugs from synthetic modifications of lead compounds to biodiversity. The unmatched availability of biodiversity provides unlimited opportunity for lead drug discovery from natural sources. Mistletoe species abound in almost all geographical localities all over the world and has enjoined celebrated fame as folkloric panacea for most common ailments of man. It has been used in traditional medicine to treat ailments like hypertension, diabetes, chronic cramp, epilepsy, headache, menopausal symptoms, infertility, arthritis, rheumatism, convulsive distemper, haemorrhages, prevention of pregnancy (berries), anticancer and a variety of nervous system disorders, stroke, stomach problems, palpitation of the heart, difficulties in breathing, hot flushes, as an antispasmodic, emetic, narcotic tonic, nervine.There has also been many scientific validations of the traditional uses of the semi-parasitic plant which has encouraged some clinical uses of the plant. In this review, an overview of the various species of the plant already described, the folkloric, ethnobotanical, pharmacological and clinical uses of the plant and its phytochemistry and toxicity is presented.

Keywords: Mistletoe, Folkloric importance, Phytochemistry, Pharmacological uses.

* Corresponding Author: E-mail: deleyele@yahoo.com.

Introduction

Natural products, either as pure compounds or as standardised plant extracts, provide unlimited opportunities for new drug leads because of the unmatched availability of chemical diversity (Paul Cos *et al.*, 2006). In fact, approximately 60 per cent of the world's population relies almost entirely on plants for medication (Bancova, 2007). With about 250 000 higher plant species, it is estimated that 35 000 to 70 000 species have, at one time or another, been used in some cultures for medicinal purposes (WHO, 1998).

Mistletoes are semi-parasitic ever-green plants which depend on their host tree for minerals and water only but photosynthesise their carbohydrate by means of its green leaves (Griggs, 1991). They grow on a variety of evergreen and deciduous trees all year round. Over 700 species of the mistletoe plants are known world-wide (Gill, 1973). The name mistletoe is used for several plants that may belong to several genera such as *Viscum* (60 species), *Loranthus, Tapinanthus* etc. and can grow on a variety of host trees.

Mistletoe plants include the European mistletoe (*Viscum album* Linn), Korean mistletoes (*Korthalsella japonica* also known as *Pseudixus japonicus)*, Japanese mistletoe (*Viscum album coloratum*), Australian or Argentine mistletoe (*Ligaria cuneifolia* R. et T.), American mistletoe (*Phoradendron flavescens* also known as *Phoradendron serotinum*), New Zealand mistletoes (*Alepis flavida, Peraxilla tetrapetela, Iloestylus micranthus, Tupeia antartica, Peraxilla colensoi*), Spanish mistletoe (*Arceuthobium oxycedri*) and African mistletoe (*Loranthus bengwensis, Viscum capense, V. rotundifolium, Moquinella rubra, V. obscurum, V. crassulae, V. minimum, Tapinanthus oleifolius, Tapinanthus vittatus, Loranthus micranthus, Viscum engleri, Viscum fischeri* and *Phragmanthera dschallensi, (*Wiens and Barlow, 1975; Gill, 1973; Osadebe *et al.*, 2004*)*

Each species of mistletoe can grow on a variety of host trees. Several host trees of mistletoe have been cited around the world. *Viscum album* Linn. grows on several host trees including fir, pine, apple, oak, wild pear, willow, maple, elm, birch, spruce, populus, rubber, apricot, and eucalyptus among others (Kast *et al.*, 1990; Jung *et al.*, 1996; Becker, 1986; Popova *et al.*, 1990; Ziolinski, J., 1997; Barney *et al.*, 1998). *V. album* mostly parasitizes the Rosaceae family (Barney *et al.*, 1998).

The host trees of Japanese mistletoe, *V. album* var. *coloratum*, include *Quercus mongolica* var. *grosseserrata, Prunus jamasa cura, Quercus serrata, Fagus crenata, Acer palmatum* var. *palmatum, Fagus japonica, Quercus acutissimma, Prunus mume, Pyrus pyrifolia, Alnus japonica, Celtis sinensis* var. *japonica and Populus nigra* var. *italica.*

The host trees of the African mistletoe include cocoa, coffee, custard, apple, guava, hevea, shea tree and citrus fruits. The Northern Nigerian species, *L. bengwensis*, may parasitize *Citrus limon, Vernonia amygdalina, Jatropha curcas* and guava (Obatomi *et al.*, 1994; Obatomi *et al.*, 1997). Other host trees of the African mistletoe include *Bauhinia monandra, Cassia siamea, Ficus benjamina, Callistemon rigidus, Jacaranda mimosifolia, Nerium oleander, Punica granatum, Schinus molle, Diplorhynchus condylocarpon, T. ciliata, Bauhinia monandra Kurz, Callistemon rigidus R. Br., Cassia siamea Lam., Ficus benjamina L.*(Benjamin fig*), Jacaranda mimosifolia D. Don, Nerium oleander L.* (ornamental oleander*), Punica granatum L.* (pomegranate), *Schinus molle, F. benjamina, N. oleander, and J. mimosifolia, Acrocarpus fraxinifolius Arn., Casuarina equisetifolia L., Cupressus arizonica E. Greene, Grevillea robusta Cunn,* black wattle tree, *Acacia mollissima Willd., Carissa edulis Vahl, Juniperus sp., Olea africana Mill., Prunus spp., Rhus natalensis Bernh. Ex Krauss, Acacia nebrownii, Catophractes alexandri, Grewia flava Ziziphus mucronata, Acacia karroo, Euphorbia virosa, Salvadora persica and Tamarix usneoides* (Omuyin *et al.*, 1996; Popp *et al.*, 1995; Johnson *et al.*, 1996; Dalziel, 1937).

Traditional Names of Mistletoe

Mistletoe has several traditional names in different parts of the world. These include:

1. Ibo (Nigeria): Owube or Awurisi
2. Yoruba (Nigeria): Afomo onisana
3. Hausa (Nigeria): Kauchin
4. Mende (Sierra Leone): Ngulu-ngolo-ei
5. Temne (Sierra Leone): E-Lifa
6. English (United Kingdom): Childrens' matches or golden bough

Folkloric Uses

Mistletoe has been used in different cultures for centuries in a variety of medicinal and non-medicinal purposes (American Cancer Society, 1983; Hauser, 1991; Dalziel, 1955; Warren-Davis, 1988). Mistletoe was described as an all-purpose plant (Kafaru, 1993). Both the Celtic Druids and the Norseman hold mistletoe sacred. It was also the plant of peace in Scandinavian antiquity, among whom it was believed that if enemies met by chance beneath it in a forest; they laid down their arms and maintained a truce until the next day. The Druid priesthood in a very special ceremony used mistletoe. The plant is distributed to the people, who hung them over doorways as protection against thunder, lightning and other evils. The folklore, and the magical powers of this plant, blossomed over the centuries. A sprig placed in a baby's cradle would protect the child from fairies. Giving a sprig to the first cow calving after New Year would protect the entire herd. Kissing under the mistletoe is an ancient English custom, originating from the Norse mythology.

Mistletoe is the state flower of Oklahoma in the United States of America, reportedly chosen because it was once used to decorate a settler's gravesite when no other flowers were available (Geobiological Survey, 2001). Magical preparations are prepared by Hausa hunters from the ground berries, Shear butter and a kind of rock salt (Hausa gallo). Eating of the magical preparation every morning is believed to make the hunted game drowsy and easy to kill.

In French Guinea, a species with hairy leaves is used for skin diseases. In Senegal, mistletoe growing on *Acacia seyal* is used to treat chest diseases. The leaves are regarded as purgative, beneficial in colds and chest complaints, especially if collected from *Detarium senegalense*. In Gold Coast, pregnant women are given decoctions of mistletoe. In Sierra Leone, the treatment for rheumatism and boils consists of grinding up the ashes of the plant with palm oil. Some fowl droppings are added before burning the mistletoe to ashes. The preparation is applied to the skin. In Hausa communities, Loranthus parasitic on Shear butter (Kauchin Ka'de) or *Vitex cienkowskii* (Kauchin 'Dunya) are used in prescriptions for Leprosy along with washings of the Koran (drunk along). In the Benue region of Nigeria, Loranthus parasitic on *Calotropis* is specially valued. *Loranthus ophiodes* that grows chiefly on symphonia is a violent poison. (Dalziel, 1955). In Nigeria and some other parts of Africa, it is believed that the aqueous extract of mistletoe (Loranthus) species consumed over a long time will bid farewell to the cause of hypertension, diabetes and other metabolic diseases (Obatomi *et al.*, 1994; Dalziel, 1955; Ofem *et al.*, 2007). It is used in folk medicine to cure many ills. North American Indians used it for toothache, measles and dog bites.

The ethnobotanical uses of mistletoe include the treatment of hypertension, diabetes mellitus, chronic cramp, epilepsy, headache, menopausal symptoms, infertility, arthritis, rheumatism, convulsive distemper, haemorrhages, prevention of pregnancy (berries), anticancer and a variety of nervous system disorders, stroke, stomach problems, palpitation of the heart, difficulties in breathing, hot flushes, as an antispasmodic, emetic, narcotic tonic, nervine (Kafaru, 1994). It is therefore no surprise that mistletoe appears in legends and folklore as a cure all (panacea).

Phytochemistry

Several chemical substances have been isolated and identified in mistletoe plants. These include ML1, ML11, ML111 and *Viscum album* chitin binding agglutinins, isolable from *V. album* (Timoshenko and Gabius, 1993). The complete amino acid sequence of the alpha chain of *V. album's* Lectin 1 has been determined (Soler *et al.*, 1996). Fernandez *et al.*, 1998 identified the flavonoids (quecertin free, quercetin glycosylated and proanthocyanidins corresponding to cyanidin monomers) and protein constituents in *Ligaria cuneifolia*. Comparative studies of *L. cuneifolia* and *V. album* shows that whereas *L. cuneifolia* produces quercetin and its glycosides (quercetin-3-o xyloside, quercetin-3-o rhmnoside, foeniculin, aviculavin) Leuco (catechin, epicatechin, flavan-4-β-ol) and proanthcyanidins (dimers, oligomers and polymers of flavan-4-β-ol), *V. album* produces quercetin methyl derivatives but no proanthocyanidins. Each extract showed a characteristic protein pattern and a differential immunogenic capacity (Wagner *et al.*, 1996).

Two new flavonoid glycosides (rhmnazin-3,4-di-o-glucoside, (2S)-homoeriodictyol-7-o–[apiosyl (102)] glucoside and two known flavonoid glycosides (flavoyadorinin-B and homo-flavoyadorinin-B) were isolated from butanol extract by Fukunaga *et al.* (1989). The authors did not find flavonoid glycosides common to Japanese and European mistletoes. Ursolic acid has been isolated from the European mistletoe (methanolic extract), previously extracted with petroleum ether (Popova and Murzveva, 1990).

Analysis of the fleshly part of *T. leendertziae* showed that aspartic acid was the most abundant amino acid present in the berries (Godschalk, 1983). Other compounds that have been isolated include 2-hydroxy-4, 6-dimethoxychalcon-4-glucoside, syringin, syringarasinol-4, 4-di-o-glucoside, syringaresinolmono-o-glucoside, α–and β-carotenoids, eloxanthin, violaxanthin, β-amyrin, lupeol, stigmasterol, sterol A, ergosterol, galacturonic acid, galactose, arabinose, xylose, fructose, glucose, sucrose, raffinose, rhamnose, palmitic acid, oleic acid, stearic acid, linoleic acid, sinapic acid, caffeic acid, fenilic acid, ascorbic acid, vanilic acid, syringic acid, p-hydroxyphenylacetic acid, protocatechuric acid, quinic acid, shikinic acid, β-phenylethylamine, tyramine, histamine, acetylcholine, propionylcholine and choline (Petricic *et al.*, 1980; Becker *et al.*, 1979; Neamtu and Bodea, 1970; Krzaczek *et al.*, 1976; Krzaczek *et al.*, 1977; Ergun and Didem, 1996).

Pharmacological Activities

Scientific studies, especially of the European mistletoe have shown that composition or activities of mistletoe are host tree, species and harvesting period dependent. (Fukunaga *et al.*, 1989; Obatomi *et al.*, 1994; Osadebe *et al.*, 2004; 2006; Scheer *et al.*, 1992; Wagner *et al.*, 1996). The macromolecular and micromolecular components of different mistletoes species sourced from different host trees may also vary.

The use of the European mistletoe (*Viscum album*) as an anticancer is well documented. Extracts derived from *V. album* have been shown by several authors to kill cancer cells *in vitro* (Hulsen and Mechelke, 1987; Janssen *et al.*, 1993; Jung *et al.*, 1990; Khwaja *et al.*, 1986; Kuttan *et al.*, 1990; Ribereau *et al.*, 1986; Stirpe *et al.*, 1982; Walzel *et al.*, 1990; Schaller *et al.*, 1996). The cell-killing activity has been attributed to the alkaloids (Khwaja *et al.*, 1986), viscotoxins (Scaller *et al.*, 1996; Stein *et al.*, 1999; Stein *et al.*, 1999) and lectins (Walzel *et al.*, 1990; Stirpe *et al.*, 1982; Bussing *et al.*, 1996; Beuth *et al.*, 1992).

Some researchers have identified four different mistletoe lectins: ML1. ML11, ML111 and Viscum album chitin-binding agglutinins. It is proposed that ML1, also called viscumin may be responsible for the many biologic effects of mistletoes since its removal from mistletoe leads to a loss of cytotoxic activities (Janssen *et al.*, 1993; Stirpe *et al.*, 1982). It is most probable that the combination of the alkaloids, lectins and viscotoxins is responsible for mistletoe's effects (Khwaja *et al.*, 1986). Panossian *et al.* (1998) suggested the inhibition of protein kinase as a possible reason for the antitumor effect of *V. album*.

V. album extracts are known to stimulate the immune system cells both *in vitro* and *in vivo* (Hajto *et al.*, 1989; Timonshenko and Gabius, 1993; Bloksma *et al.*, 1982). Mistletoe has therefore been classified as a type of biological response modifier. The immune response is mainly attributed to a stimulation of the mononuclear phagocytic system and to an induction of inflammation by macrophage-derived cytokines (Yesilada *et al.*, 1998). It has also been attributed to stabilisation of the DNA in white blood cells (WBC), including WBC that have been exposed to DNA-damaging chemotherapy agents (Bussing *et al.*, 1995; Bussing *et al.*, 1994). The immune system modulation has also been attributed to the lectin, ML1. Argentine mistletoe, Ligaria cuneifolia, has been demonstrated to exert an immunomodulatory effect on the mouse immune system (Fernandez *et al.*, 1998). Yoon *et al.* (1998) demonstrated that the prophylactic effect of Korean mistletoe extract on tumour metastasis was mediated by enhancement of NK cell activity.

The antihypertensive activities of mistletoe have been documented. The significant reduction of mean arterial pressure by the Northern Nigerian species of the African mistletoe was demonstrated by Obatomi *et al.* (1996) in both normotensive ($P< 0.01$) and spontaneously hypertensive ($P<0.001$) rats. Recently, the antihypertensive property of the south eastern version of mistletoe was reported (Ofem *et al.*, 2007). There was significant reduction of mean arterial pressure of hypertensive rats but not normotensive ones.

The antidiabetic activity of the European mistletoe has not been extensively studied. One research group has documented the antidiabetic activities of the Europoean mistletoe, *Viscum album* (Gray and Flatt, 1999). The researchers also showed that the mechanism of action of the plant extract may be due to stimulation of insulin secretion. The ability of the extract to enhance insulin secretion did not depend upon the use of heat during extract preparation and was therefore not mediated by lectins.

Mistletoe however enjoys folkloric popularity especially in developing countries as an antidiabetic plant. Obatomi *et al.* (1994) showed that the Northern Nigerian species of the African mistletoe (*Loranthus bengwensis*) possess anti-diabetic effects. Infusions of mistletoe parasitic on *Citrus limon* and guava trees significantly decreased serum glucose levels. However, extract of Loranthus bengwensis parasitic on *Jatropha curcas* did not significantly reduce serum glucose. Also, Ohiri *et al.* (2003), reported the hypoglycaemic activity of *Loranthus micranthus*, which was called *Viscum album* in the paper. The host tree variation of antidiabetic activities of *Loranthus micranthus* have also been reported, thus validating the folkloric use of the leaves *of L. micranthus* as an antidiabetic drug (Osadebe *et al.*, 2004). The study showed that *L. micranthus* harvested from *K. acuminata* and *A. indica* host trees exhibited comparatively better antihyperglycemic activities among the tested host trees. A follow-up study by demonstrated that the antidiabetic activities may be attributable to the flavonoids of the powdered leaves (Osadebe *et al.*, 2006).

Anti-inflammatory activities of mistletoe have also been reported. Moderate to weak anti-inflammatory activities has been linked to the less polar components of three Turkish subspecies of *V. album*. Ethanolic extracts are not beneficial for anti-inflammatory purposes probably due to the partial extraction of the low molecular weight polypeptides *e.g.* viscotoxins, which induce an inflammatory response (Yesilida *et al.*, 1998). Preliminary studies on the Eastern Nigerian species, *Loranthus micranthus* showed that the non-polar constituents are potentially anti-inflammatory. This finding is consistent with the studies on the Turkish subspecies of *Viscum album* by Yesilida *et al.* (1998).

Detailed antimicrobial activity of *Viscum album* has not been scientifically documented. Ergun *et al.* (1997) investigated the antifungal activities of the ethanolic extracts of *V. album*. The antimicrobial activities of *L. micranthus* has been reported (Osadebe and Ukwueze, 2004; Osadebe and Akabogu, 2005). The study by Osadebe and Akabogu showed that methanol, ethanol, chloroform and petroleum extracts exhibit antibacterial activities. Only the petroleum extract showed antifungal activities.

Other studies on the plant show that the plant possesses antimotility activities (Osadebe and Uzochukwu, 2006). Recently too, the free radicals scavenging potential of mistletoe has been reported (Nwanjo, 2007). The study suggests that aqueous extract of mistletoe has pronounced antioxidant property, a function that could make mistletoe good for fighting stress and thereby reduce the speed of ageing.

Clinical Uses

Mistletoe is used mainly in Europe and Asia, where mistletoes are commercially available. Brands such as Iscador®, Eurixor®, Helixor®, Isorel®, Vysorel® and Adnobaviscum® are widely used for the management of cancers (Complementary and Alternative Medicine Review, 2000). At the present, there is no official preparation of mistletoe in the Nigerian Drug market and this is the target of my research group.

Toxicity

Mistletoes have been used for centuries without adverse effect. Safety of the plant has been studied (Obatomi *et al.*, 1994; Osadebe *et. al.*, 2004). These studies show that the plant is generally safe. LD_{50} of 5900 to 11650 mg/kg are reported for *L. micranthus* parasitic on some host trees (Osadebe *et al.*, 2004)

Conclusion

Mistletoe plant has been used for many medicinal purposes and can contribute in the solution to many chronic diseases of man if fully exploited.

References

American Cancer Society (1983). Unproven methods of cancer management: Iscador. *CA-A. Cancer Journal for Clinicians*, 33(3): 186-188.

Barney, C. W., Hawksworth, F. G. and Geils, B. W. (1998). Hosts of *Viscum album*. *European Journal of Forest Pathology*, 28(3): 187-208.

Bankova, V. (2007). Natural products chemistry in the third millennium. *Chemistry Central Journal*, 1:1

Becker, H. (1986). Botany of European mistletoe (*Viscum album* L.). *Oncology*, 43(1): 2-7.

Becker, H., Exner, J. and Schilling, G. (1979). Isolation and identification of 2-Hydroxyl-4, 6-dimethoxychalcone-40glycoside of *Viscum album*. *Plant Biochem.*, 90:313.

Bloksma, N., Schmiermann, P., De Reuver, M. *et al.* (1982). Stimulation of humoral and cellular immunity by *Viscum* preparations. *Planta Medica*, 46(4): 221-227.

Boussim, J., Salle, G. and Raynal-Roques, A. (1991). Identification, distribution and biology of *Tapinanthus* species parasitizing Shea trees in Burkina Faso: In proceedings of the fifth international symposium of parasitic weeds. Cimmyt, Nairobi, Kenya, 527.

Bussing, A., Azhari, T., Ostendorp, H. *et al.* (1994). *Viscum album* L. extracts reduce sister chromatid exchanges in cultured peripheral blood mononuclear cells. *European Journal of Cancer*, 30A (12): 1836-1841.

Bussing, A. Regnery, A., Schweizer, K. (1995). Effects of *Viscum album* L. on cyclophosphamide-treated peripheral blood mononuclear cells *in vitro*: sister chromatid exchanges and activation/ proliferation marker expression. *Cancer Letters*, 94(20): 199-205.

Dalziel, J. M. (1937). The useful plants of tropical West Africa, being an appendix to the flora of tropical Africa. Crown agent for Oversea Governments and Administrations, London, 1-612.

Ergun, F. and Didem, D. (1996). HPLC analysis of ascorbic acid in *Viscum album* L. samples. *Journal of Faculty of Pharmacy of Gazi University*, 13(2): 121-125.

Ergun, F. and Didem, D., Berrin, O. and Ufuk, A. (1997). Screening of antifungal activities of various *Viscum album* L. samples. *Journal of Faculty of Pharmacy of Gazi University*, 14(1): 1-4.

Fernandez, T., Marcelo, L. W., Beatriz, G. V., Rafeal, A. R., Silvia, E. H., Alberto, A. G. and Elida A. (1998). Study of an Argentine mistletoe, the hemiparasite, *Ligaria cuneifolia* (R. et. P.) Tiegh. (Loranthaceae). *Journal of Ethnopharmacology*, 62(1): 25-34.

Fukunaga, T., Kajikawa, I., Nishiya, K., Takeya, K. and Itokawa, H. (1989). Studies on the constituents of the Japanese mistletoe, *Viscum album* L. var coloratum Ohwi grown on different host trees. *Chemical and Pharmaceutical Bulletin*, 37(5): 1333-1303.

Geobiological Survey (2001). Oklahoma's State flower: Mistletoe (*Phoradendron flavescens*), USA:1

Gill, F. B (1973). The Machiavellian Frontiers, 38 (2): 2-5.

Godschalk, S. K. B. (1983). A biochemical analysis of the fruit of *Tapinanthus leenderrtziae*. *S. African J. Bot.*, 2: 42-45.

Gray, A. M. and Flatt, P. R. (1999). Insulin secreting activity of the traditional antidiabetic plant, *Viscum album* (mistletoe). *Journal of Endocrinology*, 160: 409-414.

Griggs, P. (1991). Mistletoe, myth, magic and medicine. *The Biochemist*, 13:3-4.

Hajto, T., Hostanska, K. and Gabius, H. J. (1989). Modulatory potency of the beta-galactoside specific lectin from mistletoe extract (Iscador) on host defence system *in vivo* in rabbits and patients. *Cancer Research*, 49(17): 4803-4808.

Hulsen, H. and Mechelke, F. (1987). *In vitro* effectiveness of mistletoe preparation on cytostatic drug resistant human keukemia cells. *Naturwissenschaften*, 74(3): 144-145.

Janssen, O., Scheffler, A. and kabelitz, D. (1993). *In vitro* effects of mistletoe extracts and mistletoe lectins: cytotoxicity towards tumour cells due to the induction of programmed cell death (apotosis). *Progress in Drug Research*, 43(11): 1221-1227.

Johnson, J. M. and Choinski, J. S. (1993). Photosynthesis in the *Tapinanthus diplorhychus* mistletoe host relationship. *Annals of Botany, 72(2):* 117-122.

Jung, M. L., Baudino, S., Ribereau-Gayon, G. *et al.* (1990). Characterization of cytotoxic proteins from mistletoe (*Viscum album*). *Cancer Letters*, 51(2): 103-108.

Kafaru, E. (1993). Mistletoe–an example of an all-purpose herb, herbal remedies, *Guardian Newspapers*, 3rd June: 11

Khwaja, T. A., Dias, C. B. and Pentecost, S. (1986). Recent studies on the anticancer activities of mistletoe (*Viscum album*) and its alkaloids. *Oncology*, 43(1): 42-50.

Kinmonth A. L., Woodcock A., Griffin S., Spiegal N, Campbell M. J. (1998). Randomised controlled trial of patient centred care of diabetes in general practice: impact on current wellbeing and future disease risk. The Diabetes Care from Diagnosis Research Team. *B. M. J.*, 317(7167): 1202–1208.

Kirpichnikov, D., McFarlane, S. I. and Sowers, J. R. (2002). Metformin: An update. *Ann. Intern. Med.*, 137: 25-33.

Kuttan, G., Vasudevan, D. M. and Kuttan, R. (1990). Effect of a preparation from *Viscum album* on tumour development *in vitro* and in mice. *Journal of Ethnopharmacology*, 29(10): 35-41.

Krzaczek, T. (1976). Pharmacobotanical studies of the sub-species *Viscum album* L. 11 *Saccharide*, 31: 281-290.

Krzaczek, T. (1977). Pharmacobotanical studies of the sub-species *Viscum album* L. 111 *Terpane and Sterts*, 31: 281-290.

National Center for Complementary and Alternative Medicine (2000). mistletoe complementary and alternative medicine. NCCAM, MD, USA:1-22.

Neamtu, G. and Bodea, C. (1970). Chemotaxonomic studies on higher plants, three carotenoids of *Viscum album*. *Plant Biochemistry*, 73(13): 59-63.

Nwanjo, H.U. (2007). Free radical scavenging potential of the aqueous extract of Viscum album (Mistletoe) leaves in Diabetic wister rats Hepatocytes. The Internet Journal of Nutrition and wellness. 3 (2):

Obatomi, D. K., Aina, V. O. and Temple, V. J. (1996). Effect of African mistletoe on blood presuure in spontaneously hypertensive rats. *International Journal of Pharmacognosy*, 34 (2): 124-127.

Obatomi, A. K., Bikomo, P.O. and Temple, V.J. (1994) Anti-diabetic properties of the African mistletoe in streptozotocin-induced diabetic rats. *J. Ethnopharmacol.*, 43:13-17.

Obatomi, A. K., Oye, A. A. A. and Temple, V. J. (1997). Reduction in serum glucose and cholesterol levels in experimental diabetic rats treated with extracts of African mistletoe (*Loranthus bengwensis*). *Med. Sci. Res.*, 25: 651-654.

Ofem, O. E., Eno, A. E., Imoru, E., Nkanu, F., and Ibu, J.O. (2007). Feefects of crude aqueous extract of *Viscum album* (Mistletoe) in hypertensive rats. *Indian Journal of Pharmacology*: 39 (1): 15-19.

Ohiri F.C., Esimone O.C., Nwafor S.V., Okoli, C.O. and Ndu, O.O. (2003). Hypoglcaemic properties of *Viscum album* (Mistletoe) in Alloxan-induced Diabetic Animals. *Pharmaceutical Biology*, 41 (3): 184-187

Omuyin, M. E. and Wabule, M. N. (1996). Occurrence of African mistletoe, *Eriathemum ulugurense* on *Toona cliata* and other trees in Kenya. *Plant disease*, 80(7): 823.

Osadebe, P. O., Abana, C. V. and Uzochukwu, I. C (2006). Bioassay-guided isolation targeted studies on the crude methanol extract and fractions of the leaves of *Loranthus micranthus* Linn parasitic on *Azardirachta indica*. In *Recent Progress in Medicinal Plants* Vol 21 (in press).

Osadebe, P.O. and Akabogu, I.C. (2005). Antimicrobial activity of *Loranthus micranthus* harvested from kola nut tree. *Phytotherapia*, 77: 54-56.

Osadebe, P. O., Okide, G. B. and Akabogu, I. C. (2004). Study on anti-diabetic activities of crude methanolic extracts of *Loranthus micranthus* (Linn) sourced from five different host trees. *Journal of Ethnopharmacology*, 95: 133-138.

Osadebe, P.O. and Ukwueze, S.E. (2004). Comparative study of the antimicrobial and phytochemical properties of mistletoe leaves sourced from six host trees. *J. of Biolog. Res. and Biotech.*, 2(1): 18-23.

Osadebe, P. O. and Uzochukwu, I. C. (2006). Chromatographic and antimotility studies on the extracts of *Loranthus micranthus*. *Journal of Pharmaceutical and Allied Sciences*, 3(1): 263-268.

Panossian, A., Kocharian, A., Matinian, K., Amroyan, E., Gabrielian, E., Mayr, C. and Wagner, H. (1998). Pharmacological activity of phenylpropanoids of the mistletoe, *Viscum album* L., host: *Pyrus caucasica*. *Fed. Phytomedicines*, 5(10): 11-17.

Paul Cos, Arnold J. Vlientinck, Dirk Vanden Berghe and Louis Maes, (2006). Anti-infective potential of natural products: How to develop a stronger *in vitro* "proof-of-concept". *Journal of Ethnopharmacology*, 106: 290-302.

Popova, O. I. and Murav' eva, D. A. (1990). Ursolic acid from leafy shoots of *Viscum album*. *Chemistry of Natural Compounds*, 26(3): 346

Popp, M., Mensen, R., Richter, A., Buschmann, H. and Von Willert, D. (1995). Solutes and succulence in Southern African mistletoe trees, 9: 303-310.

Ribereau-Gayon, G., Jung, M. L., Baudino, S. et. al. (1986). Effects of mistletoe (*Viscum album* L.) extracts on cultured tumour cells. *Experientia*, 42 (6): 594-599.

Scheer, R., Scheffler, A. and Errenst, M. (1992). Two harvesting times, summer and winter: are they essential for preparing pharmaceuticals from mistletoe (*Viscum album*)? *Planta Medica*, 58(7): 594.

Soler, M. H., Stanka, S. C. S., Sabine, W., Thomas, S. and Wolfgang, V. (1996). Complete amino acid sequence of alpha chain of mistletoe lectin 1. *FEBS Letters*, 399(1-2): 153-157.

Stirpe, F., Sandvig, K., Olsnes, S. *et al.* (1982). Action of viscumin, a toxic lectin from mistletoe, on cells in culture. *Journal of Biological Chemistry*, 257(220): 13271-13277.

Wagner, M. L., Teresa F., Elida A., Rafeal A. R., Silvia, H. and Alberto, A. G. (1996). Micromolecular and macromolecular comparison of Argentina mistletoe (*Ligaria cuneifolia*) and European mistletoe (*Viscum album*). *Acta Farmaceutica Bonaerense*, 15 (2): 99–105.

Warren-Davis, D. (1988). The myth of mistletoe. *The Herbal Review*, 13: 5-10.

WHO/WPRO (1998). Guideline for the appropriate use of herbal medicines, WHO/WPRO: 1–88.

Wiens, D. and Barlow, B. A. (1975). Permanent translocation, heterozygosity and sex determination in East African mistletoes. *Science*, 187: 1208-1209.

Yesilada, E., Deliorman, D., Ergun, F. *et al.* (1998). Effects of the Turkish subspecies of *Viscum album* on macrophage-derived cytokines. *Journal of Ethnopharmacology*, 61(3): 195-200.

Ziolinski, J. (1997). The mistletoe, *Viscum album* Linn on the left bank of the river in Szczecin. *Zeszyty Naukowe Akademii Rolnictwo*, 66: 69-87.

Utilisation and Management of Medicinal Plants (2010) *Pages 183–201*
Editors: V.K. Gupta, Anil K. Verma and Sushma Koul
Published by: DAYA PUBLISHING HOUSE, NEW DELHI

Chapter 10

Comparative Assessment of Growth Productivity and Chemical Profiling of Wild and Cultivated Populations of *Withania somnifera* (L.) Dunal.

Arun Kumar[1]*, M.K. Kaul[1], Punit Kumar Khanna[2], Sushma Koul[1] and K.A. Suri[1]
[1]Indian Institute of Integrative Medicine (CSIR)
Canal Road, Jammu Tawi – 180 001, India
[2]Shri Mata Vaishno Devi University,
Udhampur – 182 121, Jammu and Kashmir, India

ABSTRACT

Morphological variation among the wild and cultivated populations of *W. somnifera* and relationship of growth characters at different phenophases was studied. Type differences existed as regards to plant height, number of secondary branches, leaf area, biomass, root yield, root characteristics and growth indices like leaf area index (LAI), specific leaf weight (SLW), crop growth rate (CGR) and net assimilation rate (NAR) along with chemical profiling in both the populations. Wild plants exhibited longer growth duration, higher dry matter production and high values for LAI, CGR and NAR at all the stages of growth than cultivated plants. Correlation studies for root yield and different characters revealed that plant height had a direct and positive association with total dry matter production, root yield and NAR in wild populations. Plant height and CGR were also significantly related with each other in both the types but LAI

* Corresponding Author: E-mail: arunsonal2001@gmail.com.

and SLW did not show any regular correlation with plant height or biomass. Phenological studies in relation to energy summation indices (environmental indices) suggested that an average of 2739 degree days are required by the plant for the initiation of seed ripening to obtain maximum dry root yield *i.e.* 17.4 and 5.5 g plant^{-1} in wild and cultivated populations respectively. Chemically both the populations showed uniformity in presence of three markers withanolides-withanolide A, withanone and withaferin A in the roots and quantitatively wild is superior than cultivated populations.

Keywords: *Correlation coefficient, Energy summation indices, Growth indices, Phenophase, Withania somnifera, Withanolides.*

Introduction

Withania somnifera (L.) Dunal (Fam. Solanaceae) is an important shrub, used in Indigenous systems of medicine since ancient times (Singh *et al.*, 1998). A great number of medicinal properties are attributed to this plant and more than hundered formulations are being sold in the market under different trade name in which ashwangadha is a major component (Tripathi *et al.*, 1996). However, recent researches have confirmed its adaptogenic and immunomodulatory value and it has acquired great prominence as anti-stress, anti-inflammatory anti-tumour, anti convulsant and CNS depresing agent (Mishra *et al.*, 2004). It is widely distributed from the southern Mediterranean region to the Canary Island and to South and East Africa; from Palestine upto North India, covering Isarel, Jordan, Egypt, Sudan, Iran, Afganistan, Baluchistan and Pakistan. In India the plant grows wild in North Western regions extending to mountaineous regions of Punjab, Himachal Pradesh and Jammu upto an altitude of 1500m. In India 5000 ha are cultivated in Rajasthan, Madhya Pradesh, Andhra Pradesh and Uttar Pradesh (Kothari *et al.*, 2003). Ashwagandha roots of commerce are obtained mostly from cultivated source of Manasa plantations in Madhya Pradesh where as some of the demand is also met from wild collections. The cultivated type is quite distinct in growth habit and other characters from wild ones (Kumar *et al.*, 2006). A survey of literature revealed that no work has been done to compare the physiological basis of variation in growth, yield and chemical profiling between cultivated and wild germplasms of this species. The present investigation was therefore undertaken to study the extent of morphophysiological variability in these two populations and also to derive a correlation between various physiological parameters, root yield and chemical profiling at different developmental stages.

Materials and Methods

Field experiments were conducted in 2006-2007 at the experimental fields of Indian Institute of Integrative Medicine, Jammu Tawi (400 m above msl, longitude (E) 74°55′, latitude (N) 32°44′). The annual rainfall is about 510mm. The average day temperature is 30.6°C and varies from 17.8°C to 45°C. The highest (45°C) day temperature being in June and lowest (3.32°C night temperature) in January. The experimental location has a subtropical climate.

The experiment was conducted in a randomized block design and seedlings at 4-6 leaf stage were transplanted at 15 × 15 cm distance during September. The net plot size was 4 × 2 m. Growth and development during 210 days life span of the plants was studied to evaluate the best stage for economy. The 210 days of life span of both the populations grouped into three stages (*i*) vegetative stage (150 DAP) (*ii*) Flowering (≥90 per cent stage 180 DAP) and seed ripening/maturity (210 DAP) and replicated 7 times.

The experimental material consisted of wild accessions (AGB 002 from wild populations of Bikaner) and cultivated populations (AGB 025) from Manasa (Madhya Pradesh).

These phonological measurements were assessed using environmental indices *viz.* calendar days, degree days and pan evaporation. The degree days were calculated from seedlings transplanting date to each phenophases according to the following formula:

$$\text{Degree Days} = \sum \frac{Tmax - Tmin}{2} - Tb$$

where

Tmax: Maximum ambient temperature

Tmin: Minimum ambient temperature

Tb: Base temperature (5°C Shahi *et al.*, 1987)

Heat use efficiency (HUE) was calculated by dividing biomass with heat units accumulated degree days (Shastry *et al.*, 1985). Observations on growth and physiological characters are recorded at successive intervals starting from vegetative stage upto seed ripening in each accessions. 20 plants from each accessions were harvested at each phenophase 150, 180 and 210 days after planting (DAP) for recording data. Physiological indices like leaf area index (LAI), specific leaf weight (SLW), crop growth rate (CGR) and net assimilation rate (NAR) at different stages of growth were calculated in each populations following Radford (1967) and data were statistically analysed (Panse and Shukhatme, 1985). Regression equations were computed between root yield as dependent variable and energy summation indices as independent variable (Patterson, 1939). The examination of three withanolides (Withanolide A, Withanone and Withaferin A) content in root was carried out by HPLC method (Khajuria *et al.*, 2004). Present phytochemical variation was carried out on the basis of 3 markers only.

Results

Quantitative Growth Analysis

AGB 025 [Cultivated Populations Figure 10.4(a)]

Morphological analysis of growth behaviour during the different developmental stages presented in Figure 10.1(a) clearly revealed that biomass production and root yield increased significantly with increase in the age of plant till maturity. Results presented in Table 10.1 revealed that plant height, number of leaves and harvest index increases with the advancement of age of the plants till flowering period (180 DAP). Later on progressive trend of increase declined in maturity (210 DAP). The average maximum plant height (40.7 cms) was recorded at flowering stage followed by vegetative stage (34.5 cms). Similar trend was observed in case of number of leaves where maximum number of leaves were recorded at flowering stage (108) followed by vegetative stage (89.8) and lowest at maturity (56.28). The average biomass production per plant during the different growth stages was 23.6g, 32.4g and 39.4g at vegetative, flowering and seed ripening stages respectively. The dry root yield per plant progressively increased with the increase in age during the course of development and were found to be associated with increase in biomass production. In case of harvest index (per cent), it decreases with the increase in age during the various developmental stages and it was observed that 14.85 per cent of harvest index was found at vegetative stage followed by 13.88 per cent and 12.69 per cent at flowering and seed ripening stage respectively (Table 10.1).

Table 10.1: Morphometric and Root Yie!d Characteristics of Wild and Cultivated Populations of *W. somnifera* during Different Phenophases*

Phenos-phase(s)	*Height (cms)*		*No. of Leaves*		*Leaf Area (cm^2)*		*Biomass (g) Dry*		*RootDry Yield (g)*		*Root Length (cm)*		*Root Dia (cm)*		*Harvest Index (per cent)*	
	AGB 002	*AGB 025*	*AGB 002*	*AGB 025*	*AGB 002*	*AGB 025*	*AGB 002*	*AGB 025*	*AGB 002*	*AGB 025*	*AGB 002*	*AGB 025*	*AGB 002*	*AGB 025*	*AGB 002*	*AGB 025*
Vegetative	44.4± 3.6	34.5± 1.77	100.2± 2.7	89.8± 1.8	17.5± 1.2	9.6± 0.8	21.2± 3.2	23.6± 2.9	5.1± 0.9	3.5± 0.03	25.3± 1.2	11.4± 0.5	1.7± 0.05	0.9± 0.03	24.05	14.83
Flowering and Fruiting	69.7± 2.8	40.7± 2.3	108.0± 4.2	110.0± 3.8	23.4± 1.7	9.5± 1.2	51.4± 4.2	32.4± 2.5	12.9± 0.5	4.5± 0.18	27.7± 0.8	12.7± 0.8	3.2± 0.01	1.5± 0.02	25.09	13.88
Seed Maturity	70.9± 3.1	36.7± 3.0	123.4± 3.9	56.2± 3.2	17.2± 2.0	9.5± 1.5	78.3± 3.8	39.4± 3.0	17.4± 1.2	5.0± 0.82	31.6± 0.9	13.4± 1.2	3.6± 0.09	2.0± 0.01	22.22	12.69

*: The Values indicate Mean±SE of 20 plants.

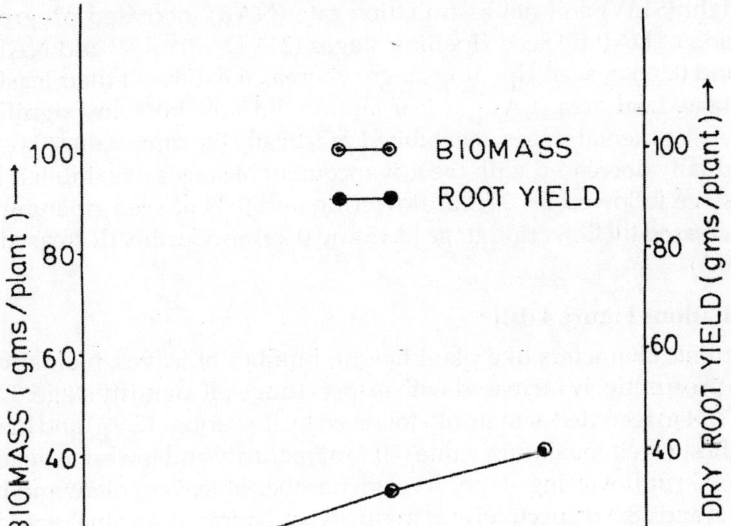

(a) AGB 025

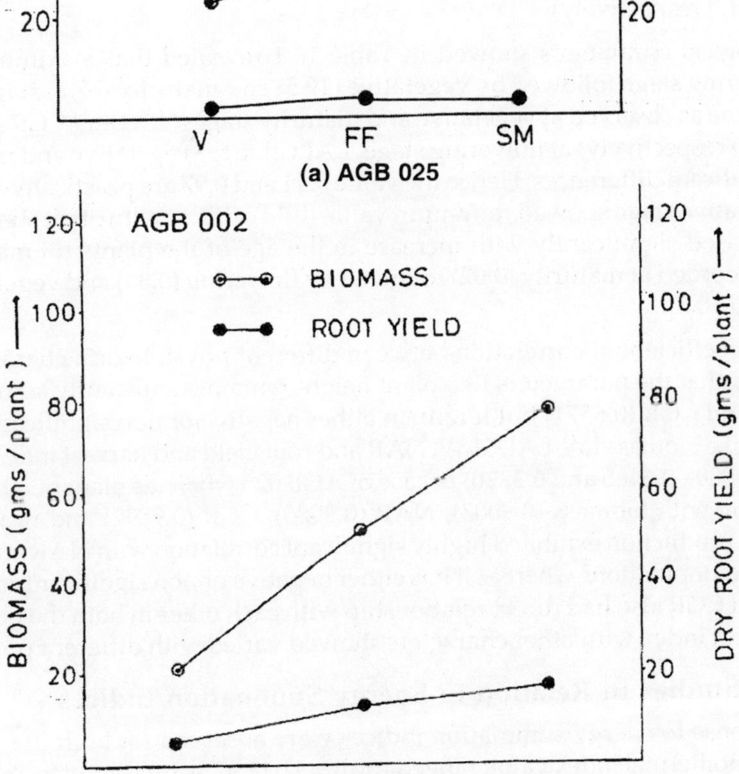

(b) AGB 002

Figure 10.1: Relationship Between Biomass and Root Yield at Various Developmental Stages
Growth Indices: SLW, LAI and NAR
V: Vegetative, FF: Flowering and Fruiting, SM: Seed Maturity

A perusal of the data presented in Figure 10.2(a) for physiological analysis and growth showed that specific leaf weight (SLW) and net assimilation rate (NAR) increased progressively with the increase in the duration of DAP till seed ripening stages (211 DAP). SLW and NAR exhibited their higher values (0.62 and 0.59) in seed ripening stage whereas it exhibited their least value (0.01 and 0.09) at vegetative stage. Leaf area (LA) per leaf lamina did not show any significant result with respect to different developmental stages. It exhibited practically the same value (9.6, 9.5 and 9.5). Leaf area index (LAI) gradually decreased with the advancement of stages. It exhibited maximum value (1.60) at vegetative stage followed by 0.63 at flowering and 0.39 at seed ripening stage. The crop growth rate (CGR) increased till flowering stage (0.15 and 0.29) and further decreased at seed ripening stage (0.23) (Figure 10.3).

AGB 002 [Wild Populations Figure 4 (b)]

The morphoeconimic characters like plant height, number of leaves, biomass production and root yield production prospectively increased with respect to age till maturity stage. Table 10.1 showed maximum root yield (17.4 g) recorded at maturity followed by flowering (12.9 g) and lowest at vegetative stage (5.1). Plant height showed maximum value (70.9) at maturity and lowest at vegetative (44.4) and intermediate value (69.7) at flowering stage. Aveage number of leaves/plant and biomass showed maximum value (123.4 and 78.3 respectively) at maturity and minimum value recorded at vegetative stage (100.2 and 21.2 respectively).

The physiological parameters showed in Table 10.1 revealed that maximum leaf area (23.4) exhibited in flowering stage followed by vegetative (19.5) and maturity (17.2) stages. Leaf area/leaf was practically same as observed at vegetative and maturity stages. LAI and CGR showed maximum value (1.19 and 1.0 respectively) at flowering stage. LAI value for vegetative and maturity stages did not show any significant differences. Hence the value 0.94 and 0.97 are practically similar where as in case of CGR vegetative stage showed minimum value (0.14) and at maturity it showed intermediate (0.90). NAR increased significantly with increase in the age of the plants till maturity. Maximum values for NAR recorded at maturity (0.92) followed by flowering (0.84) and vegetative (0.15) stages [Figure 10.2(b) and 10.3].

A perusal of coefficient of correlation between different physiological characters presented in Table 10.2 showed that the parameters like plant height remain significantly associates with leaves number (0.9124) and CGR (0.6571) but it remain either negative or non significant correlation with other parameters like biomass LA, LAI, SLW, NAR and root yield and harvest index (0.2066,–0.2471,–0.0613,–0.0775, 0.0080,–0.6465 and 0.3320) in case of AGB 025 where as plant height had a direct and positive association with biomass (0.9003), NAR (0.9985), CGR (0.9892) and root yield (0.9461) in AGB 002. Biomass production exhibited highly significant correlation with NAR and CGR in both the wild and cultivated populations whereas it has either negative or non significant correlation with LA and LAI. NAR and CGR also had direct relationship with each other in both the populations (0.7484 and 0.9798). Harvest index with other characters showed varied with different populations.

Morphological Studies in Relation to Energy Summation Indices

A linear response to energy summation indices were observed for both the populations in *W. somnifera*. The phenothermal index value ranged form 9.92-12.97 as presented in Table 10.3. Calendar days was observed from 150-211 at different developmental stages *i.e.* vegetative, flowering and maturity. An average of 2739 degree days are required by the plant for the initiation of seed ripening stage where the maximum dry root yield was observed in both the accessions. (AGB 002-17.4gm, AGB 025-5.5gm)

Table 10.2: Correlation Coefficient for Different Characters in Two Populations of *Withania somnifera* (L.) Dunal

Characters	*Population(s)*	*Biomass*	*Number of Leaves*	*LA*	*LAI*	*SLW*	*NAR*	*CGR*	*Root yield*	*HI*
Plant Height	AGB 025	–0.2066	0.9134**	–0.2471	–0.0613	–0.0775	0.008	0.6571*	–0.6465	0.332
	AGB 002	0.9003**	0.7835**	0.4264	0.5593	0.3509	0.9985**	0.9892**	0.9461**	–0.1964
Biomass	AGB 025	–	–0.5869	–0.8969	–0.9633	0.9914**	0.9800**	0.6017*	–0.6127	–0.9915
	AGB 002		0.9758**	–0.0095	0.1429	0.0913	0.9227**	0.8271**	0.9927**	–0.6034
Number of Leaves	AGB 025	–	–	0.6872*	0.1685	0.3502	–0.4765	–0.4101	0.2685	–0.9819
	AGB 002			0.2278	–0.0767	0.3067	0.8162**	0.6843*	0.9425**	–0.7554
LA	AGB 025	–	–	–	0.9823**	–0.9468	–0.9669	–0.8928	0.8990*	0.8319**
	AGB 002				0.9883**	0.3765	0.3765	0.554	0.1105	0.7970**
LAI	AGB 025	–	–	–	–	–0.9903	–0.9975	–0.7926	0.8010**	0.9211**
	AGB 002					–0.9725	0.5133	0.6744*	0.2607	0.1191
SLW	AGB 025	–	–	–	–	–	0.9975**	0.7005	–0.7104	–0.9666
	AGB 002						0.2994	–0.4840	–0.0288	–0.8491
NAR	AGB 025	–	–	–	–	–	–	0.7484**	–0.7576	–0.9444
	AGB 002							0.9798**	0.9623**	–0.2495
CGR	AGB 025	–	–	–	–	–	–	–	–0.9999	–0.5151
	AGB 002								0.8886**	–0.051
Root Yield	AGB 025	–	–	–	–	–	–	–	–	–0.8586
	AGB 002									–0.5033

*: Significant at 5 per cent (P=0.005); **: Significant at 1 per cent (P=0.01).

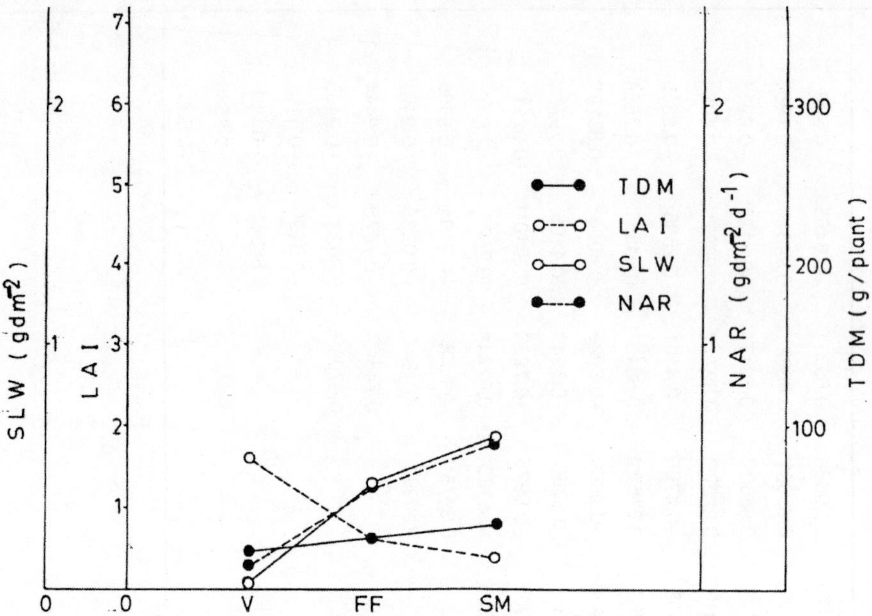

(a) AGB 025

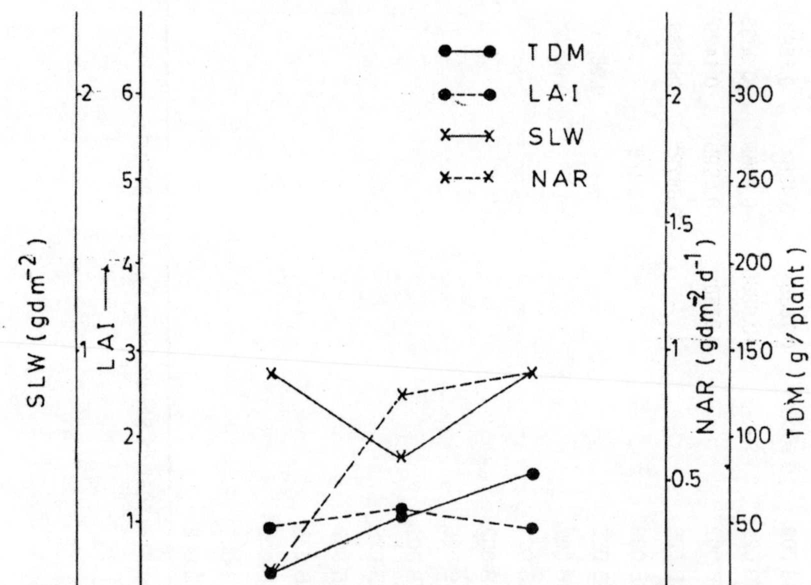

(b) AGB 002

Figure 10.2: Growth Indices and Dry Matter Production at Various Developmental Stages in *Withania somnifera* Types

Growth Indices: SLW, LAI and NAR

V: Vegetative, FF: Flowering and Fruiting, SM: Seed Maturity

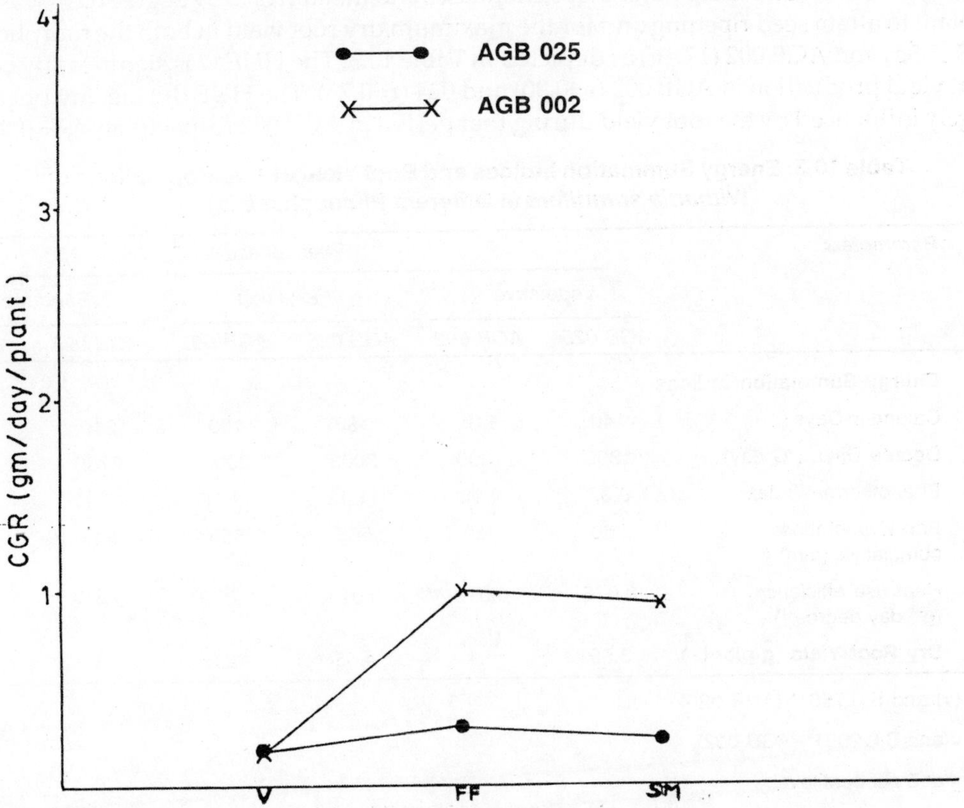

Figure 10.3: Crop Growth Rate (CGR) at Various Developmental Stages

respectively (Table 10.3). The heat use efficiency (HUE) was greatly influenced by the crop growth stage. It was less during the vegetative stage and maximum in the later stage *i.e.* seed maturing stage except 025 where HUE was less (0.012) as compared to vegetative and flowering stage (0.016 and 0.017 respectively). The HUE was significantly correlated with root yield production in both the accessions (Table 10.3). Significant correlation coefficient (r) among root yield and calendar days, degree days and pan evaporation was observed (Table 10.4). It has proved that all three parameters *viz.* calendar days, degree days and pan evaporation are equally important for production of root during the studied growing period. Therefore production of root yield to significantly correlated calendar days, degree days and pan evaporation has been presented in the form of a linear regression (Table 10.4).

A linear response to energy summation indices were observed for *Withania somnifera* to phasic developments suggesting that heat unit concept is appropriate for this medicinal crop. The phenothermal value ranged from 9.92 to 12.97 as presented in Table 10.3 indicated that the effect of varying ambient temperature along with crop age has no determental effect on production of root yield possible due to the value remained consistent around the mean value 11.7. The variability in root yield of the plant was observed during different phenophases and the sum of 2739 degree days was required by this plant to attain seed ripening and for the maximum dry root yield in both the morphotypes *i.e.* AGB 025 (5.5g) and AGB 002 (17.4g) as depicted in Table 10.3. The HUE was significantly correlated with root yield production in AGB 002 (r=0.90) and 024 (r=0.75). The HUE during any phenophases was largely influenced by the root yield during that period in AGB 002 respectively (R^2=0.81).

Table 10.3: Energy Summation Indices and Root Yield of Two Populations of *Withania somnifera* at Different Phenophase (s)

	Parameters	Phenophase (s)					
		Vegetative		Flowering		Seed Maturity	
		AGB 025	AGB 002	AGB 025	AGB 002	AGB 025	AGB 002
A.	**Energy Summation indices**						
(i)	Calendar Days	140	140	180	180	210	210
(ii)	Degree Days (°C day)	1390	1390	2003	2003	2739	2739
(iii)	Phenothermal Index	9.92	9.92	11.12	11.12	12.97	12.97
(iv)	Pan Evaporation cumulative (mm)	360	360	565	565	844	844
(v)	Heat use efficiency (g^{-1} day $degree^{-1}$)	0.016	0.015	0.017	0.029	0.012	0.028
B.	**Dry Root Yield (g $plant^{-1}$)**	3.55	5.1	4.55	12.9	5	17.4

r between (v) and B 0.7561* (AGB 025)

r between v and B 0.9091* (AGB 002)

* Significant at 5 per cent level.

Table 10.4: Linear Descriptive Statistics Between Root Yield (Dependent Variable) Calendar Days, Degree Days and Pan Evaporation in Two Populations

Parameter	Statistics				
	Correlation Coefficient (r)* Y and X_1, X_2 and X_3	Coefficient Determination (r^2 x 100)	Regression Constant (a)	Regression Coefficient (b)	Regression Equation
	Root yield (y) (g $plant^{-1}$)				
(i) Calendar Days (CD) (X_1)	(i) 0.9900 (ii) 0.9812	(i) 98.01 (ii) 96.27	(i) –1.266 (ii) –24.50	(i) 0.031 (ii) 0.201	(i) Y_{CD}=-1.266 + 0.031 X_1 (ii) Y_{CD}=-24.50 + 0.201 X_1
(ii) Degree Days (DD) (X_2)	(i) 0.9993 (ii) 0.9760	(i) 99.86 (ii) 95.52	(i) 1.406 (ii) –7.032	(i) 0.0015 (ii) 0.009	(i) Y_{DD}=1.406 + 0.0015 X_2 (ii) Y_{DD}=-7.032 + 0.009 X_2
(iii) Pan Evaporation (PE) (X_3)	(i) 0.9956 (ii) 0.9696	(i) 99.12 (ii) 94.01	(i) 2.063 (ii) –11.107	(i) 0.004 (ii) 0.047	(i) Y_{PE}=2.063 + 0.004 X_3 (ii) Y_{PE}=-11.107 + 0.047 X_3

Abbreviation: (i): AGB 025; (ii): AGB 002.

* Significant at 5 per cent probability level.

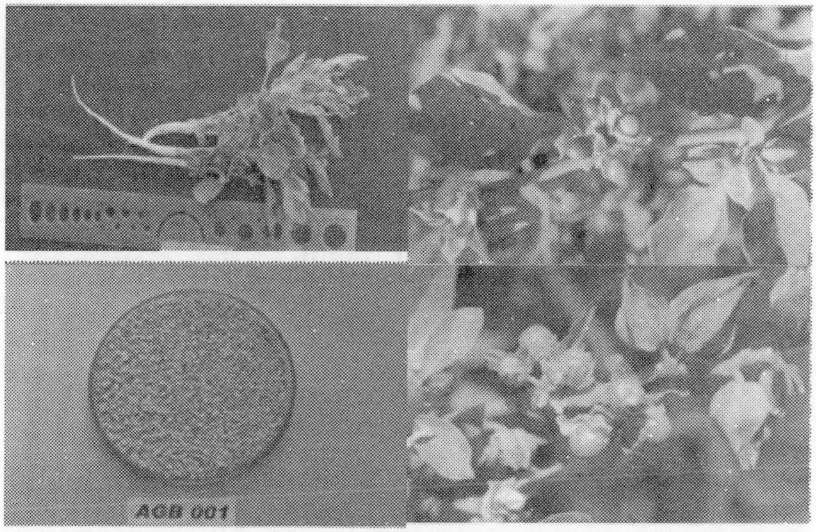

(a) AGB 025

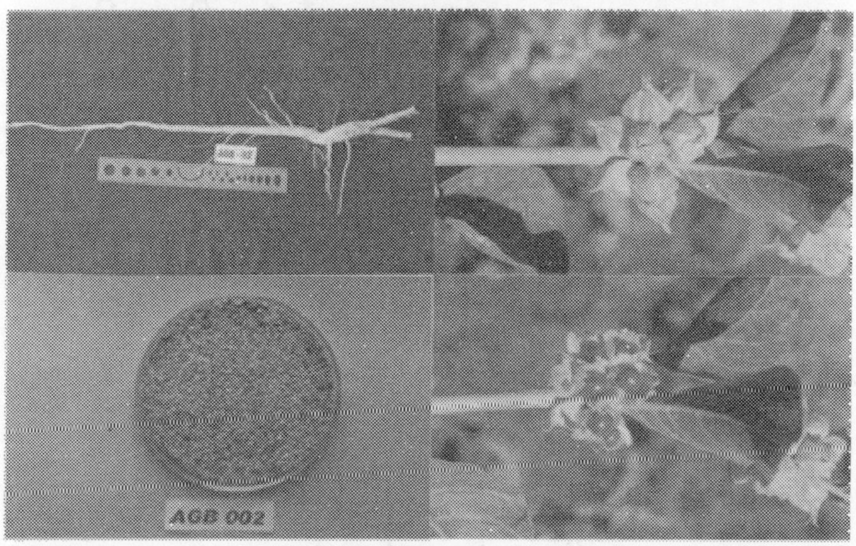

(b) AGB 002

Figure 10.4: Wild Population (AGB 002) and Cultivated Population (AGB 025) of *Withania somnifera*

Phenological Studies in Relation to Root Yield and Chemical Constituents

A linear increase in root yield and its associated characters was observed in both the accessions in accordance with various phenophases as depicted in Table 10.1. Maximum root yield was obtained at seed maturation stage irrespective to different populations. AGB 002 and AGB 025 populations exhibited maximum root yield (17.4 g plant^{-1}, 5g plant^{-1}) at seed maturity stage. Although no marked

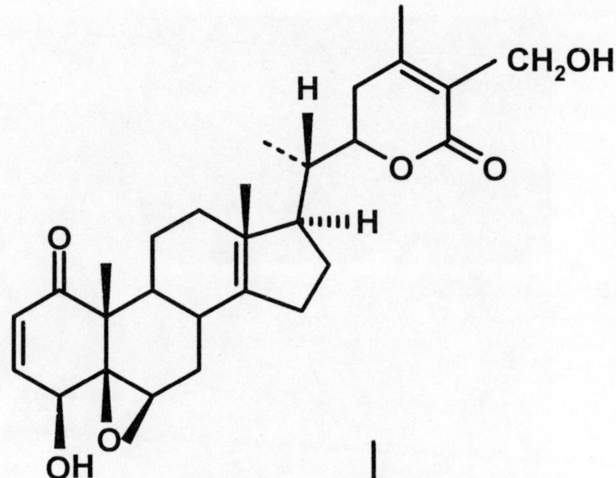

Withaferin A

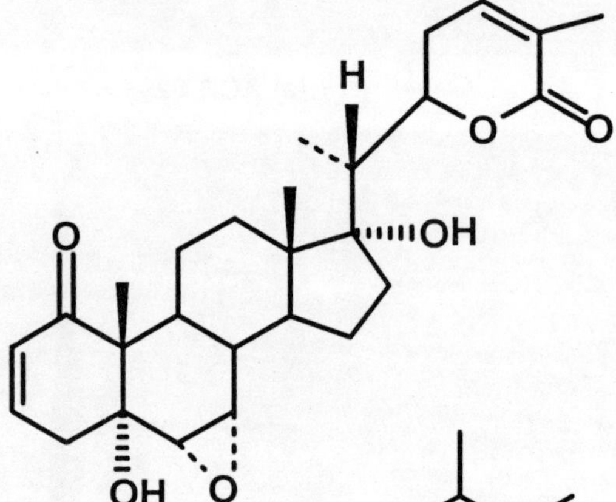

Withanone

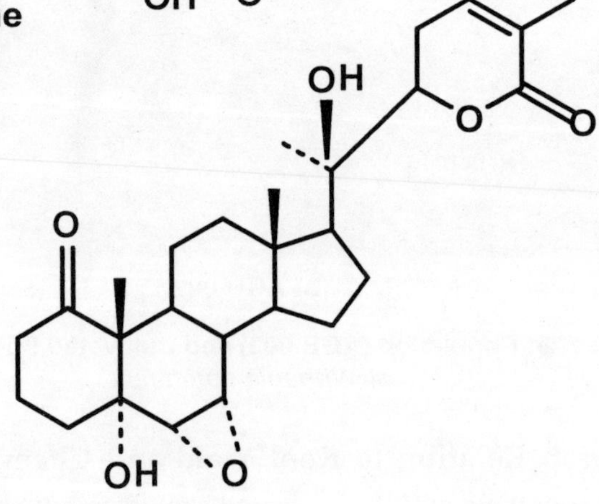

Withanolide A

Figure 10.5: Chemical Structure of Three Withanolide Markers

differences were observed in tap root length and secondary root numbers in the studied two populations in relation to root yield but tap root diameter exhibited progressive increase. Chemical profiling (Figure 10.5) of roots at different phenophases of the wild and cultivated populations showed that Withanolide A and Withanone increases gradually with the advancement of age where as withaferin A content decreases. AGB 002 possessed higher withanolide A content during all the phenophases (0.12, 0.016 and 0.115 g/100g) as compared to AGB 025 (0.008, 0.13 and 0.018 g/100g). Withaferin A content was maximum at vegetative stage followed by flowering and fruiting stage in both the populations. There were no significant difference in withanone content between AGB 002 and AGB 025 (Table 10.5).

Table 10.5: Withanolides Content in Roots of AGB 002 and AGB 025 at Different Phenophases

Phenophases	*Withanolide content (g/100g)**					
	Withanolide A		*Withanone*		*Withaferin A*	
	AGB 025	*AGB 002*	*AGB 025*	*AGB 002*	*AGB 025*	*AGB 002*
Vegetative	0.008±0.002	0.012±0.003	0.012±0.001	0.010±0.001	0.017±0.0001	0.029±0.0005
Flowering Fruiting	0.013±0.003	0.016±0.004	0.015±0.0001	0.025±0.003	0.010±0.0002	0.015±0.0001
Seed Maturity	0.018±0.002	0.115±0.002	0.006±0.0003	0.076±0.002	0.008±0.0005	0.006±0.0001

* Mean of 3 replicates.

Discussion

Present experiment reveals that wild populations (AGB002) having longer duration of growth produced higher dry matter than short duration type AGB025 (cultivated) populations [Figures 10.1(a) and (b)]. Similarly minimum biomass produced in the latter was traced to lowest values of LAI, NAR, and CGR (Figure 10.2(a). This suggests that differences in total dry matter production are linked directly with LAI, NAR and CGR. Such observations have been recorded in a number of crops like soyabean (Nirmala and Balasubramanian, 1990) and Pea (Sharma and Garg, 1984). The optimum peak value LAI varies between 0.39 to 1.60 in AGB025 and 0.94 to 1.19 in AGB002. In cereals the optimum value of LAI varies between 4 and 6 (Hipps *et al.*, 1983). Rahangdale *et al.*, 1987 reported that in newly germinated crop, LAI remains below 1.0; reaches maximum value (2-8) as crop develops. Since environmental conditions effect growth and development, LAI values are also reflected with environment. In the present study the LAI at vegetative stage below 1 due to developmental stage [Figures 10.2(a) and (b)]. LAI was found to have no significant association with plant height and biomass in AGB002 and negative correlation in AGB 025. It was observed that SLW did not show any positive correlation with root yield in any populations. From the above discussion on leaf characters it can be inferred that the yield with respect to biomass production and root yield was affected through the assimilate supply to the seed and is governed by the size of photosynthetic system active over a longer period of time would translate more dry matter to the seed. In this regard, the low yielding populations of *Withania somnifera* (AGB025) showed a predominant source limitations to the root yield and biomass production in having fewer leaves, lower leaf area and specific leaf weight.

Correlation studies for NAR and different physiological characters showed that biomass and CGR had a direct positive association with NAR in both the populations AGB025 and AGB002 where as plant height and root yield has also positive correlation with NAR in AGB002 except AGB025. Out of 9 coefficient of correlations between various characters with NAR, 5 were found significant in AGB002 except AGB025 (Table 10.2; Figure 10.3).

In the context of physiological growth ratio in the plant species, which have a high growth rate *viz.*, CGR and NAR in the early part of the growing stage might be of great interest and is worth further considerations and could be better harvested for dry matter productions, possibly resulting in an important yield potential *i.e.* a higher generative sink capacity and in higher phytomass production. Even in the present context the physiological growth rates have shown an increase significantly till maturity period in both the populations studied herewith and declined in rest stages of growth excluding crop growth rate. The frequencies of these growth rates have been observed to be less in dormancy period (December to January) due to inference with the photosynthetic process. The frequency differences in both the populations at various growth staged was not at per as suggested by Yoshida (1972) in various cereals. Concerning the goal of overall increased NAR and CGR; Day and Chalabi (1988) showed a simple mathematical model that a 10 per cent increase in maximum photosynthetic rate corresponded to a mere 2.5 per cent increase in canopy photosynthesis and hence crop growth. Even this marginal benefit would disappear if the increase in the photosynthetic rates were to be associated with the decreased leaf size as has been observed in several crop species (Planchon and Fesquet, 1982; Bhagsari and Brown, 1986). Similar to NAR, the crop growth rate (CGR) also followed the same pattern but the frequencies were found to be specific to both populations and it resumed the pattern of increasing with the advancement of age. Present studies are in conformity with the earlier workers like Kumar *et al.* (2008).

The evaluation of correlation between phytomass and associated parameters revealed that SLW, NAR, LA and HI were found to have significant correlations with biomass root yield production (Table 10.2). These associations were only limited to higher productivity shown during the various growth stages while in low productive populations these correlations were not significant. The pooled analysis of physiological and coefficients of correlation between the different characters showed that high yielding AGB 002 was found superior to all the characters as compared to AGB 025 (Cultivated populations). On the basis of results discussed it is clear that plant height, SLW, LAI, NAR, CGR, biomass and root yield can be used as important markers in the selection of high yielding strain of *Withania somnifera*.

The role of climatic factors chiefly ambient temperature, pan evaporation and heat use efficiency (HUE) in relation to root yield at different phenophases of the *Withania somnifera* was studied. Living system are influenced by the environment which includes both external and internal factors. The internal environment is stable and its effects are slow and subtle. The external environment is the climate which regulates and determines the growth and development of crop plants (Mavi, 1986). Climate of an area is a major ecological factor determining the types of plants that could occur there. Climo-vegetation relationship is one of the best parameters for understanding the performance, occurrence and stability of the plant in a community within the existing climatic conditions.

Ambient temperature is one of the important climatic factor as heat energy affects the growth and distribution of plants. Growth of plant is virtually inhibited near 0°C. Growth of plants is stopped and damaged at low temperature just below 15°C in a large number of plants in tropical and sub-tropical region. Temperature, through its effect on rates of germination, emergence and leaf growth, influences the plant to attain a leaf area index of 4 (at which most incoming radiation are intercepted). These rates vary greatly between species and also to some extent within species. The leaf extension of sorghum nearly ceases around 10°C (Johnson, 1967), whereas even at 3°C barley leave continue to grow slowly. Thus, rates of most biological processes are affected by temperature. Reaumur's assumption that thermometric constant expressed the amount of heat required for a plant to reach a given stage of maturity (Nuttonson, 1955) gave rise to the heat unit system of today. The heat unit approach is used for studying plant temperature relationship by the accumulation of daily temperature during the growing season. In other words heat unit is a mathematical expression of plant and temperature relationship expressed as degree days or growing degree days. Growing degree days, heat units, effective heat units or growth units are a simple means of relating plant growth, development and maturity to air temperature (Vittum *et al.*,1965). It holds that the growth of the plant is dependent upon the amount of heat to which it was subjected during its life time.

Heat unit system has found use in vegetables (Peas), wheat, sorghum, corn and fruit plants for predicting the dates of harvest and for the timing of successive planting (Katz, 1952; Gilmore and Rogers, 1958; Warnick, 1973; Chakravarty and Sastry, 1983; Ghadekar *et al.*, 1985). Degree day accumulation can be used by growers to monitor the development of biological processes and thus can be used in crop and pest management. The adaptations and use of degree days by individual growers and agricultural advisors, however have been limited partly because of computational difficulties involved in the derivation of degree days. Snyder (1985) has described a method for the calculation of degree days with any threshold temperatures using simple arithmetic operations and a table of normalized areas from the trigonometric sine curve method of calculating degree days.

The simplicity of the degree day method has made it widely popular in guiding agricultural operation and planning and use. Most applications of the growing degree day concept are for the forecast of crop harvest dates, yield and quality. It also helps in forecasting labour needs for factory and to reduce harvesting and factory cost (Mavi, 1986). The concept is also applied to plants other than crop plants and to the problems of growth and development in insects, plant pathogens, birds and other animals (Hord and Spell, 1962). A potential area of its application lies in estimating the likelihood of the successful growth of a plant in an area in which it has not been grown earlier. It also helps in selection of one variety from several varieties of plants to be grown in a new area. It has practical utility to plant breeders who are concerned with labeling newly developed hybrids with the best possible estimate of relative maturity, as studied by Gilmore and Roger (1958) while working on corn. As a result of this, farmers desire to choose hybrids with the right maturity to match on existing environment. This study is also beneficial for estimating corn growth yield (Swan *et al.*, 1987).

Year to year variation in range of herbage yield has been attributed to variations in precipitation (Sneva and Hyder, 1962). Pitt and Heady (1978) identified 5 annual range weather variables that explained 73 per cent of the variation in standing crop. George *et al.* (1988) explained that the accumulated degree days accounted for 74 to 91 per cent of the variation in seasonal herbage yield while accumulated days accounted for 64 to 86 per cent of the variation on winter annual range lands of California.

Heat units is a mathematical expression of plant and temperature relationship expressed as Degree Days or Growing Degree Days (GDD). It holds that the growth of plant is dependent upon the amount of heat to which it was subjected during the life time. Knowledge of the average number of heat units required to reach various phenological stages may aid in the modeling of plant development, scheduling of planting and harvesting dates. Several workers have pointed out that the dates of phenological events in plants when correctly interpreted, are the best indices of the bioclimatic characters of an area/region. On the basis of phenological pattern, a phenothermal index relates to plant climate interactions. It has also practical utility to plant breeders who are concerned with leveling newly developed hybrids with the best possible estimate of relative maturity.

A linear response to energy summation indices were observed for *Withania somnifera* to phasic developments suggesting that heat unit concept is appropriate for this medicinal crop. The phenothermal index value ranged from 9.92 to 12.97 as presented in Table 10.3, indicated that the effect of varying ambient temperature alongwith crop age had no determental effect on production of root yield possible due to the value remained consistent around the mean value 11.17. The variability in root yield of this plant was observed during different phenophases and the sum of 2739 degree days was required by this plant to attain seed ripening stage and for the maximum dry root yield in different populations AGB 025 (5.50g) and AGB 002 (17.4g) as depicted in Table 10.3. The Heat use efficiency (HUE) was greatly influenced by the crop growth stages. The HUE was significantly correlated with root yield production in AGB 002. The HUE and CGR facilitate relative assessment of different growth stages (Singh *et al.*,1991; Kumar *et al.*, 2001). Significant correlation coefficient (r) among root yield and calendar days, degree days and pan evaporation was observed in both populations studied (Table 10.4). It has proved that all the three parameters *viz.* calendar days, degree days and pan evaporation are equally important for production of root yield during the studied growing period. Therefore, prediction of root yield to significantly correlated calendar days, degree days and pan evaporation has been presented into the form of a linear regression equation (Table 10.4).

The study based on meteorological time scale seems to be good predictor of harvest management practices for getting optimal root yield under specific envionrment. Thus accurate and reliable simulations of crop phenophases help in judging the optimum period of harvest to get maximum root yield. Similar finding were also reported from other crops *viz.* wheat an sorghum (Chakravarty *et al.*, 1983; Ghadekar *et al.*, 1985).

Phenological description provide ecologically valuable informations about the average duration of the growing and foliated periods of the plant species. Phenology is not limited to the describe dating of events, but also to clarify that influence of climatic factors (Larcher, 1983). Phenology relates to the periodical phenomena of plant life with a series of quantitative estimates of environmental factors. Due to large number of factors involved in any vital approach, most of the phenological studies have been studied.

Phenological studies in relation to root yield and chemical constituents have been studied on this medicinal plant in relation to crop management. A linear increase in root yield and its associated characters was observed in all the four morphotypes in accordance with various phenophases as depicted in Table 10.1. Maximum root yield was obtained at seed maturation stage irrespective to morphotype suggested that we can get optimum yield of *Withania somnifera* when it harvested at seed maturation stage. The root yield of AGB 002 populations exhibited maximum root yield 17.40g plant^{-1} at seed maturation stage followed by flowering (12.90 g plant^{-1}) and vegetative stage (5.10 g plant^{-1}). Where as AGB 025 populations showed lowest root yield as compare to AGB 002 but it also exhibited maximum root yield at seed maturation stage *i.e.*, 5.00 g plant^{-1} followed by flowering (4.55g plant^{-1}) and vegetative stage (3.55g plant^{-1}).

Although, no marked differences were observed in tap root length and secondary root numbers in the studied morphotypes in relation to root yield but tap root diameter exhibited a progressive increase (Table 10.1). Root diameter ranged from 1.5 to 3.0 cms was found most suitable in terms of root chemical composition having less fibre content. Delayed harvesting might result in poor root chemical composition and higher production of fibrous content.

Ontogenetic changes in alkaloidal and withanolide content were reported by Kumar *et al.* (2001) that total alkaloid and withanolide content gradually decreases with the advancement of crop age while studying with four morphotypes of *Withania somnifera*.

Declining trend in Withaferin A content was observed in both the populations with passage of time and at maturity exhibited minimum value for its content. In case of withanolide A and withanone content AGB 002 (0.012, 0.016 and 0.115/0.010, 0.025, 0.076) showed superiority over AGB 025 (0.008, 0.13, 0.18/0.012, 0.015 and 0.006) but the pattern is in reverse order *i.e.* its content gradually increased with the advancement of age. Active constituents like total alkaloid and withanolide are also reported to be higher in leaves of *Withania somnifera* at vegetative stage but there was no qualitative changes of these constituents during the different developmental stages (Abraham *et al.*, 1968). Although, root yield in both populations of *Withania somnifera* was found higher at seed ripening stage but Withaferin A content were low, probably due to increase in fibrous content of the roots which also decreased chemical constituents of the roots. From the above mentioned results, it has been concluded that crop should be harvested at full blooming stage to get optimum root yield production and better root chemical composition irrespective to any populations in *Withania somnifera*.

Acknowledgements

The author are thankful to Director, IIIM, Jammu for providing facilities and Sh. Madan Lal for his technical assistance and field work.

References

Abraham, A., Kirson, I., Glotter, E. and Lavie, D. (1968). Chemotoxanomic study of *Withania somnifera* (L.) Dunal. *Phytochemistry*, 7: 957-962.

Bhagsari, A. S. and Brown, R. H. (1986). Leaf photosynthesis and its correlation with leaf area. *Crop Science*, 26: 127-132.

Chakravarty, N. V. K. and Sastry, P. S. N. (1983). Phenology and accumulated heat unit relationship in wheat under different planting dates in the Delhi region. *Agricultural Science Progress*, 1: 33-43.

Day, W. and Chalabi, Z. S. (1988). Use of models to investigate the link between the modification of photosynthetic characteristics and improved root yields. *Plant Physiol. Biochem.*, 26: 511-517.

George, M. R., Raguse, C. A., Clawson, W. J., Wilson, C. B., Milloughby, R. L., Mcdougald, N. K., Duncan, D. A. and Murphy, A. H. (1988). Correlation of degree days with annual herbage yield and livestock gains. *J. Range Manage*, 41: 193-197.

Ghadekar, R. S., Chipde, D. L. and Sethi, H. N. (1985). Growth and yield and heat unit accumulation in Sorghum hybrids in wet season on the vertisole of Nagpur. *Ind. J. Agric. Sci.*, 55: 487-490.

Gilmore, E. C. and Rogers, J. S. (1958). Heat unit as a method of measuring maturity in Corn. *Agron. J.*, 50: 611:615.

Hipps, L. E., Asper, G. and Kanemasu, E. T. (1983). Assessing the interception of Photosynthetically active radiation in winter wheat. *Agric. Meteor.*, 28: 253-259.

Hord, N. H. V. and Spell, D. P. (1962). Temperature as a basis for forecasting banana production. *Trop. Agric.*, 39: 219-223.

Johnson, W. C. (1967). Diurnal variation in growth rate of grain sorghum. *Agron. J.*, 59: 41-44.

Kartz, Y. H. (1952). The relationship between heat unit accumulation and planting harvesting of unit accumulation and planting harvesting of canning Peas. *Agron. J.*, 44: 74-78.

Khajuria, R. K., Suri, K. A., Gupta, R. K., Satti, N. K., Amina, M., Suri. O. P. and Qazi, G. N. (2004). Separation, identification and quantification of selected withanolides in plant extracts of *Withania somnifera* by HPLC-UV (DAD)-positive ion electroscopy ionization-mass spectrometry. *J. Sep. Sci.*, 27(7-8): 541-546.

Kothari, S. K., Singh, C. P., Kumar, Y. V. and Singh, K. (2003). Morphology, yield and quality of ashwagandha (*Withania somnifera* L. Dunal) roots and its cultivation economics as influenced by tillage depth and plant population density. *J. Hortic. Sci. Biotechnol.*,78(3): 422-425.

Kumar, A., Kaul, B. L. and Verma, H. K. (2000). Correlation of root yield and yield component in different morphotypes of *Withania somnifera* (L.) Dunal. *Int. J. Mendal.*, 17(1-2): 21-22.

Kumar, A., Kaul, B. L. and Verma, H. K. (2001). Phenological observations on root yield and chemical composition in different morphotypes of *Withania somnifera* (L.) Dunal. Journal of *Medicinal and Aromatic Plant Sciences*, 23: 21-23.

Kumar, A., Kaul, M. K., Bhan, M. K., Khanna, P. K. and Suri, K. A. (2007). Morphological and chemical variation in 25 collections of the Indian Medicinal Plant, *Withania somnifera* (L.) Dunal (Solanaceae). *Genet. Resour. Crop. Evol.*, 54: 655-660.

Kumar. A., Kaul., B. L. and Verma, H. K. (2001). Adaptability of *Withania somnifera* (L.) Dunal under subtropical environment of Jammu. *Int. J. Mendel.*, 18(1): 25-26.

Larcher, W. (1983). Physiological Plant Ecology. Springer Verlag. Berlin.

Mavi, H. S. (1986). Introduction to agrometeorology. Oxford and IBH Publishing Company, New Delhi.

Mishra, L. C., Singh, B. B. and Dagenais, S. (2000). Scientific basis for the therapeutic use of *Withania somnifera* (Ashwagandha). A review. *Altern. Med. Rev.* 5(4): 334-46.

Nirmala, K. A. and Balasubramanian, M. (1990). Physiological analysis of growth in soyabean. *Ind. J. Plant Physiol.*, XXXIII(3): 248-252.

Nuttunson, M. Y. (1955). Heat climate relationship and use of phenology in ascertaining the thermal and photothermal requirements of wheat. *Am. Inst. Crop Eco.* Washington DC.

Panse, V. G. and Shukhatme, P. V. (1985). Statistical methods for agricultural workers. ICAR. New Delhi.

Patterson, D. D. (1939). Statistical technique in agricultural research. Mc. Graw Hill Book company. Inc. New York.

Pitt, M. D. and Heady, H. P. (1978). Responses of annual vegetation to temperature and rainfall patterns in Northern California. *Ecology*, 58: 336-350.

Planchon, C. and Fesquet, J. (1982). Effect of the D genome and of selection on photosynthesis in wheat. Theor. *Appl. Genet.*, 61: 359-365.

Radford, P. J. (1967). Growth analysis formula their use and abuse. *Crop Science*, 7: 171-175.

Rahangdale, S. L., Dhopte, A. M. and Desmukh, S. M. (1987). Physiological basis of varietal differences in productivity of early tall and dwarf upland rice (*Oryza sativa*). *Ann. Plant Physiol.*, 1(1): 19-35.

Sastry, P. S. N., Chakravarty, N. V. K. and Rajput, R. P. (1985). Suggested index for characterization of crop response to thermal environment. Int. J. Eco. Environ. Sci. 2: 25-30.

Shahi, A. K. and Singh, A. (1987). The significance of heat unit system for crop management practices in aromatic plants: An introductory study on *Mentha arvensis*. *Indian Perfumer*, 31: 100-108.

Sharma, A. N. and Garg, O. K. (1984). Physiological analysis of yield variation in Pea (*Pisum sativum* L.) genotypes. *Ind. J. Plant Physiol.*, XXVII (1): 108-111.

Singh, R. S., Rao, A. S. and Ramakarishna, Y. S. (1991). Growth characteristics of mustard crop in response to thermal environment under arid conditions. Mausam. 2: 409-418.

Singh, S., Kumar, S. (1998). *Withania somnifera*. The Indian Ginseng ashwagandha. CIMAP, Lucknow, India.

Sneva, F. A. and Hyder, D. N. (1962). Estimating herbage production on semi-arid ranges in the intermountain region. *J. Range Manage.*, 15: 88-93.

Snyder, R. L. (1985). Hand calculating degree days. *Agricultural and forest meteorology*, 25: 656-658.

Swan, J. B., Schneider, E. C., Moncrief, J. F., Paulson, W. N. and Peterson, A. E. (1987). Estimating corn growth yield and grain moisture from air growing degree days and residue over. *Agron. J.*, 79: 53-60.

Tripathi, A. K., Sukla, Y. N. and Kumar, S. (1996). Ashwagandha *Withania somnifera* Dunal (solanaceae): A status report. *Journal of Medicinal and Aromatic Plant Sciences*, 23: 21-23.

Vittum, M. T., Dethier, B. E. and Lesser, R. C. (1965). Estimating growing degree days. *Proc. Am. Soc. Hort. Sci.*, 87: 449-452.

Warnick, S. J. (1973). Tomato development in California in relation to heat unit accumulation. *Hort. Sci.*, 8: 6-8.

Yoshida, S. (1972). Physiological aspects of grain yield. Ann. Rev. Plant Physiol. 23: 437-464.

Utilisation and Management of Medicinal Plants (2010) *Pages 202–216*
Editors: **V.K. Gupta, Anil K. Verma and Sushma Koul**
Published by: **DAYA PUBLISHING HOUSE, NEW DELHI**

Chapter 11

Bioprospecting: A Move from Land to the Seas

Kushal Qanungo*
Department of Applied Sciences and Humanities,
Faculty of Engineering and Technology,
Mody Institute of Technology and Science (Deemed University),
Lakshmangargh, Dist. Sikar – 332 311, Rajasthan, India

ABSTRACT

Marine bio-prospecting, i.e. looking for possible drug leads and other beneficial properties in plant and animal life in seas began merely as scientific curiosity. It is based on the premise that if terrestrial plant and animal life could yield a myriad of chemicals, marine flora and fauna could do so as well; and the sponges, snails and sea weeds washed ashore provided scientists the first samples for analysis. Marine bio-prospecting in the shallow coastal seas started in the fifties and sixties, and slowly gathered momentum when its economic potential was realized in the eighties and nineties. The technological advances in the last fifteen years have allowed scientists to explore the biological richness of the deep seas more effectively. This paper seeks to answer several questions, as to why the marine biodiversity has been largely un-prospected? In which seas do the marine bio-prospectors' operate? Who owns the marine genetic resources and controls access to it? The relevant international laws, the United Nations Convention on the Law of Seas vis-a-vis the Convention of Biological Diversity is critically examined. A survey of marine derived drugs in clinical trails worldwide and other bio-products is presented followed by the Indian scenario in marine biotechnology.

Keywords: Marine bioprospecting, UNCLOS, EEZ, Drug development, Marine derived drugs.

* E-mail: kushalq@redffmail.com; kushalq@hotmail.com; kushalq@mitsuniversity.ac.in.

Introduction

Foundation of Treatment of Human Diseases: Drugs from Natural Sources

Thousands of years ago early societies learned through trial and error that many plants contained substances with significant curative properties. Even today 80 per cent of the African population relies on traditional medicines for primary health care (Bagozi, 2003). Over the years the natural products became used in more refined ways leading ultimately to the use of pure single component 'active ingredient' as drugs. Aspirin, widely used all over the world as a mild pain killer, was originally discovered from the bark of the willow tree and found early use in curing tooth ache; morphine a strong pain killer was discovered from the opium poppy, opium being used for centuries as a drug, are examples of how modern drug have traditional medicine in its roots. Even in cancer therapy, naturally derived chemotherapeutic agent, Taxol has documented use of in the form of *Taxus baccata* in Indian traditional medicine (Agrawal, 2008).

On the other hand penicillin originally discovered in bread mould has no history of traditional use. Similarly there are hundreds of examples of other antibiotics and other drugs which have been discovered through searching for possible cures for diseases in plants and animal life. Termed, as bio-prospecting, this searching for cures involves sampling and screening of living organisms for substances of medicinal value. These substances can either be used directly as medicines, or as leads for making improved semi-synthetic or synthetic drugs. Bio-prospecting is now a multibillion-dollar industry world over (Chin, *et al.*, 2006). Natural products or related substances accounted for 40 per cent, 24 per cent, and 26 per cent, respectively, of the top 35 worldwide ethical drug sales from 2000, 2001, and 2002 (Chin, *et al.*, 2006). Though modern pharmaceutical industry can design and synthesize many new drugs, millions of complex compound exists in nature, many with potential therapeutic properties, because of the evolutionary time scale has been long enough for a diversity of molecules to be formed (the natures laboratory has been 'working at it' for million of years, in comparison to the modern day chemical drug synthesis of say 100 years). Therefore modern medicine in its own interest relies on compounds from nature to provide new drug leads (Butler, 2005). To quote, 'modern medicine has come to a full circle to see nature as the best place for cures that ails us' (Tooth, 2001).

Unfortunately many of the historically successful pharmaceuticals are becoming ineffective as pathogenic microbes develop multi-drug resistance capabilities (Capon, 1998). This is another strong reason to discover safer and more effective drugs against a wider selection of diseases, therefore continue to explore all available repositories of molecular diversity.

Why Turn to the Seas for Looking for Drug Leads?

In recent decades the search for new drug leads have been compelling because, drug resistant strains of bacteria and viruses arise almost daily and to search for cures for yet incurable diseases. With the terrestrial biodiversity largely bioprospected, thus it was inevitable that scientists eventually turned to the seas. In a more realistic view, however, marine bio-prospecting for drugs, *i.e.* looking for possible drug leads in the plant and animal life in the seas began merely as scientific curiosity. The premise was that if terrestrial plant and animal life could yield a myriad of chemicals, marine flora and fauna would do so as well; and sponges, snails, sea weeds washed ashore provided scientists easy sample to start with.

Marine bio-prospecting started in the 1950's and 1960's but picked momentum when the economic potential was realised in the 1980's and 1990's. In addition technological advances in the last fifteen years have allowed scientists to explore the biological richness more aggressively. It is now considered as the sunrise amongst the sunrises of biotechnology, pharmaceutical and the IT (Aldridge, 2006).

In 2002, global sales of marine biotechnology products reached $2.4 billion (Avery, 2007). According to one estimate the sales of marine biotechnology related products worldwide is 100 billion USD, the annual profits from sales a compound to treat herpes which was originally derived from a sea sponge is 50 million to 100 million USD, and anti-cancer agents are valued at 1 billion USD a year from marine organisms (Collins, *et al.*, 2005).

Cures from Marine Organisms: The Underlying Philosophy

Oceans occupy over 70 per cent of the earth's surface and it contains a large number of plants and animals yet unknown to man. It is estimated that 80 per cent of all earth's life forms inhabit the oceans. The bulk of animal categories or phyla are represented in the sea; 33 of the 34 animal phyla that exist today are of marine origin and of these 13 are exclusively marine.

Many organisms spend their life anchored to the seabed and have evolved elaborate defence mechanisms to ward off preys like fishes (Kijjoa and Sawangwong, 2004). Usually two types of defences are seen:

1. Physical defences like spines, shells, claws, fangs and,
2. Chemical defences like toxins which kill or make them unpalatable to the prey,
3. Some have both, poisonous spines for their survival.

In an evolutionary perspective these toxins (secondary metabolites, secondary metabolites are compounds that are not involved in primary metabolic processes like NADP etc, but are used for protection etc), have helped them to survive against competing organisms. It is the poisonous toxins which are the most sought after as cures against cancer and other diseases etc. It is thought that the same mechanisms with which these toxins are able to harm the predators (without harming the organisms itself), could be used to treat cancer (Kijjoa and Sawangwong, 2004). For example, killing cancerous cells selectively while not harming healthy cells, or killing pathogenic bacteria without killing the host. Sometimes marine organisms have signalling mechanisms, which attract other organisms to grow with them or induce mating responses.

Many molecules found in marine organisms have totally different patterns of construction from the molecules of medicinal value found in terrestrial plants and animals (Fenical, 2006). These marine compounds can lead to new mechanisms of action in the human body, and thus opening up the possibility of treating drug resistance diseases (Capon, 1998).

Why Ocean Biodiversity has been Largely Un-prospected?

Pliny (The Elder) in 60 AD, described the toxic properties of sea hares of the genus *Dolabella* in his comprehensive book, Historia Naturalis (Pettit, 1983). There is little documented history of traditional use of marine organisms in herbal medicines (Hunt and Vincent, 2004). Any use, either traditional or modern would come from knowledge about these organisms, which in turn would depend upon their availability, and marine flora and fauna has been less explored primarily because the organisms were not easily accessible. Terrestrial plants and other life forms can be easily reached and a continuous supply can be had. In contrast accessing marine organism would require an expedition, a repeat sampling another expedition and so on, incurring huge costs and specialised logistics (Tangley, 1996; Benkendorff, 2002).

Table 11.1: Examples of Marine Derived Drugs in Clinical Trails Worldwide (HBML, 2008)

Drug	*Activity*	*Source*	*Origin*	*Status*
Contignasterol		Sponge, *Petrosia contignata* (Porifera)	Off the coast of Papua New Guinea	Phase II
Debromohy-menialdisine	Anti-Alzheimer Agent; Treatment Against Osteoarthritis	Sponge *Stylotella aurantium* (porifera)	Off the Coast of Palau Island (near Phillipines)	Phase I
Discodermolide	Pancreatic and Lung Cancer	The Caribbean Deep-Sea Sponge *Discodermia dissoluta* (porifera)	Caribbean Sea	Phase I
Halochondrin	Anticancer	The Japanese Sponge *Halichondria okadai* (porifera)	Japan	Phase I
Krn7000	Antitumour, Immuno-stimulator	Analog derived Sponge, *Agelas mauritianus*	Japan	Phase I
Pseudopterosins	Anti-Inflammatory and Analgesic agent	Caribbean Sea Whip *Pseudopterogorgia elisabethae* (cnidaria)	Caribbean	Commercial
Anabaseine	Anti-Alzheimer Agent	Various Nemertine Worms, Esp. *Paranemertes peregrina* (Nemertea)	Friday Harbour, Washington State, USA	Phase I
Dolastatins	Anticancer	Indian Ocean Sea Hare *Dollabella auricularia* (Mollusca)	Indian Ocean	Phase 1
Kahalalide F	Anticancer	Hawaiian Sacoglossan *Elysia rufescens* (Mollusca)	Hawai	Phase II
Spisulosine (Es-285)	Anticancer	*Bivalve spisula* (=Mactromeris) Polynyma (Mollusca)	Arctic	Phase I
Ziconotide	Analgesic, for Treatment of Severe Pain (for Example in Cancer)	Derivative of a Conotoxide of Cone Snails *Conus geographicus*, *Conus magus* (mollusca)	Phillipines	FDA-Approved (SNX-111) Prialt® 2004
Bryostatin 1	Anti-Cancer and Immuno Suppressive	The Bryozoan *Bugula meritina* (Ectoprocta)	Gulf of California and Gulf of Mexico	Phase Ii
Aplidine (Aplidin®, Dehydrodidemnin B)	Anti-Cancer Agent via Apoptosis Induction	The Tunicate *Aplidium albicans* (Chordata)	Mediterranean	Phase II
Ecteinascidin 743 (Yondelis®, ET-743)	Anti-Cancer Agent via Apoptosis Induction	The Tunicate *Ecteinascidia turbinata* (chordata)	Caribbean Sea	Phase II Clinical Trials, European Orphan Drug Designation Against Soft Tissue Sarcoma
Squalamine	Anti-Tumor Agent; Anti-Angiogenic Agent	The Shark *Squalus acanthus* (Chordata)	New England Coastal Waters	Phase II Clinical Trials; also sold as A Non FDA-Approved Dietary Supplement

Contd...

Table 11.1–Contd...

Drug	Activity	Source	Origin	Status
Hemiasterlins	Anti Cancer, Cytotoxic and Tubulin Interactive Agents	Sponges of Genus *Auletta, siphonochalin* (Porifera)	South Africa	Phase 1
Ara-A (Attaway, and Zaborsky, 1993)	Anti Viral, populuar drug for Herpes, Largely been Replaced by Acyclovir	Sponge *Cryptotethya crpta* (Discovered in 1955)	Sea off the Coast of Florida	Currently manufactured by Parke-Davies and King Pharmaceuticals, Popular Drug
Ara-C	Anti Cancer	Sponge *Cryptotethya crpta* (First Reported in 1969)	Sea off the coast of Florida	Currently manufactured by Pharmacia-Upjohn

The average depth of the earth's oceans is 3800 m, with 98-99 per cent of the ocean floor is within 6000-7000 m from the oceans surface (Meer, 2008), the rest having depths upto 11 kms.

Marine organisms in relatively shallow waters near the shores can be collected by scuba diving. Nearly every developed country is pursuing this form of sample collection. Scuba diving without pressure suits is generally limited to depths of about 100 m because the problems the divers face in decompression when they rise to the surface. The divers have to be trained marine biologists otherwise there would be too many repeat collections. Another advantage of having trained biologists is that the region's seabed biodiversity would be mapped. This would open up potential for future bioprospectors. The main problem of exploring marine biodiversity other than its difficult accessibility, is that the marine biodiversity is not yet mapped (accessibility is one strong reason why it is not yet mapped). According to one estimate only 300,000 of marine species have been described, but one has to recall that biodiversity mapping is knowing what species occur where, together with the interdependencies of species, and not merely cataloguing them (Sala, 2007; Kenchington, 2002; Pomponi, 1999).

For bio-prospecting in depths below 100 metres, dredging and trawling have to be undertaken, these are not selective, *i.e.* it is not possible by these methods to choose a particular organism for collection and bio-prospectors have to be content with whatever comes up from the sea bed. These methods are limited by depths of upto 1000 meters.

Deep sea submersibles cost generally between 25miliion USD to 60 million USD. Cheaper submersibles which can dive upto depths of 1000 meters costs upto 2 million USD. Since submersibles have be launched from specialised support ships operating costs is nearly 50,000 USD per day (USSUBS, 2008).

According to the National Cancer Institute USA (NCI), the average cost of collecting 1 kilogram of marine invertebrates (sponge, clam, sea hare etc) works out 1000 USD, a prohibitively expensive amount (Green, 2003).

Among the various marine organisms the sponges have been one of the most promising ones (Narsinh, 2004). In addition to the pharmaceutical value of macro-organisms, there is a huge biodiversity of the micro-organisms, bacteria, algae, plankton etc. in the sea remaining to be explored. For example a tea spoon of sea water typically contains 10,000 to 100,000 bacteria or perhaps 1000 different types most of them never identified and much less studied (MBL 1995). Therefore, despite the vast potential marine bioprospecting has lagged behind land based bioprospecting because it is more complex, more dangerous and more expensive (Sabal, 2007). Marine micro-organisms have also proved in recent years to be extremely valuable marine resource.

In Which Seas Do Marine Bio-prospectors Operate?

It is widely accepted that the coastal waters in the tropical oceans and seas are teeming with life, the 'biodiversity rich' zones (Pratt, 2002). This is because the coastal waters are shallow, warm, with sunlight penetrating and supporting carbon dioxide fixing phytoplankton. Most of the developing nations lie in the tropics, with their territorial waters and exclusive economic zone {according to current international law (international law, is a set of rules that most countries obey when dealing with other countries} each country has an EEZ of 200 km from its shoreline, within which it is free to exploit its natural resources, both living and non-living) straddling most of the earth's oceanic biodiversity. So it makes sense both for economic and scientific reasons to bio-prospect in coastal tropical waters *e.g.* the Arabian Sea, Bay of Bengal, Indian Ocean, Gulf of Mexico, Caribbean, Mediterranean, coastal Tropical Africa, seas off Malayan and Sumatran Peninsula, Oceania, and seas off Latin America etc. From what is known of the marine biodiversity at present, it is believed that the tropical seas have as much potential if not more potential for discovery of new drugs as tropical rainforests (there are various economic models which put a monetary value to a particular region say rain forests or coral reefs (Spurgeon, 2001). Recently however the Arctic (Leary, 2008), Antarctica (Herber, 2006) and the deep seas (Collins, 2005) have also identified as promising grounds for marine bioprospecting (Glowka, 2003; Leary, 2008).

Who Owns the Seas?

Countries have usually claimed some part of the seas further than their coast as a part of their territory as a zone of security against smugglers, warships, and other intruders. The history of territorial rights over seas is very interesting. It was believed in the 16th century till the 18th century that those who rule the seas ruled the earth. The Pope Alexander XI in 1494 issued a Papal Bull separating the world's oceans, by a line drawn in the middle of the Atlantic Ocean, between the two great naval powers of those times, Spain and Portugal. The seas to the right were assigned to the Portuguese and to the left of the line were Spanish! Ever since, the rights over seas have been a conflict of interests of the different states naval and economic prowess. Those states which did not have big naval or merchant ship presence favoured extensive territorial waters in order to guard their own coastal waters from the states that did.

Another principle developed gradually during the 17th and 18th centuries that the coverage of the territorial sea should be measured by the military might of the shore based ruler. The 'cannon shot rule' commonly acknowledged in 18th century Europe, was the territorial boundary of the country over the sea. This was measured by the firing range of a shore based cannon of that era, of one marine league. The cannon shot rule became the origin of the three nautical mile territorial sea limit of the twentieth century. The sea outside the limit that was open to all for navigation and is famously known as the 'Freedom of Seas Doctrine' (Division of Ocean Affarirs, 1998).

The discovery and development of oil fields off the coast of Florida in the US after the World War II dealt the first most important blow to the Freedom of Seas Doctrine. Domestic economic and political demands forced the US to unilaterally expand the American authority over all natural resources on its continental shelf. No mention was however made of the sea above it (because none realised its potential).

After the World War II, Egypt, Ethiopia, Saudi Arabia, Libya, Venezuela and some East European countries, claimed a 12 nautical mile sea limit. In 1946, Argentina staked its claim on its continental shelf and the sea above it, and subsequently Chile in 1947 and Peru and Ecuador in 1950, claimed rights to seas upto 200 miles from its shores. The intention of Chile, Peru and Ecuador to set the limits, was to keep off the big American and Japanese fishing trawlers from fishing near South America's western coastline (there is a continuous upwelling of the ocean currents off the coast of Chile and Peru bringing up mineral rich waters which support a high growth of phytoplanktons, zooplanktons and eventually marine life. The sea is very rich in anchovies there). A two hundred mile nautical limit was claimed by all Caribbean countries by the Santiago, Montevideo and the Lima Declarations

In determining the extent of sea rights of a country, security, fishing and oil and natural gas became the three main reasons in the latter half of the twentieth century. There was depletion of the fishing stocks due to over-fishing by big flotilla of long range trawlers the all over the world. Sophisticated fish factories with big flotillas of vessels mainly from Japan, the US, Portugal, Spain, the UK, and the Scandinavian countries roamed the high seas in search of fish and many a time they would fish in waters claimed by traditional fishermen.

Fish in economic parlance is considered to be a common property resource, (CPR) (other examples of common property resource being, grazing land, forests, water etc). To solve the problem of over-fishing and fishing disputes between nations, and also since the fishing stocks are limited, many countries especially in Europe have evolved the system of Total Allowable Catch (TAC) for each country which is then divided into Individual Tradable Quota (ITQ) (Hanneson, 1991). The ITQ can be freely traded in some countries. Marine organisms could also be treated as a CPR in principle, but it needs to be understood that unlike fishing it has is intellectual property and a knowledge associated with it, and not a consumptive property. Also the 'tragedy of commons principle', which holds good for grazing land forests, fishing etc would be applicable only in a very limited way in the case of marine organisms.

Another common resource which caused much debate among international policy makers in the sixties was the deep sea mineral nodules. Although first discovered in 1874 in the seas between Hawaii and Tahiti, it was only in the sixties that serious exploratory research into the spatial extent of these nodules rich in nickel, cobalt and copper were made, and its economic potential realised. It was found that these occurred in what is now known as the 'Clarion Clipperton Zone', extending few degrees north and south of the equator occupying an area of 1.35 million square miles of the Pacific between Mexico and Hawaii. (It is only in the eighties that India found nodules in the Indian Ocean). By 1970 the nodules economic importance had gained wide publicity and a conflict of interest rose between nations (developed countries) who had the technological capability to mine them and nations (developing countries) who did not.

In an effort to resolve the conflict, the United Nations Conference on the Law of Sea in 1982 (UNCLOS) sometime referred to as the Law of Sea, agreed among other things (Leary, 2008), that the territorial limits of coastal nations would be three nautical miles from the shoreline, an exclusive economic zone (EEZ) of 200 nautical miles from the shoreline within which a coastal state is free to exploit its natural resource, given that its actions do not harm their neighbours, if the continental shelf extends beyond 200 nautical miles, then the coastal state, could exploit that regions resources, but has to share income with other states through an international authority, designates the ocean floor (beyond the continental shelf) the sea bed and the subsoil as the 'Area' and its resources as the 'common heritage of the mankind', sets up an International Sea Bed Authority (ISA), a special regime and institutional structure to control prospecting, exploitation and exploration of the 'Areas' mineral resources.

The UNCLOS is silent about non-mineral resources in the Area, and ISA's authority is to look after the Area's resources an international property and exploit it for the 'benefit of the mankind'.

Who Own the Marine Genetic Resources and Controls Access to it?

A scrutiny of customary international law would place marine genetic resources under two international treaties, the UNCLOS and the CBD.

The UNCLOS empowers nations to exploit natural resources, (marine genetic resources come under natural resources logically) in a nation's EEZ. It therefore follows legally and logically that marine organism in a nation's EEZ is its property and therefore can regulate its access. For marine scientific research in another nation's jurisdiction, permission has to be taken from the country prior to conducting research, which is to be granted under normal conditions. Consent is presumed unless the coastal state has a reason to suppose that the proposed study is directly significant to commercial exploration and exploitation of natural resources both living and non living (article 446.3 of UNCLOS). When marine research is not for commercial purposes, the researching nation is to ensure the involvement of scientists from the coastal sate and exchange all research results upon request. The UNCLOS also places on the coastal states, the responsibility of 'managing its living resources'. Beyond the national jurisdiction however, the UNCLOS is quiet about the marine genetic resources, both on its research and utilisation aspects. ISA's administration is only on the exploitation of the deep sea nodules.

An examination of CBD (CBD, 1992) would also point that the marine genetic resource within EEZ is under the national jurisdiction of the coastal state (one of the fundamental premises of the CBD is that it confers the national jurisdiction over all the states genetic resources). It is clearly mentioned in the CBD (article 22) that in respect to marine genetic resources, its directive should not run contrary to the Law of Sea. It, also as in UNCLOS asks parties to seek prior informed consent from competent authorities of a state, before researching or collecting samples and that the consent is not be denied under normal circumstances, but facilitated.

A coastal country might reject commercial marine bio-prospecting companies consent to bio-prospect in its EEZ under UNCLOS, though has to facilitate its right to access under CBD obligations. In principle, one could extend this denial, for marine scientific research also, since marine scientific research; especially sample collection for screening for potentially medicinal compounds has huge commercial value.

Beyond natural jurisdiction CBD is silent on who has the jurisdiction over the marine genetic resources (Hansen, and LaMotte, 2006). Quite logically it follows that 'the high seas belongs to nobody' and 'belongs to everybody who is able to appropriate it', a free for all in the present time (Fontaubert, 2001).

The Role of UN so far

In recent years recognising the importance of marine bioprospecting there has been renewed interest in this issue by the international policy makers (Collins, 2005)(Ocean Studies Board, 1999). The UN has been holding a series of 'ad hoc open-ended informal working group to study issues relating to the conservation and sustainable use of marine biological diversity beyond areas of national jurisdiction' (Office of Ocean Affairs, 2007).

It has been also been holding yearly meetings since 2004 called, 'a regular process for the global reporting and assessment of the state of the marine environment, including socio-economic aspects' (Office of Ocean Affairs, 2006).

The key report conclusions (UNO) summarized below from the analysis of the report of the United Nations University and UNESCO's, Man and Biosphere Programme on the United Nations Informal Consultative Process on Oceans and the Law of the Sea Eight Meeting United Nations, New York, 25-29 June 2007. The UN study acknowledges that the current policy regime for marine genetic resources may be inadequate and the information base on marine genetic resources is growing but scattered. There has been a steady increase in scientific research publications on marine genetic resources. The number of patents on marine genetic research is also increasing. The perspectives of the scientific community on marine genetic resources should be clarified and how the research should be carried out in future should be sorted out.

Indian Scenario in Marine Biotechnology

In India Marine Bio-prospecting began in 1991 as the National Project on Development of Potential Drugs from the (Annual Report, 1991) Sea. The Central Drug Research Institute, Lucknow coordinates the activity together with several other collaborating institutes and universities all over India. Others are the Central Salt and Marine Chemicals Research Institute, Bhavnagar; Post Graduate Institute of Medical Sciences, Calcutta, University College of Science, Calcutta; Indian Institute of Chemical Technology, Hyderabad, ALMPG Institute of Basic Medical Sciences, University of Madras; Regional Research Laboratory, Bhubaneswar; Andhra University Vishakhapatnam, and the National Institute of Oceanography, Goa etc.. Organisms from the long Indian mainland coastline, the Andaman and Nicobar Islands etc are identified, screened and specimens stored at the National Repository, at The National Institute of Oceanography, Goa. The following bioactivities are being looked for, anticancer, immunomodulatory, anti-helminthic, wound healing, antifungal, anti-protozoal, anti-fungal, antibacterial, anti-inflammatory, anti-viral, anti-fertility; antihyperglycemic, anti-hyperlipidemic, apasmolytic, CNS, pesticidal and antiallergic. Till 2007 some 6500 samples have been collected and screened. An antidiabetic compound (CDR-134-D-123) has entered into Phase II of Clinical Trials. Two more compounds having combined potentials for anti-hyperglycemic-cum-anti-hyperlipidemic activities, are poised to enter clinical trials as well. A quarterly newsletter 'Ocean Drug Alert' is being published from CDRI since (Mullick, 2008) 1992.

Both the Government of India and various state governments (coastal states) are encouraging marine biotechnology industry by setting up marine biotech parks and, establishing centers to monitor and conduct research activities and generate trained manpower. Public private R&D joint ventures have resulted in NIO, Goa, joining hands with Nicholas Piramal Research Centre (Vishwakarma, 2007). There has been also some activity in IPR issues in marine biotechnology (Kumaram, 2007) and general biotech issues marine (Jain and Tiwari, 2007; Qanungo, 2002, 2005, 2008).

In the private R&D sector the sector, the Chennai based Geomarine Biotechnologies limited has the following techhnologies ready for transfer, a new immunostimulant for shrimps, a new all herbal ammonia adsorbent for aquaculture, protein hydrolyzate from marine wastes. Their ongoing research in includes probiotics of marine origin, probiotics for marine aquarium in aquaculture and value added products from marine wastes and luciferine and luciferase production etc. (Geomarine Biotechnologies, 2008).

ABL Biotechnologies Limited (ABL), based in Chennai, India, is a pioneer in the Indian Marine biotechnology. ABL's Research and Development facility located at Vishakapatnam and the Microbial

Metabolites Laboratory is located at Chennai. Among other products it markets, 'Poly Carotene' which is vegetable oil suspension of naturally occurring mixture of carotenoids extracted and concentrated from the marine green alga *Dunailiella salina*. (ABL Biotechnologies, 2008).

The biotech policy of Tamil Nadu mentions marine biotechnology as one of the main thrust areas. A marine biotechnology park would be set up near Mandapam, Tamil Nadu. The Marine Biotechnology Park will function in close coordination with the Gulf of Mannar Biosphere Trust (Government of Tamil Nadu, 2007).

The Andhra Pradesh Government is establishing a marine biotech park in Parwada near Visakhapatnam (Singh, 2004), of 218 acre area, where Celgen Biologicals (a wholly owned subsidiary of ABL Pharmaceuticals) is setting up India's first facility for the production of the essential fatty acid DHA. It would also produce beta carotene. The Government is supporting the development of a Centre of Excellence in Marine Biotech Resources Development at the Andhra University, Visakhapatnam(Department of Industries, 2008). The University of Agricultural Sciences, Dharwad, Karnataka together with the Department of Fisheries proposes to establish a marine biotech park at Karwar for promoting research in marine biotechnology.

The University of Science and Technology at Cochin (CUSAT), Kerala, is establishing establish a Centre for Marine Biotechnology (Gujrat State Biotech Mission, 2006). Advanced training is being offered in marine biotechnology by the School of Environmental Studies at National Centre for Aquatic Animal Health, CUSAT (NCAAH, 2008).

Maharashtra's biotechnology policy (2001) includes efforts to exploit the marine organisms along its coastline(MBP, 2001); Karnataka Millennium Biotech Policy, (2000) plans to set up a marine biotech park at Karwar to promote marine biotech (Bangalore Bio, 2008). Marine bioprospecting is a major theme of Kerala's biotechnology policy (Kerala Govt., 2008). The Central Marine Fisheries Research Institute, Ernakulam, would be the nodal centre to coordinate the R&D efforts with other academic and research institutions of the state. For example, the Bharathidasan University, Trichy hosts the National Facility for Marine Cynobacteria. The Biotechnology Park to be set up at Cochin would have marine biotechnology as the thrust area. Orissa draft biotechnology policy 2005 has plans for a marine biotechnology park at Chandrabhaga near Konarak (Orrissa Govt., 2008). However recently the Orrisa Govt. has announced that a special marine biotech park would be set up in Ganjam district of the state (WebIndia123, 2008).

The production and processing of marine bioproducts, like nutraceuticals can be easily located in coastal areas. 'High value products can be obtained through relatively small-scale operations' (Benkendorff, 2001). 'Support should also be available to all bioprospecting startup companies to facilitate market analyses and the development of business plans when appropriate' (WebIndia123, 2008).

Conclusion

The importance of marine organisms as the source of medicine and other health related products is unfolding. The next few decades would see many exciting discoveries of health related products from the oceans (Fenical, 2006). Marine bioprospecting is a challenging job because of the complexity of the sample identification, collection and expense of operations in the deep seas. As the economic potential of the world oceans become clear questions are being raised in the civil society across the world as to the ownership of marine genetic resources. The United Nations has acknowledged that there is need to address this important issue.

India has also forayed into marine bioprospecting in a modest way with the involvement of several national laboratories, universities and some private enterprises. Marine Biotech parks are being set up by the government in the coastal regions to support the industry.

At the end of my article I would like to draw attention to the recent concept of marine biotechnology as 'Blue-Green Capitalism' which has been introduced by an anthropologist at Harvard, (Stefan Helmreich, 2007) who eloquently describes his ideas as: 'where blue stands for a vision of the freedom of the open ocean and for speculative sky-high promise, and green for belief in ecological sustainability as well as biological fecundity.'

Acknowledgements

The author thanks the Dean of Faculty of Engineering and Technology and Head, Dept. of Applied Sciences and Humanities, MITS, Lakshsmangarh, Rajasthan, India for encouragement and support.

References

ABL Biotechnologies (2008) http://www.ablbiotechnologies.com/Products.htm (date accessed 22, June 2008).

Agrawal, D.P., Himalayan Medicine System and Its Materia Medica, *http://www.indianscience.org/essays/20–per cent 20E—Himalayan per cent 20Medicine per cent 20System per cent 20fine12.pdf* (date accessed 19th June 2008).

Aldridge, S. (2006). Marine Bioprospecting for Novel Drugs, Dipping into the Sea to Discover Therapies for Cancer and Infections, *Genetic Engineering and Biotechnology News*, 26. (21), Dec1, http://www.genengnews.com/articles/chitem.aspx?aid=1958&chid=4 (date accessed 19th June 2008).

Attaway, D.H., Zaborsky O.R (1993). Marine Biotechnology, Vol. 1, Pharmaceuticals and Bioactive Natural Products, Plenum Press, New York, 1993.

Annual Report (1991). Ministry of Earth Sciences, Govt. of India, from 1990 till present. http://moes.gov.in/ann0607.pdf http://moes.gov.in/ar05-06.pdf (date accessed 22, June 2008).

Avery, K. (2007). Marine Genetic Resources Show Potential for Human Health and Industry, *UN Chronicle Online Edition.*

Bagozi, D. (2003). Traditional medicine, WHO, Programmes and Projects, Media Centre, Fact Sheet No 134, *http://www.who.int/mediacentre/factsheets/fs134/en/*(date accessed 19th June, 2008).

Benkendorff, K. (2001) Submission Regarding The Inquiry Into The Development Of High Technology Industries In Regional Australia Based on Bioprospecting and references cited therein. http://www.aph.gov.au/HOUSE/committee/primind/bioinq/sub38e.pdf (date accessed 19th June, 2008).

Benkendorff, K. (2002) Potential conservation benefits and problems associated with bioprospecting in the marine environment. *In:* A Zoological Revolution: Using native fauna to assist in its own survival. Ed. by D. Lunney and C. Dickman. Royal Zoological Society of New South Wales and Australian Museum, Australia, 90-100.

Bangalore Bio, (2008) http://164.164.128.27/GovtInfo/biotechpolicy.htm (date accessed 19th June, 2008).

Butler, M. S. (2005). Natural Product to Drug: Natural Product Derived Compounds in Clinical Trails, *Nat. Prod. Rep.*, 22, 162-195.

Capon R.J. (1998). Bioprospecting: Plumbing the Depths, Today's Life Science, 10 (4) 16-19.

CBD, (1992) Convention on Biological Diversity http://www.cbd.int/(date accessed 22, June 2008.

Chin Y-W, Balunas, M.J., Chai, H.B., Kinghorn, A.D. (2006). Drug Discovery from Natural Sources, *AAPS Journal*, 8, 239-253.

Collins, T., Ray, R., Borromeo, M. (2005). Vast Genetic Treasure on Sea Beds, Clear Rules Needed to Govern Deep Sea, Research, Avoid Unfettered Bioprospecting Gold Rush: UNU, United Nations University, Yokohama, Japan. NoMR/E16/05, 8 June, Press Release, http://www.unu.edu/media/archives/2005/mre16-05.doc (date accessed 19th June 2008).

Committee on Biological Diversity in Marine Systems (1995). Undererstanding Marine Biodiversity, A Research Agenda for the Nation, Oceans Studies Board, National Academy Press, Washington D.C. Department of Industries, Govt. of Andhra Pradesh, (2005) Dept of Industries, Specialised Parks http://www.apind.gov.in/marinebio.html (date accessed 19th June, 2008).

Fenical, W. (2006). Marine Pharmaceuticals Past, Present, and Future, *Oceanography*, 19(2): 111-119.

Fontaubert, D. (2001). Legal and Political Considerations, *In*: The Status of The Natural Resources on the High Seas, Eds. WWF/IUCN WWF/IUCN, Gland, Switzerland.

Glowka, L. (2003). Putting Marine Scientific Research on a Sustainable Footing at Hydrothermal Vents. *Marine Policy*, 27 303-312.

Government of Tamil Nadu (2007)Government of Tamil Nadu, Industries Department, Biotechnology Policy, http://www.tn.gov.in/policynotes/archives/policy/indbiopol-e.htm (date accessed 19th June, 2008).

Green, J.J. (2003). Report of the Workshop on Bioprospecting in the High Seas, Interm Summary, *In*: Proceedings of the Deep Sea 2003 Conference, 1-5 December 2003, 29-36, Queenstown, New Zealand. Geomarine Biotechnologies, (2008) www.geomarinebiotech.com (date accessed 22, June 2008).

Gujrat State Biotech Mission (2006). http://btm.gujarat.gov.in/Biotech per cent 20Sector/marine/Indian per cent 20Marine per cent 20Biotechnology.html (date accessed 19th June, 2008).

Hanneson, (1991). From Common Fish to Rights Based Fishing: Fisheries Management and the Evolution of Exclusive Rights to Fish, *European Economic Review*, 35, 397-407.

Hansen, K.M., and LaMotte, K.R. (2006) Trends In Commercial Development Of Ocean Resources: New Laws And Policies Present Opportunies And Risks–Part II, *The Metropolitan Corporate Counsel*, 21, Mountainside, NJ, USA. http://www.metrocorpcounsel.com/pdf/2006/May/21.pdf (date accessed 22, June 2008).

Helmreich, S. (2007). Blue-green Capital, Biotechnological Circulation and an Oceanic Imaginary: A Critique of Biopolitical Economy, *BioSocieties*, 2, 287–302.

Herber, B.P. (2006). Bioprospecting in Antarctica: the Search for a Policy Regime, Polar Record, 42, 139-146.

HBML (2008) Adapted from Drugs from the Sea Index http://www.marinebiotech.org/dfsindex.html (date accessed 19th June, 2008).

Hunt, B., and Vincent, A.C.J. (2004). The Use of Marine Organisms in Traditional and Allopathic Medicines, *Proceedings of a Global Synthesis Workshop on 'Biodiversity Loss and Species Extinctions: Managing Risks in a Changing World', Sub Theme : Conserving Medicinal Species and Securing a Healthy Future,* 3rd IUCN World Conservation Congress, Bangkok Thailand, Novemver17-25.

http://www.iucn.org/congress/2004/documents/outputs/biodiversity-loss/use-marine-organisms-hunt-vincent.pdf (date accessed 19th June 2008).

Jain, R., and Tiwari, A (2007). Sponges: An Invertebrate Of Bioactive Potential, Current Science, 93, 4, 444-445, http://www.ias.ac.in/currsci/aug252007/444.pdf (date accessed 22, June 2008).

Kenchington, E. (2002) The Effects of Fishing on Species and Genetic Diversity, The Reykjavik Conference on Responsible Fisheries in the Marine Ecosystem, October 1-4, Reykjavik, Iceland. *In:* M. Sinclair and G. Valdimarson (eds.). Responsible fisheries in the marine ecosystem. CAB International. From Center for Marine Biodiversity, Marine Species http://www.marinebiodiversity.ca/cmb/research/discovery-corridor/marine-species (date accessed 19th June 2008).

Kijjoa, A., and Sawangwong, P. (2004), Drugs and Cosmetics from the Sea, *Mar. Drugs*, 2,73-82.

Kerala Govt. (2008) http://nmcc-vikas.gov.in/PolicyGovernance/PDF/BioTech per cent 20Policy-Kerala.pdf. http://www.kerala.gov.in/annualprofile/biotech.htm#mar (date accessed 19th June, 2008).

Kumaran, L.M. (2007) IPR issues in Marine Biotechnology, International Symposium on New Fronties in Marine Natural Product Research, National Institute of Oceanography, Goa, India 23–24 February, 2007. http://www.nio.org/past_events/NFMNPR/session_IV.jsp (date accessed 22, June 2008).

Leary, D. (2008). UNU-IAS Report, Bioprospecting in the Arctic, United Nations University Institute of Advanced Studies, David Leary, Yokohama, Japan. http://www.ias.unu.edu/sub_page.aspx?catID=111&ddlID=674 (date accessed 22, June 2008).

Leary, D. (2008). Bi-Polar Disorder? Is Bioprospecting an Emerging Issue for the Arctic as well as for Antarctica? Reciel 17, 1,.

Meer (2008) The World's Ocean Basin Depths, http://www.meer.org/M2.htm (date accessed 19th June 2008).

MBL, (1995) Prospecting in New England Waters, An MBL biologist looks for Antibiotics and Anti-Cancer Drugs in the World of Marine MicrobesLab Notes Fall 95, Vol. 5, No. 4., Marine Biological laboratory, Woods Hole Oceanographic Instititution, Woods Hole, Masschusets, USA. http://www.mbl.edu/publications/pub_archive/labnotes/5.3/bioprospecting.html (date accessed 19th June 2008).

MBP, (2001) http://www.mahabiotech.org/modules/home/page1.pdf (date accessed 19th June, 2008).

Mullick, (2008). Personal communication from Dr. Summan Mullick, CDRI, Lucknow.

Narsinh, L., Thakur, N.L., and Müller, W.*E.G.* (2004) Biotechnological Potential of Marine Sponges, *Current Science*, 86,11, 1506-1512. http://www.ias.ac.in/currsci/jun102004/1506.pdf (date accessed 19th June 2008).

NCAAH, (2008) http://www.ncaah.org/pdf/mTechMarineBiotechnology.pdf (date accessed 19th June, 2008).

Oceans and the Law of the Sea, The United Nations Convention of the Law of the Sea (A Historical Perspective)–Overview of Convention and Related Agreements, United Nations, 2001. Division for Ocean Affairs and the Law of the Sea, Office of Legal Affairs, United Nations. http://www.un.org/Depts/los/convention_agreements/convention_historical_perspective.htm (date accessed 22, June 2008).

Office of Ocean Affairs (2007). http://www.un.org/Depts/los/biodiversityworkinggroup/biodiversityworkinggroup.htm (date accessed 22, June 2008).

Office of Ocean Affairs (2006). http://www.un.org/Depts/los/global_reporting/global_reporting.htm (date accessed 22, June 2008).

Ocean Studies Board (1999). Understanding the Oceans Role in Human Health, Committee on Ocean Role in Human Health, Ocean Studies Board, Commission on Geosciences, Environment and Resources, National Research Council, National Academy Press, Washington, DC, USA.

Orrisa Govt. (2008)http://orissagov.nic.in/biotechnology per cent 20policy-2005-circulated per cent 20copy.pdf (date accessed 19th June, 2008).

Pettit, G. R. (1983). Cell Growth Inhibitory Substances United States, University Patents, Inc. Tempe, Arizona, USA *US Patent No. 4414205*, http://www.freepatentsonline.com/4414205.html (date accessed 19th June 2008).

Pomponi, S.A. (1999). The Bioprocess-Technology Potential of the Sea, *Journal of Biotechnology*, 70, 5-13.

Prat, A.R. M. (2002). The Impact of TRIPS and the CBD on Coastal Communities, 2002, International Collective in Support of Fishworkers (ICSF), Catalunya, Spain, 1-55 http://www.icsf.net/icsf2006/uploads/publications/occpaper/pdf/english/issue_1/ALL.pdf (date accessed 19th June 2008).

Qanungo, K (2002) Time for a New Deal in Marine Bioprospecting,., SciDev.Net 17th January, 2002. (date accessed 22, June 2008).

Qanungo, K. (2008) Equitable Sharing of Marine Genetic Resources, Current Science, v94, No.1, 9-10,. http://www.ias.ac.in/currsci/jan102008/8a.pdf (date accessed 22, June 2008).

Qanungo, K. (2005) Drugs from the Ocean Beds, *The Tribune, Chandigurh*, November 25, 2005 http://www.tribuneindia.com/2005/20051125/science.htm (date accessed 22, June 2008).

Sabal, M. (2007).The Future of Marine Resources as Pharmaceutical Products, University of Miami, http://jrscience.wcp.muohio.edu/fieldcourses07/PapersMarineEcologyArticles/TheFutureofMarineResource.html (date accessed 19th June 2008).

Sala, E. and Nancy Knowlton, N., J. Emmett Duffy (2007). Global marine biodiversity trends. *In:* Encyclopedia of Earth. Eds. Cutler J. Cleveland (Environmental Information Coalition, National Council for Science and the Environment). Washington, D.C. USA. [First published in the Encyclopedia of Earth May 22, 2007; Last revised June 20, 2007. http://www.eoearth.org/article/Global_marine_biodiversity_trends (date accessed 19th June 2008).

Singh, N. (2004) New Entrants in Genome Valley, Biospectrum, http://biospectrumindia.ciol.com/content/BioAsia/104031109.asp (date accessed 19th June, 2008).

Spurgeon, J. (2001). Valuation of Coral Reefs: The Next Ten Years, Spurgeon, J., Paper presented at "Economic Valuation and Policy Priorities for Sustainable Management of Coral Reefs" an

International Consultative Workshop, Organised by ICLARM, in Penang, Malaysia. December 2001. http://www.icriforum.org/docs/Valuation_CR.pdf (date accessed 19th June 2008).

Tangley, L. (1996). Ground Rules Emerge for Marine Bioprospectors, *BioScience.* 46, 4, 245-249.

Tooth G. (2001).Bioprospecting in Queensland: Oceans of Opportunity, Forests of Concern, 27 May, *ABC National Radio Background Breifing, Program Transcript*, http://www.abc.net.au/rn/talks/bbing/stories/s303991.htm (date accessed 19th June 2008).

UNU-IAS, (2007) http://www.un.org/Pubs/chronicle/2007/webArticles/062807_marine_genetic.htm (date accessed 19th June 2008.

USSUBS (2008) FAQs http://www.ussubs.com/faq/deep.php3 (date accessed 19th June 2008).

Vishwakarma, R. (2007), Natural Products as Sources of New Chemical Entities: Experience at Nicholas Piramal Research Centre, International Symposium on New Fronties in Marine Natural Product Research, National Institute of Oceanography, Goa, India 23–24 February, 2007. http://www.nio.org/past_events/NFMNPR/session_IV.jsp (date accessed 22, June 2008).

WebIndia 123, (2008) http://news.webindia123.com/news/Articles/India/20080528/964077.html (date accessed 19th June, 2008).

Utilisation and Management of Medicinal Plants (2010) *Pages 217–227*
Editors: **V.K. Gupta, Anil K. Verma and Sushma Koul**
Published by: **DAYA PUBLISHING HOUSE, NEW DELHI**

Chapter 12

The Genus *Mentha*: A Versatile Plant

Amrita Chakraborty, Krittika Sasmal and Sharmila Chattopadhyay*

Drug Development/Diagnostics and Biotechnology Division,
Indian Institute of Chemical Biology,
4, Raja S.C. Mullick Road, Kolkata – 700 032

ABSTRACT

Mentha (mint) is a genus of about 25 species (and many hundreds of varieties) of flowering plants in the family Lamiaceae (Mint Family). Species within the genus *Mentha* have a subcosmopolitan distribution across Europe, Africa, Asia, Australia, and North America. Several mint hybrids commonly occur. Mints are aromatic, almost exclusively perennial, rarely annual, herbs. The most common and popular mints for cultivation are peppermint (*Mentha piperita*), spearmint (*Mentha spicata*) and (more recently) pineapple mint (*Mentha suaveolens*). As an English colloquial term, mint stands for any small sugar confectionery item flavored to taste like the aforementioned plant. Mints have been known from the time immemorial as kitchen herbs and also as the pharmacopoeial herbs of the ancient human civilization. Mint was originally used as a medicinal herb to treat stomach ache and chest pains. During the Middle Ages powdered mint leaves were used to whiten teeth. Mint tea is a strong diuretic and also aids digestion. Menthol from mint essential oil (40-90 per cent) is an ingredient of cosmetics and perfumes. These oils are widely used by industries in food, pharmaceutical, flavor and/or fragrance. Owing to the diverse biological activities of the genus *Mentha* and increasing consumer interest (Mimica-Dukic *et al.*, 2003; Kumar and Chattopadhyay, 2007), genetic transformation has been attempted with limited success (Kumar *et al.*, 2008; Bhat *et al.*, 2002). Among the several mint species, *M. arvensis* L., or

* Corresponding Author: E-mail: sharmila@iicb.res.in; Phone: 91-33-2473 3491; Fax 91-33-2472-3967.

Japanese mint, is the most preferred one and covers large cultivation areas in India. This review will discuss further about the versatility of the genus with its potential and challenges for future application.

Keywords: *Mentha spp., Menthol, Mint, Kitchen herb, Bioactivity, Biotechnology, Transgenic pudina.*

Introduction

The genus *Mentha* includes about 20 true species, but because of hybridization, there are dozens, even hundreds of variations. In fact there are as many as 2,300 named variations, half of which are synonyms, however, the rest are legitimate intraspecific names (Tucker, 1980). While long thought to be a distinct species, peppermint (*Mentha piperita* L.) is now believed to be a hybrid of spearmint (*Mentha spicata* L.) and water mint (*Mentha aquatica* L.). There is substantial genetic diversity in the genus *Mentha,* but gene introgression through plant breeding has not contributed significantly to cultivar development (Harley and Brighton, 1977). Most of the commercial mint varieties are alloploids, including peppermint, a sterile allohexaploid. Crop improvement is limited by sterility of commercial varieties and ploidy differences amongst potential members of the gene pools (Tuker, 1992). Dried and fresh mint leaves and the essential oil distilled from fresh or dried leaves, are widely used in industries like pharmaceutical drugs, food additives, flavorings, cosmetics and folk medicine.

Morphology

Mints are aromatic, almost exclusively perennial, rarely annual, herbs. They have wide-spreading underground rhizomes and erect, branched stems. Mints perpetuate by runners. The leaves are arranged in opposite pairs, from simple oblong to lanceolate, often downy with a serrated margin. Leaf colors range from dark green and gray-green to purple, blue and sometimes pale yellow. The flowers are produced in clusters ('verticils') on an erect spike, white to purple, the corolla two-lipped with four subequal lobes, the upper lobe usually the largest. The fruit is a small dry capsule containing one to four seeds.

Habitat

While the species that make up the *Mentha* genus are widely distributed and can be found in many environments, but it grows best in wet environment and moist soils. Mints grow 10–120 cm tall and can spread over an indeterminate sized area.

Harvest and Storage

Harvesting of mint leaves can be done throughout the year. Fresh mint leaves should be used immediately or stored up to a couple of days in plastic bags within a refrigerator. Optionally, mint can be frozen in ice cube trays. Dried mint leaves should be stored in an airtight container placed in a cool, dark, dry area.

Uses

The leaf, fresh or dried, is the culinary source of mint. Fresh mint is usually preferred over dried mint when storage of the mint is not a problem. The leaves have a pleasant warm, fresh, aromatic, sweet flavor with a cool aftertaste. Mint leaves are used in teas, beverages, jellies, syrups, candies, and ice creams. In Middle Eastern cuisine mint is used on lamb dishes. In British cuisine, mint sauce is popular with lamb. Mint is a necessary ingredient in Touareg tea, a popular tea in northern African and Arab countries. Alcoholic drinks sometimes feature flavor of mint, namely the Mint Julep and the Mojito. Crème de menthe is a mint-flavored liqueur used in drinks such as the grasshopper (drink). Mint essential oil and menthol are extensively used as flavorings in breath fresheners, drinks, antiseptic mouth rinses, toothpaste, chewing gum, desserts and candies. The substances that give the mints their characteristic aromas and flavors are menthol (the main aroma of Spearmint, Peppermint, and Japanese Peppermint) and pulegone (in Pennyroyal and Corsican Mint). Methyl salicylate, commonly called "oil of wintergreen", is often used as a mint flavoring for foods and candies due to its mint-like flavor. Mints are used as food plants by the larvae of some Lepidoptera species including Buff Ermine.

Mint was originally used as a medicinal herb to treat stomach ache and chest pains. During the Middle Ages, powdered mint leaves were used to whiten teeth. Mint tea is a strong diuretic. Mint also aids digestion.Menthol from mint essential oil (40-90 per cent) is an ingredient of many cosmetics and some perfumes. Menthol and mint essential oil are also much used in medicine as a component of many drugs, and are very popular in aromatherapy. A common use is as an antipruritic, especially in insect bite treatments (often along with camphor). Menthol is also used in cigarettes as an additive, because it blocks out the bitter taste of tobacco and soothes the throat. Many people also believe the strong, sharp flavor and scent of mint can be used as a mild decongestant for illnesses such as the common cold.

Mint leaves are often used in many natural conditions to repel mosquitoes. It is also said that extracts from mint leaves have a particular mosquito-killing capability. Mint oil is also used as an environment-friendly insecticide for its ability to kill some common pests like wasps, hornets, ants and cockroaches.

With this background, this review will discuss further on the genus *Mentha* spp. and its future potential.

Phytochemical Analysis

Burbott and Loomis isolated menthol from *Mentha* long back in 1962 and that is the starting point of chemical analysis of this genus. The distribution of secondary metabolites in plants is far more restricted than that of primary metabolite (Sasson, 1991). The conversion of monoterpene was studied in details with *Mentha* species (Werrmann and Knorr, 1993). Two new monoterpenoid glycosides, spicatoside A and spicatoside B, were isolated from the whole herbs of *M. spicata* L., which have anti-inflammatory and hemostatic activities. Their structures have been determined on the basis of spectral and chemical analysis (Zheng *et al.*, 2003). Electrophoretic analysis of the partially purified carveol dehydrogenase from extracts of both the glands and the leaves of *M. spicata* following gland removal indicated the presence of a unique carveol dehydrogenase species in the glandular trichomes, suggesting that the other dehydrogenase found throughout the leaf probably utilizes carveol only as an adventitious substrate. These results demonstrate that carvone biosynthesis takes place exclusively in the glandular trichomes in which this natural product accumulates (Gershenzon *et al.*, 1989). A simple and accurate reversed phase HPLC procedure is proposed for the determination of 19 phenolic compounds (flavonoids, phenolic acids, and coumarins) in seven medicinal species including *M. piperita*. The sample preparation involved extraction, alkaline and acid hydrolysis and purification through a Bond-Elut C18 column. A diode-array detector monitored the effluent and chromatograms were recorded. The optimized methodology seems to be useful for the phytochemical analysis of plant extracts. A close correlation between the phenolic compound patterns and the botanical origin of plants was found (Andarde *et al.*, 1998). UV-A radiation (360 nm) affects the photomorphogenesis and essential oil chemical composition of *M. piperita*. Total phenols and chlorophyll *b* are also affected by UV-A. UV-A irradiation during the night period induces a typical shade-avoidance syndrome, with stem elongation, decreased leaf area and leaf-area index, decreased protein and total phenol content, and decreased essential oil and menthol content (Mafeii *et al.*, 1999). It is demonstrated by Fowler *et al.* (1999) that linalyl acetate is biosynthesized *via* non-mevalonate (l-deoxyxylulose phosphate) terpene pathway in the plant *M. citrata*. The incorporation of isotopically labeled DL-[3-2H3]-alanine and [6,6-2H2]-D-glucose has revealed that five of the deuterium atoms of 1-deoxyxylulose phosphate are retained during the biosynthesis of linalyl acetate. Measurement was done for the accumulation of monoterpenes, a model group of constitutive defenses, in peppermint (*M. piperita* L.) leaves and investigated several physiological processes that could regulate their accumulation, the rate of biosynthesis, the rate of metabolic loss and the rate of volatilization (Gershenzon *et al.*, 2000). A wide range of compounds such as terpenoids, iridiods, phenolic compounds and flavonoids have been reported from *Mentha* spp. (Zegorka and Glowniak, 2001). Chromatographic separation of eight phenolic acids and four flavonoids methylated via the PTC derivatization step was achieved in *M. spicata*. The detection limits for the described GC–MS (SIM) method of analysis ranged between 2 and 40 ng/ml whereas limits of quantitation fall in the range 5–118 ng/ml, with flavonoids accounting for the lowest sensitivity due to their multiple reaction behavior. Four aquatic infusions from commercially available *M. spicata*, were analyzed with other plants (Fiamegos *et al.*, 2004).

Bioactivity Profile

The effect of *M. longifolia* crude ethanol extract (F1), as well as fractions rich in luteolin glycosides (F2), apigenin glycosides (F3) and phenolic acids (F4) on intestine motility, spontaneous motility, pentobarbital induced sleep and bile secretion have been investigated. The crude ethanol extract was effective only on intestinal motility, apigenin and luteolin glycosides active on spontaneous motility. Phenolic acids were found to possess significant spasmodic, choleretic and CNS stimulative effects (Mimica-Dukiç *et al.*, 1996). Linarin (acacetin-7-O-β-D-rutinoside) from the flower extract of *M. arvensis* showed selective dose dependent inhibitory effect on acetylcholinesterase. Cholinesterase inhibitors enhance the signal transmission in nerve synapses by prolonging the effect of acetylcholine thereby have been used as symptomatic medication for Alzheimer's disease and myasthenia gravis (Jokela *et al.*, 2006). The main aromatic constituents of essential oils (EO) of *M. suaveolens* as characterized by IR, NMR and MS studies *i.e.* pulegone, piperitenone oxide (PEO) and piperitone oxide (PO) occurring in different amounts depending on the subspecies confirmed antimicrobial activity against gram +ve, gram–ve as well as fungi (Oumzil *et al.*, 2002). Pulegone-rich essential oil inhibited efficiently all the microorganisms. s-Carvone extracted from *M. spicata* have been shown to posess considerable antioxidant activity compared to α-tocopherol using the thiocyanate method in the linoleic acid system (Elmasta *et al.*, 2006). The flavonoid glycosides (Figure 12.1), eriocitrin (1), narirutin (2), hesperidin (3), luteolin-7-*O*-rutinoside (4), isorhoifolin (5), diosmin (6), rosmarinic acid (7) and 5,7-dihydroxycromone-7-*O*-rutinoside (8), were isolated from the aerial part of *M. piperita* L. Among these compounds, compound 4 showed a potent inhibitory effect on histamine release induced by compound 48/80 and antigen-antibody reaction. Luteolin-7-*O*-rutinoside caused a dose-related inhibition of the antigen-induced nasal response at about 100 and 300 mg/kg indicating its clinical importance as an antihistamine and in treating allergic Rhinitis (Inoue, 2002). n-Butanol soluble fraction derived from methanol extract of *M. spicata* Linn. exhibited significant protecting activity against DNA strand scission by $^{\bullet}$OH on pBluescript II SK(–) DNA (Kumar and Chattopadhyay, 2007).

From *in vitro* studies on Chromosomal aberration (CA) and sister chromatid exchange (SCE) of human lymphocytes it was concluded that peppermint oil unlike essential oil extracted from Dill

	1	2	3		4	5	6
R_1	rut	-rut	-rut	R_4	-rut	-rut	-rut
R_2	-OH	-H	-OH	R_5	-OH	-H	-OH
R_3	-OH	-OH	-OMe	R_6	-OH	-OH	-OMe

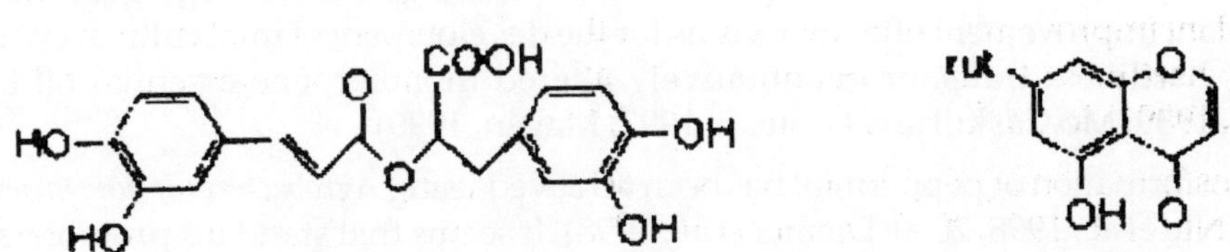

7 8

Figure 12.1: The Chemical Structure of Compounds 1–8

(*Anethum graveolens*) seeds and herb; pine needles were genotoxic in dose dependent manner. SMART test in *Drosophila* species also showed a dose dependent increase in mutation frequency whereas dill seeds were almost inactive in inducing mutation (Lazutka and Mierauskiene, 2000).

In vitro Propagation

Efficient and reliable plant regeneration of peppermint has been achieved by manipulating adventitious organogenesis (Faure *et al.*, 1998; Niu *et al.*, 1998; Li *et al.*, 1999) Shoot organogenesis of both *M. piperita* and *M. arvensis* occurs from leaf disk explants cultured on to medium supplemented with NAA, BAP, cytokonin, thidiazuron. Immature leaf explant of peppermint is most responsive morphogenetically. Suspension cultures of *M. piperita* were able to synthesize limonene as well as oxygenated, acetylated, or glucosilated monoterpenes. *Mentha* spp. suspension cultures metabolized exogenous monoterpenes ketones and monoterpene alcohols within 24h and glucosilation occurred (Dörnunburg and Knorr, 1995). Two-phase cultures of *M. piperita* have been studied to improve the production of essential oil. RP-8 has been used in the second phase to improve the production (Kim *et al.*, 1996). Chang *et al.* (1998), has reported that using optimum concentration of 200 mg/l of chitosan gives 166mg/l menthol after 12 days. Chitosan elicitation may activate the conversion of pulegone to menthol. The impact of several parameters, independently and in combination, on the stimulation of menthol production in the cell suspension culture of *M. piperita* was studied. Synergistic potentiation effect of menthone feeding, and γ-cyclodextrin treatment followed by in situ adsorption with RP-8 also showed potential stimulation of menthol production in *M. piperita* cell culture. Fungal elicitor treatment showed enhanced production level in comparison to that of control. Further studies were carried out with the establishment of *Agrobacterium tumefaciens* (Ach5) gall mediated calli and consequently cell suspension culture and results showed the significant enhancement of menthol yield (Chakraborty and Chattopadhyay, 2008).

Molecular Genetics and Biotechnology

Essential oils synthesized and stored in leaf glandular trichomes of the *Mentha* spp. are valuated commercially as additives for food products, cosmetics and pharmaceuticals. Mint production and oil yeild is attenuated by both biotic and abiotic stress. Consequently, there is need for development of cultivars with pest resistance and stable oil quality. Mint cultivars mainly are propagated vegetatively. Crop improvement is limited by sterility of commercial varieties and ploidy differences amongst potential members of the gene pools (Tucker, 1992). Weed problem in mint production must be addressed in a more effective and enviormentally acceptable way, however, molecular engineering for herbicide resistance is a plausible aprroach (Mazur and Falco, 1989). Resistance to broad–spectrum and enviormentally more acceptible heribicides like glyphosate (Nida *et al.*, 1995) and glufosinate (Botterman and Leemans, 1989) has been achieved for numerous crops using biotechnology. Biotechnolgy based approaches to plant improvement offer new vistas for the development of mint cultivars with enhanced pest resistance, hardiness traits, or quantitatively altered monoterpene essential oil biosynthesis (Dempsey *et al.*, 1989; Mc-Caskill and Croteau, 1997; Martin, 1999).

Genetic transformation of peppermint has been achieved using *Agrobacterium tumefaciens* mediated DNA delivery (Niu *et al.*, 1998, 2000; Diemer *et al.*, 1998). It seems that standard promoters like CaMV 35S-driven expression are not adequate for mint (Niu *et al.*, 1998). Recent analysis indicates maximal 35S–driven expression of tobacco osmotin in transgenic mint plants was only about 0.5 per cent of total leaf protein (Niu *et al.*, 2000) relative to 2.0 per cent maximal accumulation in potato and leaves using an analogous expression cassette (Liu *et al.*, 1994). Higher transgene expression in peppermint is driven by chimeric promoter in the pBISNI vector (Narasimhulu *et al.*, 1996). Somatic hybrid plants of Black Mitcham were obtained after protoplast fusion (Krasnyanski *et al.*, 1998).

Shoot cultures, derived by transformation of two *Mentha* spp. *M. citrata* and *M. piperita,* with *Agrobacterium*-based vectors, grew actively as axenic cultures in simple media, lacking plant growth substances. They produce a range of monoterpenes which reflect the qualitative composition of essential oils from their respective parent plants. In *M. citrata* the transformed shoot cultures were derived from wild-type nopaline strains of *A. tumefaciens* and produce an essential oil in which linalool and linalyl acetate constitute over 90 per cent and in this respect closely resemble the parent plant. However, the cultures were more effective in the acetylation reaction than the parent plant and linalyl acetate was a more dominant component in the oil from the culture. *M. piperita* shoot cultures were derived from two routes; using either the nopaline strains of *A. tumefaciens,* or using disarmed strains of *A. tumefaciens* carrying a binary vector with the ipt (isopentenyl transferase) coding sequence under the control of the powerful CaMV 35S promoter. In transgenic cultures derived from either route, menthol was the major component in the essential oil as in the parent plant, but all cultures produced lower levels of menthone and greater levels of menthofuran than the parent plant. Maximum oil production in these cultures approached 10 mg per flask over seven-week culture period. These transgenic shoot cultures have been stable in monoterpene production for over two years (Spencer *et al.*, 1993). The pioneering efforts of the Rodney Croteau's group provide key information about essential oil biosynthesis in mint including genes that encode enzymes of key regulatory steps (Colbey *et al.*, 1993; Bohlmann *et al.*, 1998; Lange and Croteau, 1999). Limonene synthase then converts the aliphatic GPP to the cyclic intermediate limonene, which is considered a committed and 'rate-limiting' step in mint oil biosynthesis. (Kjonaas and Croteau, 1983; Colbey *et al.*, 1993). This is a branch point in the biosynthesis of peppermint or spearmint oil. Over expression, in the native plant, of genes encoding key regulatory enzymes of oil biosynthesis is predicted to enhance the biosynthesis of the most desirable monoterpenes (Mc Caskill and Croteau, 1997). The oxygenation pattern of the cyclic monoterpenoids of commercial mint (*Mentha*) species is determined by regiospecific cytochrome P450-catalyzed hydroxylation of the common olefinic precursor (2)-4*S*-limonene. In peppermint (*M. piperita*), C3–allylic hydroxylation leads to (2)-*trans*-isopiperitenol, whereas in spearmint, C6-allylic hydroxylation leads to (2)-*trans*-carveol. The microsomal limonene-6-hydroxylase was purified from the oil glands of spearmint and amino acid sequences from the homogeneous enzyme were used to design PCR primers with which a 500-bp amplicon was prepared. This nondegenerate probe was employed to screen a spearmint oil gland cDNA library from which the corresponding full-length cDNA was isolated and subsequently confirmed as the C6-hydroxylase by functional expression using the baculovirus–*Spodoptera* system (Lupin *et al.*, 1999). Another transgenic approach to modulate yield of mint oil based on increasing the density of leaf glandular trichomes (Mc Caskill and Croteau, 1999). Mint monoterpenes are produced in glandular trichomes (Fahn, 1979; Gershenzon *et al.*, 1992) which are, anatomically, modified epidermal hairs consisting of a cluster of secretary cells surmounted with an oil droplet enclosed by the cuticle layer and an underlying stalk and basal cell (Fahn, 1979). Polyphenoloxidase (PPO) of peppermint leaves (*M. piperita*) was isolated by $(NH_4)_2SO_4$ precipitation and dialysis (Kavrayan and Aydemir, 2001). Isolation and bacterial expression of a sesquiterpene synthase cDNA clone from peppermint (*M. piperita* L.) that produces the aphid alarm pheromone (*E*)-b-farnesene was also by Croteau group. Regiospecific hydroxylation of (2)-4S-limonene at C3 or C6 exclusively is catalysed by two distinct cytochrome P450 in peppermint and spearmint respectively. Exchange of a single residue (F363I) in the spearmint limonene-6 hydroxylase led to its regiospecificity to be converted to C-6 hydroxylase. (Schalk and Croteau, 2000). The rate of accumulation of essential oil under ambient low light conditions were considerably lower than that predicted by mathematical kinetic modeling for prediction of biosynthetic processes involving its synthesis. This anomaly indicates the role of menthofuran and pulegone, which accumulates under such lighting conditions to be a potential inhibitor of the branch-point enzyme pulegone reductase (Rios-Estepa *et al.*, 2008). In our laboratory, true to mother type transgenic mint (*Mentha arvensis* L.) expressing bacterial glutathione synthetase gene has been developed. Transformed plants were obtained by co cultivation of leaf disks with *Agrobacterium tumefaciens* strain LBA 4404 harbouring a binary vector that carried *E. coli* glutathione synthetase (*GS*), *b*-glucuronidase as reporter gene and *npt*II as selective marker gene for kanamycin resistance. Transgenic plants were successfully acclimatized in the greenhouse conditions. An overall transformation frequency of 15 per cent was achieved in approximately 3 months of time period. These results are discussed in relation to heavy metal trafficking pathways in higher plants and to the interest of using plastid expression of *PCS* for the biotechnological applications (Kumar *et al.*, 2008).

Conclusion

Commercial mint varieties are perennial plants propagated vegetatively from disease-free (state certified) rootstocks or underground runners (*i.e.* stolons). After introduction into fields, mint is managed initially as a row crop, but the runners spread rapidly creating a meadow field during the second year. Mint production and oil yield is attenuated by both biotic and abiotic stresses. Consequently, there is need for development of cultivars with pest resistances and stable oil quality. Pest problems are often magnified because of the long-term perennial monoculture system. Major pests of mint can be categorized as weeds, insects and diseases (including nematodes). Weeds substantially affect production due to costs associated with eradication and reduced oil quality. A number of insects adversely affect mint production with relative impact depending on geographic location and season. Effective control requires knowledge of the insect pest life cycle, effective scouting to assess potential crop damage, and timely application of approved insecticides.

Bioactivity profile and chemical analysis of the mint family has been worked out from time to time. Biotechnology offers tremendous potential for vegetatively propagated plants like mint that are not amendable to genetic introgression through breeding. Genetic transformation systems of high efficiency are available for peppermint so improvement of this crop through biotechnology is very feasible. Applications of biotechnology for mint crop improvement will involve transformation with genes for herbicide, disease, insect, cold and drought resistance and modulation of the oil production biosynthetic pathways. Progress in all these areas will be possible as more information is generated relating to genes affecting these plant responses and how gene expression can be modulated to improve the agricultural characteristics of mint. Metabolic engineering of monoterpene biosynthesis in plants is an active area of research for last decades. The feasibility of increasing monoterpene yield and altering metabolite composition in essential oil plants has been demonstrated and lots of work yet to be done, and the transgenic production of monoterpenes to enhance scent and flavor in flowers and fruits is a ongoing challenge. Similar approaches to engineer these pathways for the purpose of importing terpenoid based plant defenses or to exploit allelopathic interactions can be readily envisioned. However, limitations might arise in the transplantation of monoterpene biosynthetic pathways into normally nonproducing hosts because of the absence of secretary structures and their associated transport and storage machinery. Research over the past decade has yielded substantial insight into the metabolism of monoterpenes in this genus. The biosynthetic pathways for many commercially important monoterpenes have been established and the genes encoding key pathway enzymes have been cloned from several species. The availability of appropriate molecular tools and the economic importance of monoterpenes have prompted a recent surge of interest in engineering these pathways in mint family. Finally, wide availability and acceptability, easy cultivation parameters and vegetative propagation of this popular herb along with its wide spectrum of bioactivity for the benefit of human health needs a concerted effort to develop further as dietary supplement and/or neutraceutical as well as a natural resource of menthol, an essential oil of commercially importance, chiefly for pharmaceutical industry.

Acknowledgements

Authors wish to acknowledge support from Council of Scientific and Industrial Research, Government of India. Part of this work received financial support from Department of Biotechnology, New Delhi.

References

Andrade, P.B., Seabra, R.M., Valentão, P., Areia, F. (1998). Simultaneous Determination of Flavonoids, Phenolic Acids, and Coumarins in Seven Medicinal Species by HPLC/DIODE-Array Detector. *Journal of Liquid Chromatography and Related Technologies*, 21: 2813–2820.

Bhat, S., Maheshwari, P., Kumar, S., Kumar, A. (2002). *Mentha* species: In vitro Regeneration and Genetic Transformation. *Molecular Biology Today*, 3: 11-23.

Bohlmann, J., Meyer-Gauen, G., Croteau, R. (1998). Plant terpenoid synthases: molecular biology and phylogenetic analysis. *Proceedings of the National Academy of Science USA*, 95: 4126-4133.

Botterman, J., Leemans, J. (1989). Discovery, transfer to crops, expression and biologically significance of a bialophos resistance gene. *British Crop Protection Council-Monograph*, 42: 63-68.

Chakraborty, A., Chattopadhyay, S. (2008). Stimulation of menthol production in *Mentha piperita* cell culture. *In Vitro Cell Developmental Biology Plant, In Press (Accepted on 28th April 2008).*

Chang, J.H., Shin, J.H., Chung, I.S., Lee, H.J. (1998). Improved menthol production from chitosan-elicited suspension culture of *Mentha piperita. Biotechnology Letters*, 20:1097-1099.

Colby, S.M., Alonso, W.R., Katahira, E.J., McGarvey, D.J., Croteau, R. (1993). 4-S limonene synthase from the oil glands of spearmint (*Mentha spicata*). *Journal of Biological Chemis*try, 268: 23016-23024.

Dempsey, D.A., Silva, H., Klessig, D.F. (1998). Engineering disease and pest resistance in plants. *Trends in Microbio*logy, 6: 54-61.

Diemer, F.F., Faure, O., Moja, S., Colson, M., Matthys-Roschon., Caissard, J.C. (1998). High efficiency transformation of peppermint (*Mentha* x *piperita* L.) with *Agrobacterium tumefaciens*. *Plant Science*, 136: 101-108.

Dörnenburg, H., Knorr, D. (1995). Strategies for the improvement of secondary metabolite production in plant cell cultures. *Enzyme and Microbial Technology*, 17: 674-684.

Elmasta, M., Dermirtas, I., Isildak, O., Aboul, H.Y.(2006). Antioxidant Activity of S-Carvone isolated from Spearmint (*Mentha spicata L.* Fam. Lamiaceae*). Journal of Liquid Chromatography and Related Technologies*, 29: 1465–1475.

Estepa, R.R., Turner, G.W., Lee, J.M., Croteau, R.B., Lange, B.M. (2008). A systems biology approach identifies the biochemical mechanisms regulating monoterpenoid

essential oil composition in peppermint. *Proceedings of the National Academy of Science USA*, 105: 2818-2823.

Fahn, A. (1979). Secretory tissues in plants. Academic Press, London.

Faure, O., Diemer, F., Moja, S., Jullien, F. (1998). Mannitol and thidiazuron improve *in vitro* shoot regeneration from spearmint and peppermint leaf disks. *Plant Cell Tissue and Organ Culture*, 52: 209-212.

Fiamegos, Y.C., Nanos, C.G., Vervoort, J., Stalikas, C.D. (2004). Analytical procedure for the in-vial derivatization–extraction of phenolic acids and flavonoids in methanolic and aqueous plant extracts followed by gas chromatography with mass-selective detection. *Journal of Chromatography A*, 1041: 11–18.

Fowler, D.J., Hamilton, J.T.G., Humphrey, A.J., O'Hagan, D. (1999). Plant terpene biosynthesis. The biosynthesis of linalyl acetate in *Mentha citrata. Tetrahedron Letters*, 40: 3803-3806.

Gershenzon, J., McCaskill, D., Rajaonarivony, J.I.M., Mihaliak, C., Karp, F.,Croteau, R. (1992). Isolation of secretory cells from plant glandular trichomes and their use in biosynthetic studies of monoterpenes and other gland products. *Biochemistry*, 200: 130-138.

Gershenzon, J., McConkey, M.E., Croteau, R.B.(2000). Regulation of Monoterpene Accumulation in Leaves of Peppermint. *Plant Physiology*, 122: 205–214.

Harley, R.M., Brighton, C.A. (1977). Chromosome numbers in the genus *Mentha*. *Botanical Journal of the Linnean Society*, 74:71–96.

Inoue, T., Sugimoto, Y., Masuda, H., Kamei, C. (2002). Antiallergic Effect of Flavonoid Glycosides Obtained from *Mentha piperita* L. *Biological and Pharmaceutical Bulletin*, 25: 256-259.

Gershenzon, J., McConkey, M.E., Croteau, R.B. (2000). Regulation of Monoterpene Accumulation in Leaves of Peppermint. *Plant Physiology*, 122:205–213.

Kim, T., Kim, T.Y., Bae, G.W., Lee, H.J., Chae, Y.A., Chung, I.S. (1996). Improved production of essential oils by two-phase culture of *Mentha piperita* cells. *Plant Cell Tissue and Organ Culture*, 13:189-192.

Kjonaas, R., Croteau, R. (1983). Demonstration that limonene is the first cycle intermediate in the biosynthesis of oxygenated pmenthane monoterpenes in *Mentha piperita* and other *Mentha* species. *Archives of Biochemistry and Biophysics*, 220: 79-89.

Krasnyansky, S., Ball, T.M., Sink, K.C. (1998). Somatic hybridization in mint: identification and characterization of *Mentha piperita* (+) *M. spicata* hybrids plants. *Theoritical and Applied Genetics*, 96: 683-687.

Kumar, A., Chattopadhyay, S. (2007). DNA damage protecting activity and antioxidant potential of pudina extract. *Food Chemistry*, 100: 1377-1384.

Kumar, A., Chakraborty, A., Ghanta, S., Chattopadhyay, S. (2008) *Agrobacterium*–mediated genetic transformation of mint with *E. coli* glutathione synthetase gene. *Plant Cell Tissue and Organ Culture*, (In Press)

Lange, B.M., Croteau, R. (1999). Genetic engineering of essential oil production in mint. *Current Opinion in Plant biology*, 2: 139-144.

Liu, D., Raghothama, P.M., Hasegawa, P.M., Bressan, R.A. (1994). Osmotin overexpression in potato delays development of disease symptoms. *Proceedings of the National Academy of Science USA*, 91: 1888-1892.

Li, X., Niu, X., Bressan, RA., Weller, S.C., Hasegawa, M.P. (1999). Efficient plant regeneration of native spearmint (*Mentha spicata* L.). *In Vitro Cell Developmental Biology-Plant*, 35: 333–338.

Lupien, S., Karp F., Wildung, M., Croteau, R.(1999). Regiospecific cytochrome P450 limonene hydroxylases from mint (*Mentha*) species: cDNA isolation, characterization, and functional expression of (-)-4S-limonene-3-hydroxylase and (-)-4S-limonene-6-hydroxylase. *Archives of Biochemistry and Biophysics*, 368: 181-92.

Maffei, M., Canova, D., Bertea, C. M., Scannerini, S. (1999). UV-A effects on photomorphogenesis and essential-oil composition in *Mentha piperita*. *Journal Of Photochemistry and Photobiology B: Biology*, 52: 105-110.

McCaskill, D., Croteau, R. (1995). Monoterpene and sequiterpene biosynthesis in glandular trichomes of peppermint (*Mentha* x *piperita*) rely exclusively on plastid-derived isopentenyl diphosphate. *Planta*, 197: 49-56.

McCaskill, D., Croteau, R. (1997). Prospects for the bioengineering of isoprenoid biosynthesis. In: Berger R (ed) Advances in Biochemical Engineering/Biotechnology, pp 107-146.

McCaskill, D., Croteau, R. (1999). Strategies for bioengineering the development and metabolism of glandular tissues in plants. *Nature Biotechnology*, 17: 31–36.

Martin, GB. (1999). Functional analysis of plant disease resistance genes and their downstream effectors. *Current Opinion Plant Biology*, 2: 273-279.

Mimica-Dukic, N., Jakovljevi, V., Mira, P., Gasi, O., Szabo, A. (1996). Pharmacological Study of *Mentha longifolia* Phenolic Extracts. *Pharmaceutical Biology*, 34: 359–364.

Mimica-Dukic, N., Bozin, B., Sokovic, M., Mihajlovic, B., Matavulj, M. (2003). Antimicrobial and antioxidant activities of three *Mentha* species essential oils, *Planta Medica*, 69: 413–419.

Narasimhulu, SB., Deng, XB., Sarria, R., Gelvin, S.B. (1996). Early transcription of *Agrobacterium* T-DNA genes in tobacco and maize. *The Plant Cell*, 8: 873-886.

Nida, DL., Kolacz, KH., Delannay, X., Re, D.B. (1995). Glyphosatetolerant Cotton: genetic characterization and protein expression. *Journal of Agricultural and Food Chemistry*, 44: 1960–1966.

Niu, X., Lin, K., Hasegawa, P.M., Bressan, R. A.,Weller, S.C. (1998). Transgenic peppermint (*Mentha piperita* L.) plants obtained by cocultivation with *Agrobacterium tumefaciens*. *Plant Cell Reports*, 17: 165–171.

Niu, X., Li, X, Veronese, P., Bressan, R.A., Weller, S.C., Hasegawa, P.M. (2000). Factors affecting *Agrobacterium tumefaciens*-mediated transformation of peppermint. *Plant Cell Reports*, 19: 304-310.

Oumzil, H., Ghoulami, S., Rhajaoui, M., Ilidrissi, A., Fkih-Tetouani, S., Faid, M., Benjouad, A. (2002). Antibacterial and antifungal activity of essential oils of *Mentha suaveolens*. *Phytotherapy Research*. 16: 727-731.

Oinonen, P.P., Jokela, J.K, Hatakka, A.I., Vuorela, P.M. (2006). Linarin, a selective acetylcholinesterase inhibitor from *Mentha arvensis*. *Fitoterapia*, 77: 429-434.

Sasson, A. (1991). Production of useful biochemicals by higher-plant cell cultures: biotechnological and economic aspects. *CIHEAM-IAMZ, Options Méditerranéennes–Série Séminaires*, 14: 59–74.

Schalk, M., Croteau, R. (2000). A single amino acid substitution (F363I) converts the regiochemistry of the spearmint (?)-limonene hydroxylase from a C6–to a C3-hydroxylase. *Proceedings of the National Academy of Science USA*, 97: 11948-11953.

Spencer, A., Hamill, J.D., Rodes, M.J.C. (1993). *In vitro* biosynthesis of monoterpens by *Agrobacterium* transformed shoot cultures of two *Mentha* species. *Phytochemistry*, 32:911-919.

Tucker, A.O., Harley, R.M., Fairbrothers, D.E. (1980). The Linnaean Types of *Mentha* (Lamiaceae). *Taxon*, 29: 233-255.

Turker, A.O. (1992). The truth about mints. *Herb Companion*, 4: 51–52.

Werrmann, U., Knur, D. (1999). Conversion of Menthyl Acetate or Neomenthyl Acetate into Menthol or Neomenthol by Cell Suspension Cultures of *Mentha canadensis* and *Mentha piperita*. *Journal of Agricultural and Food Chemistry*, 41: 517-520.

Zegorka, G., Glowniak, K. (2001). Variation of free phenolic acids in medicinal plants belonging to the Lamiaceae family. *Journal of Pharmaceutical and Biomedical Analysis*, 26: 179-187.

Zheng, J., Wu, L., Zheng, L., Wu, B., Song, A. (2003). Two new monoterpenoid glycosides from *Mentha spicata* L. *Journal of Asian Natural Products Research*, 5: 69-73.

Utilisation and Management of Medicinal Plants (2010) *Pages 228–243*
Editors: **V.K. Gupta, Anil K. Verma and Sushma Koul**
Published by: **DAYA PUBLISHING HOUSE, NEW DELHI**

Chapter 13

Medicinal and Aromatic Potentialities of *Ocimums* and their Efficacy in Traditional Systems of Medicine

M.K. Khosla* and V.K.Gupta
Indian Institute of Integrative medicine (CSIR), Canal Road, Jammu Tawi – 180 001, India

ABSTRACT

Ocimums (Fam. Lamiaceae) popularly known as Tulsi and collectively as basil is ranked among the few wonder herbs, which has a versatile role to play in traditional systems of medicine. Many of its species are considered to be highly medicinal and find extensive application in indigenous systems of medicine of many Asian, African and South American countries. Several scientific studies are being conducted regarding efficacy of whole plant or its parts for the treatment of different diseases and ailments. The most ancient and fundamental medical literature of India namely Charak Samhita and Sushruta Samhita describe some wonderful curative effects of *Ocimum* species. Charak describes the 'holibasil' *O. sanctum* as curative of hiccups, cough, poison, dyspnea and plurodynea, promotive of 'Pitta and curative of 'Kapha' and 'Vatha' and eliminative of 'Fetor'. The Indian Materia Medica which is a compilation of Unani and Ayurvedic systems of medicine, also refers *Ocimum* plants as highly medicinal for having properties as alexipharmic, antiemetic, antipyretic, antiseptic, carminative, demulcent, diaphoretic, diuretic, expectorant, stimulant and therefore, recommended for the treatment of diseases like catarrh, bronchitis, gastric, and genitourinary disorders, malarial fever, rheumatism, skin diseases etc. *O. sanctum* was described by these as a plant belonging to 'Sarasadi' group of drugs most of which

* Corresponding Author: E-mail: khoslamk@rediffmail.com.

are reputed vermifuges. *O. sanctum* and *O. basilicum* are considered to be effective antidote for snake poison. *Ocimum* species also possess several important natural aroma chemicals which are of tremendous value in traditional medicines as well. The different *Ocimum* species considered for their efficacy are *O. sanctum, O. gratissimum, O. viride, O. suave, O. canum, O. americanum, O. carnosum, O. kilimandscharicum, O. micranthum* and the work details carried out in this direction have been discussed in the present communication.

Keywords: *Ocimums, Medicinal, Aromatic, Efficacy, Potentialities.*

Introduction

The medicinal and aromatic plants have remained in great demand by the mankind for curing ailments, diseases as well as for pleasant aroma chemicals since the early period of its civilization. India being the privileged country for having vast area with wide variation in climate, soil, altitudes, latitudes resulting in the extensively diversified agroclimatic conditions, thus forms a heritable emporium of many medicinal and aromatic plants. The country has one of the oldest, richest and most diverse cultural traditions associated with the use of medicinal and aromatic plants. The classical Indian literature *viz.*, RigVeda (5000 yrs B.C.), YajurVeda and AtharaVeda (4500-2500 yrs B.C.) and later Charak Samhita (700 yrs B.C.), Sushruta Samhita (200 yrs B.C.), Bag Vatta and many others produced remarkable description of the Indian medicinal plants including *Ocimum* species and has helped in compounding of drugs which are still used in classical formulations in the Ayurvedic system of medicine. *Ocimums* like many other important medicinal and aromatic plants are highly valued for both medicinal as well as aromatic properties. Their medicinal potentialities and fine aroma chemicals have been of immense use in the traditional as well as modem pharmacological system of many Asian, African and South American countries. *Ocimum* plants from ancient time till today has been treated as sacred and are worshipped and offered to God and even at present days the leaves of species like *Ocimum sanctum* are given to devotees as sacred prasad in many parts of India (Khosla, 1995a).

The genus *Ocimum* (Fam. Lamiaceae) has tropical distribution, with nearly two-third of the 160 species are reported from West Africa and the remaining one third from Asia and America. Nine species have been reported from India, mainly from tropical areas and a few species from the peninsular area (Khosla, 1995b). *Ocimum* species include aromatic herbs or undershrubs yielding essential oils of various aroma chemicals. These essential oils and aroma chemicals are of tremendous value in pharmaceutical and perfume cum flavour industry besides their enormous use in confectionary, food, condiments, dental creams, mouth washes etc. and many of these therefore, are imported to meet the county's industrial demand. In recent decades pharmaceutical and clinical tests have shown that many of *Ocimum* species have potent insecticidal, insect repellant and anti-microbial properties. The present communication thus deals with the work details regarding the medicinal and aromatic potentialities along with efficacy of some *Ocimum* species *viz., O. sancium, O. gratissimum, O. viride, O. basilicum, O. americanum, O. canum, O. carnosum, O. kilimandscharicum, O. suave* and *O. micranthum.*

Medicinal and Aromatic Potentialities and Efficacy

Ocimum sanctum Linn. (Sacred Tulsi)

O. sanctum (Figure 13.1) is ranked among few wonder herbs for having enormous medicinal potentialities which acts as panacea for various ailments and diseases. The medicinal properties of *O.*

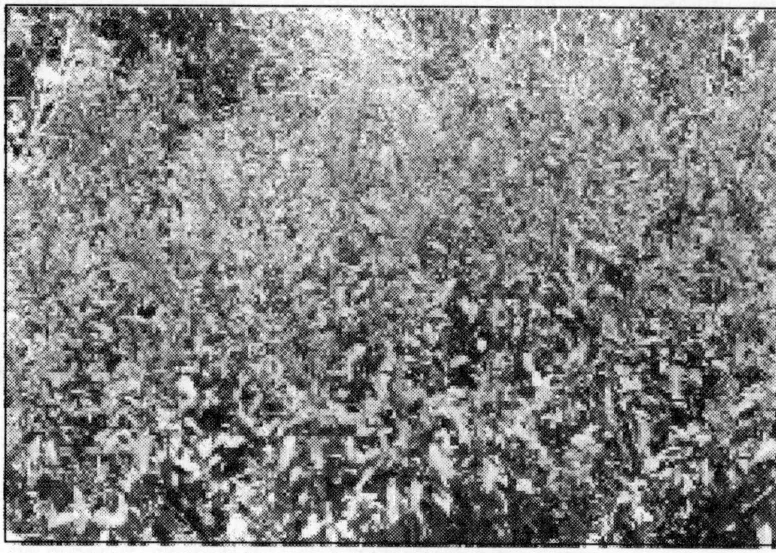

Figure 13.1: *Ocimum sanctum* Linn.

sanctum have been mentioned in most ancient and fundamental literature of Hindus describing it as curative of Kapha and Vatha. Due to its manifold curative uses, the plant is considered as highly sacred, worth worshipping and hence given the name as "Sacred Tulsi" or "Holy Basil". The plant is erect, annual or biennial, much branched with green or purplish leaves, found throughout India upto an altitude of 1800m in the Himalayas, cultivated and grown in garden and temples. The plant is propagated through fresh seeds which are globose to sub-globose, pale brown with black markings and are slightly mucilaginous on wetting. The plants has been bred and developed as a rich source of important chemical eugenol (70-75 per cent) present in its essential oil which is pale yellow with strong spicy odour (Khosla, 1981).

O. sanctum possesses tremendous medicinal properties so much so that each and every part of the plant finds its use in one form or the other. The plant is pungent, bitter in taste, hot, stomachic, cholagogue, anthelminthic, alesiteric, useful in disease of heart and blood, leucoderma, strangury, asthma, vomiting, halitosis, lumbago pains, hiccough, painful eyes, purulent discharge from the ear, in burning sensation and snake bite (Kirtikar and Basu, 1935). Santals (tribals) use the plant in fever, dropsy and anasarca, hemiplegia, vomiting, constipation, cholera, cough, postnatal complaints, haemorrhage, septicaemia and dog bite (Jain and Tarafdar, 1970). *O. sanctum* belongs to Surasad group of drugs most of which are reputed vermifuges.

The leaves of *O. sanctum* have expectorant properties and their juice is usefully applied in catarrhal bronchitis and also in throat and chest troubles. A decoction of leaves alongwith tea and milk has proved extremely useful in malaria. It is very helpful in curing cold, cough and indigestion. The dried leaves are powdered and mixed into a paste with mustard oil and used as a tooth-paste. It fights foul odours from the mouth and is useful in curing pyorrhea and other tooth troubles. The dried leaves are also employed as snuff in ozaena (offensive discharge from the nose). These are an effective means of dislodging maggots (Chopra *et al.*, 1956). Juice of fresh leaves, fresh tops and the slender roots are considered to be a good antidote against snake bite and scorpion sting. In Ceylon, the herb is used in decoction for cough and catarrh, sometimes chewed as a substitute for betel. The juice of the leaves possesses diaphoretic anti-periodic and stimulant properties (Wealth of India, 1966). Fresh leaves paste with butter is applied on the face to remove blemishes and skin wrinkles. Ring worm rashes and other skin diseases can be cured by applying leaf juice or paste which is also used in ear ache and other minor infections of the ear, eyes and nose (Dymock *et al.*, 1980). It is also believed that five tender leaves along with five black pepper seeds taken empty stomach every morning strengthens weak heart and cures and prevents all types of fevers particularly malaria. Plant leaves are also used as condiment in salad and other foods. Few fresh leaves taken with tea or milk checks vomiting, acidity of the stomach and heat burn.

The seeds of *O. sanctum* are mucilaginous and demulcent and are used in disorders of genito-urinary system whereas its seed paste about 1g reduces burning sensation of urine. The seeds also show anti-coagulase activity (Bhat and Broker, 1954). About 2g of seed taken with warm water removes constipation and when taken with cold water checks diarrhea. Fresh roots of *O. sanctum* grounded with water are applied to the stings of wasps and bees and on the bites of worms and leeches. The bruised fresh roots, stem and leaves are applied to mosquito bites.

The essential oil obtained from *O. sanctum* has been chemically analysed in detail (Lal *et al.*, 1978; Khosla, 1981). The oil is rich in eugenol, used in dental preparations, tooth ache, mouth washes, flavouring food products and in various detergents. It is applied to reduce joint pains, inflammations and body rashes; the oil also possesses significant insecticidal and larvicidal activity against house flies, blue bottle flies and especially mosquitoes (Chopra *et al.*, 1941) and antimicrobial and anti-mycotic effect *in vivo*, the former being stronger than the later (Grover and Rao, 1977).

O. sanctum plant has been studied for abortifacient and anti-fertility activity (Vohra *et al.*, 1969; Batta and Santha, 1971; Kashinathn *et al.*, 1972). The plant (dried powder) showed adaptogenic (anti-stress) activity (Bhargava and Singh, 1981). The plant prevents stress induced peptic ulcer and hyper-acidity and thus manifess a non-specific type of protection against a variety of stress induced biological changes (Wagh,1977; Seethalakshmi *et al.*, 1982). *O. sanctum* is also reported to possess anti-tuberculosis substance (Gupta and Vishwanathan, 1955), property of therapeutic effect (Gonopoti, 1952) and for lowering the blood sugar level (Luthy *et al.*, 1964). There are also reports of powerful germicidal and antiseptic properties of the plant (Nene *et al.*, 1968). Alleged anti-asthmatic potential are reported of tulsi leaves in the treatment of human bronchial asthma (Palit *et al.*, 1983; Singh and Agarwal, 1991). The plant is used as an ingredient of Teftoli, a propriety product for viral hepatitis (Rajalakshmi *et al.*, 1991). It is used to clear bilirubin from the urine and S.G.P.T. levels showing a beneficial change (Sankaran, 1980). The species is also reported to have therapeutical active constituent like anti-biotic, anti-cancerous etc. (Mhaskar and Caius, 1931; George *et al.*, 947; Joshi and Magar, 1952; Matsushiro and Nakada, 1955; Dhar *et al.*, 1968; Hartwell, 1969; Wagh, 1977).

The Smarkand Medical Research Institute, USSR and with which Indian doctors are collaborating in studies on tiredness caused by stresses have confirmed that Indian *O. sanctum* herb definitely possesses anti-stress property which can help in curing the exhaustion caused by physiological strain.

Ocimum gratissimum Linn. (Ram Tulsi)

O. gratissimum (Figure 13.2) being an indigenous South Indian perennial under shrub, 150-160 cms in height with ovate-lanceolate green leaves. Flowers are small pale yellow and bisexual, while its seeds are dark brown, rugose, sub-globose and slightly mucilaginous. The plant has been successfully

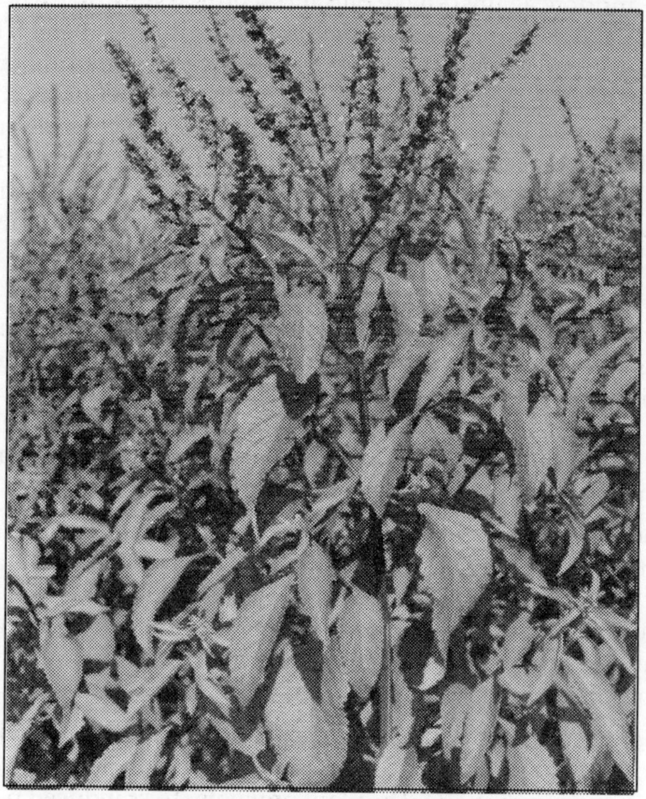

Figure 13.2: *Ocimum gratissimum* Linn.

developed as a rich source of eugenol which acts as an alternate source for clove oil, hence named as "Clocimum" (Clove scented *Ocimum)*. The essential oil is pale yellow which turns to deep yellow with brownish tinge after few weeks time. The GC of the oil revealed the presence of eugenol (8.0-85 per cent)' as major chemical constituent (Khosla *et al.*, 1988) which is widely used in perfume, flavour and pharmaceutical products. The oil serves in flavouring of all kinds of food products, meals, sausages, detergents, various dental preparations and as mosquito repellant. It is also applied on inflamed joints and other inflammatory body conditions. Eugenol is used for the synthesis of vanillin-world's mostly used flavour for all kinds of food beverages *viz.*, ice-creams, dairy products, desserts, confectionary, baked goods, cola beverages and liquors.

The plant has a bitter sharp taste, carminative, aphrodisiac; useful in diseases of the brain, heart, liver and spleen; removes foul breath, strengthens the gums; good for griping and piles (Khosla, 1981; Nandkarni and Nandkarni, 1954). Aromatic baths of fumigations prepared with the plant are given in the treatment of rheumatism and paralysis. A strong leaf decoction has been found to be effective in the aphthae of children, in cases of seminal weakness and is also as a good remedy in gonorrhea (Chopra *et al.*, 1956). It is a diaphoretic, stomachic, laxative and is good for the treatment of fevers (Said *et al.*, 1969). The seeds are given in headaches and neuralgia (Chopra *et al.*, 1956). It has been reported that *O. gratissimum* has got maximum medicinal use in Africa and the oil vapours of the plant could kill protozoa (Said *et al.*, 1969). Its essential oil also possesses anti-bacterial and anti-fungal activity'

(Grover and Rao, 1977; Sawhney *et al.*, 1977). Leaf oil of the plant is quite effective against number of plant pathogens (Thakur *et al.*, 1989; Khana *et al.*, 1989; Dixit and Shukla.1992) and the therapeutic effect of oil in the treatment of toothaches and headaches has been successfully studied (Khosla, 1986) The oil has been tested for its cytotoxic activity against P388 leukemia cells (Dubey *et al.*, 1997) The plant species has been reported to have potent antitubercular activity (Ramasway and Sirsi,1967)

Ocimum viride Willd. (Ban Tulsi)

O. *viride* (Figure 13.3) is an exotic West African species of great medicinal value and is commonly known as fever plant of Sierra Leone. The plant is a perennial, erect much branched under shrub, 145-160cm in height with elliptic-lanceolate brownish green leaves. Flowers small, pale yellow, seed globose, brownish and non mucilaginous. The species has been developed as a rich source of thymol (75-80 per cent) (Khosla *et al.*, 1989) which forms a cheap alternate source of thyme oil or ajowan oil *(Trachyspermum ammi* L.) of commerce. The essential oil is pale yellow, viscid with characteristic odour of thymol, having pungent and spicy flavour. Thymol being an important aroma chemical is extensively used in pharmaceutical, food and flavour industries, as a strong antiseptic disinfectant, antimicrobial, anti-fungal (tropical), anthelmintic, in deodorant, mouth washes, tooth pastes, gargles, preservative, as a stabilizer-antioxidant and antitoxidant. The oil when used internally acts as a laxative followed by astringent effect (Irvine, 1995). It is also used in compounding of synthetic essential oil besides as a starting material for making synthetic menthol.

The plant is extensively used in West African medicine and is sold in the market as a well known fabrifuge. The whole plant may be used as a poultice for rheumatism and lambago. It is called the mosquito plant since it is reputed to keep away mosquitoes. A pomade containing pulped leaves and sea butter is applied to itch. A decoction of leaves is used in fever and coughs and the juice is used for catarrh and as eye drops for conjunctivitis (Wealth of India, 1966). Some Europeans use the hot leaves infusion as fabrifuge and diaphoretic, being taken like tea with milk and sugar. The leaves are also

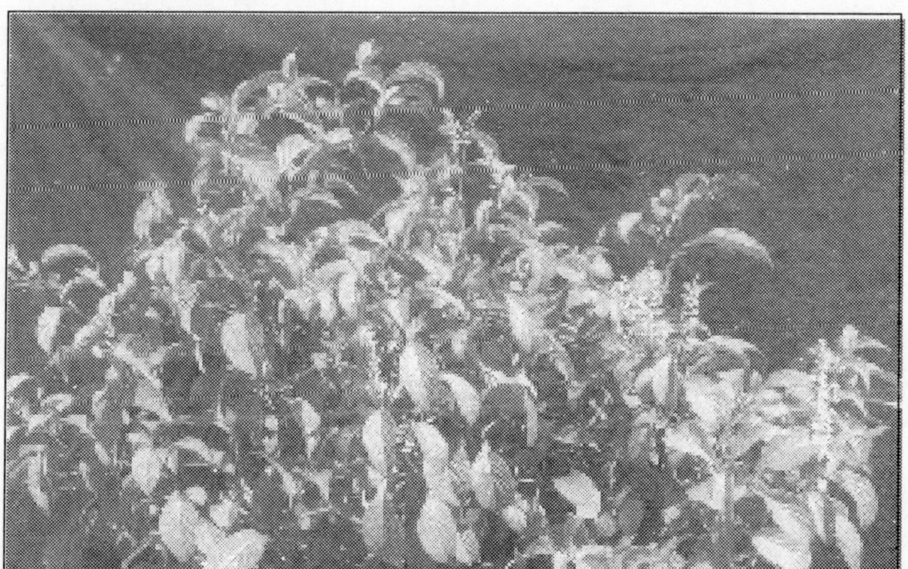

Figure 13.3: ***Ocimum viride*** **Willd.**

taken together with *Paullinia pinnata* as a remedy for dysentery. In Nigeria and Congo, the leaves are used as a stomachic and laxative or purgative. The leaves boiled with those of *Spondias* and the bark of *Funtumia elastica* are applied to the piles in Nigeria. The African natives prepare a special beverage from O. *viride* which they drink as a general tonic for health and vitality.

Ocimum basilicum Linn. (Babui Tulsi)

O. basilicum (Figure 13.4), commonly known as Indian basil, is an indigenous South Indian, erect, annual under shrub, 65-85cm high with green or purplish stem. The leaves are ovate and flowers are white pinkish or purplish. The seeds are dark brown to black, ellipsoid and mucilaginous. The plant has been developed as a rich source of methyl chavicol (80-85 per cent) (Khosla *et al.,* 1999) The essential oil is pale yellow, slightly viscid with a sweet spicy herbal odour. The oil is extensively used as flavouring agent in confectionary, baked goods, sauces, soups, catsûps tomato pastes, pickles, meats, sausages and beverages. Also used for scenting dental and oral preparations and in certain perfume compounds, notably Jasmine blends, to impart strength and smoothness. Basil oil possesses insecticidal and larvicidal activity against houseflies, blue bottle flies and particularly against mosquitoes (Chopra *et al.,* 1941; Deshpande and Tipnis, 1967). The plant is stomachic, stimulant, carminative, antipyretic, diaphoretic, expectorant, diuretic and also useful in heart, brain and blood diseases, asthma, inflammations and enlarged spleen (Kirtikar and Basu, 1935). The juice of the leaves warmed with honey is useful in the treatment of croup (Chopra *et al.,* 1956). It also forms an excellent nostrum for the cure of ringworms, scorpion sting and snake bite. It gives luster to the eyes; good for toothache, ear-ache, headache and can be mixed with camphor to stop nasal haemorrhage (Kirtikar and Basu, 1935).The seeds steeped in water and eaten are said to be cooling and very nourishing. Its infusion is given in gonorrhea, diarrhea and chronic dysentery (Chopra *et al.,* 1956). The washed and pounded seeds are used in poultices for unhealthy sores and sinuses. Also used with sharbat in habitual constipation and in internal piles. The seeds are chewed in snake-bite (Kirtikar and Basu, 1935). The flowers of the plant have stimulant, carminative, diuretic and demulcent properties (Chopra

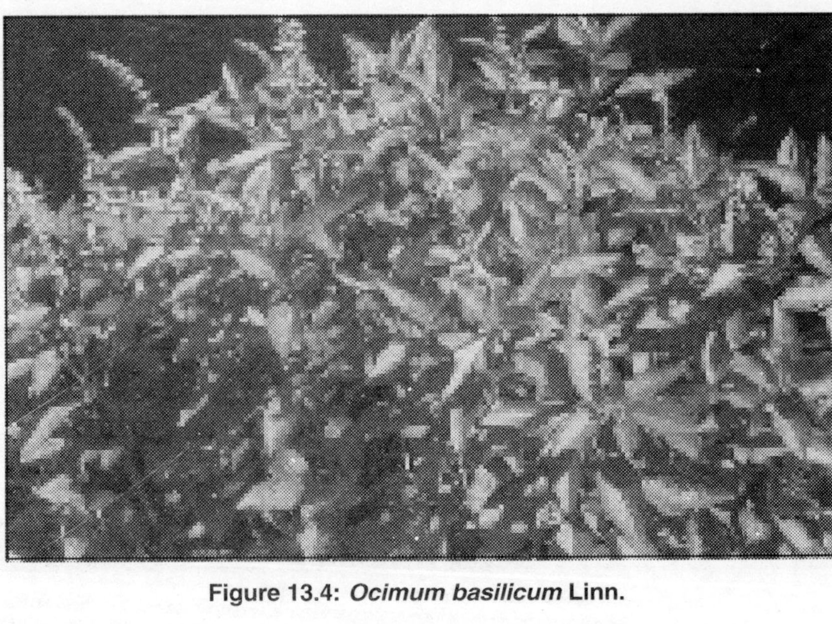

Figure 13.4: *Ocimum basilicum* Linn.

et al., 1956). A teaspoon full of seed infused in a tumbler of water with little sugar, when taken daily, acts as a demulcent in genito-urinary disease. A cold infusion of seeds is said to relieve the after pains of child birth. An infusion of seed is also given in fever (Dastur, 1970). The essential oil showed anti-bacterial and anti-fungal activity against various organisms (Khorana and Vangikar, 1950; Kaul and Nigam, 1977; Lahariya and Rao, 1979; Sawhney *et al.*, 1977; Singh *et al.*, 1983; Singh and Sharma, 1978). The roots of the plant are used for bowel complaints in children (Chopra *et al.*, 1956). The plant is used by tribals (Santals) in headache, earache, fever, dropsy, hemiplegia, epilepsy, obstetric problems, convulsions and cramps, liver complaints, fibsile delirium, collapse, cholera, rabid dog bite and snake bite (Jain and Tarafdar, 1970).

Ocimum americanum Linn. (Kala Tulsi)

O. americanum (Figure 13.5), an indigenous, erect sweet scented, pubescent annual herb, 70-80cm, high with eliptic-lanceolate leaves. The flowers are white pink or purplish in colour. The. seeds are black narrowly elliptic and mucilaginous. The essential oil is pale yellow with characteristic odour of lemon. The detailed GC of the 'oil has shown citral (80-85 per cent) as the major constituent (Pushpangadan *et al.*, 1979). The essential oil is extensively used in perfume, flavour and pharmaceutical industry, flavouring sauces, soups, salads etc. It is mainly used in the synthesis of Vit.A besides yielding important perfumery grade isolates from B-ionones. The leaves in the form of paste are used in parasitical disease of the skin and also applied to the finger and toe nails in fever during cold weather conditions. The juice of the leaves is given in cold, catarrh and bronchitis in children. The plant is said to be carminative, diaphoretic and having stimulant properties. A decoction of the plant is used for cough and that of leaves for dysentery and as a mouth wash for relieving toothache (Wealth of India, 1966; Chopra *et al.*, 1956; 1958). The plant is considered to be useful by tribals in headache,

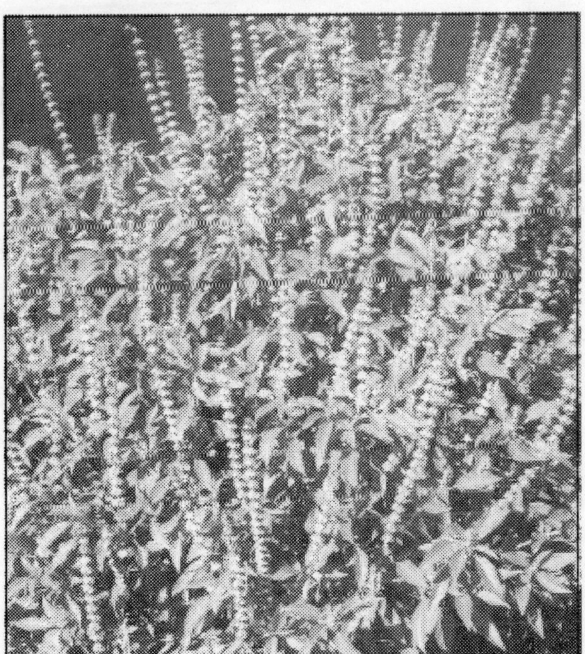

Figure 13.5: ***Ocimum americanum*** **Linn.**

convulsions and cramps, cholera, rabid dog bite and snake bite (Jain and Tarafdar, 1970). The essential oil showed anti-bacterial and anti-fungal activity (Joshi and Magar, 1952; Ramasway and Sirsi, 1967; Dhar *et al.*, 1973; Mehta *et al.*, 1978; Khosla, 1992; Singh *et al.*, 1983).

Ocimum canum Sims (a)

O. canum (Figure 13.6), an indigenous South Indian, annual herb, 70-80cm in height with elliptical, lanceolate leaves. The flowers are bisexual and pinkish white. The seeds are dark brown, narrowly ellipsoid and mucilaginous. The plant has been developed as a rich source of methyl cinnamate (80-85 per cent) (Khosla, 1992). The essential oil is of sweet basil type, straw coloured with fruity balsamic note and is much sweeter than the exotic basil and french basil oils. The oil rich in methyl cinnamate is used in composition of oriental and floral perfumes and as an excellent fixative and blender in soap perfume industry (Guenther, 1948). Methyl cinnamate obtained from the essential oil has been found to be mainly responsible for the insecticidal activity against *Tribolillm castanellm, Sitophillis aryzae, Stagobillm paniceum* and *Bruchus chinensis* (Deshpande and Tipnis, 1977).

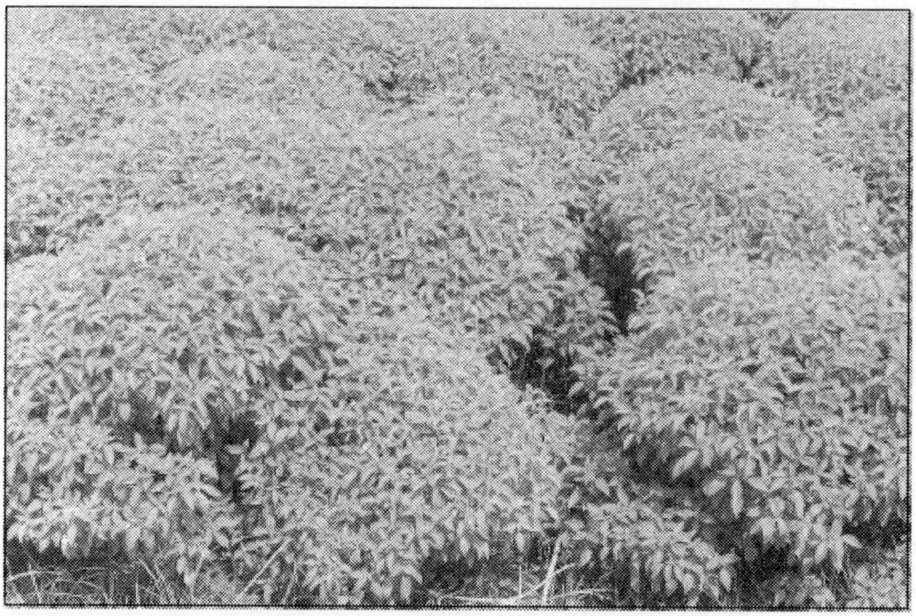

Figure 13.6: *Ocimum canum* Sims(a)

Ocimum canum Sims (a′)

O. canum (Figure 13.7), another chemotype, is an indigenous South Indian annual herb, 75-85cm high with small ovate leaves having hirtelous lamina. The flowers are small pinkish white. The seeds are ellipsoid, dark brown and mucilaginous. The plant has been developed as a rich source of linalool (70-75 per cent) (Gupta and Sobti, 1993). The essential oil is used in perfume, flavour and cosmetic industry. The plant is used to cure fever, dysentery, parasitical disease of skin and hemorrhage from the nose. The leaves and the seeds are considered as aromatic tonic, febrifuge, anticatarrhal, expectorant, sternutatory and anti-rheumatismal. Seeds are grounded in an infusion of the leaves to cure malaria. The juice and the powder obtained by pounding together the seeds and the leaves are taken as an errhine in migraine (Kirtikar and Basu,1935) The plant has also been studied for antifertility activity (Dixit and Bhat,1975), anti-biotic activity (Dhar *et al.*, 1973) and anti-cancer activity (Hartwell,1969).

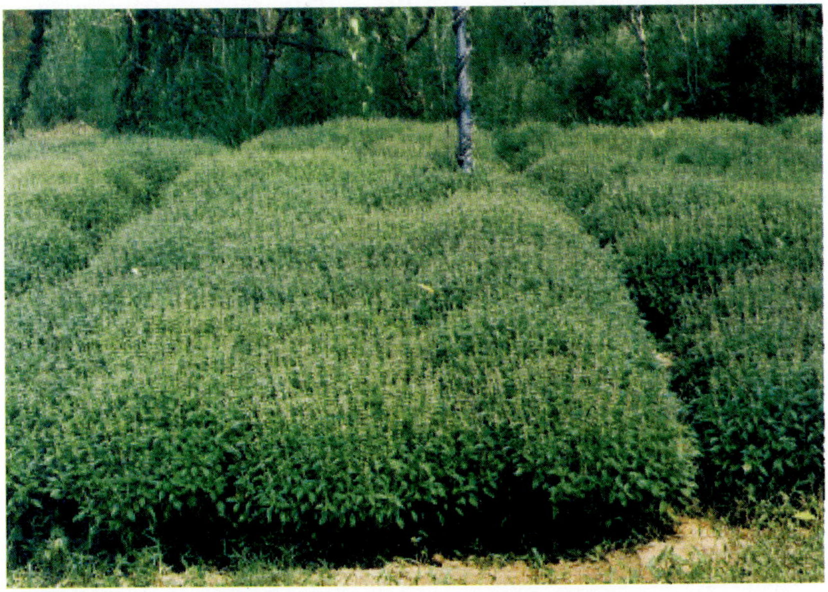

Figure 13.7: ***Ocimum canum*** **Sims(a')**

The oil is reported to possess potent anti-bacterial (Sirsi *et al.*, 1952)) and anti-fungal activity (Dixit and Bhat, 1975).

Ocimum carnosum LK. et Otto.

O. carnosum (Figure 13.8), an exotic South American species, has been successfully introduced in North India. The plant is perennial, much branched, spreading, 60-80cm in height, under shrub with simple, ovate-oblanceolate and dark green leaves. The flowers are small and purplish whereas the seeds are ellipsoid, purplish to dark brown and slightly mucilaginous. The plant has been developed as a rich source of elemicin (70-75 per cent) (Khosla,1995). On hydrodistillation of the whole herb, the plant yields light yellow, viscid oil with strong spicy earthy odour. The essential oil is highly prized for its immense pharmaceutical value besides having flavouring properties. The major oil constituent elemicin is used in the production of 3,4,5 trimethoxy-benzaldehyde which forms the starting material for the synthesis of trimethoprim, an ingredient used in the production of an important anti–bacterial drug, Septran.

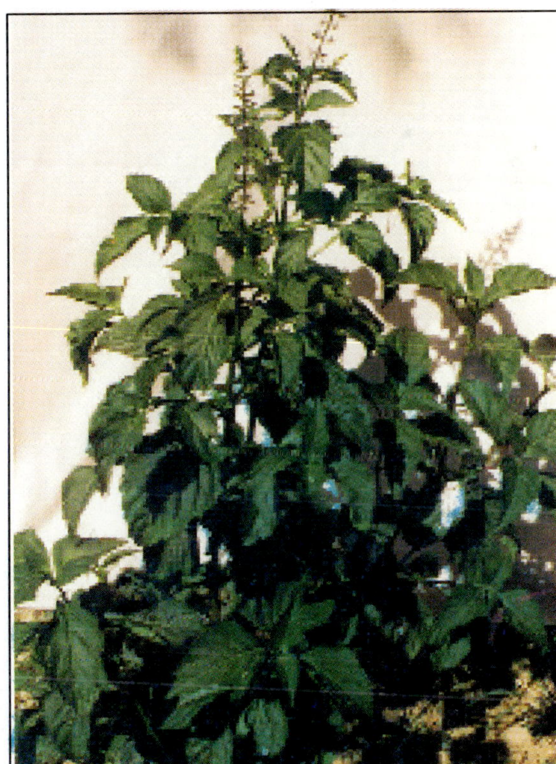

Figure 13.8: ***Ocimum carnosum*** **LK. et. Otto.**

Ocimum kilimandscharicum Guerke. (Kapur Tulsi)

O. kilimandscharicum (Figure 13.9), a West African, perennial undershrub, 70-90cm high with ovateoblong leaves. The flowers are light purplish or white. The seeds are ovoid-oblong, black to brown and mucilaginous. The essential oil is light yellow with strong odour or camphor. The detailed GC of the oil has shown camphor (75-80 per cent) as the major constituent. The oil is widely used in perfume, flavour and pharmaceutical industry. It is used in the preparations for local application on sprains, certain types of diarrhea, as cardiac stimulant, antipyretic, carminative and in various dental and oral preparations. The oil possesses anti-bacterial and anti-fungal activity against various organisms (Ramasway and Sirsi, 1967; Suri and Thind, 1978; Thind and Suri, 1979; Singh *et al.*, 1980)

Ocimum suave Willd.

O. suave, a West African exotic species, extensively grown in Tanzania, much branched, highly pubescent, perennial undershrub, 60-80cm high with ribbed stem. The leaves are ovate to ovate-Ianceolate with bluntly serrated margin, grey green in colour. The flowers are small, pinkish white, borne in whorls. The seeds are small, globose, dark brown and non-mucilaginous. The plant has been developed as a rich source of sesquiterpene alcohols (44.90 per cent) (Pushpangadan *et al.*, 1978). The

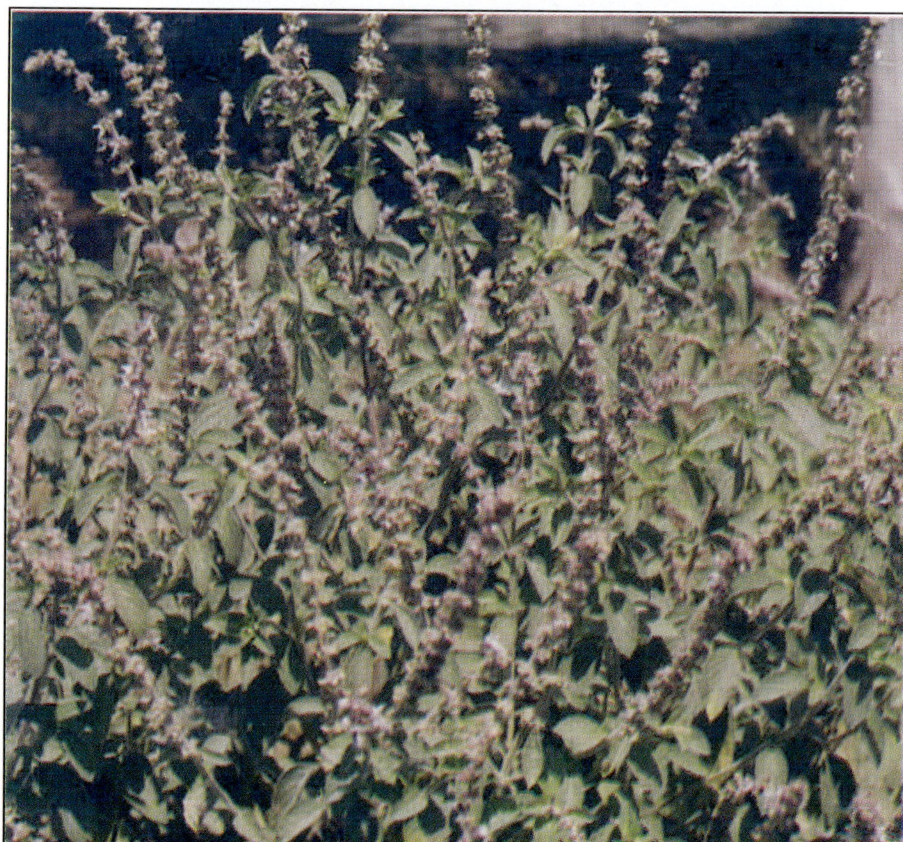

Figure 13.9: ***Ocimum kilimandscharicum*** **Guerke.**

essential oil is highly viscid, light yellow with a pleasant balsamic, woody dusty odour. The oil is mainly used in flavouring of tobacco and snuff. Also used as body perfume and a mosquito repellent (Chogo and Crank, 1981) and maize weevil repellant (Hassanali *et al.,* 1990). The plant is used as a local application for the relief of nasal congestion. Extracts of the plant have been used for the treatment of coughs, abdominal pains, ear and eye inflammation and as a gargle for mouth infections (Murice and Iwu, 1993).

Ocimum micranthum Willd.

O. micranthum (Figure 13.10), an exotic South American, evergreen, annual, undershrub, 40-60cm high with green and ovate-lanceolate leaves. The flowers are white pinkish in colour. Seeds are ellipsoid, purplish to dark brown and are slightly mucilaginous. On hydro-distillation of the whole herb, the plant yields light yellow, viscid essential oil with pleasant spicy odour. The detailed GC of the oil has shown methyl eugenol and its derivatives (67.33 per cent) as major oil constituents (Khosla *et al.,* 1980). The essential oil is used as a fixative in flavour and perfume industry. It is also used in the preparation of hallucinogenic beverage along with some other plant (Pinkley, 1969).

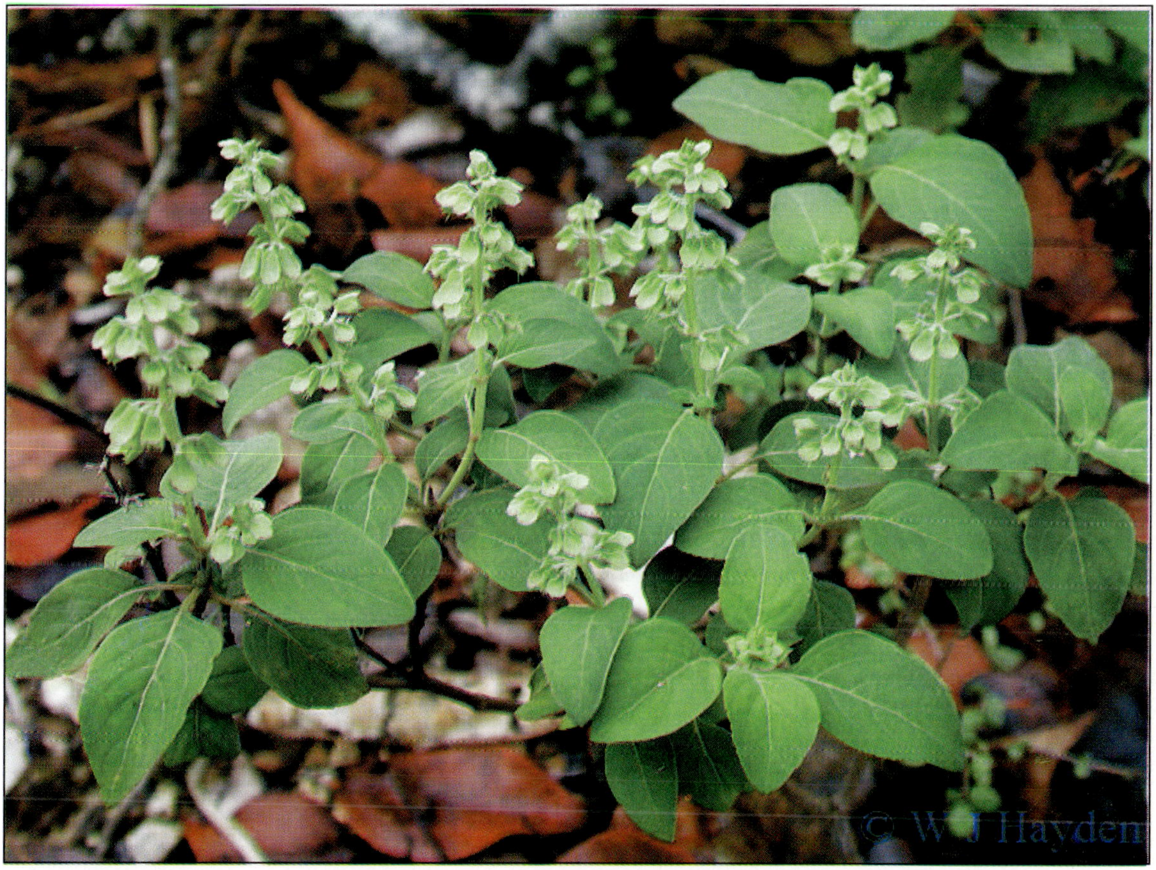

Figure 13.10: ***Ocimum micranthum*** **Willd.**

Acknowledgements

The authors are grateful to Director, Indian Institute of Integrative Medicine (CSIR), Jammu for providing facilities and his keen interest during the course of present investigations.

References

Batta, S.K and Santha Kumari, G. (1971). Antifertility effect of *Ocimum sanctum* L. *Indian J. Med. Res.*, 59:777-781.

Bhargava, K.P. and Singh, N. (1981). Antistress activity of *Ocimum sanctum* Linn. *Indian J. Med. Res.*, 73: 443.

Bhat, l.V. and Broker, R.l.(1954). Anticogulase factors in some indigenous plants. *I Sd. Ind. Res.* 13B: 305.

Chopra, R.N., Chopra, I.C., Handa, K.L. and Kapoor, L.D. (1958). Chopra's Indigenous Drugs of India. 2nd edition U.N. Dhur and Sons Pvt. Ltd. Calcutta.

Chopra, R.N., Nayar, S.L. and Chopra, l.C. (1956). Glossary of Indian Medicinal Plants, CSIR, New Delhi.

Chorpa, R.N., Roy, D.N. and Ghosh, S.M. (1941). Insecticidal and larvicidal action of the essential oils of *Ocimum basilicum* Linn. and *Ocimum sanctum* Linn. 1. *Malaria Inst. India*, 4: 109-112.

Chogo, J.B. and Crank, G. (1981). Chemical composition and biological activity of the Tanzania plant *Ocimum suave. J. Af. Nat. Prod.* 44: 308-311

Dastur, J.F. (1970). Medicinal plants of India and Pakistan. D.B. Taraporewala Sons and Co. Pvt. Ltd. Bombay.

Deshpande, R.S. and Tipnis, H.P. (1977). Insecticidal activity of *Ocimum baslicum* Linn. *Pesticides*, ll: 11-12.

Dhar, M.L., Dhar, M.M., Dhawan, B.N., Mehrotra, B.N., Srimal, R.C. and Tandon, I.S. (1973). Screening of Indian plants for biological activity. Part IV. *Indian J. Exp. BioI.* 1l: 43-54.

Dhar, M.L., Dhar, M.M., Dhawan, B.N. and Roy, C. (1968). Screening of Indian Plants for biological activity. Part IV. *Ind. J Exptl. BioI.*, 11:43-54.

Dixit, S.K. and Bhatt, G.K (1975). Folklore studies on unknown indigenous antifertility drugs. *J. Res. Ind. Med.*, 10: 77-83.

Dixit, Y. and Shukla, K (1992). Evaluation of essential oil of *Octmum gratissimum* against storage. *Indian Perfumer*, 36: 277-283.

Dubey, N.K, Kishore, N., Verma, Jaya and Lee Young, Sook. (1997). Cytotoxicity of the essential oils of *Cymbopogon citratus and Ocimllm gratissimllm. Indian J. of Pharamceuticals Sci.*, 59: 263-264.

Dymock, W., Warden, C.J.H. and Hooper, D. (1980). *Pharmacographia Indian*, 38: 67-73.

George, M., Venkataraman, P.R. and Pandalai, K.M. (1947). Investigations on plant antibiotics Part II. A search for antibiotic substances in some Indian medicinal plants *J. Sci. Industr. Res.*, 6B: 42-46

Gonopoti, R.D. (1952). Chemical composition of *Ocimum sanctum.* Congo *Lt so-espan farm*, 3: 187-191.

Grover, S.S. and Rao, J.T. (1977). Investigations on the anti-microbial efficiency of essential oils of *Ocimum sallctum* and *Ocimum gratissimum* L. *Pari Um Undo Kosmet*, 58:326-328.

Guenther, E. (1948). The essential oils. Vol. II pp. 644-645. D. Van. Hostrand Company, Incl. New York.

Gupta, K.C. and Vishwanathan, R. (1955). A short note on antitubercular substance from *Ocimum sanctum. Antibiotics chemotherpay*, 5: 22.

Gupta, S.C. and Sobti, S.N. (1993). RRL-Oc-ll, A linalool rich strain of *Ocimum canum* Sims. 37:261-266.

Hartwell, l.L. (1969). Plants used against cancer. A survey. *Lloydia*, 32: 247-296.

Hassanali, A., Lwande, W., Ole-Sitaya, N. Moreka, L., Nokoe, S. and Chapya, A (1990). *Discovery Innovation*, 2: 91-95.

Irvine, P.R. (1995). Woody plants of Ghanna of 1995. Pp. 766-767. Oxford Press. London.

Jain, S.K and Tarafdar,C.R. (1970). Medicinal Plant-lore of the Santals (A review of P.O. Bodding's work). *Eco. Bot.*, 24: 241

Joshi, C.S. and Magar, N.G. (1952). Antibiotic activity of some Indian medicinal plants. *J. Sci. Indusr. Res.*, 11B:261.

Kashinathan, S., Ramkrishnan, S. and Basu, S.L. (1972). Antifertility effect of *Ocimum sanctum Indian J. Expt.. Biol.*, 10: 23-25.

Kaul, Y.K. and Nigam, S.S. (1977). Antibacterial and antifungal studies of some essential oils. *J. Res. Ind. Med.* 12: 132-135.

Khanna, R.K, Johri, J.K, Srivastava, K.M. and Khanna, S. (1991). Screening for alternative biocides amongst plant-based essential oils. *National Academy Science Letters*, 14: 3-6.

Khosla, M.K. (1995). Sacred Tusli (*Ocimum sanctum* L.) in traditional Medicine and pharmacology. *Ancient Science of Life*, XV: 53-61

Khosla, M.K. (1995). Study on inter-relationship, phylogeny and evolutionary tendencies in genus *Ocimum*. *Indian J. Gen.* 55: 71-83.

Khosla, M.K. (1981). Cytogenetical investigations in genus *Ocimum* with special reference to the "Sanctum group". Ph.D. thesis submitted to the University of Jammu, Jammu

Khosla, M.K. (1986). A preliminary study on the therapeutic effect of "Clocimum" (New hybrid strain of *Ocimum gratissimum)* in the treatment of toothach and headaches. *J. of Scientific Research In Plants and Medicines*,7: 30-33.

Khosla, M.K. (1992). Study on genetic variability in *Ocimum*. Development of *O. canum* as a potrential source of methyl cinnamate. *Pafai*, 144: 34-36.

Khosla, M.K. (1995). Polyploidy induction in *Ocimum camosum* for improved herb,oil and elemicin content. *Indian Perfumer*, 39:133-135.

Khosla, M.K. Bhasin, Mala and Kaul, B.L. 1999. Breeding for evolving high yielding. methyl chavicol rich strain of Basil *(Ocimllm basilicllm* var. *glabratum). Fafai*, 1:17-21

Khosla, M.K., Bradu, B.L. and Gupta, S.C. (1989). Proc. 11th International congress of Essential oils, fragrances' and flavours. New Delhi, 12-16 November

Khosla, M.K., Pushpangadan P., Thappa, R.K. and Sobti, S.N. (1980). Search for new aroma chemicals from *Ocimum* species 111. Studies on genetic variability for essential oil and other allied characters of South American species *O.micranthum* Willd. *Indian Perfumer*, 24: 148-152.

Kirtikar, KR. and Basu, B.D. (1935). Indian Medicinal Plants. Vol. III 2nd Edn. Lalit Mohan Basu, Allahabad, 1959-1968.

Luthy-Nydia, Ortelio and Martinez. (1964). A study of a possible oral hypoglycemic factor in *Albabaca morada* and *Ocimum sanctum* Fortun. *J. Sci.*, 64: 223-224

Lahariya, A.K. and Rao, J.T. (1979). *In vitro* antimicrobial studies of the essential oils *of Cypeerus scarious and Ocimum basilicum. Indian Drug*, 16: 150.

Lal, R.N., Sen, T,K. and Nigam, M.C. (1978). Gas chromatography of the essential oil of *Ocimum sanctum* L. *Prafum. Undo Kosmet*, 59: 230-231.

Matsushiro, A and Nakada, D. (1955). Short note on antituberculous substance from *Ocimum sanctum. Antibitics and chemotherapy*. 5: 22-23.

Mehta, A., Chopra, S., Mehta, P. and Kharaya, M.D. (1978). Antimicrobial activity of some essential oil against certain pathogenic bacteria. *Bull. Bot. Sci. Univ. Sagar*, 14: 25-26.

Mhaskar, K.S. and Caius, J.F. (1931). Indian plant remedies used in snake bite. *Indian Med. Res. Mem.*, 19: 58.

Murice, M., Iwu (1993). Handbook of Afiican Medicinal Plants, pp.215-216.

Nandkarni, G.B. and Nandkarni, K.M. (1954). Indian Materia Medica, Popular Book Depot Bombay.

Nene, Y.L., Thapliyal, P.N. and Kumar, Krishna Labdev. (1968). Screening of some plant extract for antifungal properties. *J. Sci. Technoi*. 68: 226-228.

Palit, G., Singh, S.P., Singh, N., Kohli, R.P. and Bhargava, K.P. (1983). An experimental evaluation of anti-asthmatic plant drugs from the ancient ayurvedic medicine. Aspects. *Allergy Immunol,*, 16:39.

Pinkley, H.V. (1969). Plant admixtures to Ayahuasca the South American Hallucinogenic drink. *Lyoydia*, 32: 305-314.

Pushpangadan, P., Sobti, S.N., Khosla, M.K. and Thappa, R.K. (1978). A search for new aroma chemicals from *Ocimum* species 1. Essential oil of West African species *O. suave.*

Pushpangadan, P., Sobti, S.N. and Thappa, R.K. (1979). Genetic improvement and physico-chemical evaluation of a citral type strain of *Ocimum americanum* L. *Indian Perfumer*, 23: 21-24.

Rajalakshmi, G., Sivanandam, G. and Veluchamy, G.l (1988). *Res. Ayur. Sidha*, IX: 118-123.

Ramasway, A.S. and Sirsi,.M. (1967). Antitubercular activity of some natural products. *Indian J. Phar.* 29: 157-159.

Rao, B.G.,V.N. Rao and P. Subba. (1972). The efficacy of some essential oils on pathogene fungi. II. *The Flavour Industry*, 3: 368-370.

Said, E.F., Sofowava, E.A, Malcom, S.A and Hofor, A (1969).Investigation into *Ocimum gratissimum* as used in Nigerian native medium. *Planta Medica*, 17:195-200.

Sankaran, l.R. (1980). T efToli in the management of viral hepatitis. *Antiseptic*, 77:643.

Sawhney, S.S., Suri, R.K and Thind, T.S. (1977). Anti-microbial efficacy of some essential oils *in vitro. Indian Drug*. 15: 30-32.

Seethalakshmi, B., Narasappa, A.P. and Kenchaveerappa, S. (1982). Protective effect of *Ocimum sanctum* in experimental liver injury in albino rats. Proc. Indian Pharmacol Soc. XIV Ann. Conf. Bombay, Dec. 29-31, 1981. *Indian J. Pharmacol.*, 14: 63.

Singh, S. and Agarwal, S.S. (1991). Antiasthmatic and anti-inflammatory activity of *Ocimum sanctum*. *Int. J. Pharmacognosy*, 29: 306-310.

Singh, AK., Dixit, A, Sharma, M.L. and Dixit, S.N. (1980). Fungitoxic activity of some essential oils. *Eco. Bot.* 34: 186.

Singh, L. and Sharma, M. (1978). Antifungal properties of some plant extracts. *Indian Drugs Pharmaceut. Ind.*, 14: 25.

Singh, S.P., Singh, S.K and Tripathi, S.C. (1983). Antifungal activity of essential oils of some Labiatae plants against dermatophytes. *Indian Perfumer*, 27: 171.

Sirsi, M., Kole, L.N. Natarajan, S. and Nayak, U.B. (1952). Studies on the antimicrobial activity and pharmacological properties of some essential oils, extracted from locally cultivated plants. *J. Indian Inst. Sci.* 34A: 261-267.

Suri, R.K. and Thind, T.S. (1978). Antibacterial activities of some essential oils.*Indian Drugs. Pharmaceut Ind.*, 13: 25-28.

Suri, RK. and Thind, T.S. (1979). *In vitro* antifungal efficacy of some essential oils. *East Pharm.*, 22: 109.

Thakur, R.N.Singh, P. and Khosla, M.K. (1989). *In vitro* studies on antifungal activities of some aromatic oils. *Indian Perfumer*, 33: 257-260.

Thind, T.S.and Suri, R.K. (1979). *In vitro* antifungal efficacy of some essential oils. *Indian Perfumer*, 23: 138-140.

Vohra, S.B., Garg, S.K. and Choudhary, R.R. (1969). Antifertility screening of plants Part III, Effect of six indigenous plants on early pregnancy in albino rats. *Ind. J. Med. Res.*, 57: 893-899.

Wagh, S.Y. (1977). Hyperacidity and peptic ulcer–A review of Ayurvedic drugs. *Maharashtra Med. J.*, 24: 223-227.

Wealth of India (1966). Raw materials, VIII: 89.

Utilisation and Management of Medicinal Plants (2010) *Pages 244–277*
Editors: **V.K. Gupta, Anil K. Verma and Sushma Koul**
Published by: **DAYA PUBLISHING HOUSE, NEW DELHI**

Chapter 14

Herbs that can Compact Noise Stress: A Mini Review

R. Sheeladevi*
Department of Physiology, Dr. ALM. P.G.I.B.M.S. University of Madras, Taramani Campus, Chennai – 600 113, India

ABSTRACT

Sound and hearing are important mechanisms for communication. However, sound that is beyond 90db is a definite stressor. Noise is an unavoidable phenomenon in the modern world which affects both auditory and extra auditory systems in the body, hence a remedy is required. The marked elevated cortisol level even after 15 days of noise exposure indicated that stress is not yet adapted. After exposure to noise (100dB white noise for 4 h/day–for 15 days) the herbal preparations under human consumption like *Acorus calamus* (AC), *Ocimum sanctum* (OS) and Triphala were analysed for the efficacy in various parameters in Wistar strain of albino rats. Triphala crude powder (equal proportion of *Terminalia chebula*, *Terminalia bellerica* and *Emblica officinalis)* was administered orally whereas the extracts of AC and OS were reported to be administered intra peritoneally. The free radicals generated are assessed by the alteration in the scavenging enzymatic and non enzymatic system in various tissues by AC, OS (brain) and Triphala (lymphoid organs).Further, the ability to maintain the homeostasis of brain neurotransmitter by OS

The free radicals generated during noise stress induced changes in the brain scavenging enzymatic (superoxide dismutase, catalase, glutathione peroxidase, as well as in the non enzymatic systems such as reduced glutathione, vitamin K were almost prevented by AC as well as by OS during noise exposure. Similarly, the free radicals generated during the 15 days of noise stress

* Corresponding Author: E-mail: drsheeladevi@yahoo.com.

exposure induced changes in lymphoid organs were prevented by Triphala. These herbal preparations with full bioactive molecules are already under human consumption, this study recommends its usage pro phylactically as noise is indispensable.

Keywords: *Acorus calamus, Ocimum sanctum, Triphala, Noise stress, Adaptogen.*

Introduction

Sound is of great value as it warns of danger and appropriately arouses an individual and it also gives us the advantage of speech and language within the limit. Human ears are sensitive to the frequency range of 20 Hz to 20 kHz. Discrimination between sound and noise is difficult. Yuh-Fung *Chen et al.* (2002) reported that sound those are unwanted, unpleasant or hurtful becomes noise. Loud noise is generally considered as an environmental stress factor. The commonly used parameter for noise is the sound level in decibels (dB). However, noise exposure of any kind exceed 90 dB, becomes a stressor (Ramsey, 1982). Further, the effects of noise stress encountered vary depending on the characteristics of noise, such as intensity, frequency (Kjellberg, 1990), exposure time, form, individual age, sex and health condition. Today people are unavoidably exposed to noise ranging from high acoustic levels (Petiot *et al.*, 1992) to hazardous noise levels at work. People such as firefighters, military personnel, construction workers, factory workers, truck and bus operators are exposed to over 90 dB and some up to 140 dB. The World Health Organization (WHO) has declared "Noise to be an International Health Problem" as it could not be avoided or eliminated in the modern way of living.

Effect of Noise on Auditory System

It has been postulated that noise acts as an environmental stressor (Passchier-Vermeer, 1993; Berglund and Lindvall, 1995). The brain is the key organ involved in interpreting and responding to potential stressors (McEwen, 2000). Researchers have also found that the auditory system has the fastest metabolic rate in the brain (Hudspeth and Konishi, 2000). After exposure to high noise level the threshold shift (hearing loss) may be temporary, if the organ of Corti is able to recover or it may be permanent (Saunders *et al.*, 1985) when the hair cells or neurons die (Borg, 1995). Pathology of noise-induced hearing impairment (Kawada, 2004) includes the degeneration and loss of the outer hair cells in the organ of Corti of the Cochlea, or the degeneration of the intracellular organelles within the hair cells (Vlajkovic *et al.*, 2004). Further, the changes in the presynaptic region of the outer hair cells apposing the afferent nerve endings also have been reported (Canlon *et al.*, 1993). Usually noise-induced hearing impairment is accompanied by an abnormal loudness perception, which is known as loudness recruitment (Berglund and Lindvall, 1995). With a considerable loss of auditory sensitivity, some sounds may be perceived as distorted (paracusis). Another sensory effect that results from noise exposure is tinnitus. Commonly, tinnitus is referred to as sounds that are emitted by the inner ear itself (physiological tinnitus).

Effect of Noise on Non-Auditory System

Noise stress can induce not only acoustic disorders, but also cardiovascular, nervous, and endocrine alterations (Alario *et al.*, 1987). Different noises may also have different information content and this also could affect physiological threshold and noise-response relationships (Edworthy and Hellier, 2000). Environmental noise impairs a number of cognitive and motivational parameters in children (Hygge *et al.*, 2002). Haines *et al.* (2001) reported that poorer auditory discrimination and speech perception decrease in memory and reduced reading ability in children exposed to high levels of environmental noise. It has also been observed that in the night the total time spent in rapid eye movement sleep (REM), REM onset latency and slow wave sleep were significantly decreased after the exposure to noise (Vallet *et al.*, 1983). Exposure to high levels of occupational environmental noise has been associated with the development of neurosis, irritability and deteriorated mental health (Stansfeld *et al.*, 2000). Noise can therefore, influence perceptual, motor, and cognitive behavior, and also trigger glandular, cardiovascular, and gastrointestinal changes by means of the autonomic nervous system (Suter, 1991). The non-auditory effects reported include the reduction in stroke volume and cardiac output (Andren *et al.*, 1980), hypertension due to peripheral vasoconstriction. Behavioral alteration in monkeys with slow reaction and delayed response to events were also observed (Arnsten and Goldman-Rakic, 1998). But the assumed causal linkages between environmental noises, primary and secondary effects on the one hand and the hypothesized final outcomes on the other hand remain to be determined (Porter *et al.*, 2000).

Multiple Noise Stress Mediators: Corticosteroids

Stress is a state of threatened homeostasis by disturbing the normal physiological equilibrium or homeostasis leads to allostatic load. According to Sapolsky (2000), the stress hormones, such as glucocorticoids, trigger the fight-or-flight response that is intended to save human beings when they are confronted by danger. It has been reported that in real life even moderate environmental noise exposure can increase the acute release of stress hormones (Ising *et al.*, 1990). According to Babisch (2002), noise activates the pituitary–adrenal–cortical axis and the sympathetic–adrenal–medullary axis. Noise levels above 120 dB are also reported to increase cortisol level in humans (Ising *et al.*, 1990). It has been well established that the corticosterone level is an indicator of stress intensity and greater HPA axis activation in response to stress (Sandstrom, 2005). Increased hippocampal glucocorticoid receptor binding in response to noise was observed in pigs (Kanitz *et al.*, 2004). Too much cortisol can prevent the brain from laying down a new memory, or from accessing already existing memories. Noise exposure leads to behavioral suppression and causes time-dependent alterations in noise-induced plasma catecholamine, ACTH and cortisol concentrations (Otten *et al.*, 2004). Spreng (2000) reported that the short-term effects of glucocorticoids are essential whereas the long-term effects lead to immunosuppression, along with the insulin resistance, catabolism and intestinal problems. Moreover, glucocorticoids also trigger a curious cascading death of the very brain cells these hormones are meant to protect.

One day noise stress has been shown to significantly elevate the plasma corticosterone level in rats (Sembulingam *et al.*, 1997). There was a sustained increase in corticosterone levels even after 30 days noise stress (Manikandan *et al.*, 2005a) indicating even after prolonged exposure noise stress is not yet adopted. Based on the corticosteroid levels it can be understood that noise stress can become a chronic stressor.

Selye (1952) has shown that if adaptation to stress fails, circulating corticosteroid levels will remain elevated for a prolonged period of time after the stress exposure. This may be due to the changes in the glucocorticoid receptor levels, which were associated with the altered glucocorticoid negative feed back sensitivity in rats (Meaney *et al.*, 1996). This sustained elevation in circulating corticosterone has been recognized as the prime factor that mediates the neuropathological effects and the negative health consequences of chronic stress (Sapolsky, 1996).

Free Radicals: One Another Mediator Released during Noise Stress

In the auditory system, the noise-induced temporary threshold shift as well as hair cell damage and death which are mediated by reactive oxygen species (Henderson *et al.*, 1999). Researchers have confirmed the role of oxidative stress in the potentiation of noise-induced hearing loss (Fechter, 2005). The term 'Free radicals' was defined as, "It is an atom or group of atoms possessing one or more unpaired electrons" (Leigh, 1990). Any molecule can become a free radical by either losing or gaining an electron. Brain cells are the most vulnerable to free radical damage, because they are relatively deficient in the protective mechanisms compared with other organ systems (Olanow, 1990; Skaper, 1999; Contestabile, 2001).

Native Defence in the Body against Free Radicals

Stress itself is not an illness, it is simply a fact of life and always has been. The stressors have changed over the years, but human physiology has remained the same because of the native protecting mechanisms against such free radicals. In normal cells, a balance exists between oxidative products and antioxidant protection. The enzymatic superoxide dismutase (SOD, EC 1.15.1.1), catalase (CAT, EC 1.11.1.6), glutathione peroxidase (GPx, EC 1.11.1.9, and G6PD) and non-enzymatic (reduced glutathione [GSH], vitamin C, vitamin E) antioxidant systems are present to neutralize the reactive oxygen species (ROS). The GPx and catalase are the two essential enzymes involved in the cytosolic defence against reactive oxygen metabolites. Vitamin C is a well-known water-soluble keto-acetone and plays a crucial role in the suppression of superoxide radicals (Cadet and Brannock, 1997). The intracellular antioxidants GSH, vitamins C and E are interrelated with each other and they can be recycled.

The antioxidant mechanism fails due to either overproduction of free radicals or decreased activities of scavenging enzymes, or both causing lipid peroxidation. When the production of free radicals is faster than their neutralization by antioxidative mechanisms, oxidative stress is induced (Sies, 1991). Since lipid peroxidation is a self-propagating chain reaction, the initial oxidation of only a few lipid molecules can result in significant tissue damage and disease, especially so in polyunsaturated fatty acids rich brain tissues. The oxygen radicals can attack proteins, nucleic acids and lipid membranes, thereby disrupting cellular functions and integrity. Brain is a major target of ROS toxicity due to its high oxygen consumption (Skaper *et al.*, 1999). Brain is the tissue most vulnerable to oxidative damage, because of its high content of polyunsaturated fatty acids, relatively low antioxidant levels, non-replicatory nature of neuronal cells, and high levels of iron and copper (Floyd and Carney, 1992). Aravind kumar *et al.* (1998) reported that acute loud noise exposure generates excessive free radicals and causes disorders involving extra-auditory organs such as nervous, endocrine and cardiovascular systems.

Preventive Measures

Prevention is always better than cure. Various legislation, regulation and policy frameworks have been used for noise management internationally. The noise control legislations licensed or regulated under relevant State and Territory environmental statutes include the Noise Control Ordinance 1988. Other such legislations employed in US are Noise Control Act of 1972, Aviation Safety and Noise Abatement Act of 1979, Airport Noise and Capacity Act of 1990, Federal Interagency Committee on Aviation Noise founded in 1993. However, a combination of three options represents much of international 'best practice' in the management of noise. They are:

1. Elimination or reduction of noise at the source.
2. Elimination or disruption of the transmission path.
3. Isolation or insulation of the receiver from the noise or compensatory treatment to eliminate its effects (Carroll, 2004).

Since noise could not be completely removed from the environment, the only remedy is to find an antidote. In recent years, drug development has rediscovered the potential value of phytopharmaceuticals and their incorporation into medical care has been encouraged by the World Health Organization's Traditional Medicines Strategy (WHO, 2001). There has been a worldwide move towards the use of traditional medicines because of its efficacy and being free from serious toxic effects (WHO, 2002). Herbal medicine has now become an integral part of our standard healthcare. Studies have shown that herbal medicine plays an important role by helping the body to adapt stress, by reducing the damage of the stress response and maintain homeostasis (Azmathulla *et al.*, 2006; Riley *et al.*, 2006;). Pharmacological effects of the medicinal plants are related to its free radical scavenging properties which include the inhibition of lipid peroxidation, maintaining integrity and permeability of the cell wall (Stoll *et al.*, 1996) as well as protection of neurons against oxidative stress (Seif-el-Nasr and El-Fattah, 1995; Oyama, 1996).

Noise Stress Induction

During the experiment, the noise level peaked at 100 dB immediately after the generator (produced by a loudspeaker 15 W), installed at a distance of 30cms above the cage and driven by a white-noise generator emitting all the frequencies in the range 0-26 kHz) was switched on and lasted 4 h. Control animals were sham exposed by placing them in the exposure chamber with the noise generator turned off to take care of the handling and the environment induced changes (Archana and Namasivayam, 2000).

Indigenous System of Herbal Medicine Selected

The free radicals generated as well as the neurotransmitter changes during noise exposure, the efficacy of *Acorus calamus* to prevent the free radical induced changes, the efficacy *Ocimum sanctum* to prevent free radical induced changes as well as the neurotransmitter changes in the brain regions whereas Triphala for its efficacy to prevent the alteration in lymphoid organs and the immune functions.

Acorus calamus Linn. (AC)

Roots and rhizomes of *A. calamus*, also commonly known as sweet flag or sweet cane (family: Araceae) have been used in the Indian and Chinese systems of the medicine for hundreds of years for its beneficial effects on learning performance, and anti-aging effect (Nishiyama *et al.*, 1998; Zhang *et al.*, 1994). The other names are rat root, sweet sedge, flag root, sweet calomel, sweet myrtle, sweet cane, sweet rush, beewort, muskrat root, pine root, racha, vacha, vasambu (India), cinnamon sedge, myrtle flag, myrtle grass, myrtle sedge, shih-ch'angpu (China). From the volatile oil of *A. calamus*, Baxter *et al.* (1960) isolated three active substances namely asarone, trans and cis forms of α-asarone and β-asarone, of 2,4,5-trimethoxy-1-propenyl benzene. Dandiya *et al.* (1959) reported that AC oil is containing phenol, aldehyde and alcohol contents. *A. calamus* contains glucoside acorin ($C_{36}H_{60}O_6$) crystalline alkaloid, calamine, trimethyl amine and choline to exist in calamus root. A higher content of some aliphatic and oxygenated mono terpenes was found in oils of the leaves at their earliest growth phase (May), while the β-asarone content was at its lowest level (Venskutonis and Dagilyte, 2003).

It could be ideal remedy for noise stress, as it helps to manage a wide range of symptoms including neuralgia, epilepsy, memory loss and shock. It is also reported to rejuvenate the brain, promote cerebral circulation, stimulate nervine and anti-spasmodic (Nadkerani, 1976; Nishiyama *et al.*, 1994 a,b; Zhang *et al.*, 1994).

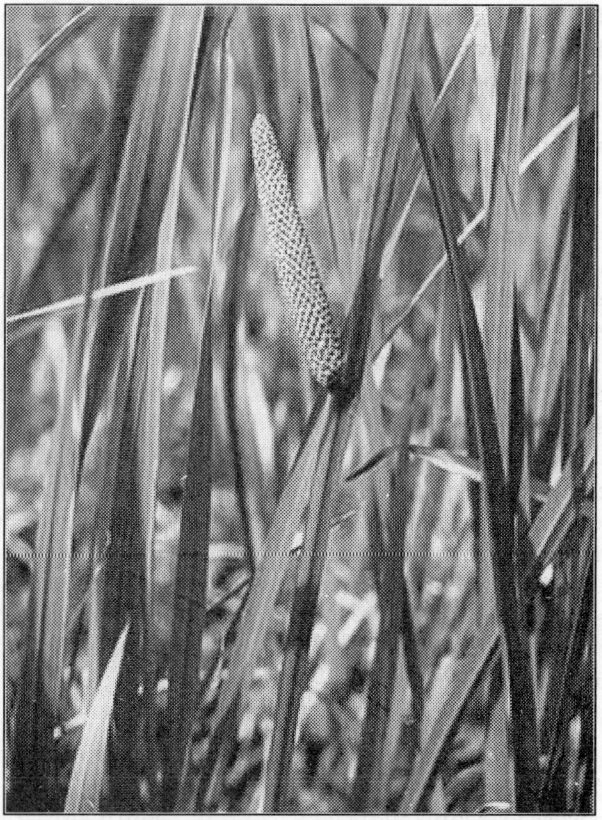

Figure 14.1: *Acorus calamus* Linn. (AC)

Noise Stress Effects on Brain

Lipid peroxidation (LPO) serves as a marker of oxidative stress. Neural tissue is especially sensitive to oxidative stress due to the fact that brain cells are most vulnerable to free radical damage caused by lipid peroxidation compared to other tissues, owing to their highest percentage of unsaturated fats (Antonio, 2001). Exposure of noise stress for 30 days significantly increased the lipid peroxidation in all the regions of the brain (cerebral cortex, cerebellum, pons medulla, midbrain, hippocampus and hypo thalamus) (Manikandan *et al.*, 2005a). The increase in lipid peroxidation after different stressors had been reported (Bhattacharya *et al.*, 2001). Chronic stress induced increase in corticosterone has been hypothesized to act on the brain in an excitatory rather than an inhibitory fashion and this would be expected to decrease the level of discomfort and anxiety induced by chronic stress (Dallman *et al.*, 2004). A study by Lin *et al.* (2004) revealed that chronic dietary supplementation of corticosteroids could result in a significantly enhanced plasma LPO, suggesting that corticosteroids may be one of the reasons for the augmented production of reactive oxygen species during chronic stress. Considering these observations together, one can understand that the elevation of corticosterone in chronic noise stress may not be beneficial.

After an acute noise stress exposure, a significant increase in SOD, catalase, GPx levels in acute noise stress has been observed. The increased SOD activity is an indication that the brain's antioxidant machinery is activated in response to excessive generation of free radicals (Bannister *et al.*, 1987). Animal studies have shown an increase in gene expression of glutathione and catalase synthesis after a noise stress exposure (Jacono *et al.*, 1998) with an increase in the cochlear glutathione synthesis (Yamasoba *et al.*, 1998).

Protein thiolation is apparently induced by different mechanisms that involve thiol/disulfide exchange or one or two electron oxidations of cysteinyl residue (Costa *et al.*, 2003; Giles *et al.*, 2003). The protein thiol levels in noise-stressed animals showed a marked decrease in all the brain regions studied (Samson *et al.*, 2005) indicating the inadequate scavenging activity. It is also justified by the decreased level of one of the major thiol substances, GSH. Similar results showing decreased protein thiols in brain due to oxidative damage, has been reported by Patsoukis *et al.* (2004). Decreased protein thiols in brain are due to oxidative damage. Mandavilli and Rao (1996) reported that regions like cortex, hypothalamus, hippocampus and striatum are more susceptible to oxidative damage when compared to cerebellum. However, Manikandan *et al.* (2005a) observed that cerebellum, midbrain and pons medulla were also equally susceptible to oxidative damage induced by noise stress.

Possible Actions of *A. calamus*

In an *in vitro* study, the ethanolic extract of *A. calamus* has been reported to possess antioxidant activity (Acuna *et al.*, 2002). However, Manikandan *et al.* (2005a) reported after an *in vivo* study the ethyl acetate extract of *A. calamus* was found to be more potent in scavenging activity than the methanolic extract of *A. calamus*. Manikandan *et al.* (2005a) reported that administration of ethyl acetate extract of *A. calamus* could effectively decrease the LPO levels observed in all the brain regions studied after 30 days of noise-stressed animals. This is indicating the effectiveness of *A. calamus* extracts in reducing the oxidative stress. There is a direct correlation between plasma CORT and LPO level (Ohtsuka *et al.*, 1998). In Manikandan *et al.* (2005a,b) study treatment with ethyl acetate extract of *A. calamus*, methanolic extract (methyl acetate) and α-Asarone normalized the plasma corticosterone level. However, LPO level in all the brain regions as well as the plasma LPO was markedly decreased, but not normalized indicating that few more factors other than corticosterone may be responsible for the increase in the LPO. Although few regions could not show the normal LPO level even after treatment with *A. calamus* extracts, indicating that the stress-induced free radical formation may be faster than the scavenging system and also the difference in regional distribution of antioxidant enzyme in the various parts of the brain. This was well in agreement with Manoli *et al.* (2000) and Baek *et al.* (1999) where the vulnerability to oxidative stress in the brain is reported to be region specific.

After the chronic repeated exposure to noise stress, an increase in SOD activity with the concomitant decrease in the activities of CAT, GPx, levels of GSH, vitamin C, vitamin E and protein thiols were observed (Manikandan *et al.*, 2005a). There were earlier reports, wherein different stressors have been reported to induce similar changes in frontal cortex and striatum in similar parameters (Bhattacharya *et al.*, 2001). Enhanced SOD activity catalyses the conversion of Superoxide ($O_2\bullet$) to hydrogen peroxide ($H_2O_2\bullet$), which is more toxic than the oxygen-derived free radicals and requires to be scavenged further by tissue thiols (glutathione redox pathway) and catalase (Fridovich, 1995). The ROS scavenging activity of SOD is effective only when it is followed by the actions of CAT and GPx, because the dismutase activity of SOD generates H_2O_2 and requires to be scavenged further by CAT and GPx (Bhattacharya *et al.*, 2001). However, the decreased activity of CAT and glutathione levels in the 30 days noise-stressed animals may be the cause behind the decrease in protein thiols and increase in the LPO levels (Manikandan *et al.*, 2005a). According to the study of Halliwell and Gutteridge (1999) antioxidant enzymes are inactivated by excess of lipid peroxides and ROS. Manikandan *et al.* (2005a) observations revealed that administration of ethyl acetate extract of AC could normalize the activities of SOD, CAT and GPx in almost all brain regions of noise-exposed animals. Manikandan *et al.* (2005a) observations are in agreement with Xuejiang *et al.* (1999), Shah and Vohora (2002) and Salim *et al.* (2003) who have shown that the treatment of rats with herbal formulations/or plants extract resulted in the increased activity of these enzymes because of the ROS scavenging activity of these traditional drugs which might lead to the restoration of the depleted enzymes.

Normally the glutathione status of a cell could be taken as the most accurate single indicator of the health of the cell. The GSH depletion accompanied by a decrease in vitamins C and E levels established the vulnerability to oxidant attack during the 30 days of noise-stress exposure. To such noise-stressed animals, administration of ethyl acetate extract of AC causes significant increase in the levels of these vitamins and GSH (Manikandan *et al.,* 2005a). From their observation, they could conclude that the anti-stressor effect might be due to an increase in brain antioxidative capacity by protecting the decrease in GSH, vitamins C and E levels which in turn restore the free radical scavenger's enzymatic activity.

In addition, Manikandan *et al.* (2005b) in another study reported that α-asarone, the major constituent of *A. calamus* was found to posses the antioxidant activity and 9 mg/kg body weight was found to be more useful in preventing than the other two doses (3 mg/kg and 6 mg/kg) used. Further, they added that this 9 mg/kg was found to be non-toxic as the cortex of the animals, which received the drug α-asarone (9 mg/kg) along with noise stress showed normal histological features and the alterations observed in noise-stress group rat cortex were not present in these brain sections. Moreover, the cortex of the animals (not exposed to noise stress) which were treated only with the drug α-asarone (9 mg/kg) did not show any change and they were very similar to cortex of the control animals.

Ocimum sanctum Linn. (Tulsi)

A widely used medicinal herb among the basils is *O. sanctum* Linn.(OS), which has been recently named as *Ocimum tenuiflorum* and known as Holy Basil or "Tulsi" Basils (Ocimum spp., Lamiaceae) contain a wide range of essential oils rich in phenolic compounds (Phippen and Simon, 2000) and a wide array of other natural products including polyphenols such as flavonoids and anthocyanins. The main components are tannins (4.6 per cent) and essential oil (up to 2 per cent). The major constituent is believed to be Eugenol (up to 62 per cent), methyl eugenol (up to 86 per cent), and α- and β-caryophyllene (up to 42 per cent). Other constituents with likely pharmacological activity include the triterpenoid, ursolic acid, rosmarinic acid, linoleic acid, gallic acid, caffeic acid, vanillic acid, alkaloids, saponins, isothymusin, isothymosin, flavonoids (including apigenin, orientin, vicenin and luteolin and glycosides) and phenylpropane glucosides (Kelm *et al.,* 2000). It is relevant to point out the recent

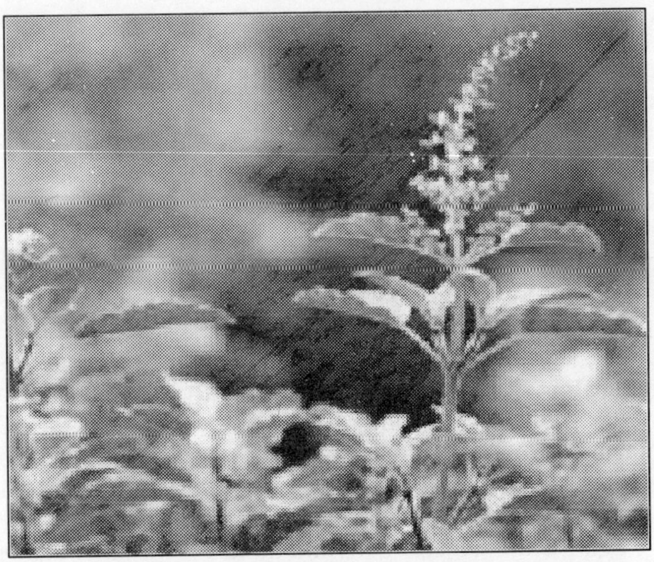

Figure 14.2: ***Ocimum sanctum*** **Linn. (Tulsi)**

study, which has indicated that the antioxidant property of *O. sanctum* is more in phenolic compounds rather than the essential oil (Juliani and Simson, 2002).

Oxidative Stress During Noise

During the generation of ATP energy using oxygen, a small percentage (2–3 per cent or less) of oxygen in mitochondria is inadvertently converted to superoxide radical (SOR) (Beckman and Ames, 1998). This explains the reason for the increased generation of free radicals in noise stress. Sokolovski *et al.* (1987) reported that alterations in the glutathione system occur, when rats were exposed to noise of 90 dB. GPx is a major antioxidative enzyme in many tissues and has been speculated to be a major antioxidative mechanism in the brain (Barlow-Walden *et al.*, 1995). In addition, Storey (1996) also suggests that the ratio of reduced/oxidized glutathione in the cell is a good indicator of the level of oxidative stress. The GSH levels are significantly reduced and GSSG levels are markedly increased in noise-exposed animals indicating the oxidative stress occurring in the discrete regions of brain (Samson *et al.*, 2007). Moreover, these scientists also expressed that the regions associated with the neuroanatomical auditory and physiological stress response pathway such as the hypothalamus, hippocampus and pons medulla show more alterations when compared to other regions indicating a predominant role for these regions in determining the effects of noise stress. *O. sanctum* pre-treatment significantly increased the GSH/GSSG ratio from their corresponding noise-exposed levels, even though it could not completely attenuate the noise-induced alteration (Samson *et al.*, 2007). *O.sanctum* on its own, has been reported to increase endogenous GSH levels in liver within 60 min after its administration (Devi and Ganasoundari, 1999). Deficiency of glutathione has been linked to increased susceptibility to noise-induced damage, while replenishing tissue glutathione stores reduces its susceptibility (Yamasoba *et al.*, 1998; Henderson *et al.*, 1999). In chronic noise stress, the regions like cerebellum, pons medulla, hypothalamus showed an increase in GPx levels whereas catalase levels did not show any variation in these regions, whereas increase in catalase levels in cerebral cortex and midbrain was observed. This reflects the fact that GPx and catalase substitute for each other (Ralf and Bernd, 1997).

The Possible Compound Responsible for the Antistressor Activity

The central nervous system plays an important role in the development of stress-induced ulcers and *O. sanctum* was found to prevent the development of ulcers during stress conditions (Bhargava and Singh, 1981). It appears that the pharmacological action of *O. sanctum* is due to its various constituents. Active principles present in *Ocimum* species such as rosmarinic acid, lithospermic acid, phenolics and flavonoids have been attributed to be responsible for their diverse medicinal activities (Kelm *et al.*, 2000; Hase *et al.*, 1997; Juliani and Simson, 2002). Balanehru and Nagarajan (1992) had reported the reduction in the free radical level by the *O. sanctum* component such as ursolic acid. Studies have shown that phenolic compounds, particularly flavanoids and catechins, are important antioxidants and superoxide scavengers. Their scavenging efficiency depends on the concentration of phenol and the numbers and location of the hydroxyl groups (Benavente-Garia *et al.*, 2002).The estimation of phytochemicals in *O. sanctum* has revealed that 1 g of ethanolic extract contains 9766 mg of phenolics, 786 mg of flavanoids and 358 mg of carotenoids (Samson *et al.*, 2007). This is supported by the report of Phippen and Simon (2000) who also reported that Basils (Ocimum spp., Lamiaceae) contain a wide range of essential oils rich in phenolic compound. Kelm *et al.* (2000) also accounted the presence of phenols and flavonoids in *O. sanctum*. Flavonoids have been reported as potential exogenous agents in protecting the aging brain, other organs and tissues of the body against free radical induced damage (Blaylock, 1999). Flavonoids have been shown to scavenge various reactive oxygen species and have been implicated as inhibitors of lipid peroxidation (Mora *et al.*, 1990). The flavonoids present in plant are found to enhance free radicals scavenging enzyme activities like GPx and CAT or were capable of preventing the stress-induced decrease of enzyme levels (Al-Qirim *et al.*, 2002).

Geetha *et al.* (2004) showed that *O. sanctum* extracts contain powerful anti-lipid per oxidative effect (*in vivo* as well as *in vitro*). Apart from this, *O. sanctum* has been reported to have a strong superoxide anion scavenging activity, Fe^{2+} chelating activity and reducing power in a concentration-dependent manner (Juntachote and Berghofer, 2005).

Neurotransmitter and *O. sanctum*

Lopez *et al.* (1999) reported that the brain regions activated by the acute stressors includes neocortex, allocortex, hippocampus, nucleus accumbens, lateral septum, several hypothalamic nuclei, medial and cortical amygdaloid nuclei, dorsal raphe, locus coeruleus, and several brain stem nuclei. According to them these brain regions are activated largely irrespective of the type of acute stressor administered, perhaps indicating that these structures are involved in a more "general" integrative stress response. Exposure to noise stress (100 dB) for 30 min caused a significant reduction in total acetylcholine content (Sembulingam *et al.*, 1996, 1999) and increase in the activity of acetylcholinesterase in cerebral cortex, corpus striatum, hypothalamus and hippocampus of brain (Sembulingam *et al.*, 2003). Pre-treatment of the animals with ethanol extract of *O. sanctum* leaves for 7 days prevented the noise-induced changes in these cholinergic systems in the areas of brain studied. Administration of *O. sanctum* extract alone or PG (vehicle control) alone did not alter the base line values of ACh content or AChE activity in any brain area (Sembulingam *et al.*, 2005). On the basis of such observations, these authors suggest that *O. sanctum* fulfills the criteria to be called an adaptogen as suggested by the pioneer scientists like Lazarev, Brekhman and Dardymov about the adaptogenic agents (Sembulingam *et al.*, 1997).

Ravindran *et al.* (2005) reported that after sub-acute (15 days) noise stress exposure all the brain regions, significantly showed an increase in the norepinephrine, epinephrine, and dopamine levels, whereas the 5-HT levels showed a significant increase only in regions like cerebellum, hypothalamus, pons and corpus striatum from the controls. They also confirmed that *O. sanctum* is an adaptogen, as it never alters the normal levels of neurotransmitter when administered to control rats. According to Singh *et al.* (1991), dopamine levels in the brain elevate as a compensatory mechanism and as a precursor for the synthesis of more epinephrine and norepinephrine to cope with the increased demand. The altered epinephrine and norepinephrine level and dopamine level (except pons and striatum where it showed normal level) though showed a marked decrease from stress level, it did not return to the normal level in any of the regions with *O. sanctum* pre-treatment which indicates the need for different dosage testing (Ravindran *et al.*, 2005). However, *O. sanctum* could modify the enzyme activity, which gets altered during stress exposure. It is note worthy that *O. sanctum* can bring the monoamine oxidase (MAO) level back to the normal level, which decreased during the swimming stress (Singh *et al.*, 1991).

Samson *et al.* (2006) reported that in chronic noise exposures (4 h daily for 30 days) the biogenic amine levels were significantly altered only in certain regions. Their observation also revealed that the noise-induced alterations in neurotransmitters are not confined to specific regions in the brain. The ethanol extract of *O. sanctum* leaves was found to prevent the reduction in adrenergic neurotransmitters in brain of rats exposed to swimming stress and gravitational stress (Singh *et al.*, 1991). It is also further reported that *O. sanctum* normalized the stress-induced membrane changes in the hippocampus and sensory motor cortex (Sen *et al.*, 1992).

Possible Mechanism

O. sanctum has been suspected to involve the endogenous opioids and central noradrenaline in its analgesic activity (Khanna and Bhatia, 2003). In such case, the animal's threshold for stress may be altered and thereby the animal may not be affected by the stress. If *O. sanctum* acts in such a way, then it may be beneficial to the individuals who react more for even small events. It is also possible that *O. sanctum* action may be due to the mechanism through which buspirone, ipsapirone and eight OH-DPAT suppress the effect of stress on the secretions of hormones which is mediated by reducing the firing rate of serotonergic neurons in the dorsal raphe (Jorgensen *et al.*, 2001). Since the LD50 of the ethanolic extract of *O. sanctum* was found to be 4508 ± 80 mg/kg when administered orally (Bhargava and Singh, 1981) in small animals, the dosage used by these reporters are much far away (*e. g.* Samson *et al.* (2006) and Ravindran *et al.* (2005)–100 mg/kg b.wt.), which reflects the feasible use of *O. sanctum* as an antidote for noise stress.

Triphala

Triphala is a traditional Ayurvedic herbal formulation consisting of the powder of dried fruits mixed in equal proportions of three medicinal plants, *Terminalia chebula*, *Terminalia belerica*, and *Emblica officinalis* also known as the 'three myrobalans'. Triphala means 'three' tri) fruits' (phala).

Triphala, is considered as a 'tridoshic rasayan', having balancing and rejuvenating effects on the three constitutional elements that govern human life, *i.e.*, Vata, Pitta and Kapha by Charka (1500 B.C.) in the Charak Samhita (Sharma and Dash, 1998). *T. chebula* governs Vata which regulates the nervous

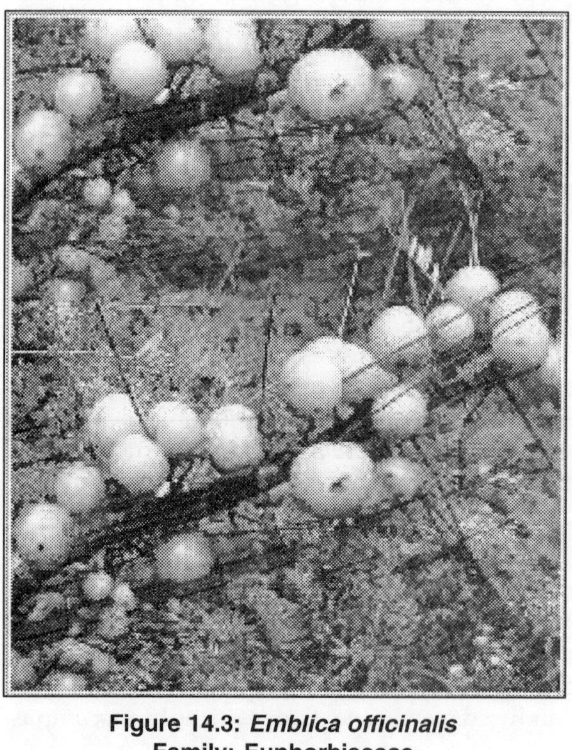

Figure 14.3: *Emblica officinalis*
Family: Euphorbiaceae

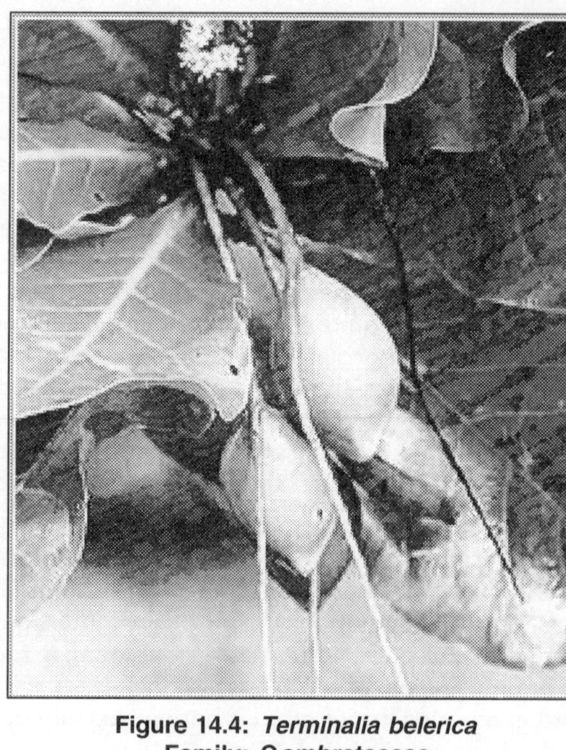

Figure 14.4: *Terminalia belerica*
Family: *Combretaceae*

system, *E. officinalis* governs Pitta which maintains metabolic process and *T. belerica* governs Kapha which supports structural integrity. It is an antioxidant rich herbal formulation (Naiwu *et al.*, 1992; Jose and Kuttan, 1995; Takagi and Sanashiro, 1996; Vaidya *et al.*, 1998). Triphala has been reported to treat anemia, jaundice, constipation, cough, asthma, fever, eye diseases, chronic ulcers, leucorrhoea, pyorrhea (Nadkarni, 1976).

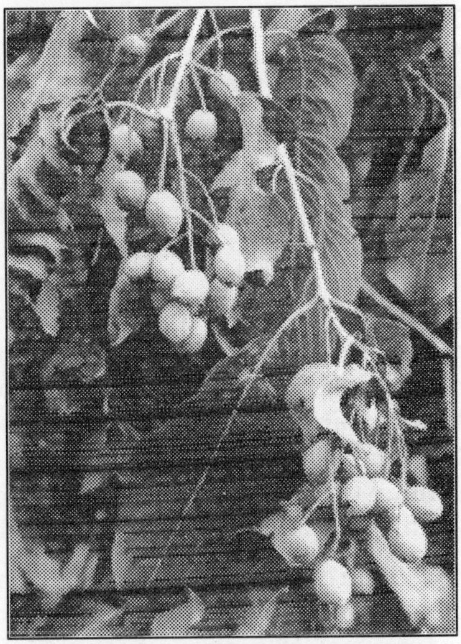

Figure 14.5: *Terminalia chebula*
Family: *Combretaceae*

Studies on stress-associated immune deregulations have interested both clinicians and scientists in the field of psychoneuroimmunology. The effects of noise on the immune status have also been reported (Archana and Namasivayam, 2000). Immunostimulants are the substances, which enhance the non-specific defence mechanism and provide resistance during the pathogen invasion or during stress. After exposure to the noise stress, the neutrophil functions like adherence phagocytic index, avidity index and killing ability were significantly suppressed and in these animals there was a significant increase in the corticosterone levels were observed. These noise-stress induced changes were significantly prevented by Triphala administration in the immunized as well as unimmunized groups. Based on the increased in the adherence and the avidity index of Triphala fed controls they suggested that non-specific immunity could be improved by Triphala (Srikumar *et al.*, 2005).

LPO and corticosterone level in both plasma and lymphoid tissues (thymus and spleen) showed a significant increase after 15 days of noise stress exposure (Srikumar *et al.*, 2006). Further, they also reported that when the animals are challenged with an antigenic response and treated with Triphala and exposed to noise stress, the LPO levels were similar to immunized control animals indicating the efficacy of Triphala.

During stress, limbic system of the brain triggers the hypothalamus to secrete corticotropin-releasing hormone (CRH) (Carpenter and Gruen, 1982) The CRH triggers the pituitary gland to secrete adreno-corticotropic hormone, which activates the adrenal glands to release corticosterone secretion in the blood stream (Britton *et al.*, 1992). Triphala-treated stressed animals as well as Triphala-treated immunized animals showed normal level corticosteroids than the stressed and immunized stressed animals.

Possible Antistressor Effect

An extract of *Emblica* fruits has been reported to contain 2 per cent vitamin C as determined by HPLC (Kim *et al.*, 2005). According to Cinar *et al.* (2006), ACTH may be inhibited by vitamin C, and decreases the release of glucocorticoids and mineralocorticoids in the adrenal gland. Further, they suggested that ascorbic acid may functionally inhibit ACTH-mediated steroidogenesis by altering cell membrane lipid composition/structure and thus influencing ACTH binding to its membrane-bound receptor. Further, it is strengthened by Campbell (1999) who report that vitamin C significantly reduced stress-hormone levels in the rats' blood and also reduced other indicators of physical and emotional stress, including enlarged adrenal glands and changes in the thymus and spleen, which help produce immune cells. Raghu *et al.* (2007)'s investigation revealed that dried *Emblica* fruits contained 34–

38 mg vitamin C equivalent to 100 g of fresh weight. This may be due to the ascorbic acid content in *E. officinalis* which is also available in most stable form. Further, an important antioxidant is also found to be reducing the corticotrophin-releasing hormone levels in the blood stream and allow the immune system to work more efficiently (Kojo *et al.*, 1999).

A significant decrease in the antioxidant status (decrease in SOD, GPx and vitamin C level) in the plasma, thymus, and spleen of noise-stressed animals were observed whereas administration of Triphala for 48 days did not show such changes (Srikumar *et al.*, 2006). Ascorbic acid content in *E. officinalis* available in most stable form and also an important antioxidant found to be reducing the corticotrophin releasing hormone levels in the bloodstream which allow the immune system to work more efficiently (Kojo *et al.*, 1999). Ghosal *et al.* (1996) reported that *Emblica* fruits (one of the constituent of Triphala contain two hydrolysable tannins of low molecular weight, namely, Emblicanin A and Emblicanin B, and other tannins such as punigluconin and pedunclagin. They also added that the two Emblicanins are shown to exhibit a very strong antioxidant action. Triphala was reported to contain compounds such as ascorbic acid, gallic acid and total polyphenols with antioxidant activity (Vani *et al.*, 1997). Gallic acid reported to be a strong antioxidant (Haslam, 1996).

Sabu *et al.* (2002) also confirmed 'Triphala' with strong antioxidant activity and it was due to its constituents (*T. chebula*, *T. belerica* and *E. officinalis*) and these components may be partially responsible for many of the biological properties manifested by these drugs. According to them *T. belerica* was the most active antioxidant followed by *E. officinalis* and *T. chebula*. Further, they listed the major ingredients responsible for the antioxidant activity in them. For *T. belerica* it is the ellagic and gallic acid. For *E. officinalis* it is having several gallic acid derivatives including epigallocatachin gallate whereas in the *T. chebula* it is only the gallic acid. However, Saleem *et al.* (2001) differ in their opinion and they reported that among 37 medicinal plants extracts, *T. chebula* fruit (a component of Triphala) extract has higher phenolic content and stronger *in vitro* lipid peroxidation inhibition capability. This is further added by Naik *et al.* (2004) who analysed the phytochemicals responsible for the antioxidant activity of *T. chebula* using HPLC analysis showed the presence of compounds such as ascorbate, gallic acid and ellagic acid. This difference in the report may partially attribute to the components of Triphala from where they are procured for their analysis. As the environmental factors as well as the time of collection are known to alter the concentration of the different ingredients in the herbs, this variation may be attributed to these factors also. Triphala components are known to clear these free radicals as it posse's more than one antioxidant compound. Hence, no free radical is left free to alter these available free radical scavenging enzymes.

The adaptogenic activity is also reported by few scientists because any anti stressor plant material substance that cause a state of nonspecific increased resistance are known as adaptogens (Breckhman and Dardymov, 1969). Therefore, this study reinforces the popular belief that daily consumption of these in small quantities is both harmless and will be beneficial to all mankind, particularly to those who are exposed to noise stress in this modern era of urbanized life style. Further, it also indicates that the comprehensive action of these herbs may due to the multiple active natural compounds present in it, to tackle the various biological changes occurring during stress.

Acknowledgements

I greatly acknowledge the research work done by Dr.R.Ravindran, Dr. J.Samson and Dr.S. Manikandan under my supervision and also the financial assistance given by UGC and ICMR of India.

References

Acuna, U.M., Atha, D.E., Ma, J., Nee, M.H., Kennelly, E.J.(2002). Antioxidant capacities of ten edible North American plants. *Phytotherapy Research,* 16:63–5.

Aebi, H.(1984). Catalse in vitro. *In:* Methods in Enzymology, (Packer L, ed),Newyork, Academic, pp. 121-126.

Agrawal, P., Rai, V., Singh, R.B. (1996). Randomized, placebo-controlled, single-blind trial of holy basil leaves in patients with noninsulin-dependent diabetes mellitus. *International Journal of Clinical Pharmacology and Therapeutics*, 34:406–409.

Akbar, M.T., Wells, D.J., Latchman, D.S., DeBelleroche, J. (2001). Heat shock protein 27 shows a distinctive widespread spatial and temporal pattern of induction in CNS glial and neuronal cells compared to heat shock protein 70 and caspase 3 following kainite administration. *Molecular Brain Research*, 93:148-163.

Alario, P., Gamallo, A., Villanua, M.A., Trancho, G. (1987). Chronic noise stress and dexamethasone administration on blood pressure elevation in the rat. *Journal of Steroid Biochemistry*, 28:433-436.

Al-Qirim, T.M., Shahwan, M., Zaidi, K.R., Uddin, Q., Banu, N. (2002). Effect of khat, its constituents and restraint stress on free radical metabolism of rats. *Journal of Ethnopharmacology*, 83:245-250.

Ananthan, J., Goldberg, A.L., Voellmy, R. (1986). Abnormal proteins serve as eukaryotic stress signals and trigger the activation of heath shock genes. *Science*, 232:522-524.

Anisman, H., Zacharko, R.M. (1990). Multiple neurochemical and behavioral consequences of stressors: implications for depression. *Pharmacological Therapeutics*, 46:119-136.

Andren, L., Hansson, L., Bjorkman, M., Jonsson, A. (1980). Noise as a contributory factor in the development of elevated arterial pressure. A study of the mechanisms by which noise may raise blood pressure in man. *Acta Medica Scandinavica*, 207:493-498.

Antonio, C. (2001). Oxidative stress in neurodegeneration: mechanism and therapeutic perspectives. Current Topics in Medicinal Chemistry, 1, 553–568.

Arnsten, A.F., Goldman-Rakic, P.S. (1998). Noise stress impairs prefrontal cortical cognitive function in monkeys: Evidence for a hyperdopaminergic mechanism. *Archives of General Psychiatry*, 55:362-368.

Aravindkumar, N., Mathangi, D.C., Namasivayam, A. (1998). Noise induced changes in free radical scavenging enzymes in the blood and brain of albino rats. *Medical Science Research, 26:* 811-812.

Archana, R., Namasivayam, A. (2000). Effect of *Ocimum sanctum* on noise induced changes in neutrophil functions. *Journal of Ethnopharmacology*, 73: 81-85.

Archana, R., Namasivayam, A. (2000). Effect of *Ocimum sanctum* on noise induced changes in immune parameters. *Pharmacy and Pharmacological Communications*, 6:145-147.

Areso, M.P., Frazer, A. (1991). Effect of repeated administration of novel stressors on central beta adrenoceptors. *Journal of Neural Transmission*, 86:229-35.

Atsumi T, Fujisawa S, Tonosaki K (2005). A comparative study of the antioxidant/prooxidant activities of eugenol and isoeugenol with various concentrations and oxidation conditions. *Toxicology In Vitro*, 16, [Epub ahead of print].

Auddy, B., Ferreira, M., Balsina, F. (2003). Screening antioxidant activity of three Indian medicinal plants traditionally used for the management of neurodegenerative diseases. *Journal of Ethnopharmacology*, 4:131.

Azmathulla, S., Hule, A., Naik, S.R. (2006). Evaluation of adaptogenic activity profile of herbal preparation. *Indian Journal of Experimental Biology*, 44:574-579.

Babisch, W. (2000). Traffic noise and cardiovascular disease: epidemiological review and synthesis. *Noise and Health*, 8:9-32.

Babisch, W. (2002). The Noise/Stress Concept, Risk Assessment and Research Needs. *Noise and Health*, 4:1-11.

Backer, C.A., Backhuisen van den Brink, R.C. (1965). Eds. Flora of Java. Vol. 2. Noordhof, NVP.

Baek, B.S., Kwon, H.J., Lee, K.H., Yoo, M.A., Kim, K.W., Ikeno, Y., Yu, B.P., Chung, H.Y. (1999). Regional difference of ROS generation, lipid peroxidation, and antioxidant enzyme activity in rat brain and their dietary modulation. *Archives of Pharmocological* Research, 22:361-366.

Bagchi, D., Carryl, O.R., Tran, M.X., Bagchi, M., Garg, A., Milnes, M.M. (1999). Acute and chronic stress-induced oxidative gastrointestinal mucosal injury in rats and protection by bismuth subsalicylate. *Molecular and Cellular Biochemistry*, 196:109–116.

Bagdy, G., Calogero, A.E., Murphy, D.L., Szemeredi, K. (1989). Serotonin agonists cause parallel activation of the sympathoadreno medullary system and the hypothalamo-pituitary–adrenocortical axis in conscious rats. *Endocrinology*, 125:2664–2669.

Balanehru, S., Nagarajan, B. (1991). Protective effect of oleanolic acid and ursolic acid against lipid peroxidation. *Biochemistry International*, 24:981-990.

Ballentine, R., Burford, D.D. (1957).Determination of metals. *In:* "Methods in Enzymology", By Colowick, S.P., and Kaplan, N.O., Eds, Academic press, Inc. Newyork, 3: 1002-1035.

Banerjee, S., Prashar, R., Kumar, A., Rao, A.R. (1996). Modulatory influence of alcoholic extract of Ocimum leaves on carcinogen-metabolizing enzyme activities and reduced glutathione levels in mouse. *Nutrition and Cancer*, 25:205-217.

Bannister, J.V., Bannister, W.H., Rotillio, G. (1987). Aspects of structure, function and application of superoxide dismutase. *Critical Reviews in Biochemistry*, 22:111-180.

Barlow-Walden, L.R., Reiter, R.J., Abe, M. (1995), Melatonin stimulates brain glutation peroxidase activity. *Neurochemistry International*, 26:497-502.

Baumgarten, H.G., Grozdanovic, Z. (1997). Anatomy of the central serotoninergic projection systems. *In:* Serotoninergic Neurons and 5-HT Receptors in the CNS, edited by H.G. Baumgarten and M. Gothert. Berlin, Germany: Springer-Verlag, pp. 41–89.

Baxter, R.M., Dandiya, P.C., Kandel, S.I., Okany, A., Walker, G.C. (1960). Separating of hypnotic potentiating principles from the essential oil of *Acorus calamus* Linn. of Indian origin by gas liquid chromatography. *Nature*, 185:466-467.

Beckman, K., Ames, B. (1998). The free radical theory of aging matures. *Physiological Review*, 78:548-581.

Belojevic, G., Saric-Tanaskovic, M. (2002). Prevalence of arterial hypertension and myocardial infarction in relation to subjective ratings of traffic noise exposure. *Noise and Health*, 4:33-37.

Benavente-Garcia, O., Castillo, J., Lorente, J., Alcaraz, M. (2002). Radioprotective effects *in vivo* of phenolics extracted from *Olea europaea* Linn. leaves against X-ray-induced chromosomal damage: comparative study versus several flavonoids and sulfur-containing compounds. *Journal of Medicinal Food*, 5:125-35.

Berglund, B., Lindvall, T. (1995). Community noise. *Archives of the Center for Sensory Research*, 2:1-195.

Bernardis, Bellinger. (1998). The dorsomedial hypothalamic nucleus revisited: 1998 update. *Proceedings of the Society for Experimental Biology and Medicine*, 218:284-306.

Bhargava, K.P., Singh, N. (1981). Antistress activity of *Ocimum sanctum* Linn. *Indian Journal of Medical Research*, 73:443-451.

Bhattacharya, A., Ghosal, S., Bhattacharya, S.K. (2001). Antioxidant effect of *Withania somnifera* glycowithanolides in chronic foot shock stress-induced perturbations of oxidative free radical scavenging enzymes and lipid peroxidation in rat frontal cortex and striatum. *Journal of Ethanopharmacology*, 74:1-6.

Bhattacharya, S.K., Muruganandam, A.V. (2003). Adaptogenic activity of *Withania somnifera*: an experimental study using a rat model of chronic stress. *Pharmacology Biochemistry and Behaviour*, 75:547-555.

Blake, D.R., Allen, R.E., Lunec, J. (1987). Free radicals in biological systems–a review orientated to inflammatory processes. *British Medical Bulletin*, 43:371-385.

Blanchard, R.J., McKittrick, C.R., Blanchard, D.C. (2001). Animal models of social stress: Effects on behaviour and brain neurochemical systems. *Physiology and Behavior*, 73:261-271.

Blane, G.D., Harve, H., Simon, H., Lisoprowski, A., Glowinski, J., Tassiin, J.P. (1980). Response to stress of mesocorticofrontal dopaminergic neurons in rats after long term isolation. *Nature*, 284:265-267.

Blaylock, R.L. (1999). Neurodegeneration and aging of the central nervous system: prevention and treatment by phytochemicals and metabolic nutrients. *Integrative Medicine*, 1:117-133.

Blondeau, N., Plamondon, H., Richelme, C., Heurteaux, C., Lazdunski, M. (2000). KATP Channel openers, Adensine Agonists and Epileptic Preconditioning are stress signals inducing Hippocmapal Neuroprotection. *Neuroscience*, 100:465-474.

Bohne, B., Harding, G.W. (2000). Degeneration in the cochlea after noise damage: primary versus secondary events. *American Journal of Otolaryngology*, 21:505-509.

Borg, E. (1995). Noise-induced hearing loss-literature review and experiments in rabbits-morphological and electrophysiological features, exposure parameters and temporal factors, variability and interactions. *Scandinavian Audiology*, 24:6–147.

Breckhman, I.L., Dardymov, I.V. (1969). New substances of plant origin which increase non specific resistance. *Annual Reviews in Pharmacloogy*, 9:419-430.

Bremner, J.D., Krystal, J.H., Southwick, S.M., Charney, D.S. (1996). Noradrenergic mechanisms in stress and anxiety: II. Clinical studies. *Synapse*, 23:39-51.

Breschi, M.C., Scatizzi, R., Martinotti, E. (1994). Morphofunctional changes in the noradrenergic innervation of the rat cardiovascular system after varying duration of noise stress. *International journal of Neuroscience*, 75:73-81.

Britton, K.T., Segal, D.S., Kuczenski, R. (1992). Dissociation between in vivo hippocampal norepinephrine response and behavioral/neuroendocrine response to noise stress in rats. *Brain Research*, 574:125-130.

Britton, K.T., McLeod, S., Koob, G.F., Hauger, R. (1992). Pregnane steroid alphaxalone attenuates anxiogenic behavioral effects of corticotropin releasing factor and stress. *Pharmacology and Biochemical Behavior*, 41:399-403.

Cabib, S., Puglisi-Allegra S. (1996). Stress, depression and the mesolimbic dopamine system. *Psychopharmacology*, 128: 331–342.

Cadet, J.L., Brannock, C. (1997). Invited Review–Free radicals and the pathbiology of brain dopamine systems. *Neurochemistry International*, 32:117-131.

Calabrese, V., Renis, M., Calderone, A., Russo, A., Reale, S., Barcellona, ML., Rizza, V. (1998). Stress proteina and SH-groups in oxidant-induced cellular injury after chronic ethanol administration in rat. *Free radical biology and medicine*, 24: 1159-1167.

Campbell, S.P. (1999). Vitamin C lowers stress hormone in rats. *Science News*, 156(10):158.

Canlon, B., Lofstrand, P., Borg, E. (1993). Ultrastructual changes in the presynaptic regions of outer hair cells after acoustic stimulation. *Neuroscience Letters*, 150:103-106.

Carlsson, P., Laer, LV., Borg, E., Bondeson, ML., Thys, M., Fransen, E., Camp, GV. (2005). The influence of genetic variation in oxidative stress genes on human noise susceptibility. *Hearing Research*, 202: 87–96.

Carpenter, W.T Jr., Gruen,PH. (1982). Cortisol's effects on human mental functioning. *Journal of Clinical Psychopharmacology*, April;2(2):91-101.

Carroll, A. (2004). The health effects of environmental noise–other than hearing loss. *In:* The Health council, commonwealth of Australia, 3311: 39-50.

Cassens,G., Roffman, M., Kuruc, A., Schildkraut, JJ. (1980).Alterations in brain norepinephrine metabolism induced by environmental stimuli previously paired with inescapable shock. *Science*, 209: 1138–1140.

Chance, B., Sies, H., Boveris, A. (1979). Hydroperoxide metabolism in mammalian organs. *Physiological Reviews*, 59: 527-605.

Chattopadhyay, R.R. (1993). Hypoglycemic effect of Ocimum sanctum leaf extract in normal and streptozocin-diabetic rats. *Indian Journal of Experimental Biology*, 31: 891–893.

Chattopadhyay, R.R. (1994). A comparative evaluation of some anti-inflammatory agents of plant origin. *Fitoterapia*, 65:146–148.

Chericoni, S., Prieto, J.M., Iacopini, P., Cioni, P., Morelli, I. (2005). *In vitro* activity of the essential oil of *Cinnamomum zeylanicum* and eugenol in peroxynitrite-induced oxidative processes. *Journal of Agricultural and Food Chemistry*, 53(12): 4762-5.

Cinar, A., Belge, F., Donmez, N., Tas, A., SelCuk, M., and Tatar, M. (2006). Effects of stress produced by adrenocorticotropin (ACTH) on ECG and some blood parameters in vitamin C treated and non-treated chickens. *Veterinarski Arhiv, 76* (3), 227-235.

Conner, J.M., Lauterborn, J.C., Yan, Q., Gall, C.M., Varon, S. (1997). Distribution of brain-derived neurotrophic factor (BDNF) protein and mRNA in the normal adult rat CNS: evidence for anterograde axonal transport. *Journal of Neuroscience*, 17: 2295-313.

Contestabile, A. (2001). Oxidative stress in neurodegeneration: mechanisms and therapeutic perspectives. *Current Topics in Medical Chemistry*, 1:553-568.

Costa, N.J., Dahm, C.C., Hurrel, F., Taylor, E.R., Murphy, M.P.(2003). Interaction of mitochondrial thiols with nitric oxide. *Antioxidant and Redox Signalling*, 5:291-305.

Cotgreave, I.A., Gerdes, R.G. (1998). Recent trends in glutathione biochemistry glutathione-protein interactions: a molecular link between oxidative stress and cell proliferation? *Biochemical and Biophysical Research Communications*, 242: 1-9.

Dallman, M.F., Akana, S.F., Strack, A.M., Scribner, K.S., Pecoraro, N., La Fleur S.E., Houshyar, H., Gomez, F. (2004). Chronic stress-induced effects of corticosterone on brain: direct and indirect. *Annals of Newyork Academy of Sciences*, 1018:141-50.

Damier, P., Hirsch, EC., Zhang, P., Agid Y, Javoy-Agid F (1993). Glutathione peroxidase, glial cells and Parkinson's disease. *Neuroscience*, 52: 1-6.

Dandiya, P.C., Baxter, R.M., Walker, G.C., Cullumbine, H. (1959). Studies on *Acorus calamus*. II. Investigation of volatile oil. *Journal of Pharmacy and Pharmacology*, 11:163-168.

De Boer, S.F., Slangen, J.L., van der Gugten, J. (1988).Adaptation of plasma catecholamine and corticosterone responses to short-term repeated noise stress in rats. *Physiology and Behaviour* 44:273-80.

Decker, E.A. (1995). The Role of Phenolics, Conjugated Linolenic Acid, Carnosine and Pyrroloqinoline Quinone as Nonessential Dietary Antioxidants. *Nutrition Reviews*,53 (3): 49–58.

Desagher, S., Glowinski, J., Premont, J. (1996). Astrocytes protect neurons from hydrogen peroxide toxicity. *Journal of Neuroscience*, 16, 2553-2562.

DeSouza., VanLoon.(1986).Brain serotonin and catecholamine responses to repeated stress in rats. *Brain Research* 367:77-86.

Deutch, A.Y., Roth, R.H.(1990).The determinants of stress-induced activation of the prefrontal cortical dopamine system. *Progress in Brain Research*, 85: 367–402.

Devasagayam, T.P.A., Tarachand, V. (1987). Decreased LPO in rat kidney during gestation. *Biochemical and Biophysics Research Communications*, 145: 134-138.

Devi,PU.,Bisht,K.S.,Vinitha,M. (1998). A comparative study of radioprotection by Ocimum flavonoids and synthetic aminothiol protectors in the mouse. *British Journal of Radiology*,71: 782-784.

Devi,P.U.,Ganasoundari,A. (1998). Modulation of glutathione and antioxidant enzymes by *Ocimum sanctum* and its role in protection against radiation injury. *Indian Journal of Experimental Biology*,37(3): 262-8.

Devi,P.U.((2000).Radio protective anticancerogenic and antioxidant properties of the Indian holy basil, *Ocimum sanctum* (Tulasi). *Indian JournaBiol* 39: 185-90.

Devi, U.P., Ganasoundari, A., Vrinda, B., Srinivasan, K.K., Unnikrishnan, M.K. (2000). Radiation protection by the ocimum flavonoids orientin and vicenin: mechanisms of action. *Radiation Research*, 154(4): 455-60.

Dinan, T.G. (1996). Serotonin and the regulation of hypothalamicpituitary-adrenal axis function. *Life Science*, 58: 1683–1694.

Dringen, R., Hamprecht, B(1997.). Involvement of glutathione peroxidase and catalase in the disposal of exogenous hydrogen peroxide in culture astroglial cells. *Brain Research*, 759, 67-75,

Drukarch, B., Schepens, E., Stoof, J.C., Langeveld, C.H., van Muiswinkel, F.L. (1998). Astrocyte-enhanced neuronal survival is mediated by scavenging of extracellular reactive oxygen species. *Free Radical Biology and Medicine*, 25: 217-220.

Edworthy, J., Hellier, E. (2000). "Auditory warnings in noisy environments," *Noise and Health*, 6: 27-39.

Engeland, W.C., Miller. P., Gann, D.S. (1990). Pituitary-adrenal and adrenomedullary responses to noise in awake dogs. *American Journal of Physiology*, 258: 672-7.

Fechter, L.D. (2005). Oxidative stress: a potential basis for potentiation of noise-induced hearing loss. *Environmental Toxicology and Pharmacology*, 19:543-546.

Fillenz, M. (1993). Neurochemistry of stress: introduction to techniques. *In:* From synapse to syndrome, By Stanford, S.C., Salmon, P., editors, London, Academic Press, pp. 247-79.

Fisher. (1989). Corticotropin-releasing factor: endocrine and autonomic integration of responses to stress. *Trends in Pharmacological Sciences*, 10: 189-192.

Floyd, R.A., Carney, J.M. (1992). Free radical damage to protein and DNA: mechanism involved and relevant observation on brain undergoing oxidative stress. *Annals of Neurology*, 32: 22-27.

Foote, S.L., Bloom, F.E., Aston-Jones, G. (1983). Nucleus locus coeruleus: new evidence of anatomical and physiological specificity. *Physiological Reviews*, 63 :844–914.

Fridovich, I. (1995). Superoxide radical and superoxide dismutases. *Annual Review of Biochemistry*, 64, 97-112.

Gamaro, G.D., Manoli, L.P., Torres, I.L., Silveira, R., Dalmaz, C. (2003). Effects of chronic variate stress on feeding behavior and on monoamine levels in different rat brain structures. *Neurochemistry International*, 42(2): 107-14.

Ganasoundari, A., Devi, PU., Rao, B.S. (1998).Enhancement of bone marrow radioprotection and reduction of WR-2721 toxicity by *Ocimum sanctum*. *Mutation Research*, 397: 303-312.

Ganong, W.F. (2001). Synaptic and junctional transmission. *In:* Review of medical physiology, 20th edition, The McGraw-Hill companies, Inc. pp. 110.

Geetanjali, B., Ananth, R. (2003). Effect of Acute exposure to loud occupational noise during daytime on nocturnal sleep architecture, heart rate and cortisol secretion in healthy volunteers. *Journal of Occupational Health*, 45: 146-152.

Geethaa, R., Kedlayab., Vasudevan, D.M. (2004). Inhibition of lipid peroxidation by botanical extracts of *Ocimum sanctum*: *In vivo* and *in vitro* studies. *Life Sciences*, 76: 21–28.

Giles, N.M., Watts, A.B., Giles, G.I., Fry, F.H, Littlechild, J.A., Jacob, C. (2003). Metal and redox modulation of cysteine protein function. *Chemistry and Biology*, 10:677-693.

Glowinski, J., Iverson, L.L. (1966). Regional studies of catecholamines in the rat brain-I. *Journal of Neurochemistry*, 13: 655-669.

Godhwani, S., Godhwani, J.L., Vyas, D.S. (1988). *Ocimum sanctum*: A preliminary study evaluating its immunoregulatory profile in albino rats. *Journal of Ethnopharmacology*, 24: 193-198.

Godhwani, S., Godhwani, J.L., Vyas, D.S. (1987). *Ocimum sanctum*: An experimental study evaluating its antiinflammatory, analgesic and antipyretic activity in animals. *Journal of Ethnopharmacology*, 21: 152-163.

Grayer, R.J., Kite, G.C., Veitch, N.C., Eckert, M.R., Marin, P.D., Senanayake, P, Paton, A.J. (2002). Leaf flavonoid glycosides as chemosystematic characters in Ocimum. *Biochemical Systematics and Ecology*, 30: 327–342.

Gupta, K.C., Viswanathan, R. (1955). A short note on antitubercular substance from *Ocimum sanctum*. *Antibiotics and Chemotherapy*, 5: 22–23.

Gupta, S.K., Prakash, J., Srivastava, S. (2002).Validation of traditional claim of Tulsi, *Ocimum sanctum* Linn, as a medicinal plant. *Indian Journal of Experimental Biology*, 40: 765-773.

Gutteridge, J.M. (1995). Lipid peroxidation and antioxidants as biomarkers of tissue damage. *Clinical Chemistry*, 41: 1819-28.

Habib, K.E., Gold, P.W., Chrousos, G.P. (2001). Neuroendocrinology of stress. *Endocrinology Metabolism Clinics of North America*, 30: 695–728.

Haines, M.M., Stansfeld, S.A., Brentnall, S., Head, J., Berry, B., Jiggins, M., Hygge, S. (2001). 'West London Schools Study: the effects of aircraft noise exposure on child performance and health'. *Psychological Medicine*,. 31:. 1385–96.

Halliwel, B., Gutteridge, J.M., Aruoma, O.I. (1987). The deoxyribose method: A simple test tube assay determination of rate constants for reactions of hydroxyl radicals. *Annals of Biochemistry*, 165: 215.

Halliwell, B., Gutteridge, J.M.C. (1989). Free radicals in biology and medicine, 2nd edition,Oxford, Claredon press.

Halliwell, B. (1992). Reactive oxygen species and the central nervous system. *Journal of Neurochemistry*, 59: 1609-1623.

Halliwell, B., Gutteridge, J.M.C. (1996). *In:* Free radicals in biology and medicine, By Halliwell, B., Gutteridge JMC eds.. Oxford, Clarendon press, pp. 422-437.

Halliwell, B., Gutteridge, J.M.C. (1999). Free Radicals in Biology and Medicine, 3rd Ed. Clarendon Press, Oxford.

Harborne, J.B. (1975). Biochemical systematics of flavonoids. *In:* The Flavonoids By Harborne, J.B., Mabry, H., Eds., New York and Sanfrancisco, Academic press, pp. 1056-1095.

Hase, K., Kasimu, R., Basnet, P., Kadota, S., Namba, T. (1997). Preventive effect of lithospermate B from *Salvia miltiorrhiza* on experimental hepatitis induced by carbon tetrachloride or D-galactosamine: lipopolysaccharide. *Planta Medica*, 63: 22–26.

Haslam, (1996). Natural polyphenols (vegetable tannins) as drugs: possible modes of action. *Journal of Natural Products*, 59(2):205-15.

Henderson, D., McFadden, S.L., Liu, C.C., Hight, N., Zheng, X.Y. (1999). The role of antioxidants in protection from impulse noise. *Annals of Newyork Academy of Sciences*, 884:368-380.

Herman, J.P., Cullinan, W.E. (1997).Neurocircuitry of stress: central control of the hypothalamo-pituitary-adrenocortical axis. *Trends in Neuroscience*, 20, 78–84.

Hissin, P.J., Hilf, R. (1976). A Flourimetric method for determination of Oxidised and Reduced glutathione in tissues. *Annals of Biochemistry*, 74: 214-226.

Hockey, G.R., Hamilton, P. (1970). Arousal and information selection in short-term memory. *Nature*,226: 866-7.

Hudspeth, A.J., Konishi, M.(2000). Auditory neuroscience: Development, transduction and integration'. *Proceedings of the National Academy of Sciences*, 97,(22) 11690–691.

Hygge, S., Evans, G.W., Bullinger, M. (2002). 'A prospective study of some effects of aircraft noise on cognitive performance in school children'. *Psychological Science*, 13 (5). 1–6.

Ising, H., Rebentisch, E., Babisch, W., Baumgärtner, H., Curio, I., Sharp, D. (1990). Medically relevant effects of noise from military low-altitude flights–results of an interdisciplinary pilot study. *Environment International*, 1: 411-21.

Ising. H., Babisch, W., Gunther, T. (1999). Work noise as a risk factor in myocardial infarction. *Journal of Clinical Basic Cardiology*, 2: 64-68.

Ising, H., Michalak, R. (2004). Stress effects of noise in a field experiment in comparison to reactions to short term noise exposure in the laboratory. *Noise Health*, 6(24):1-7.

Ising, H., Rebentisch, E., Babisch, W., Baumgärtner, H., Curio, I., Sharp, D. (1990). Medically relevant effects of noise from military low-altitude flights–results of an interdisciplinary pilot study. *Environmental International*, 1: 411-21.

Jacobs, B.L., Azmitia, E.C. (1992). Structure and function of the brain serotonin system. *Physiological Reviews*, 72: 165-229.

Jacono, A.A., Hu, B., Kopke, R.D., Henderson, D., Van De Water, T.R., Steinman, H.M. (1998). Changes in cochlear antioxidant enzyme activity after sound conditioning and noise exposure in the chinchilla. *Hearing Research*, 117(1-2):31-8.

Jacquier-Sarlin, M.R., Polla, B.S. (1996). Dual regulation of heat-shock transcription factor (HSF) activation and DNA-binding activity by H_2O_2: role of thioredoxin. *Biochemical Journal*, 318: 187–193.

Janes, S.E., Price, C.S., Thomas, D. (2005).Essential oil poisoning: N-acetylcysteine for eugenol-induced hepatic failure and analysis of a national database. *European Journal of Pediatrics*, 14 [Epub ahead of print].

Jesberger, J,A., Richardson, J.S. (1991). Oxygen free radicals in brain dysfunction. *International Journal of Neurosciences*, 57-1-17.

Johnson, E.O., Kamilaris, T.C., Chrousos, G.P., Gold, P.W. (1992). Mechanisms of stress: a dynamic overview of hormonal and behavioral homeostasis. *Neuroscience and Bio-behavioural Reviews*, 16: 115-130.

Jorgensen, H., Kjær, A., Warberg, J., Knigge, U.(2001). Differential effect of serotonin 5-HT1A receptor antagonists on the secretion of corticotrophin and prolactin. *Neuroendocrinology*, 73: 322–333.

Jose, J.K., Joy, K.L., Kuttan, R. (1999). Effect of *Emblica officinalis*, *Phyllanthus amarus* and *Picrorrhiza kurroa* on N-nitrosodiethylamine induced hepatocarcinogenesis. *Cancer Letters*, 136:11-16.

Juliani, H.R., Simson, J.E. (2002). Antioxidant activity of basil. *In:* Trends in new corps and new uses, By Janick.J and Whipkey, A. Eds, ASHS Press, Alexandria, VA, pp. 575-579.

Juntachote, T., Berghofer, E. (2005). Antioxodative properties and stability of ethanolic extracts of Holy basil and Galangal. *Food chemistry*, 92: 193-202.

Kanitz, E., Otten, W., Tuchscherer, M. (2004). Central and peripheral effects of repeated noise stress on hypothalamic-pituitary-adrenocortical axis in pigs. *In:*Livestock production science, doi 10.1016/ j. livprodsci. 2004.12.002.

Kaplowitz, N., Fernandez-Checa, J.C., Kannan, R., Garcia-Ruiz, C., Ookhtens, M., Yi, J.R. (1996). GSH transporters: molecular characterization and role in GSH homeostasis. *Biological Chemistry,* Hoppe-Seyler. 377: 267-273.

Karthikeyan, K., Ravichandran, P., Govindasamy, S. (1999). Chemopreventive effect of *Ocimum sanctum* on DMBA-induced hamster buccal pouch carcinogenesis. *Oral Oncology,* 35: 112-119.

Kashif, S.M., Zaidi, R., Naheed Banu. (2004). Antioxidant potential of vitamins A, E and C in modulating oxidative stress in rat brain. *Clinica Chimica Acta,* 340: 229–233.

Kaul, S.C., Matsui, M., Takano, S., Sugihara, T., Mitsui, Y., Wadhwa, R. (1997). Expression analysis of mortalin, a unique member of the Hsp 70 family of proteins, in rat tissues. *Experimental Cell Research,* 232(1): 56-63.

Kaushik, S., Kaur, J. (2003). Chronic cold exposure affects the antioxidant defense system in various rat tissues. *Clinica Chemica Acta,* 333(1-2): 69-77.

Kawada, T. (2004). The effect of noise on the health of children. *Journal of Nippon Medical School,* 71(1): 5-10.

Kelm, M.A., Nair, M.G., Strasburg, G.M., DeWitt, D.L. (2000).Antioxidant and cyclooxygenase inhibitory phenolic compounds from *Ocimum sanctum* Linn. *Phytomedicine,* 7: 7-13.

Kemp, C.F., Woods, R.J., Lowry, P.J. (1998). The corticotrophin-releasing factor-binding protein: an act of several parts. *Peptides,* 19: 1119-1128.

Khanna, N., Bhatia, J. (2003). Antinociceptive action of *Ocimum sanctum* (Tulsi) in mice: possible mechanisms involved. *Journal of Ethnopharmacology,* 88: 293-296.

Khumphant, E., Lawson, D.B. (2002). Acute toxicity, mutagenicity and antimutagenicity of ethanol *Ocimum sanctum* leaf extract using rat bone marrow micronucleus assay. *Kasetsart (Natural Science),* 36: 166-174.

Kim, H.J., Yokozawa, T., Kim, H.Y., Tohda, C., Rao, T.P., Juneja, L.R. (2005). Influence of amla (*Emblica officinalis* Gaertn) on hypercholestero-lemia and lipid peroxidation in cholesterol-fed rats. *Journal of Nutitional Scence and Vitaminoogy, (Tokyo),* 51: 413-418.

Kirtikar, K.R., Basu, B.D. (1975). Indian Medicinal Plants By BSMP Singh Co, Dehradun, India. Vol 3: 1762.

Kirtikar, K.R., Basu, B.D. (1965). *Ocimum sanctum* in Indian Medicinal Plants. Allahabad, Basu, L.M., 1933; 3.

Kjellberg, A. (1990). Subjective, behavioral and psychophysiological effects of noise. *Scandinavian Journal of Work, Environment and Health,* 16 (Suppl 1): 29-38.

Kleinveld, H.A., Swaak, A.J.G., Hack, C.E., Koster, J.F. (1989). Interactions between oxygen free radicals and proteins. *Scandinavian Journal of Rheumatology,* 18: 341-352.

Konstantinov, A.A., Peskin, A.V., Popova, E.Y., Khomutov, G.B., Ruuge, E.K. (1987). Superoxide generation by the respiratory chain of tumor mitochondria. *Biochimica et Biophysica Acta,* 894: 1-10.

Kryter, K.D. (1994). The Handbook of Hearing and the Effects of Noise. *Physiology, Psychology and Public Health,* Academic Press, San Diego.

Laemmli, U.K. (1970). Cleavage of structural protein during the assembly head bacteriophage T_4. *Nature*, 227: 680-685.

Lal, R.N., Sen, T.K., Nigam, M.C. (1978). Gas chromatography of the essential oil of *Ocimum sanctum* L. *Parfümerie und Kosmetiks*, 59: 230–231.

Lamaison, J.L., Carnat, A. (1990). Teneurs en acid rosmarinique en derives hydroxycinnamiques totaux et actvites antioxydantes chez les Apiacees, les Borrabinacees et les Lamiacees medicinales. *Pharmaceutica Acta Helvetiae*, 65: 315-320.

Landfield, P.W., Eldridge, J.C. (1994). Evolving aspects of the glucocorticoid hypothesis of brain aging: hormonal modulation of neuronal calcium homeostasis. *Neurobiology of Aging*, 15: 579–88.

Latchman, D.S.(1995).Cell stress genes and neuronal protection, *NeuropathologyandApplied. Neurobiology*, 21: 475–477.

Laurence, D., Fechter. (2005).Oxidative stress: a potential basis for potentiation of noise induced hearing loss. *Environmental Toxicology and Pharmacology*, 19: 543-546.

Lazarus, H. (1998)."Noise and communication: Present state," In Noise effects '98 By Carter, N., and Job, R.F.S., Eds (Noise Effects '98 Pty Ltd, Sydney), pp. 157-162.

Lee, S.E., Ju, E.M., Kim, J.H. (2001). Free radical scavenging and antioxidant enzyme fortifying activities of extracts from Smilax china root. *Experimental and Molecular Medicine*, Vol. 33: No. 4, 263-268.

Lehotsky. J., Kaplan, P., Racay, P., Matejovicova, M., Drgova, A., Mezesova, V. (1999). Membrane ion transport systems during oxidative stress in rodent brain: protective effect of stobadine and other antioxidants. *Life Science*, 65(18-19): 1951-8.

Leigh, G.J. (1990). *In:* Nomenclature of inorganic chemistry Recommendations 1990, By Blackwell Scientific Publications, Oxford.

Lin, H., Decuypere, E., Buyse, J. (2004). Oxidative stress induced by corticosterone administration in broiler chickens (Gallus gallus domesticus) 1. Chronic exposure. *Comparative Biochemistry and Physiology*, 139:737-744.

Lopez, J.F., Huda Akil., Stanely, J. Watson. (1999). Neural circuits mediating stress. *Biological Psychiatry*, 46: 1461-1471.

Lowenstein, D.H., Chan, P.H., Miles, M.F. (1991). The stress protein response in cultured neurons: characterization and evidence for a protective role in excitotoxicity. *Neuron*, 7: 1053–1060.

Lowry, C.A., Plant, A., Shanks, N., Ingram, C.D., Lightman, S.L.(2003). Anatomical and functional evidence for a stressresponsive, monoamine-accumulating area in the dorsomedial hypothalamus of adult rat brain. *Hormones and Behavior*, 43: 254-262.

Lowry, C.A., Rodda, J.E., Lightman, S.L., Ingram, C.D.(2000).Corticotropin-releasing factor increases *in vivo* firing rates of serotonergic neurons in the rat dorsal raphe nucleus: evidence for activation of a topographically organized mesolimbocortical serotonergic system. *The Journal of Neuroscience*, 20: 7728-7736.

Lowry, O.H., Rose Brough, N.J., Farr, A.L., Randall, R.J. (1951). Protein measurement with the Folin Phenol reagent. *Journal of Biological Chemistry*, 4: 492-501.

Lundberg, I.E. (2000). The role of cytokines, chemokines, and adhesion molecules in the pathogenesis of idiopathic inflammatory myopathies. *Current Rheumatology Reports*, 2(3):216-24.

Mandal, S., Das, D.N., De, K. (1993).*Ocimum sanctum* Linn–a study on gastric ulceration and gastric secretion in rats. *Indian Journal of Physiology and Pharmacology*, 37: 91-92.

Mandavilli, B.S., Rao, K.S. (1996). Neurons in the cerebral cortex are more susceptible to DNA-damage in aging rat brain. *Biochemistry and Molecular Biology International*,40:507–14.

Manikandan,S., Srikumar, R., Jeya Parthasarathy, N and Sheela Devi, R. (2005a) Protective Effect of *Acorus calamus* LINN on free radical scavengers and lipid peroxidation in discrete regions of brain against noise stress exposed rat. *Biological and Pharmaceutical Bulletin*, 28(12) 2327–2330.

Manikandan,S., and Sheela Devi, R. (2005b). Antioxidant property of asarone against noise-stress-induced changes in different regions of rat brain. *Pharmacological Research*, 52(6): 467-74.

Manoli, L.P., Gamaro, G.D., Silveira, P.P., Dalmaz, C. (2000). Effect of chronic variate stress on thiobarbituric-acid reactive species and on total radical-trapping potential in distinct regions of rat brain. *Neurochem Res*, 25:915-921.

Marini, M., Frabetti, F., Musiani, D., Franceschi, C. (1996). Oxygen radicals induce stress proteins and tolerance to oxidative stress in human lymphocytes. International *Journal of Radiation Biology*, 70(3): 337-50.

Marklund, S., Marklund, G. (1974). Involvement of the Superoxide Anion Radical in the autooxidation of Pyrogallol and a convenient Assay for Superoxide dismutase. *Journal of Biochemistry*, 47: 469-474.

Massa, S.M., Swanson, R.A., Sharp, F.R. (1996).The stress gene response in brain, *Cerebrovascular Brain Metabolism Review*, 8: 95–158.

Mattingly, D. (1962). A simple fluorimetric method for the study of free H-Hydroxy corticosteroids in human plasma. *Journal of Clinical Pathology*, 15: 374-379.

Maulik, G., Maulik, N., Bhandari, V.E., Pakrashi, S., Das., D.K. (1997). Evaluation of antioxidant effectiveness of a few herbal plants. *Free Radical Research*, 27: 221–228.

McDuffee, A.T., Senisterra, G., Huntley, S., Lepock, J.R., Sekhar, K.R., Meredith, M.J., Borrelli, M.J., Morrow, J.D., Freeman, M.L. (1997). Proteins containing non-native disulfide bonds generated by oxidative stress can act as signals for the induction of the heat shock response. *Journal of Cell Physiology*, 171: 143–151.

McEwen, B.S. (2002). Sex, stress and the hippocampus: allostasis, allostatic load and the aging process. *Neurobiology of Aging*, 23: 921–939.

McEwen, B.S., Stellar, E. (1993). Stress and the individual: mechanisms leading to disease. *Archives of Internal Medicine*, 153: 2093–101.

McEwen, B.S. (2000). The neurobiology of stress: from serendipity to clinical relevance. *Brain Research Interactive*, 886: 172-189.

McIntosh, L.J., Sapolsky, R.M. (1996). Glucocorticoids increase the accumulation of reactive oxygen species and enhance adriamycin-induced toxicity in neuronal culture. *Experimental Neurology*, 141: 201–6.

Meaney, M.J., Diorio, J., Francis, D., Widdowson, J., La Plante, P., Caldij, C., Sharma, S., Seckl, JR., Plotsky, P.M. (1996). Early environmental regulation of forebrain glucocorticoid receptor gene expression: implications for adrenocortical responses to stress. *Development Neuroscience*, 18, 49–72.

Mediratta, P.K., Sharma, K.K., Surender Singh. (2002).Evaluation of immunomodulatory potential of *Ocimum sanctum* seed oil and its possible mechanism of action. *Journal of Ethnopharmacology*, 80: 15–20.

Mennini, T., Taddei, C., Codegoni, A., Gobbi, M., Garattini, S. (1993). Acute noise stress reduces [3H]5-hydroxytryptamine uptake in rat brain synaptosomes: protective effects of buspirone and tianeptine. *European Journal of Pharmacology*, 241: 255-60.

Miki, K., Kawamorita, K., Araga, Y., Musha, T., Sudo, A. (1998). Urinary and salivary stress hormone levels while performing arithmetic calculation in a noisy environment. *Industrial Health*, 36, 66–69.

Moberg, G.P. (2000). Biological response to stress: implications for animal welfare. *In:* The Biology of Animal Stress, By Moberg, G.P., Mench, J.A. Eds, CABI Publishing, Wallingford, pp. 1–21, 2000.

Mora, A., Paya, M., Rios, J.L., Alcaraz, M.J. (1990). Structure–activity relationships of polymethoxyflavones and other flavonoids as inhibitors of non-enzymic lipid peroxidation. *Biochemical Pharmacology*, 40:793-797.

Morimoto, R.I. (1999).Regulation of the heat shock transcriptional response: cross talk between a family of heat shock factors, molecular chaperones, and negative regulators. *Genes and Development*, 12: 3788–3796.

Mosser, D.D., Caron, A.W., Bourget, L., Denis-Larose, C., Massie, B. (1997).Role of the human heat shock protein HSP70 in protection against stress-induced apoptosis. *Molecular Cell Biology*, 17: 5317–5327.

Nadkarni, A.K. (1954). Nadkarni's Indian Materia Medica. Bombay: Popular Book Depot, pp. 868.

Nadkarni, A.K. (1976). Indian Materia Medica, 3rd edition, Popular Press Ltd. Mumbai, India. pp. 1308-1315.

Nadkarni, K.M. (1976). Indian materia medica. Mumbai, India Popular Prakashan; pp. 671.

Naiwu, F., Lanping, Q., Lei, H., Zhank, R., Chen, Y. (1992). Antioxidant action of extracts of *Terminalia chebula* and its preventive effect on DNA breaks in human white cells induced by TPA. *Chinese Traditional and Herbal Drugs*, 23:26-29.

Nankova, B., Kvetnansky, R., McMahon, A., Viskupic, E., Hiremagalur, B., Frankle, G., Fukuhara, K., Kopin, I.J., Sabban, E.L. (1994). Induction of tyrosine hydroxylase gene expression by a nonneuronal nonpituitary-mediated mechanism in immobilization stress. *Proceedings of National Academy of Sciences, U S A*, 1; 91(13): 5937-41.

Narayan reddy, K.S. (1990). Metallic poisons. *In:* The essentials of forensic medicine and toxicology, 12th edition, 394-403.

Narayanaswamy, P., Palanisami, A. (1973). Studies on yellow mosaic disease of soybean. I. Effect of virus infection on plant pigments. *Experientia*, 29: 1165-1167.

Nemeroff, C.B. (1996).The corticotropin-releasing factor (CRF) hypothesis of depression: new findings and new directions. *Molecular Psychiatry*, 1: 336-42.

Nikolaos, P., George, Z., Nikolaos, T.P., Christos, D.G., Fevronia, A., Nikolaos, A.M. (2004). Thiol redox state (TRS) and oxidative stress in the mouse hippocampus after pentylenetetrazol-induced epileptic seizure. *Neuroscience Letters*, 357, 83–86.

Nisenbaum, L.K., Zigmond, M.J., Sved, A.F., Abercrombie, E.D. (1991). Prior exposure to chronic stress results in enhanced synthesis and release of hippocampal norepinephrine in response to a novel stressor. *Journal of Neuroscience*, 11:1478–1484.

Nishiyama, N., Zhou, Y., Saito, H. (1994a). Ameliorative effects of chronic treatment using DX-9386, a traditional Chinese preparation, on learning performance and lipid peroxide content in senescence accelerated mouse. *Biological Pharmaceutical Bulletin*, 17:1481-1484.

Nishiyama, N., Zhou, Y., Takashina, K., Saito, H. (1994b). Effects of DX-9386, a traditional Chinese preparation, on passive and active avoidance performances in mice. *Biological Pharmaceutical Bulletin*, 17:1472-1476.

Ohtsuka, A., Kojima, H., Ohtani, T., Hayashi, K. (1998). Vitamin E reduces glucocorticoid-induced oxidative stress in rat skeletal muscle. *Journal of Nutritional Science and Vitaminology*, (Tokyo), 44:779-786.

Olanow, C.W. (1990). Oxidation reactions in Parkinson's disease. *Neurology*, 40:34-39.

Orrenius, S. (1995).Apoptosis: molecular mechanisms and implications for human disease. *Journal of International Medicine*, 237(6): 529-36.

Otten, W., Kanitz, E., Puppe, B., Tuchscherer, M., Brussow, K.P., Numberg, G., Stabenow, B. (2004).Acute and long term effects of chronic intermittent noise on hypothalamic-pituitary-adrenocortical and sympatho-adrenomedullary axis in pigs. *Animal Science*, 78: 271-284.

Oyama, Y., Chikahisa, L., Ueha, T., Kanemaru, K., Noda, K. (1996). Ginkgo biloba extract protects brain neurons against oxidative stress induced by hydrogen peroxide. *Brain Research*, 712:349-352.

Ozguner, M.F., Delyba, N., Tahan, V., Koyu, A., Koylu, H. (1999). Effects of industrial noise on the blood levels of superoxide dismutase, glutathione peroxidase and malondialdehyde. *Eastern Journal of Medicine*, 4 (1): 13-15.

Pacak, K., Palkovits, M., Kvetnansky, R., Yadid, G., Kopin, I.J., Goldstein. D.S. (1995a). Effects of various stressors on in vivo norepinephrine release in the hypothalamic paraventricular nucleus and on the pituitary-adrenocortical axis. *Annals of New York Academy of Sciences*, 29; 771:115-30.

Pacak, K., McCarty, R., Palkovits, M., Cizza, G., Kopin, I.J., Goldstein, D.S., Chrousos, G.P. (1995b). Decreased central and peripheral catecholaminergic activation in obese Zucker rats. *Endocrinology*. 136(10): 4360-7.

Page, M.E., Abercrombie, E.D. (1999). Discrete local application of corticotropin-releasing factor increases locus coeruleus discharge and extracellular norepinephrine in rat hippocampus. *Synapse*, 33: 304–313.

Panda, S., Kar, A. (1998). *Ocimum sanctum* leaf extract in the regulation of thyroid function in the male mouse. *Pharmacology Research*, 38: 107–110.

Paparelli, A., Soldani, P., Breschi, M.C. (1992). Effects of subacute exposure to noise on the noradrenergic innervation of the cardiovascular system in young and aged rats: a morphofunction study. *Journal of Neural Transmission Gen Sect*, 88:105-13.

Pare, W.P., Glavin, G.B. (1986). Restraint stress in biomedical research: a review. *Neuroscience and BioBehavioural Reviews*, 10(3): 339-370.

Passchier-Vermeer, W., Passchier, W.F. (2000). Noise exposure and public health. *Environmental Health Perspectives Supplements*, 108(1): 123–131.

Passchier-Vermeer, W. (1993). Noise and Health. *In*: The Hague: Health Council of the Netherlands, Publication no A93/02E.

Paton, A., Harley, R.M., Harley, M.M.(1999).Ocimum–an overview of relationships and classification. *In:* Ocimum. Medicinal and Aromatic Plants–Industrial Profiles, By Holm, Y., Hiltunen, R. Eds, Harwood Academic, Amsterdam, pp. 1–38.

Patsoukis, N., Papapostolou, I., Zervoudakis, G., Georgiou, C.D., Matsokis, N.A., Panagopoulos, N.T.(2005). Thiol redox state and oxidative stress in midbrain and striatum of weaver mutant mice, a genetic model of nigrostriatal dopamine deficiency. *Neuroscience Letters*, 7; 376(1): 24-8.

Pethkar, A.V., Gaikaiwari, R.R., Paknikar, K.M. (2001). Biosorptive removal of contaminating heavy metals from plant extracts of medicinal value. *Current Science*, 80 (9): 1216-1219.

Petiot, J.C., Parrot, J., Lobreau, J.P., Smolik, H.J. (1992). Cardiovascular effects of impulse noise, road traffic noise, and intermittent pink noise at LAeq = 75 dB, as a function of sex, age, and level of anxiety: a comparative study. II. Digital pulse level and blood pressure data. *International Archives on Occupational and Environmental Health*, 63:485-493.

Phelix, C.F., Liposits, Z., Paull, W.K. (1992).Serotonin-CRF interaction in the bed nucleus of the stria terminalis: a light microscopic double-label immunocytochemical analysis. *Brain Research Bulletin*, 28: 943–948.

Phippen, W.B., Simon, J.E. (2000). Anthocyanin inheritance and instability in purple basil (*Ocimum basilicum* L.). *Journal of Heredity*, 91, 289–296.

Plotsky, P.M., Cunningham, E.T. Jr, Widmaier, E.P. (1989). Catecholaminergic modulation of corticotropin-releasing factor and adrenocorticotropin secretion. *Endocrine Reviews*, 10(4): 437-58.

Plumier, J.C., Ross, B.M., Currie, R.W., Angelidis, C.E, Kazlaris, H., Kollias, G., Pagoulatos, G.N. (1995). Transgenic mice expressing the human heat shock protein 70 have improved post-ischemic myocardial recovery. *Journal of Clinical Investigations*, 95: 1854–1860.

Poll, R.V., Straetemans, M., Nicolson, N.A.(2001). Ambient noise in daily life: a pilot study. *In*: Proceedings of the 2001 International Congress and Exhibition on Noise Control Engineering, The Hague, vol. 4. Ed. By Boone, R. Internoise 2001, Nederlands Akoestisch Genootschap, Maastricht, pp. 1807–1810.

Porter, N.D., Flindell, I.H., Berry, B.F. (1998). Health effect based noise assessment methods: a review and feasibility study. *NPL Report CMAM* 16.

Prakash, J., Gupta, S.K. (2000). Chemopreventive activity of *Ocimum sanctum* seed oil. *Journal of Ethnopharmacology*, 72: 29-34.

Price, M.L., Hagerman, A.E., Butler, L.G. (1980). Tannin content of cow peas, chick peas, pigeon peas and mung beans. *Journal of Agriculture and Food chemistry*, 28: 459-461.

Pushpangadan, P., Bradu, B., Basil. (1995). Advances in Horticulture. *In*: Medicinal and Aromatic Plants, vol. 11. By Chadha, K.L., Gupta, R. Eds, Malhotra Publishing House, New Delhi, pp. 627–657.

Quirk, G.J., Armony, J.L., LeDoux, J.E. (1997). Fear conditioning enhances different temporal components of tone-evoked spike trains in auditory cortex and lateral amygdala. *Neuron*, 19: 613–624.

Radak, Z., Sasvari, M., Nyakas, C., Kaneko, T., Tahara, S., Ohno, H., Goto, S. (2001). Single bout of exercise eliminate the immobilization–induced oxidative stress in rat brain. *Neurochemistry International*, 39: 33-38.

Raghu, V., Kalpana Platel., Srinivasan, K. (2007). Comparison of ascorbic acid content of *Emblica officinalis* fruits determined by different analytical methods. *Journal of Food and Nutrition*, 20: 529–533.

Rai, M.K., Upadhyay, S (1988).Screening of medicinal plants of Chindwara district against Trichophyton mentagrophytes: a causal organism of *Tinea pedis*. *Hindustan Antibiotic Bulletin*, 30: 33–36.

Rai, V., Iyer, U., Mani, U.V. (1997). Effect of Tulasi (*Ocimum sanctum*) leaf powder supplementation on blood sugar levels, serum lipids and tissue lipids in diabetic rats. *Plant Foods for Human Nutrition*, 50: 9-16.

Raju, S. (2003). Noise Pollution and Automobiles. *In:* Symposium on International Automotive Technology, pp. 57-58.

Ralf, D., Bernd, H. (1997). Involvement of glutathione peroxidase and catalase in the disposal of exogenous hydrogen peroxide in culture astroglial cells. *Brain Research*, 759, 67–75.

Ramsey, J.M.(1982). Modern stress and disease process. *In:* Basic Physiology, Addison-Wesley publishing company, California, pp.177-179.

Ravindran, R., Sheela Devi, R., Samson, J., Senthilvelan, M.(2005). Noise-Stress-Induced Brain Neurotransmitter Changes and the Effect of Ocimum sanctum (Linn) Treatment in Albino Rats. *Journal of Pharmacological Sciences*, 98:354-360.

Ravishankara, M.N., Shrivastava, N., Padh, H., Rajani, M. (2002). Evaluation of antioxidant properties of root bark of *Hemidimus indicus* R. Br. (Anatmul). *Phytomedicine*, 9: 153.

Rege, N.N., Thatte, U.M., Dahanukar, S.A. (1999). Adaptogenic properties of six rasayana herbs used in Ayurvedic medicine. *Phytotherapy Research*, 13: 275-291.

Reinhardt, J.F., Mammon, W.J., Roth, R.H. (1982). Acceleration by stress of dopamine synthesis and metabolism in prefrontal cortex antagonism by diazepam. *Naunyn Schmiedeberg's Arch Pharmacology*, 318: 374–7.

Rice-Evans, C.A., Miller, N.J., Paganga, G. (1996). Structure-antioxidant activity relationships of flavonoids and phenolic acids. *Free Radical Biology*, ed 20: 933–956.

Riley, L.G., Roufogalis, B.D., Li G.Q., Weiss, A.S. (2006). A radioassay for synaptic core complex assembly: screening of herbal extracts for effectors. *Annals of Biochemistry*, 357:50-57.

Rordorf, G., Koroshetz, W.J., and Bonventre, J.V. (1991). Heat shock protects cultured neurons from glutamate toxicity. *Neuron*, 7: 1043-1052.

Rosenbaum, D.M., Kalberg, J., Kessler, J.A. (1994). Superoxide dismutase ameliorates neuronal death from hypoxia in culture. *Stroke*, 25: 857-863.

Rosenlund, M., Berglind, N., Pershagen, G., Ja¨ rup L., Bluhm, G. (2001).Increased prevalence of hypertension in a population exposed to aircraft noise. *Occupational Environmental Medicine*, 58: 769–773.

Roth, R.H., Tam, S.Y., Ida, Y., Yang, J.X., Deutch, A.Y. (1988). Stress and the mesocorticolimbic dopamine systems. *Annals of New York Academy of Sciences*, 537: 138–147.

Rotruck, JT., Pope, AC., Ganther, HE., Hafeman, DG., Hoekstra, W.G. (1973). Selenium: Biochemical role as a component of Glutathione peroxidase. *Science,* 179: 588-590.

Rylander, R. (2004). Physiological aspects of noise induced stress and annoyance. *Journal of Sound and Vibration*, 277: 471-478

Saez, G.T., Bannister, W.H., Bannister, J.V. (1990). Free radicals and thiol compounds the role of glutathione against free radical toxicity. *In:* Glutathione: Metabolism and Physiological Functions, By Vina, J. Ed. CRC Press, Boca Raton, FL, USA, pp. 237-254.

Sajdyk, T.J., Katner, J.S., Sekhar, A.(1997).Monoamines in the dorsomedial hypothalamus of rats following exposure to different tests of "anxiety." *Prog Neuropsychopharmacol Biol psychiatry*, 21(1): 193-209.

Sakina, M.R., Dandiya, P.C., Hamdard, M.E., Hameed, A. (1990). Preliminary psychopharmacological evaluation of *Ocimum sanctum* leaf extract. *Journal of Ethnopharmacology*, 28: 143-150.

Saksena, N., Tripathi, H.H.S. (1985).Plant volatiles in relation to fungistasis. *Fitoterapia*, 56:243–244.

Saleem, A., Husheem, M., Harkonen, P., Pihlaja, K.(2002). Inhibition of cancer cell growth by crude extract and the phenolics of *Terminalia chebula* retz. Fruit. *Journal of Ethnopharmacology*, 81:327-336.

Samson, J., Sheela Devi R., Ravindran, R., Senthilvelan, M. (2005).Effect of noise stress on free radical scavenging enzymes in brain. *Environmental Toxicology and Pharmacology*, 20: 142-148.

Samson, J., Sheeladevi, R., Ravindran, R., Senthilvelan, M. (2006). Biogenic amine changes in brain regions and attenuating action of *Ocimum sanctum* in noise exposure. *Pharmacology Biochemistry and Behaviour*, 83, 67–75.

Samson, J., Sheeladevi, R., Ravindran, R., Senthilvelan, M. (2007). Stress response in rat brain after different durations of noise exposure. *Neuroscience Research*, 57 143–147.

Sandstrom, N.J. (2005). Sex differences in the long-term effect of preweanling isolation stress on memory retention. *Hormones and Behavior*, 4:7 556-562.

Saphier, D., Farrar, G.E., Welch, J.E. (1995). Differential inhibition of stress induced adrenocortical responses by 5-HT1A agonists and by 5-HT2 and 5-HT3 antagonists. *Psychoneuroendocrinology*, 20: 239–257.

Sapolsky, R. (1996). Why stress is bad for your brain. *Science,* 273:749-750.

Sapolsky, R.M., Romero, L.M., Munck, A.U.(2000). How do glucocorticoids influence stress responses? Integrating permissive, suppressive, stimulatory, and preparative actions. *Endocrine Reviews*, 21: 55–89.

Sapolsky, R.M. (2000). Stress hormones: good and bad. *Neurobiology of Disease*, 7: 540–542.

Saunders, J.C., Dear, S.P., Schneider, M.E. (1985). The anatomical consequences of acoustic injury: A review and tutorial. *Journal of Acoustical Society of America*, 78: 833-860.

Scalbert, A., Williamson, G. (2000). Dietary intake and bioavailability of polyphenols. *Journal of Nutrition*, 130: 2073S–2085S.

Sedlack, J., Lindsay, R.H. (1968). Estimation of total, protein bound and non protein sulphydryl groups in the tissue with Ellman's reagent. *Analytical Biochemistry*, 25: 192-205.

Seif-El-Nasr, M., El-Fattah, A.A. (1995). Lipid peroxide, phospholipids, glutathione levels and superoxide dismutase activity in rat brain after ischemia: effect of ginko biloba extract. *Phamacological. Research*, 32:273-278.

Selye H.(1952).The Story of the Adaptation Syndrome. *Acta, Montreal.*

Selye, H. (1973). The evolution of the stress concept. *American Scientist*, 61: 692-9.

Selye, H. (1976).The three phases of the GAS, adaptation energy, aging. *In:* Stress in Health and Disease By Butterworth Publishers, Boston, pp. 1146.

Sembulingam, K., Prema Sembulingam, Namasivayam, A. (1996). Effect of acute noise stress on cholinergic neurotransmitter in corpus striatum of *albino rats. Pharmaceutical Sciences*, 2, 241–242.

Sembulingam, K., Sembulingam, P., Namasivayam, A. (1997). Effect of *Ocimum sanctum* Linn on noise induced changes in plasma corticosterone level. *Indian Journal of Physiology and Pharmacology*, 41: 139-143.

Sembulingam, K., Prema Sembulingam., Namasivayam, A. (1999). Effect of acute noise stress on acetylcholine in discrete areas of rat brain. *Journal of Environmental Biology*, 20, 289–292.

Sembulingam, K., Sembulingam, P., Namasivayam, A. (2003). Effect of acute noise stress on acetylcholinesterase activity in discrete areas of rat brain. *Indian Journal of Medical Science*, 57:487-492.

Sembulingam, K., Prema Sembulingam., Namasivayam, A. (2005). Effect of *Ocimum sanctum* Linn on the changes in central cholinergic system induced by acute noise stress. *Journal of Ethnopharmacology*, 96: 477–482.

Sen, P., Maiti,P.C., Puri, S., Ray, A. (1992). Mechanism of antistress activity of *Ocimum sanctum* Linn, eugenol and Tinospora malabarica in experimental animals. *Indian Journal of Experimental Biology*, 30: 592-596.

Shah, ZA., Vohora, S.B. (2002).Antioxidant/restorative effects of calcined gold preparations used in Indian systems of medicine against global and focal models of ischaemia. *Pharmacology and Toxicology*, 90:254-259.

Sharma, G. (1983). Antiasthmatic effect of *Ocimum sanctum*. *Sacitra Ayurveda*, 35: 665–668.

Sharma, R.K., Dash B. (1998). Carka Samhita Volume II. Chowkamba Sanskrit Series Office, Varanasi, India.

Sharma, M., Singh, O. (1989). Immunoassays. *In:* Murine and human monoclonal antibodies: production, purification and applications By Practical manual, National Institute of Immunology, New Delhi, pp. 27-29.

Sharma, P., Kulshreshtha, S., Sharma, A.L. (1998).Anti-cataract activity of *Ocimum sanctum* on experimental cataract. *Indian Journal of Pharmacology*, 30: 16-20.

Sharp, F.R., Sagar, S.M. (1994). Alterations in gene expression as an index of neuronal injury: heat shock and the immediate early gene response. *Neurotoxicology*, 15: 51–60.

Sherwin, R.S. (1978). Effect of starvation on the turnover and metabolic response to leucine. *Journal of Clinical Investigations*, 61(6): 1471-81.

Shyamala, A.C., Devaki, T. (1996). Studies on peroxidation in rats ingesting copper sulphate and effect of subsequent treatment with Ocimum sanctum. *Journal of Clinical Biochemistry and Nutrition*, 20: 113-119.

Sies, H. (1991). Oxidative Stress: Oxidants and Antioxidants. *Academic Press, New York.*

Singh, N., Mishra, N., Srivastava, A.K., Dixit, K.S., Gupta, G.P. (1991). Effect of antistress plants on biochemical changes during stress reactions. *Indian Journal of Pharmacology*, 23:137-42.

Singh, S., Agrawal, S.S. (1991). Anti-asthmatic and anti-inflammatory activity of *Ocimum sanctum*. *International Journal of Pharmacognosy*. 29: 306–310.

Singh, S., Majumdar, D.K. (1995). Analgesic activity of *Ocimum sanctum* and its possible mechanism of action. *International Journal of Pharmacognosy*, 33: 188–192.

Singh, S., Majumdar, D.K. (1997). Evaluation of antiinflammatory activity of fatty acids of *Ocimum sanctum* fixed oil. *Indian Journal of Experimental Biology*, 35: 380–383.

Singh, S., Majumdar, D.K. (1999). Evaluation of the gastric antiulcer activity of fixed oil of *Ocimum sanctum* (Holy Basil). *Journal of Ethnopharmacology*, 65: 13-19.

Singh, VB., Onaivi, E.S., Phan, T.H., Boadle-Biber, M.C. (1990). The increases in rat cortical and midbrain tryptophan hydroxylase activity in response to acute or repeated sound stress are blocked by bilateral lesions to the central nucleus of the amygdale. *Brain Research*, 530: 49-53.

Sinha, A.K. (1972). Calorimetric assay of Catalase. *Analytical Biochemistry*, 47: 389-394.

Skaper, S.D., Floreani, M., Ceccon, M., Facci, L., Giusti, P. (1999). Excitotoxicity, oxidative stress, and the neuroprotective potential of melatonin. *Annals of NewYork Academy of Sciences*, 890:107-118.

Skaper, S.D., Floreani, M., Ceccon, M., Facci, L., Giusti, P. (1999). Excitotoxicity, oxidative stress, and the neuroprotective potential of melatonin. *Annals of NewYork Academy of Sciences*, 890:107-118.

Sliwinska-Kowalska, M., Zamyslowska-Szmytke, E., Szymczak, W., Kotylo, P., Fiszer, M., Wesolowski, W., Pawlaczyk-Luszczynska, M., Bak, M., Gajda-Szadkowska, A. (2004). Effects of co exposure to noise and mixture of organic solvents on hearing in dockyard workers. *Journal of Occupational Environmental Medicine*, 46: 30–38.

Sokolovski, V.V., Goncharova, L.L., Kiseliva, N.N., Maka Radionova, L.P. (1987). The antioxidant system noise induced stress. *Journal of Medical Virology*, 33(6): 111-113.

Sorger, P.K. (1991). Heat shock factor and the heat shock response. *Cell*, 65: 363–366.

Spoendlin, H.(1971). Primary structural changes in the organ of Corti after acoustic over stimulation. *Acta Otolaryngology*, 71:166–173.

Spreng, M. (2000). Possible health effects of noise induced cortisol increase. *Noise Health*, 2(7): 59-64.

Sreejayan., Rao, M.N.(1997).Nitric oxide scavenging by curcuminoids. *Journal of Pharmacy and Pharmcology*, 49: 105.

Srikumar, R., Parthasarathy, N.J., Manikandan, S., Narayanan, G.S., Sheeladevi, R.(2006). Effect of Triphala on oxidative stress and on cell-mediated immune response against noise stress in rats. *Molecular and Cellular Biochemistry*, 283(1-2):67-74.

Srikumar, R., Jeya Parthasarathy, N., Sheela Devi R. (2005). Immunomodulatory activity of triphala on neutrophil functions. *Biological and Pharmaceutical Bulletin*, Aug;28(8):1398-403.

Stansfeld, S.A., Haines, M.M., Brown, B. (2000). Noise and Health in the Urban Environment. *Reviews on Environmental Health*,. 15 (1–2): 43–82.

Sterling, P., Eyer, J. (1988). Allostasis: a new paradigm to explain arousal pathology. *In*: Handbook of life stress, cognition and health By Fisher, S., Reason, J., editors New York, Wiley, pp. 629–49.

Stoll, S., Scheuer, K., Pohl, O., Muller, W.E. (1996). Ginkgo biloba extract (EGb 761) independently improves changes in passive avoidance learning and brain membrane fluidity in the aging mouse. *Pharmacopsychiatry*, 29:144-149.

Stoof, J.A., Winogrodzka, A., Vanmuiswinkel, E.L., Wolters, E.C., Voorn, P., Gronewegon, H.J. (1999). Leads for development of neuroprotective treatments in Parkinson's disease and brain imaging methods for estimating treatment efficacy. *European Journal of Pharmacology*, 375: 75-86.

Storey, K.B. (1996). Oxidative stress: animal adaptations in nature Animal adaptations for oxidative stress. *Brazilian Journal of Medical and Biological Research*, 29: 1715-1733.

Suter, A.H. (1991). 'Noise and its Effects'. *Administrative Conference of the United States, <www.nonoise.org/library/suter/suter.htm#> effects of noise on sleep.*

Sylvie Hebert., Philippe Paiement., Sonia, J., Lupien. (2004). A physiological correlate for the intolerance to both internal and external sounds. *Hearing Research,* 4831: 1-9.

Szafarczyk, A., Ixart, G., Gaillet, S., Siaud, P., Barbanel, G., Malaval, F., Assenmacher, I.(1993). Stress. Neurophysiologic studies. *Encephale*, 1:137-42.

Tanaka, M., Yoshida, M., Emoto, H., Ishii, H. (2000). Noradrenaline systems in the hypothalamus, amygdala and locus coeruleus are involved in the provocation of anxiety: basic studies. *European Journal of Pharmacology*, 405: 397–406.

Tao, G., Irie, Y., Li, D.J., Keung, W.M. (2005). Eugenol and its structural analogs inhibit monoamine oxidase A and exhibit antidepressant-like activity. *Bioorganic and Medicinal Chemistry,* 1 [Epub ahead of print].

Thomas, J., Connor., Padraig Kelliher., Andrew Harkin., John, P., Kelly, Brian, E., Leonard. (1999). Reboxetine attenuates forced swim test-induced behavioural and neurochemical alterations in the rat. *European Journal of Pharmacology*, 379: 125–133.

Towbin, H., Staehelin, T., Gordin, J. (1979). Electrophoretic transfer of proteins from polyacylamide gels to nitrocellulose sheets. *Procedures and some application*,76: 4350-4354.

Tseng, CF., Iwakami, S., Mikajiri, A., Shibuya, M., Hanaoka, F., Ebizuka, Y., Padmawinata, K., Sankawa, U. (1992). Inhibition of *in vitro* prostaglandin and leukotriene biosynthesis by cinnamoyl-b-phenethylamine and N-acyldopamine derivatives. *Chemical and Pharmaceutical Bulletin*, 40: 396–400.

Turrens, JF., Freeman, BA., Levitt, JG., Crapo, JD. (1982). The effect of hyperoxia on superoxide production by lung submitochondrial particles. *Archives of Biochemistry and Biophysics*, 217: 401-410.

Tytell, M., Barbe, MF., Brown, IR. (1993). Stress heat shock protein accumulation in the central nervous system: its relationship to cell stress and damage. *In:* Advances in Neurology, Vol. 59, Ed. By F.J. Seil, Raven Press, New York, pp. 292–303.

Ushakova, T., Melkonyan, H., Nikonova, L., Mudrik, N., Gogvadze, V., Zhukova, A., Gaziev, AI., Bradbury, R.(1996).The effect of dietary supplements on gene expression in mice tissues. *Free Radical Biology and Medicine*, 20: 279-284.

Vaidya, A.D,B., Pillai, D.M., Ramachandran, R., Ghaisis, S., Pandita, N., Bhide, S.V. (1998). Antioxidants in context of medicinal plants. *In:*Current perspectives on food antioxidants in health, Krishnaswamy, P. R, Ed. Proceedings of Scientific meeting organized by the Brooke Bond and Health Information Centre, Bangalore, India, pp. 15-21.

Vale, W., Spies, J., Rivier, C., Rivier, J. (1981).Characterization of a 41-residue ovine hypothalamic peptide that stimulates secretion of corticotrophin and beta-endorphin. *Science*, 213: 1394–1397.

Vallet, M., Gagneaux, J., Clainet, J.M. (1983). Heart rate reactivity to aircraft noise after a long-term exposure. *In:* G Rossi Noise as a Public Health Problem, Ed. Centro Recherche Studio Amplifon, Milan.

Van de Kar, LD., Blair, M.L. (1999). Forebrain pathways mediating stress induced hormone secretion. *Frontiers in Neuroendocrinology*, 20: 1–48.

Vani, T., Rajani, M., Sarkar, S., Shishoo, C.J. (1997).Antioxidant properties of Ayurvedic formulations triphala and its constituents. *International Journal of Pharmacology*, 35: 313.

Venarucci, D., Catalini, P., Scendoni, P., Venarucci, V., Casado, A., De La Torre, R.(1994). Evaluation of certain immunity parameters in rheumatoid arthritis, treated with cortisone. *Panminerva Medicine*, 36(4): 188-91.

Venskutonis, P.R., Dagilyte, A. (2003). Composition of Essential Oil of Sweet Flag (*Acorus calamus* L.) Leaves at Different Growing Phases. *Journal of Essential Oil Research*, 15:313-318.

Vernon, J.A., Moller, A.R. (1995). Models of tinnitus: generation, perception, clinical implications. In: Vernon J.A, Moller A.R, eds.by Mechanisms of tinnitus. Boston: Allyn and Bacon, pp. 57-72.

Vicente-Torres, M.A., Gil-Loyzaga, P., Carricondo, F., Bartolome, M.V. (2002). Simultaneous HPLC quantification of monoamines and metabolites in the blood-free rat cochlea. *Journal of Neuroscience Methods*, 15;119(1): 31-6.

Vincent, J.B. (2000). Quest for the molecular mechanism of chromium action and its relationship to diabetes. *Nutrition Reviews*, 58: 67-72.

Vlajkovic, S.M., Housley, G.D., Munoz, D.J.B., Robson, SC., Se´ Vigny, J., Wanga, C.J.H., Thornea, P.R.(2004). Noise exposure induces up-regulation of ecto-nucleoside triphosphate diphosphohydrolases 1 and 2 in rat cochlea. *Neuroscience*, 126: 763–773.

Voronych, N.M., Iemel'ianenko, I.V. (1994).Lipid peroxidation and antioxidant system activity in the brain, stomach and heart tissues and blood serum of rats under stress. *Fiziol Zh*, 40(5/6): 114–7.

Wagner, H., Nörr, H., Winterhoff, H. (1994). Plant adaptogens. *Phytomedicine*, 1: 63-76.

Wagner, J., Vitali, P., Palfreyman, M.G., Zariaka, M., Huot, S. (1982).Simultaneous determination of 3,4-dihydroxy phenyl alanine, 5 hydroxy tryphtophan, dopamine, 4-hydroxy 3-methoxy phenyl alanine, norepinephrine, 3,4 dihydroxy phenylacetic acid, homovanillic acid, serotonin and 5 hydroxy indole acetic acid in rat cerebrospinal fluid and brain by high performance liquid chromatography with electrochemical detection. *Journal of Neurochemistry*, 38: 1241-1254.

Wallenius, M.A. (2004). The interaction of noise stress and personal project stress on subjective health. *Journal of Environmental Psychology*, 24: 167–177.

World Health Organization, Geneva (WHO), (2002). Traditional medicine: growing needs and potential. WHO Policy Perspectives on Medicines.

Winterbourn, C.C., Metodiewa, D. (1994). The reactions of superoxide with reduced glutathione. *Archives of Biochemistry and Biophysics*, 314: 284-290.

Xuejiang, W., Magara, T., Konishi, T.(1999). Prevention and repair of cerebral ischemia-reperfusion injury by Chinese herbal medicine, shengmai san, in rats. *Free Radicals Research*, 31:449–455.

Yamasoba, T., Nuttall, AL., Harris, C., Raphael, Y., Miller, J.M. (1998). Role of glutathione in protection against noise-induced hearing loss. *Brain Research*,784: 82-90.

Yenari, M.A., Fink, S.L., Hua Sun, G., Chang, L.K., Patel, M.K., Kunis, D.M., Onley, D., Ho DY., Sapolsky, R.M., Steinburg, G.K.(1998). Gene therapy with Hsp72 is neuroprotective in rat models of stroke and epilepsy. *Annals of Neurology*, 44: 584–591.

Yoo, CB., Han, KT., Cho, K.S., Ha, J., Park, H.J., Nam, J.H., Kil, U.H., Lee, K.T. (2005). Eugenol isolated from the essential oil of Eugenia caryophyllata induces a reactive oxygen species-mediated apoptosis in HL-60 human promyelocytic leukemia cells. *Cancer Letters*, 8; 225(1):41-52.

Yuh-Fung Chen., Hsiu-Mei Chiang., Tzu-Wei Tan., Jim-Shoung Lai., Huei-Yann Tsai1. (2002).The Influence of Noise Stress-Induced Pain-Threshold Increase on Central Monoaminergic Neurons. *Mid Taiwan Journal of Medicine*, 7: 135-45.

Yuh-Shyang., Chen., Fen-Yu Tseng., Tien-Chen Liu., Shoei Yn Lin-Shiau., Chuan-Jen Hsu. (2005). Involvement of nitric oxide generation in noise-induced temporary threshold shift in guinea pigs. *Hearing Research*, 203, (1-2*): 94-100.*

Zhang, Y., Takashina, K., Saito, H., Nishiyama, N.(1994). Anti-aging effects of DX-9386 in senescence-accelerated mouse. Biological and Pharmaceutical Bulletin, 17:866-868.

Ziegler, D.R., Cass, W.A., Herman, J.P. (1999).Excitatory influence of the locus coeruleus in hypothalamic-pituitary-adrenocortical axis responses to stress. *Journal of Neuroendocrinology*,11: 361–369.

Utilisation and Management of Medicinal Plants (2010) *Pages 278–293*
Editors: **V.K. Gupta, Anil K. Verma and Sushma Koul**
Published by: **DAYA PUBLISHING HOUSE, NEW DELHI**

Chapter 15

Bioactive Compounds from *Annona* Species

Beena Joy*
Agroprocessing and Natural Products Division,
National Institute for Interdisciplinary Science and Technology,
Thiruvananthapuram – 695 019, India

ABSTRACT

The Annonaceae is a very large family of plants comprising about 120 genera and more than 2000 species. On the basis of morphology and habitat, it is a very homogenous family as source of edible fruits and oils. The Annonaceae seems to be one of the least chemically as well as pharmacologically known families compared with its large size. The chemical and pharmacological features of some of the groups of compounds from Annonaceae tempt chemists and pharmacologists to examine these plants. Hence, we were engaged in the bioactivity directed fractionation, isolation of active principle from the pericarp of *Annona squamosa and Annona reticulata* and yielded different kauranes like, (-)–Ent–kaur-17-acetoxy, 19-oic acid, 16a, 17-Dihydroxy-ent-kauran-19-oic acid and (-)–Ent-Kaur-17, 19-dioic acid etc. These compounds showed antibacterial, anti-inflammatory and antitumor effects. The anti-bacterial, anti-inflammatory and anti-tumor effects of these compounds were studied. The fixed oils of *Annona squamosa, A. reticulata* and *A. muricata* (*Annonaceae*) were found to possess anti-inflammatory activity against carrageenan induced paw oedema in albino rats.

Keywords: Bioactive natural products, Annonaceae, Annona squamosa, Annona reticulata, Annona muricata, Pericarp, Anti-bacterial activity, Anti-inflammatory activity, Anti-tumor effects.

* E-mail: bjoy39@yahoo.co.in.

Introduction

Medicinal plants play a key role in the human health care and the use of plants in curing and healing is as old as man himself. Recent investigations on medicinally important members of families like Annonaceae, Meliaceae, Rubiaceae, Asteraceae, Apocynaceae, Acanthaceae etc. resulted in the emergence of several compounds. Annonaceae seems to be one of the least chemically as well as pharmacologically known families compared with its large size. Annonaceae is a very large family of plants comprising about 120 genera and more than 2000 species. On the basis of morphology and habitat it is a very homogenous family. As source of edible fruits and oils, this family has economic importance. Seed oils of certain Annonaceae plants are used in soap production and as edible oil. Flowers of some Annonaceae plants are used in perfumery and many members of this family are used in folk medicine to treat various types of tumors and cancers. Annonaceae seems to be one of the least chemically as well as pharmacologically investigated families compared with its large size.

The earlier studies on *Annona* species showed that this family is a potent source of a wide variety of secondary metabolites belonging to several categories. Parthasaradhy *et al.* (2005) have studied the effect of organic and aqueous extracts obtained from the defatted seeds of *Annona squamosa* on different tumour cell lines and reported that the two extracts from *A. squamosa* seeds induced apoptotic features like formation of apoptotic bodies, DNA fragmentation and phosphotidyl serine externalization by Annexin V staining in MCF-7 breast carcinoma and K-562 erythroleukemic cells. A large number of Annonaceae plants are fragrant due to the presence of essential oils. The essential oil of *Annona squamosa* leaves were studied and were reported to have β–cedrene (23 per cent) and β–caryophyllene (14 per cent) as major compounds (Beena *et al.*, 1997). Ent-kaur-16-en-19-oic acid and their derivatives were known to have plant growth stimulating activity and also have other biological activities including antibiotic, antitumor, tryptanosomicidal and anti-HIV virus (Silva *et al.*, 1999).

There were reports on fatty acids with unusually high molecular weight from the seeds of some of the Annonaceae species with toxic and insecticidal properties. The important fatty acids identified from the seed oils of Annonaceae are oleic acid, linoleic acid, myristic acid, palmitic acid, stearic acid, arachidic acid and unsaturated acids like palmitoleic and linolenic acids etc

(Hufford *et al.*, 1976, 1978). A number of Annonaceae plants are found to contain polyphenols. Phenolic acids such as caffeic acid, p–hydroxy benzoic acid, p-coumaric acid, vanillic acid etc. are present in many Annonaceae plants. The common flavanoids like quercetin, quercitrin, rutin etc. are present in the leaves of many Annonaceae plants (Chang *et al.*, 1998).

Ent–kauran-16-en-19-oic acid had the strongest termite antifeedant activity among the ent kauranes isolated. A dimeric kaurine diterpenoid, Annoglabayin, isolated from the fruits of annona glabra has been studied by (Chen *et al.*, 2004). The kaurane, methyl 16 α–hydro–19-al–ent–kauran-17-oate isolated from *Annona glabra* reported to have mild activity against HIV replication in H9 lymphocyte cells (Chang *et al.*, 1998). And the 16α-17-hydroxy–ent-kauran–19-oic acids showed significant inhibition of HIV reverse transcriptase. Over the past few years, investigation on some species in the genera such as Uvaria, Rollinia, Annona, Goniothalamus have resulted in the isolation and characterization of several novel acetogenins which are now referred to as Annonaceous acetogenins. They exhibit a broad range of bioactivities such as cytotoxicity, antitumor, antihelmintic, antimalaral, antioxidant, antiplatelet, antimicrobial, immunosuppressant, antifeedant, pesticidal and other miscellaneous activities (Shirwaikar *et al.*, 2004, Yang *et al.*, 2002, Kotkar *et al.*, 2002). These compounds have attracted much because of their interesting structural features. Many Annonaceae plants and their extracts have been extensively used in folk medicine as pesticides, antitumor agents, emetics etc. Undoubtedly many of these claims can be attributed to the compounds called acetogenins and the earlier reports also strengthened this view (Wu *et al.*, 1996; Colmansaizarbitoria *et al.*, 1998).

Numerous Annonaceous acetogenins have been shown to possess cytotoxic, pesticidal, antimalarial, cell growth inhibitory, antiparasitic and antimicrobial activities (Oberlies *et al.*, 1997; Chih *et al.*, 2001). Bullatacin is one such compound that possessed antitumoural and pesticidal activity *in vivo* (Ahmmadsahib *et al.*, 1993). Methanolic extracts of *Annona muricata* and *A. cherimola* seeds have been shown to have antiparasitic activity (Bories *et al.*, 1991). Six more Annonaceous acetogenins isolated from the seeds of *Annona atemoya* exhibited potent cytotoxicity against HepG2, KB, CCM2 and CEM cancer cell lines (Fong-Rong *et al.*, 1999). Squamocin, another Annonaceous acetogenin has been reported to exert antiproliferative effects on HL-60 cancer cells via activation of caspase-3 (Xiao-Feng *et al.*, 2002).

The chemistry and anti-inflammatory effects of the seed oils of *Annona squamosa* have been studied. (Beena *et al.*, 2006,1997). Anti-bacterial and anti-inflammatory kaurane type diterpenes were also identified in the extracts of fruit pericarp of *Annona squamosa* (Beena *et al.*, 2004, 2006, 2007). The pesticide activity of extracts and their formulations of Annonaceae were tested against a wide spectrum of pests of national importance (Santhosh and Beena., 1996, 1998). An Indian patent has also been allotted for this finding with IP No.180517, IPA No.637/DEL/dated 20-5-94. "A patent for new natural and environmentally safe bio pesticide formulation for teak defoliator and some other insects" (Patent, 1994). In our earlier studies we have identified biologically active kauranes from the fruit pericarp of *Annona squamosa* and *Annona reticulata*. The chemistry and anti-inflammatroy effects of seed oils of *Annona squamosa* were also studied against Carrageenan induced paw edema in albino rats (Beena *et al.*, 2004, 2006).

Materials and Methods

Chemical Examination of the Fruit Pericarp of *Annona squamosa*

Annona squamosa fruit was collected from a tree near Pappanamcode. It was identified (by Mrs.Valsala, Taxonomist) in the Department of Botany, University of Kerala, Karyavattom, Kerala. The fruit pericarp were separated, shade dried, powdered and extracted successively with hexane, chloroform and methanol in Soxhlet extraction apparatus for 48 hours in the case of each solvents. Since both the hexane and chloroform extract were similar in TLC, the extracts were mixed and subjected to column chromatography.

Chromatographic Separation of the Combined Hexane and Chloroform Extract

The combined yellowish extract (12g) was dissolved in ether (30 ml) and 40 gm silica gel was added. The ether was removed under vacuum and the powder was transferred to a column of silica gel (240 g) set in hexane. The column was successively eluted with hexane, hexane : ethyl acetate mixtures in the order of increasing polarity (95 : 5, 90 : 10, 80 : 20, 70 : 30, 50 : 50), ethyl acetate and methanol. 100ml of fractions were collected and concentrated. All fractions were monitored by TLC and grouped (Table 15.1).

Chemical Examination of the Fruit Pericarp of *Annona reticulata*

The fruit pericarp was separated, shade dried, powdered (dry weight 300g) and extracted successively with Petroleum ether and chloroform in a soxhlet extraction apparatus for 48 hours in each case. As both the extracts behaved similarly in TLC, they were mixed and subjected to column chromatography.

Table 15.1: Chromatographic Separation of the Combined Hexane and Chloroform Extract of *Annona squamosa*

Eluant	*Fraction No.*	*Group No.*	*Compound*
Petroleum ether	1–8	I	–
Petroleum ether: Ethyl acetate(95:5)	9–14	II	–
Petroleum ether : Ethyl acetate(90:10)	15–17	III	A
Petroleum ether : Ethyl acetate(90:10)	18–38	IV	–
Petroleum ether : Ethyl acetate(90:10)	39–45	V	C
Petroleum ether : Ethyl acetate(80:20)	46–52	VI	–
Petroleum ether : Ethyl acetate(80:20)	53–54	VII	B
Petroleum ether : Ethyl acetate(80:20)	55–61	VIII	D
Petroleum ether : Ethyl acetate(50:50)	62–75	IX	E

Chromatographic Separation of the Petroleum Ether and Chloroform Extracts

The yellowish Petroleum ether and Chloroform extract (10 g) were mixed and dissolved in diethyl ether (30 ml) and silica gel 30 g was added. It was evaporated under vacuum and the powder was transferred to a column of silica gel (240 g) set in hexane. The column was eluted successively with hexane : ethyl acetate mixtures in the increasing order of polarity (hexane, 95 : 5, 90 :10, 80 : 20, 70 : 30) and finally with ethyl acetate. Fractions of 100ml were collected and concentrated. All fractions were monitored and grouped (Table 15.2)

Table 15.2: Chromatographic Separation of the Petroleum Ether and Chloroform Extracts of *Annona reticulata*

Eluant	*Fraction No.*	*Group No.*	*Compound*
Hexane	1–6	I	–
Hexane : Ethyl acetate (95:5)	7–9	II	F
Hexane : Ethyl acetate (95:5)	10–18	III	–
Hexane : Ethyl acetate (90:10)	19–60	IV	–
Hexane : Ethyl acetate (90:10)	61–89	V	G
Hexane : Ethyl acetate (80:20)	90–105	VI	H
Hexane : Ethyl acetate (70:30)	106–118	VII	I
Ethyl acetate (100 per cent)	119–136	VIII	-

Extraction of Crude Oil from *Annona squamosa* and *Annona reticulata*

The seeds of *Annona squamosa* and *Annona reticulata* were grinded separately into fine powdered form. They were extracted separately with hexane (40–60 °C) at 30±2 °C for five days using soxhlet apparatus. The solvent was removed under vacuum under reduced pressure in a rotary evaporator. Both the oils were dissolved in minimum acetone and Tween 20, as an emulsifier. The four concentrations (0.6 per cent, 1.2 per cent, 2.5 per cent and 5 per cent) were prepared in water to which Tween 20 (0.2 per cent) was added as an emulsifier.

Effect of Crude Oils of *Annona squamosa* and *Annona reticulata* on Feeding and Development of *Spodoptera lithura* Larvae

Third instar larvae of *Spodoptera lithura* was taken as the test insect. The larvae were reared in the laboratory at specified conditions of temperature (26±1 ºC), at relative humidity (RH 75±5ºC) in Caster. Leaf discs with 4cm diameter soaked with each of the specific concentration of the solution were placed in identical petridishes and the larvae were released into it. After 24 hours, the leaves were replaced with freshly treated ones and allowed the larvae to feed for next 24 hr. The feacal pellets were collected after 24 and 48 hr, dried and weighed. The control larvae were released to leaf discs of same diameter, treated with solution without the oils. Four replication of each concentration were kept for experimental purpose.

Percentage of feeding inhibition was calculated using the following formula: (C-T)/C x 100, where 'C' is the weight of the feacal pellets of the control larvae, T is the weight of the feacal pellets of the experimental larvae. The number of dead larvae, pupae and emerged adults were also recorded.

Acute Toxicity Studies of the Crude Extracts from the Seeds of *Annona squamosa, Annona reticulata* and *Annona muricata*

The seeds were separated, washed, dried and reduced to 60 mesh size. The powder was then extracted successively with Petroleum ether, chloroform and methanol. These extracts were used for pharmacological studies.

Male Wister albino rats weighing between 200 to 250g were used for the study. They were housed in polypropylene cages in an adequately ventilated room. The rats were given standard rat feed and water *ad libitum* through out the course of the study. The animals were divided into 6 groups of five each. The test extracts of *Annona squamosa* and *Annona reticulata* and *Annona muricata* seeds were administered orally to different groups in increasing dose levels of 125,250, 500, 1000 and 2000mg/kg body weight. The animals were then observed continuously for 1 hour and then frequently for 24 hours and thereafter once daily for 14 days. During this period the animals were observed for gross behavioral and morphological profiles.

Anti-inflammatory Studies of the Crude Extracts from the Seeds of *Annona squamosa, Annona reticulata* and *Annona muricata* by Carragennan Induced *Paw oedema*

48 albino rats of either sex ranging from 150 to 200 g were randomly selected and fasted for 18 hours before the experiment, but had free access to water. The animals were divided into six groups of six each.The three extracts were administered orally to six groups of six rats in doses of 250 mg and 500mg/kg body weight. The control rats received 5 per cent *Acacia* solution in a volume of 1ml/100g body weight. Standard drug given was Indomethacin at a dose of 20mg/kg of body weight in a volume of 1ml/100g body weight.One hour after the oral administration of the extracts, control and standard, 0.1ml of each of 1 per cent carrageenan in normal saline was injected into the plantar aponeurosis of the left hind paw of the rat. The thickness of the paw was measured by using the Vernier Calipers and recorded.

The hind paw thickness of the each albino rats were again measured after three hours of the carrageenan injection. The difference in initial and final thickness of the paw indicates the increase in paw volume due to oedema. The activity of the drug was compared with that of standard Indomethacin 20mg/kg body weight. The results are summarized in Table 15.4.

Table 15.3: Anti-inflammatory Effect of Seed Oils of *Annona squamosa*, *Annona reticulata* and *Annona muricata*

Groups	Dose	Initial Thickness of the Paw (in mm)	Final Thickness of the Paw (in mm)	Mean Increase in Paw Thickness± S.D (in mm)	Reduction in the Paw Thickness (in mm)	Inhibition of Oedema	P Value
1	Control 5 per cent Acacia solution	5.294	6.79	1.496±0.284	–	–	–
2	*Annona squamosa* seed oil 250 mg/kg	5.31	6.408	1.098±0.0879	0.398	26.6 per cent	<0.05
3	*Annona.squamosa* seed oil 500mg/kg	5.442	6.358	0.916±0.0786	0.58	38.77 per cent	< 0.05
4	*Annona reticulata* seed oil 250 mg/kg	6.5868	6.9394	0.3526±0.0378	1.4414	80.35 per cent	<0.001
5	*Anonna reticulata* seed oil 500mg/kg	6.4532	6.6868	0.2336±0.06688	1.5604	86.98 per cent	<0.001
6	*Annona muricata* seedoil 250mg/kg	5.714	6.478	0.764±0.266	0.732	48.93 per cent	<0.01
7	*Annona muricata* seed oil 500 mg/kg	5.112	5.998	0.886±0.4866	0.61	40.78 per cent	<0.05
8	Indomethacin 20 mg/kg	6.234	6.7528	0.5188±0.1129	1.275	71.07 per cent	<0.001

Table 15.4: Anti-inflammatory Effect of (-)–Ent kaur–17,–19–dioic acid and 16α, 17 Dihydroxykaur–19–oic Acid on Carrageenan Induced Paw Oedema

Groups/Dose	Mean Increase in Thickness±S.D (mm)	Reduction in the Paw Volume	% Inhibition of Oedema	P Value
Control 5 per cent acacia solution	1.794±0.3944	–	–	–
(-)–Ent–kaur–17,–19–dioic acid 100 mg/kg	0.3526±0.0378	1.4414	80.35	<0.001
16α, 17–Dihydroxy, kaur–19–oic acid 100 mg/kg	0.02336±0.0668	1.5604	86.98	< 0.001
Indomethacin 20 mg/kg	0.5188±0.1129	1.275	71.07	<0.001

Isolation of the Active Anti-inflammatory Compounds

The pericarp was separated, dried and reduced to coarse powder. This was then subjected to successive solvent extraction using petroleum ether, chloroform and methanol. The combined petroleum ether and chloroform extracts of *Annona squamosa* and *Annona reticulata* fruit pericarp were screened for anti–inflammatory activity. Both the petroleum ether and chloroform extracts behaved similar in TLC and hence they were combined and fractionated with hexane, 80 : 20 hexane and ethyl acetate, 50:50 hexane and ethyl acetate and 100 per cent ethyl acetate and methanol. The fractions were screened for anti-inflammatory activity.

Table 15.5: Antibacterial Activity of Kauranes from *Annonaceae*

Sl.No.	*Sample*		*Staphylococcus aureus Zone of Inhibition (mm)*	*Average*	*E. Coli Zone of Inhibition (mm)*	*Average*
1.	Ampicillin		–	–	20	20
	1000 μ gm				20	
2.	Gentamycin 850 μ gm		26 26	26	-	-
3.	16α,17-Di hydroxy–ent–kauran-19-oic acid	100 μ gm	4 4	4	10 11	10.5
		500 μ gm	9 9	9	17 18	17.5
4.	(-)–Ent–kaur–17-acetoxy,19–oic acid	100 μ gm	6 6	6	8 8	8
		500 μ gm	9 8	8.5	10 10	10
5.	(-)–Ent–kaur 17, 19–dioic acid	100 μ gm	6 6	6	8 9	8.5
		500 μ gm	9 9	9	17 17	17

Anti-bacterial Study of the Pure Compounds Isolated from the Pericarp of *Annona squamosa* and *Annona reticulata*

The detection of the anti-bacterial activity of the pure compounds isolated from the extracts of *Annona squamosa* and *Annona reticulata* were made by observing their effects on growing cultures of bacteria. Nutrient agar was used for anti bacterial study. The culture of *Eschrichia coli* and *Staphylococus aureus* were used for the study. The bacteria were sub cultured on sterile nutrient agar slants prepared in test tubes incubated at 37°C±0.5°C for 24 hours.

Two concentrations of the test samples, (-)–Ent–kaur–17-acetoxy,19–oic acid, 16α,17-Dihydroxy–ent–kauran-19-oic acid and (-)–Ent-Kaur 17,19-dioic acid (10 mg/ml and 50 mg/ml) were dissolved in methanol disc of 6mm were cut from Whatmann filter paper No. 1 and sterilized in the autoclave. 100 filter paper discs were placed in 1ml each of the test samples so that they contained 100 μgm and 500 μgm respectively. 100 discs were placed in 1ml of methanol to be treated as the control. The numbers 1-6 were marked on the bottom of the petri-dishes. 1000 μ gm disc of Ampicillin and 850 μ gm disc of Gentamycin were used as standard. They were placed in the medium in the petridishes, where it was labeled as 1 and 2 respectively. Then the disc of each of the test samples were placed in the appropriate marked area in the dish. The control disc was also placed in the appropriate marked area. Plates were prepared for each organism similarly and incubated at 37°C±0.5 °C for 24 hours. The presence of a definite zone of inhibition of any size surrounding the paper disc would indicate antibacterial activity. The results were summarized in Table 15.6.

Table 15.6: Composition of *Annona squamosa* Leaf Oil

Sl.No.	*Compound*	*Retention Time*
1.	β–Ocimene	16.97
2.	α–Terpinene	17.34
3.	Thymol	24.75
4.	Methyl eugenol	26.65
5.	Geranyl acetate	27.47
6.	α–Copane	28.02
7.	β–Elemene	28.32
8.	β–Caryophyllene	28.97
9.	β–cedrene	29.48
10.	A–Humulene	30.02
11.	Allo–aromadendrene	30.43
12.	Germacrene D	30.85
13.	α–Bisabolene	31.41
14.	β–Bisabolene	31.45
15.	Calamencene	31.58
16.	Cadina–1, 4–diene	32.11
17.	Elemol	32.57
18.	(E)–nerolidol	32.72
19.	Caryophyllene alcohol	32.85
20.	Caryophyllene oxide	33.16
21.	B–Cedrene epoxide	33.98
22.	Humulene epoxide	34.19
23.	β–Eudesmol	35.48
24.	α–Cadinol	35.70
25.	α–Bisabolol	36.00
26.	Cedrol	34.38
27	(Z, E)–Farnesol	37.64
28.	(E, E)–Farnesol	40.8

Cell Viability Assay by MTT [3-(4,5-Dimethylthiazol-2-yl)-2,5 Diphenyltetrazolium bromide] on Dalton's Lymphoma Ascites Cells (DLA)

Five thousand cells were plated in 100 µl of the medium (Dulbecco's Modified Eagle's Medium (DMEM) with 10 per cent Foetal Bovine Serum (FBS) in 96-well Corning plates in the presence or absence of various concentrations of the extracts for 24, 48, and 72 h. Media-treated cells were taken as a negative control. At the end of incubation, 25 µl of MTT solution (5 mg/ml in phosphate buffered saline (PBS) was added to each well. After a 2 h incubation at 37°C, 100µl of the extraction buffer was added (20 per cent sodium dodecyl sulfate) in 50 per cent dimethylformamide. After a 4-h incubation, the optical density (OD) at 570 nm was taken using a multiwell plate reader with the extraction buffer as a blank (Scudiero *et al.*, 1988). The percentage of cytotoxicity was calculated as:

$$\% \text{ cell cytotoxicity} = \frac{100\text{–TreatedOD}}{\text{Control OD}} \times 100$$

Extraction of Essential Oil from the Leaves of *Annona squamosa* and *Annona reticulata*

The leaves of *Annona squamosa* and *Annona reticulata* were collected locally from,Trivandrum and were shade dried. Both the plants were identified by the Taxonomist of University of Kerala and a voucher specimen is kept at Department of Botany, University of Kerala. Essential oils from both the plants were extracted by Clevenger distillation method.

Capillary GC and GC-MS Analysis

Hewlett Packard 5980 A and HP 5890 FID gas chromatographs equipped with a fused silica capillary column (50m x 0.25 mm) coated methyl silicone (thickness 0.17mm) were used for the GC analysis of the essential oils. GC conditions used were nitrogen as carrier gas with a flow rate of (1ml/min), split ratio 1:75, injection temp. 250°C, FID temp 300 °C and the column temperature was programmed from 80°C to 200°C at the rate of 5 °C/min. GC–MS analysis was conducted using a Hewlett Packard 5995 GC-MS equipped with the same capillary column under same GC conditions. The MS conditions used were electron impact, ionizing voltage 70 e V with source temperature 150°C, electron multiplier at 2000eV, scan speed at 690amu/second and scan range 40–500 amu.Compound identification was made by using a combination of Kovats indices followed by co-injection with authentic samples (wherever possible) or from the mass spectral fragmentation pattern of compounds. In mass spectral analysis the constituents were identified by matching the mass spectra with those of authentic standards held in the NBS Library on Flavour and Fragrance and also the library generated in our laboratory. Only similarity indices of 0.95 or higher were taken as proof identity.

Results and Discussion

Compounds from *Annona squamosa*

The pale yellow residue from the hexane and chloroform extracts of the pericarp of *Annona squamosa* yielded five crystalline compounds A, B, C, D and E. The structures of the compounds are given below (Figures 15.1–15.5).

Compound A : (-)–Ent–kaur–16-en–19-oic acid

The compound A was identified as (-)–Ent–kaur–16-en–19-oic acid. It was crystallized from hexane : ethyl acetate (95 : 5) mixture as white blocks, m.p 170°C (Lit m.p 167–171 °C) [37].

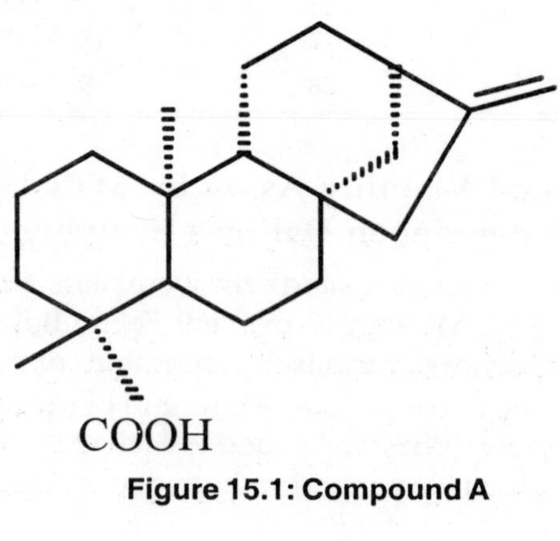

Figure 15.1: Compound A

Compound B : (-)–Ent–kaur–17-hydroxy–19-al

The Compound B was identified as (-)–Ent–Kaur–17-hydroxy–19-al. The compound was crystallized from hexane: ethyl acetate (90: 10) as white needles, with (α) =–49 (c = 0.6, $CHCl_3$) and m. p 170–172 °C (Lit 174–176 °C).

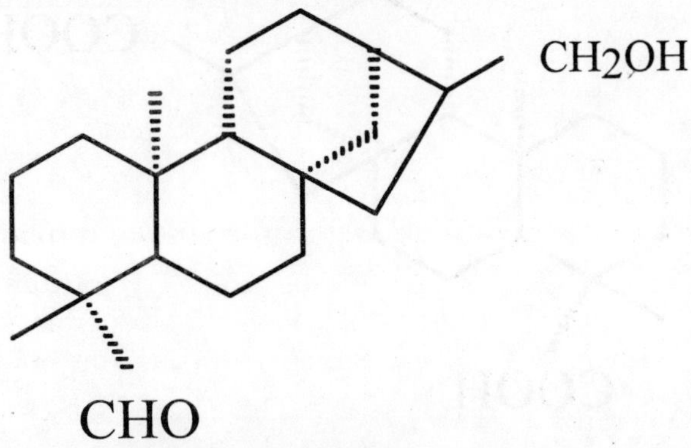

Figure 15.2: Compound B

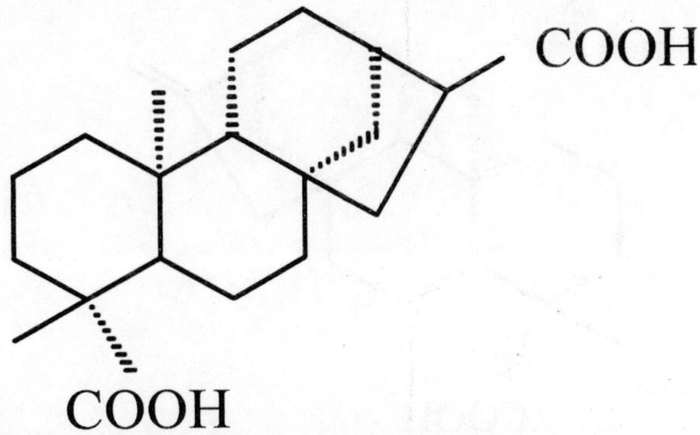

Figure 15.3: Compound C

Compound C: (-)–Ent–kaur–17,19–dioic acid

The Compound C is identified as (-)–Ent–kaur–17, 19–dioic acid, crystallized from ethyl acetate and traces of hexane as white amorphous powder (40 mg) m.p. 222°C.

Compound D: (-)–Ent–Kaur–17-acetoxy–19-oic acid

The Compound D was identified as (-)–Ent–Kaur–17-acetoxy–19-oic acid, crystallised from ethyl acetate as white amorphous powder with m.p 200°C (40 mg).

Compound E : 16 α, 17–Dihydroxy–ent–kauran 19-oic acid

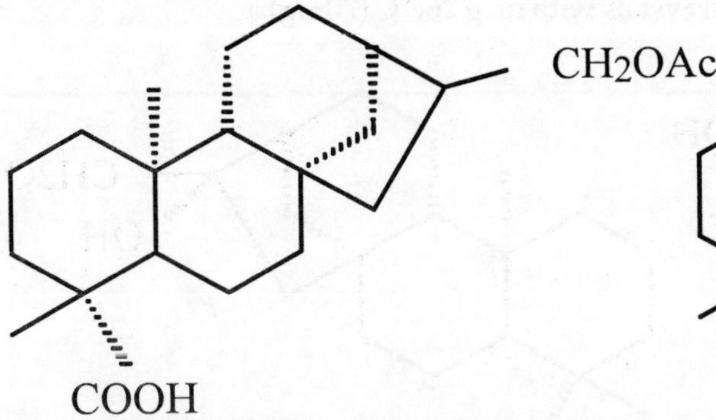

Figure 15.4: Compound D

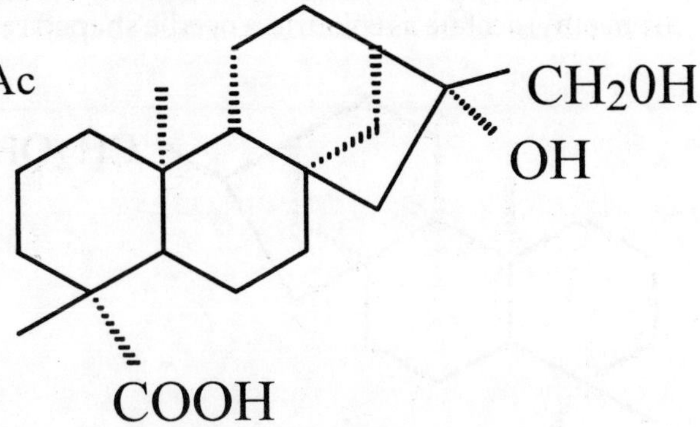

Figure 15.5: Compound E

Compounds from *Annona reticulate*

The pale yellowish residue obtained from the hexane extract and chloroform extract behaved identically in TLC. The mixed extracts were chromatographed and four compounds, Compound F, G, H and I were isolated and characterized (Figures 15.6–15.9).

Compound F

The Compound F is identified as (-)–Ent–kauran–16-en–19-oic acid. It was crystallized from hexane as colourless blocks (40 mg) m.p. 171°C with $[\alpha]_{D-}$112°C (c,0.3, $CHCl_3$).

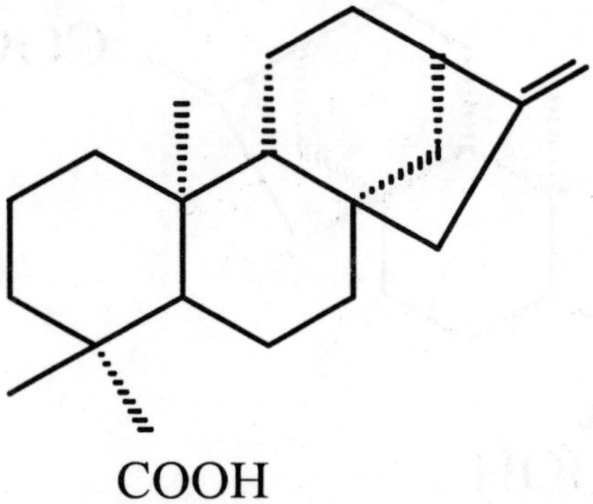

Figure 15.6: Compound F

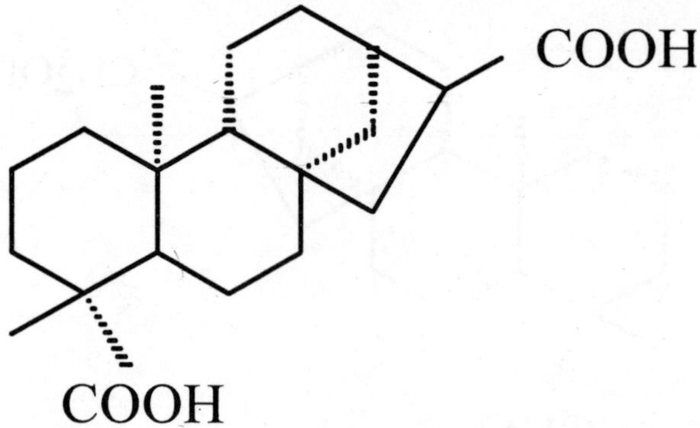

Figure 15.7: Compound G

Compound G: (-)–Ent–kauran–17,19–dioic acid

The Compound G is identified as (-)–Ent–kauran–17,19-dioic acid and was crystallized from hexane : ethyl acetate mixture as colourless blocks m.p. 222°C.

Compound H: (-)–Ent–19–carbomethoxy–kauran-17-ol

The Compound H is identified as (-)–Ent–19–carbomethoxy–kauran–17-ol and was crystallized from ethyl acetate : hexane mixture as a white amorphous powder with m.p. 165 °C (45 mg).

Compound I: Methyl, 16α, 17–dihydroxy–(-)–kauran–19–oate

The Compound I is identified as Methyl,16 α,17-dihydroxy–(-)–kauran-19-oate. It was crystallized from ethyl acetate as colourless needle shaped crystals with m. p 266°C (70mg).

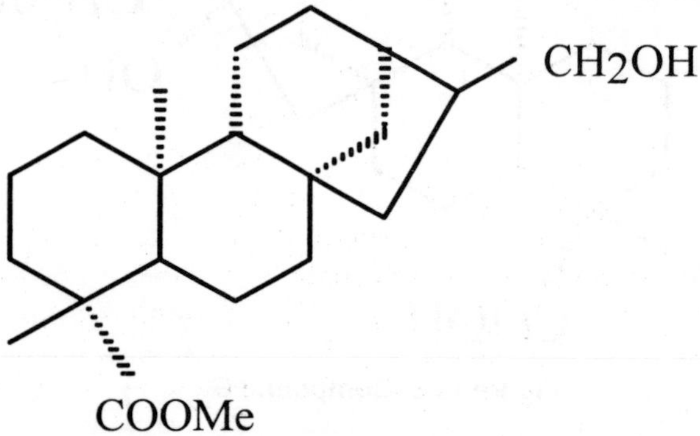

Figure 15.8: Compound H

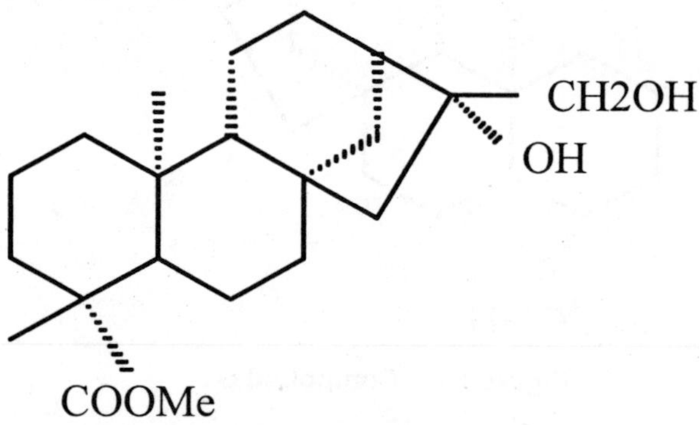

Figure 15.9: Compound I

Effect of Crude Oils of *Annona squamosa* and *Annona reticulata* on Feeding and Development of *Spodoptera lithura* Larvae

After 24 hours of feeding with 2.5 and 5 per cent oil treated leaves, a significant reduction in the weight of the feacal pellets was observed. The amount of feacal pellets was increased except at 5 per cent concentration level treatment. At 2.5 and 5 per cent concentrations, the oils show feed deterrent effect also. The mortality rate was not affected within 48 hours, and which was appreciable above 50 per cent concentrations.And in the case of larvae and pupae stages mortality rate was affected at 5 per cent concentrations. Pupation and pupal weight were not affected except at 5 per cent concentration where the formation of the pupae was observed for both oils. The adult emergence was pronounced when treated with extracts of *Annona reticulata.* The results thus indicated that the oils of *Annona squamosa* and *Annona reticulata* at higher concentrations like 2.5 and 5 per cent caused feeding deterrence and also caused death of the larvae of *Spodoptera lithura*. The study revealed the effectiveness of the seed oils of *Annona reticulata* and *Annona squamosa* as a feeding deterrent against the *Spodoptera lithura* larvae.

Acute Toxicity Studies

The acute toxicity studies of the hexane extracts (seed oils) of *Annona squamosa, Annona reticulata* and *Annona muricata* up to a dose level of 2000 mg/kg of body weight showed no mortality. Morphological profiles were also noticed for the animals.

Anti-inflammatory Studies

Anti-inflammatory studies revealed significant activity for the three extracts studied. The hexane extract of *Annona reticulata* showed very significant inhibition of oedema when compared to Indomethacin, the standard imparting the same activity. *Annona squamosa* hexane extract (seed oil) is showing only minimum activity, *i.e.* when *Annona reticulata* seed oil showed 80-86 per cent of inhibition of oedema and 40-48 per cent was exhibited by *Annona muricata* seed oil,only 27-39 per cent of inhibition was exhibited by *Annona squamosa* seed oil. Here in *Annona muricata* the activity is not dose dependent. But in *Annona reticulata* seed oil it is more dose dependent. This study therefore revealed that the three seed oils of Annona *squamosa, Annona reticulata* and *Annona muricata* were anti–inflammatory and the seed oil of *Annona reticulata* being the powerful one (Table 15.3).

Isolation of Active Anti-inflammatory Compounds from *Annona Squamosa* and *Annona reticulata*

The 50: 50 hexane ethyl acetate fraction of *Annona squamosa* was the most significant fraction giving anti-inflammatory activity and 80 : 20 fraction in the case of *Annona reticulata*. These particular fractions were chromatographed and two compounds were isolated and identified as kauranes, 16α, 17-Dihydroxy, kaur-19-oic acid and (-)-Ent–kaur–17, 19–dioic acid respectively. Both the compound showed very significant anti-inflammatory activity comparable to Indomethacin as illustrated in the Table 15.4. The compound, 16α, 17-Dihydroxy,kaur 19-oic acid isolated from *Annona squamosa* fruit pericarp is found to be much more active than the other. The compound, 16α, 17-Dihydroxy,kaur 19-oic acid showed 86.98 per cent of inhibition of oedema when compared to the control. Whereas the compound, (-)–Ent–kaur–17,19-dioic acid Showed 80.35 per cent of inhibition of oedema only compared to Indomethacin 20mg/kg of body weight.

Acute Toxicity Studies of the of the Two Compounds, (-)–Ent–kaur–17,19-dioic Acid and 16α, 17-Dihydroxy, Kaur 19-oic Acid

Acute toxicity studies of the of the two compounds, (-)–Ent–kaur–17,19-dioic acid and 16α, 17-Dihydroxy,kaur 19-oic acid showed no mortality up to 400 mg/kg body weight but the maximum dose showed depression in the animal after a period of 45 minutes.

These studies therefore provide a basis for further detailed investigations on the therapeutic efficacy of these two kauranes isolated from *Annona squamosa* fruit pericarp and *Annona reticulata* fruit pericarp by conducting clinical trials to ascertain their anti-inflammatory potential in the indigenous system of medicine.

Table 15.7: Composition of the Essential oil of *Annona reticulata* Leaf

Sl.No	*Retention Time*	*Compound*
1	9.5	2-methyl pentene
2	13.73	β-myrecene
3	16.9	Linalool
4	20.62	α-terpineol
5	20.75	β–elemene
6	21.6	β–caryophyllene
7	22.24	α–humulene
8	22.47	α–farnescene
9	22.8	β–farnescene
10	22.95	calarene
11	23.34	aromadendrene
12	23.6	Logipinene epoxide
13	24.9	spathulenol
14	25.3	farnesol
15	26.5	Δ-cadinol
17	26.9	nerolidol

Antibacterial Activity of the Compounds from *Annona squamosa* and *Annona reticulata*

Compounds,16α,17-Dihydroxy–ent-kauran-19-oicacid, (-)–Ent–kaur-17-acetoxy, 19-oic acid and (-)–Ent–kaur–17,19-oic acid obtained from the fruit pericarp of *Annona squamosa* and *Annona reticulata* were screened for their anti-bacterial studies with Ampicillin and Gentamycin as standards at concentrations of 1000 μ gm and 850 μ gm respectively. The zone of inhibition produced by the compounds on comparison with the standards were found to be very significant. This could be established from the Table 15.5. When Ampicillin showed a zone of inhibition 20mm against *E. coli*, 16α,17-Dihydroxy-ent–kauran-19-oic acid showed 10.5 and 17.5 mm of zone of inhibition at 100 and 500 μ gm concentrations, which is double the effect as the standard. The compound, (-)–Ent-kaur-17-acetoxy, 19-oic acid showed a zone of inhibition 8 and 10mm for the two concentrations respectively. The compound (-)–Ent–kaur-17,19-dioic acid showed a zone of inhibition 8.5 and 17 mm at 100 and 500 μ gm concentrations. But with *Staphylococous aureus* these compounds are not exhibiting much activity.

Cytotoxicity Assays

Bioactivity-guided fractionation and isolation yielded two crystalline compounds.

Compound 1 (-)-entkaur-16-en-19-oic acid and Compound 2 16a,17–dihydroxy-ent-kauran-19-oic acid were found to be the active compounds which exhibited cytotoxicity against DLA cells.

There was an increase in the percentage cytotoxicity with increasing concentrations of the fraction containing the compounds (Figures 15.10 and 15.11). However a slight decrease in activity with

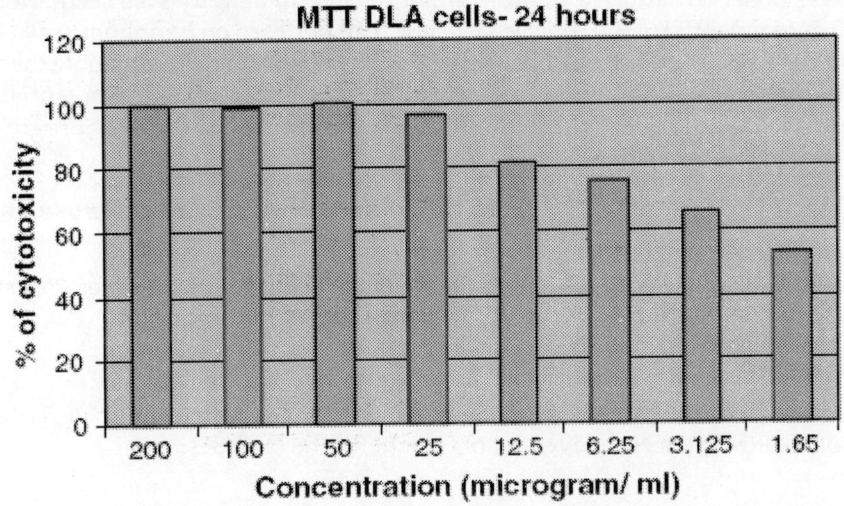

Figure 15.10: MTT Assay–Per cent of Cytotoxicity on DLA Cells–24 Hours

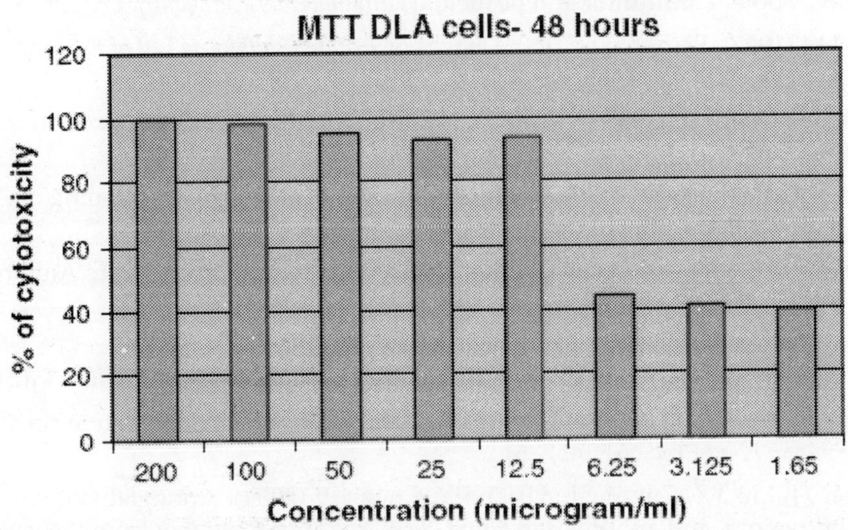

Figure 15.11: MTT Assay–Per cent of Cytotoxicity on DLA Cells–48 Hours

increasing incubation time was noted, which implies that the compound has very high cytotoxicity even after 24 h of incubation. Even at a concentration of 1.65 g/ml, the compounds exhibited more than 50 per cent cytotoxicity after 24 h. The highest activity was noted after 24 h, which implies that the efficacy of secondary metabolites as cytotoxic agents at a low dose and a short duration. The search for new chemopreventive and antitumor agents that are more effective and less toxic has kindled great interest in phytochemicals. This is the first report of antitumor agents from *Annona squamosa* fruit. Almost 100 per cent cytotoxicity was observed against DLA cells treated with 50 µg/ml of the active fraction containing the compounds after a short time interval of 24 h. Almost the same level of activity was observed after 48 h, but a slight decline in activity was seen after 72 h. This suggests the antitumor potential of the *Annona squamosa* fruit pericarp on lymphoma cells specifically. More extensive studies are needed to be done with the active compounds to elucidate the mechanism of action of the compounds against cancer cells and apoptosis. This reveals the potential of the fruit pericarp as a pharmacologically effective antitumor agent and *in vivo* studies are in progress to further explore their efficacy in this regard.

GC-MS Analysis of the Essential Oil from the Leaves of *Annona squamosa* and *Annona reticulata*

The percentage composition for each of the components of both the plant leaves are listed in Table 6 and 7 in the order of their elution from the GC column. (Tables 15.6 and 15.7)

Acknowledgements

The author would like to acknowledge the Director NIIST, Trivandrum and Dr. T.Vijayakumar, Director, School of Health Sciences, University of Calicut for the facilities.

References

Ahmmadsahib K I, Hollingworth R M, McGovren J P, Hui Y and McLaughlin J L(1993). Mode of action of bullatacin: A potent antitumor and pesticidal *Annonaceous acetogenin*. *Life Sci.*, 53: 1113–1120.

Beena Joy, Rao J M.(1997). Essential oil of the leaves of *Annona squamosa* L. *J of Essential Oil Research*, 9:349–51.

Beena Joy, Sr. Molly Mathew, Gopi TV (2004). Antiinflammatory effects of some Annona seed oils. *Indian Drugs*, 41:10

Beena Joy, Gopi TV., Sobhana D (2006). Chemistry and pharmacological screening of Annona seed oils. *Asian J. of Chemistry*, 18: 1125.

Beena Joy, Sobhana D (2007). Asian J Of Chemistry, Antibacterial Kauranes from Annonaceae. *Asian J of Chemistry*, 19: 4, 2773.

Bories C, Loiseau P, Cortes D, Myint S H, Hocquemiller R, Gayral P, Cave A and Laurens A (1991). Antiparasitic activity of *Annona muricata* and *Annona cherimolia* seeds. *Planta Med*.. 57 434–436.

Chang F. R, Yang P. Y, Lin, J. Y, Lee, K. H, Wu, Y. C.(1998) Antiplatelet aggregation constituents from *Annona purpurea*. *J Nat Prod.*, 61:1457–61.

Chen CH, Hsieh TJ, Liu TZ, Chern CL, Hsieh PY, Chen CY (2004). Annoglabayin a novel dimeric kaurane diterpenoid, and apoptosis in Hep G2 cells of annomontacin from the fruits of *Annona glabra*. *J Nat Prod.*, 67: 1942-6.

Chih H W, Chiu H F, Tang K S, Chang F r AND Wu Y C.(2001). Bullatacin, a potent antitumour Annonaceous acetogenin, inhibits proliferation of human hepatocarcinoma cell line 2.2.15 by apoptosis induction. *Life Sci.*, 69: 1321-1331

Colman Saizarbitoria, T, Johnson, H. A, Alali F. Q, Hopp D. C. Rogers, L. L., McLaughlin, J.L (1998). Annojahnin from *Annona jahnii*: a possible precursor of mono-tetrahydrofuran acetogenins. *Phytochemistry*, 49 : 1609.

Fong-Rong C, Jien-Lin C, Chih-Yuan L, Hui-Fen C, Ming-Jung W and Yang-Chang W (1999). Bioactive acetogenins from the seeds of *Annona atemoya*. *Phytochemistry*, 51: 883–889.

Hufford C. D, LassWell W. L (1976). Uvaretin and isouvaretin. Two novel cytotoxic c-benzylflavanones from *Uvaria chamae. J. Org. Chem.*, 41:1297.

Hufford C D, LassWell W L (1978). Antimicrobial activities of constituents of *Uvaria chama. J. Lloydia*, 41. 156.

Kotkar HM, Mendki PS, Sadan SV, Jha SR, Upasani SM,Maheshwari VL (2002). Antimicrobial and pesticidal activity of partially purified flavonoids of *Annona squamosa, Pest Manag Sci.*, 58(1):33-37.

Patent. A Process for new natural and environmentally safe biopesticide formulation for teak defoliator and some other insects. No.637/DEL/dated 24-3-94.

Pardhasaradhi B V V, Madhurima Reddy, Mubarak Ali A, Leela Kumari A and Ashok Khar. (2005) Differential cytotoxic effects of *Annona squamosa* seedd extracts on human tumour cell lines: Role of reactive oxygen species and glutathione. *J. Biosci.*, 30: 237–244.

Oberlies N H, Chang c J, McLaughlin J L. (1997). Structure-activity relationships of Diverse Annonaceous acetogenins against multidrug resistant human mammary adenocarcinoma (MCF-7/Adr) cells. *J Med Chem.*, 40: 2102-2106.

Santhosh P B, Rao J M and Beena Joy (1996). Evaluation of some plant extracts as feeding deterrents against adult *Longitarsus nigripennis. Mots. Entomon.*, 21: 291.

Santhosh.PB, Rao JM, and Beena Joy (1998). Effect of Crude Oils of *Annona squamosa* and *Annona reticulata* on feeding and development of *Spodoptera lithura* Larvae. *J.of Insect Science*, 11: 184.

Shirwaikar A, Rajendran K, Kumar CD.(2004). *In vitro* antioxidant studies of *Annona squamosa* Linn. Leaves. *Indian J Exp Biol.*, 42(8): 803-7.

Silva E. A, Takahashi J.A, Boaventura M. A. D, Oliveira, A. B (1999).The biotransformation of ent-kaur-16-en-19-oic acid by *Rhizopus stolonifer. Phytochemistry*, 52 : 397.

Xiao-Feng Z, Zong-Chao L, Bin-Fen X, Zhi-Ming L, Gong–Kan F, Hai-Hui X, Shu-Jun W, Ren-Zhou Y, Xiao-Yi W and Yi-Xin Z (2002). Involvement of caspase-3 activation in squamocin–induced apoptosis in leukemia cell line HL-60. *Life Sci.*, 70: 1259–1269.

Utilisation and Management of Medicinal Plants (2010) *Pages 294–305*
Editors: **V.K. Gupta, Anil K. Verma and Sushma Koul**
Published by: **DAYA PUBLISHING HOUSE, NEW DELHI**

Chapter 16

Saffron: A High Value Crop

Sushma Koul[1]*, Esha Abrol[1], Bilal A. Mir[1] and A.K. Koul[2]
[1]Indian Institute of Integrative Medicine,
Canal Road, Jammu – 180 001, India
[2]Baba Gulam Badshaw University
Rajouri, Jammu, India

ABSTRACT

Saffron or *Crocus sativus*, world's most expensive spice, is obtained from the stigmas of the flower of *Crocus sativus* Linn., commonly known as Rose of Saffron. *Crocus sativus* belongs to the family Iridaceae and is characterized for having a purple flower with red stigmas and yellow stamens. The flower of *Crocus sativus* is sterile, because it is a hybrid that has been maintained for centuries because of the value of its stigmas. The reproduction of this plant is done with bulbs. Each flower of *Crocus sativus* has three stigmas of saffron, also called filaments, which are joined by the style. The stigmas are of trumpet shape, they are bright red gradually changing to yellow in the style. The history of introduction of saffron is not well documented; however, some evidences suggest that saffron was available in Kashmir about 500 B.C. Saffron fields of Pampore existed even when Kalidas wrote his literary masterpiece. The spice is so expensive because it must be harvested by hand, and it takes more than 4,000 of tiny flower stigmas to yield about 28g of saffron. Put another way, an acre of established planting yields 4-5 kg of the spice. This paper reviews botany, utility, chemical composition and pharmacological activities of saffron (*Crocus sativus*).

***Keywords**: Saffron, Crocus sativus, Zeaxanthin, Crocin, Picrocrocin, Crocetin, Iridaceae.*

* Corresponding Author: E-mail: koul_sushma@rediffmail.com.

Introduction

Saffron is a spice derived from the dried stigma of the flower of the saffron (Crocus sativus), a species of crocus in the family Iridaceae. The flower has three stigmas, which are the distal ends of the plant's carpels. Saffron is characterised by a bitter taste and an iodoform–or hay-like fragrance; these are caused by the chemicals picrocrocin and safranal. It also contains a carotenoid dye, crocin, that gives food a rich golden-yellow hue. These traits make saffron a much-sought ingredient in many foods worldwide. Saffron also has medicinal applications. The word saffron originated from the 12th-century Old French term safran, which is derived from the Latin word safranum. Safranum is also related to the Italian zafferano and Spanish azafrán. Safranum comes from the Arabic word as far which means "yellow," via the Persian paronymous zafaran. The deep orange-red stigma is best described by its Sanskrit name, 'Agni shikha'. Stigma of no other plant is as elegant and valuable as that autumn crocus. "Kong-tehej", as the dry stigma lobe of *C. sativus* is called in Kashmiri, symbolizes feminine grace and elegance

Botany

Saffron, *Crocus sativus* Linnaeus, is a stern less perennial grass plant with a round sub-soil corm of 3-5cm diameter. Each corn produces 6 to 8 leaves similar to grass weeds. The short sprinkle roots grow at the base and circumference of the corm. The first part to appear in early autumn is the flower. However, in the first year after planting, because the corms are too weak and not properly established in the deep soil yet, the flower buds are not strong enough to develop and even the leaves come out later than usual. The flower consists of three sepals and three petals of the same lilac color which makes them hardly distinguishable. There are three stamens with filaments twice as long as the anthers. Out of the single-ovule ovary in the center of the flower grows a long thin style of a light yellow color, which ends in a bright orange red color triple stigma of 2-3 cm length.

Distribution

Saffron is grown mostly in a belt of land ranging from the Mediterranean in the west to Kashmir in the east. The entire genus lies within the range longitude 10°W to 80°E, latitude 30°N to 50°N. Iran ranks first in the world production of saffron, with more than 94 percent of the world yield. Other minor producers of saffron are Spain, India, Greece, Azerbaijan, Morocco, and Italy. In India major cultivation of saffron is confined to Jammu and Kashmir state, with Anantnag, Badgam, Baramulla and Pulwama as the major producer districts of Kashmir. In Jammu division saffron is cultivated on approximately 140 hectares at Kishtwar of district Doda. The total land area devoted to saffron cultivation in the Jammu and Kashmir state is 6,000 hectares (Mir, 1984). Attempts made to extend saffron cultivation to Kumaon, Joshi Math, Biser, Bharsar, Uttarakhand and Chaubathia, all in U. P., and to Kinnaur-district of Himachal Pradesh have been successful (Srivastava, 1964; Mathur, 1973). Today, saffron is cultivated from the Western Mediterranean (Spain) to India (Kashmir). Spain and Iran are the largest producers, accounting together for more than 80 per cent of the world's production, which is approximately 300 tons per year. In Europe, saffron production is almost limited to the Mediterranean. Spanish (La Mancha) saffron is generally considered the best. In much smaller scale, saffron is also cultivated in Italy and Greece (Crete).

History

The history of saffron cultivation reaches back-to more than 3,000 years. The wild precursor of domesticated saffron crocus was *Crocus cartwrightianus*. Human cultivators bred wild specimens by selecting for unusually long stigmas. Thus, a sterile mutant form of *C. cartwrightianus*, *C. sativus*, emerged in late Bronze Age Crete. Experts believe saffron was first documented in a 7th century BC Assyrian botanical reference compiled under Ashurbanipal. Since then, documentation of saffron's use over the span of 4,000 years in the treatment of some 90 illnesses has been uncovered.

Although the origin of saffron is confusing, we can almost confirm that it comes from Orient, because its cultivation was widely spread in Minor Asia far before the birth of Chirst. One of the most historic references to the use of saffron comes from Ancient Egypt, where it was used by eoptra and other Pharaons as an aromatic and seductive essence and to make ablutions in temples and sacred places.

Cultivation and Harvesting

The saffron crocus thrives in climates similar to that of the Mediterranean maquis or the North American chaparral, where hot, dry summer breezes blow across arid and semi-arid lands. Nevertheless, the plant can tolerate cold winters, surviving frosts as cold as 10 °C (14 °F) and short periods of snow cover. However, if not grown in wet environments like Kashmir (where rainfall averages 1000–1500 mm annually), irrigation is needed–this is true in the saffron-growing regions of Greece (500 mm of rainfall annually) and Spain (400 mm).The cultivation of saffron needs an extreme climate; hot and dry weather in summer and cold in winter. The land must be dry, calcareous, aired, flat and without trees. The soil must be equilibrated in organic material in order to avoid risks of erosion, and have some depth that allows the water to drain so that the bulb is not damaged. Raised beds are traditionally used to promote good drainage. Historically, soil organic content was boosted via application of some 20–30 tones of manure per hectare. Afterwards–and with no further manure application–corms were planted.

Rainfall timing is also key: generous spring rains followed by relatively dry summers are optimal. In addition, rainfall occurring immediately prior to flowering also boosts saffron yield; nevertheless, rainy or cold weather occurring during flowering promotes disease, thereby reducing yield. Persistently damp and hot conditions also harm yield. Digging actions of rabbits, rats, and birds, parasites such as nematodes, leaf rusts, and corm rot pose significant threats to saffron cultivation.

Saffron plants grow best in strong and direct sunlight, and fare poorly in shady conditions. Thus, planting is best done in fields that slope towards the sunlight (*i.e.* south-sloping in the Northern Hemisphere). In the Northern Hemisphere, planting is mostly done in June, with corms planted some 7–15 cm deep. Planting depth and corm spacing–along with climate–are critical factors impacting plant yield. Thus, mother corms planted more deeply yield higher-quality saffron, although they produce fewer flower buds and daughter corms. With such knowledge, Italian growers have found that planting corms 15 centimeters (5.9 in) deep and in rows spaced 2–3 cm apart optimizes threads yield, whereas planting depths of 8–10 cm optimizes flower and corm production. Meanwhile, Greek, Moroccan, and Spanish growers have devised different depths and spacing to suit their own climates.

After a period of dormancy through the summer, the corms send up their narrow leaves and begin to bud in early autumn. Only in mid-autumn do the plants begin to flower. Harvesting of flowers is by necessity a speedy affair: after their flowering at dawn, flowers quickly wilt as the day passes. Furthermore, saffron bloom within a narrow window spanning one or two weeks. The rose of saffron blooms at dawn and should stay the least possible time in the plant because it withers quickly and the stigmas loose color and aroma. This is why they are gathered between dawn and 10 am.

Once the flowers are gathered, stigmas are separated from the rest of the flower. Yields per plant are extremely low, about 4000 stigmas yield 25g of saffron. Saffron is the world's most expensive spice, it takes 150,000 flowers and 400 hours work to produce 1 kilo of dried saffron. About 25 kilos of styles can be harvested from a hectare of the plant. The stigmas of saffron have a high level of moisture, so it is necessary to dry them for its good preservation. This is the process of roasting, in which the stigmas get it definitive aspect: bright red, rigid and without wrinkles. After the process of roasting, the stigmas of saffron would have 1/5 of their original size. This means that from one kg of raw stigmas we will obtain 200 g of saffron ready for consumption. For its perfect preservation, saffron is stored in big wooden trunks lined with metal plate inside protecting it from heat, cold and especially moisture. Good saffron has very long self-life, as long as it is stored in air tight containers, shielded from light.

Adultrants

Because of the cost, saffron is frequently adulterated with cheaper substitutes such as marigold flowers and Safflower petals (which produce the color but not the flavor of saffron), or of being cheated by an unscrupulous supplier who adulterates his product. For this reason it is best to buy it in the form of dried threads rather than a powder. Saffron cheating is as old as saffron trade, and will persist as long as saffron is traded. There is a multitude of possibilities how to cheat: Crude methods include selling something that is not saffron at all–artificially coloured grass flowers. Safflower and Calendula flowers being obvious candidates. The common mislabeling of turmeric as "Indian saffron" also borders fraud (after all, there is saffron production in India!). People unaware of the taste of good saffron may be persuaded to buy an old or over dried product. Even large spice companies sometimes sell products that, although deriving from the right plant, have no or even a false aroma. Increasing the weight of saffron by coating the stigma with a non-volatile liquid (fatty oil or glycerol, which gives a sweet taste as untrained customer might even regard as sign of quality) is also very common. To ensure a reasonable quality, saffron should always be bought whole; no self-respecting vendor sells ground saffron, so if ever saffron powder is sold, it is probably not worth trying it.

Quality of Saffron

In the present time, saffron exists on the market in powdered form or as threads. Like most all spices and herbs, "whole" is more powerful than "ground.The I.S.O. (International Standard Organization) defines in its norm 3632-2. 1994 the different qualities of saffron in filament and powder based on their chemical properties (Table 16.1).

Cytology

Cytological Status of *C. sativus*

Leaving aside reports of the clones of *C. sativus* with 2n=14, 15 (Mather, 1932), 16 (Karasawa, 1940) and 40 (Karasawa, 1942) all cultivated clones of saffron studied from various countries by different workers have 2n=24. It is considered an autotriploid, based on x = 8, for more than one reason, chiefly similarity of the three constituent chromosome complements, formation of as many as 8 III's during Pmc meiosis and the resultant sterility (Ghaffari, 1986).

The fair uncommon chromosome counts, 2n=14, 15, 16 and 40 have never been recovered after they were reported once, which creates doubts about their validity. Nevertheless, search for such clones should continue. The clone which is required the most is the one with 2n=16 because it can serve to restore fertility in the exclusively asexual *C. sativus*, which is required for widening its genetic base. On grounds of karyological studies conducted till date on *C. sativus*, Chichirocco (1999) has asserted variation between European and Asiatic populations and heteromorphism in populations from Majorea, Spain and L. Aqrulla, Italy.

Table 16.1: Quality of Saffron

Characteristics	Requirements		Test Method
	Saffron Threads	Saffron Powder	
Moisture and volatile matter, per cent (m/m), max.	12	10	ISO 3632-2 CLAUSE 9
Total ash, per cent (m/m) on dry basis, max.	8	8	ISO 928 and ISO 3632-2 CLAUSE 10
Acid-insoluble ash, per cent (m/m), on dry basis, max.			
Categories I and II	1.0	1.0	ISO 930 and
Categories III	1.5	1.5	ISO 3632-2 CLAUSE 11
Solubility in cold water, per cent (m/m), on dry basis, max.	65	65	ISO 941
Bitterness, expressed as direct reading of the absorbance of picrocrocine at about 257 nm, on dry basis, min.			
Categorie I	70		ISO 3632-2 CLAUSE 13
Categorie II	55		
Categorie III	40		
Safranal, expressed as direct reading of the absorbance at about 330 nm, on dry basis. All categories			
Min.	20		ISO 3632-2 CLAUSE 13
Max.	50		
Colouring strength, expressed as direct reading of the absorbance of crocine at about 440 nm, on dry basis, min.			
Categorie I	190	190	ISO 3632-2 CLAUSE 13
Categorie II	150	150	
Categorie III	100	100	
Total nitrogen, per cent (m/m), on dry basis, max.	3.0	3.0	ISO 1871
Crude fibre, per cent (m/m), on dry basis, max.	6	6	ISO 5498

Phylogeny and Genome Constitution

Expect for a few publications which describe Kashmir crocus as *C. cashmeriana*, all cultivated crocus, including the one cultivated in Kashmir is *C. sativus* Linn. The species belongs to what Mathew (1977, 1999) has called the *C. sativus* aggregate. The 7 species comprising this aggregate are: *C. sativus* Linn, *C. nivevs*, *C. cartwightianus* Herb., *C. hadriaticus* Herb., *C. thomassi* Ten., *C. dispathacea* Bowles and *C. pallassii* Ancestry of C. sativus and its phylogenetic kinship have to be sought within this aggregate by using conventional and molecular techniques of genome analysis.

The chromosome constitution of *C. sativus* hints at strong phylogenetic kinship among *C. sativus*, *C. thomassi* and *C. cartwightianus*. The monoploid complement in all three species consists of 2 long acrocentric chromosomes, 4 metacentric chromosomes and 2 small acrocentric chromosomes. One of the two long acrocentric chromosomes carries a small satellite on the long arm (Brighton, 1977). The only difference is that *C. sativus* is triploid (2n=3x=24) while *C. thomassii* and *C. cartwightianus* are both diploid (Brighton, 1997). *C. cartwightianus* shares another similarly with *C. sativus*, it is abundant at Athens where it grows wild. The locals there use it in place of *C. sativus* for flavouring their food.

Crossability

Genomic relationship of *C. sativus* with *C. thomassii* and *C. cartwightianus* considered the putative progenitors of cultivated saffron can best be tested by raising interspecific hybrids. *C. sativus* and *C. thomassii* cross easily. The hybrid seed is viable and germinates well. Hybrid seedlings, which could reflect the genomic constitution of the interspecific hybrids have never been studied. This, and other crosses involving remaining 5 species of the *C. sativus* aggregate need to be undertaken in the coming years. Such work will not be of academic interest alone, more than that, it will help in identifying the donor species which can be tapped for borrowing desirable genes for incorporation into *C. sativus* genome.

Uses

Saffron finds a variety of uses in India and abroad. In India, it is used as a herb in Ayurvedic medicines which heal a variety of diseases ranging from Arthritis to Impotence and Infertility. It is known to have aphrodisiac properties and is widely used in Asia and the Middle East as such. Chinese and Tibetan Medicine also find many uses of this exotic herb

Edible Uses

Saffron is valued for its exotic colour and flavour which makes it the most expensive spice of the world. It is often said that saffron's flavour can neither be duplicated nor described in words. That is not surprising considering the fact that not even one additive can be substituted for saffron. "Saffron aroma enveloping a Kitchen is really appeasing"..In the food industry it is used as a colourant in sausages, margarine, butter, cheese, ice-cream, desserts, alcoholic and non-alcoholic beverages Saffron is used for several Mediterranean dishes, often in connection with fish and seafood. The flower styles are commonly used as a flavouring and yellow colouring for various foods such as bread, soups, sauces, rice and puddings. Saffron is more important in Central Asia and Northern India, where it is used extensively for rice dishes. It is an essential commodity in high quality milk/cream based confectioneries and Mughlai dishes in India wherein it imparts a rich colour and distinctive flavour. The fact is that Indians in general are crazy about this exotic spice.

Commercial Uses

The unique coloring and aromatic properties make saffron ideal for various bakery and confectionery preparations. Saffron is used as a flavoring agent in a number of dairy products like flavored milk, deserts, ice creams, butter and cheese. It is one of the crucial ingredients used in preparing products like wine, drinks, jellies, candies, cakes and cookies. Saffron is an important ingredient of cosmetic products particularly in fairness creams. Further, owing to its unique fragrance, saffron is used in perfumes and body fragrance products. Furthermore, saffron is a natural colorant and is used for coloring strings in weaving industry. It has a special significance in dye industry.

Culinary Uses

Saffron is used as a spice to add color, taste and aroma of the food. Considered to be the spice of Royalties, saffron used to be the chef's most preferred choice for delicacies and culinary. Particularly in Mughlai and other continental dishes, saffron not only adds the beautiful golden hue but also the aroma and flavor of the preparation is significantly enhanced. It is also used in desserts as well as curries. Moreover, saffron has traditionally been used in India and Europe to garnish delicacies on special occasions.

Dye

The yellow dye obtained from the stigmas has been used for many centuries to colour cloth. It is the favoured colouring for the cloth of Indian swamis who have renounced the material world.

Medicinal Uses

It is by far one of the oldest herbs ever used for medicinal purposes in the history of mankind. Major uses of saffron include the following: Saffron is also considered sovering remedy in traditional medicine, unparalleled in virtue by any drug in Materia Medica (Nandkarni, 1982). These qualities are vested largely in the stigma, and to a lesser degree in style, stamens and accessory parts of the flowers. Saffron reached the peak of popularity as a drug in the hands of the Arabs. In ancient times and even during the Middle ages it enjoyed great popularity; several therapeutic uses were ascribed to it. Over the period of time the medicinal use of saffron has dwindled. Folch (1957) has analysed the reasons in his well researched article entitled, "A drug which is gradually disappearing from the medical armamentarium". Nevertheless, it continues as an important ingredient of Ayurveda, Sidha, Unani, Chinese and Tibetan systems of medicine. It is a common belief that if saffron is regularly fed to expecting mothers, the baby born is beautiful, intelligent and fair complexioned. Its regular use is also believed to prolong life span. In Spain, areas where people consume saffron daily show a very low incidence of cardiovascular diseases.

In Ayurveda, saffron is used for curing chronic diseases such as asthma and arthritis. Dripping water of boiled saffron in nose is good for curing headache and insomnia. It is widely used for the treatment of cough and cold. Ayurvedic medicines with saffron as its ingredient are used to treat acne and other skin diseases. The paste of saffron can be used for dressing bruises and superficial sores. About 50 mg of Saffron dissolved in a glass of 200ml milk and a spoonful of sugar makes a very tasty drink which is also a health tonic. A regular intake of this every day for a period of time enables the body to build resistance against a lot of common diseases such as Asthma, Common colds, claim Ayurvedic Practitioners. Furthermore, Saffron contributes as an excellent cure for stomach ailment and is an antispasmodic as well. It also has digestive properties and helps in relieving tension as well. Since ancient time, saffron was considered to have strong aphrodisiac properties. It is also considered to be beneficial in specific gynaecological ailments. Even in modern pharmacopoeias, saffron is used to color medicines or as a cordial adjunct. The best evidence for medicinal effects of saffron involve treatment of depression. (Akhondzadeh *et al.*, 2005; Noorbala, 2005; Moshiri, 2006) Test-tube and animal studies hint that saffron and its constituents may help prevent or treat cancer, (Abdullaev Jafarova *et al.*, 2003; Abdullaev, 2003, 2004; Garcia-Olmo *et al.*, 2000) reduce cholesterol levels, protect against side effects of the drug cisplatin, (el Daly, 1998) and enhance mental function. (Abe and Saito, 2000)

Some studies have shown that saffron extract or its active constituents, crocetin and crocin may have benefits on people suffering from neurodegenerative disorders accompanying memory impairment (Hosseinzadeh, 2005). In traditional Chinese system, saffron was used as an agent to improve blood circulation and cure the bruises (Deng *et al.*, 2002). Researchers believe that crocin prevents atherosclerosis in hyperlipemia, via inhibition of both proliferation of smooth muscle cells and activation of p38MAPK (Xu *et al.*, 2005). It is also reported to posses anti-inflammatory (Hosseinzadeh and Younesi, 2002) activity and prevent cardiovascular disorders (Grisolla, 1974).In the western world it is used primarily as a spice. But it is also discovering its uses as a health tonic which naturally does not have side effects.

Religious Uses

When Budha renounced the world, his body was covered with special robe dyed in saffron. Ever since, Buddhist monk has adopted saffron as the colour that can help them achieve their goal of 'moksha'.Tibetan Monks use saffron for prayer and blessing, calligraphers have also used saffron as ink to write holy books like the Koran. Saffron is omnipresent in almost all the religions. It is a colour that flutters over Temples and Gurudwaras. For sikhs, it means a rebellion against prevailing injustice and for hindus–a religous fundamentalism. The precious spice is believed to bring power to religious practices. Calligraphers have also used saffron as ink to write holy books like the 'Koran'. In India, Tibet and China, saffron is also used to produce the yellow-red colour of robes for Hindu and Buddhist monks

Chemical Composition

The saffron stigma, which is what basically forms commercial saffron has a distinct, unique color, flavor and aroma. Saffron contains more than 150 volatile and aroma-yielding compounds. It also has many nonvolatile active components, many of which are carotenoids, including zeaxanthin, lycopene, and various α- and β-carotenes. Some of the groups of chemical compounds responsible for each of these properties have now been identified

Color

Saffron's coloring power is mainly produced by crocin (C44H64024) This crocin is trans-crocetin di-(β-D-gentiobiosyl) ester (8,8-diapo-8,8-carotenoic acid). This means that the crocin underlying saffron's aroma is a digentiobiose ester of the carotenoid crocetin (Escribano, 1996). Which is one of the few naturally occurring carotenoids easily soluble in water. This water solubility is one of the reasons for its widely preferred application in food and medicine. In addition to crocin saffron contains aglicon Crocetin as a free agent and small amounts of the pigment anthocyanin. There are also oil soluble pigments including alphacarotene, betacarotene and zegxantin. One of the most important parameters in evaluating the quality of saffron is its coloring power, which is determined by spectrophotometer the amount of coloring factors present at 443 nanometers. However, saffron's golden yellow-orange colour is primarily the result of α-crocin (443 nm). The styles are extremely rich in riboflavin (Bouvier *et al.*, 2003)

Flavor

The principal element giving saffron its special "bitter" flavor is the glycoside picrocrocin (c16 H26 07). This bitter tasting substance can be crystallized and produces glucose and the aldehyde safranal by hydrolysis The bitter glucoside picrocrocin is responsible for saffron's flavour. Picrocrocin (chemical formula: $C_{16}H_{26}O_7$; systematic name: 4-(β-D-glucopyranosyloxy)-2,6,6–trimethylcyclohex-1-ene-1-carboxaldehyde) is a union of an aldehyde sub-element known as safranal (systematic name: 2,6,6-trimethylcyclohexa-1,3-diene-1–carboxaldehyde) and a carbohydrate. Significantly, picrocrocin is a truncated version (produced via oxidative cleavage) of the carotenoid zeaxanthin and is the glycoside of the terpene aldehyde safranal.

Aroma

Saffron has a strong aroma, which is produced by certain special volatile oils and essences. The main aroma factor in saffron is safranal (Hosseinzadeh, 2005), which comprises about 60 per cent of the volatile components of saffron. In fresh saffron this substance exists as stable picrocrocin but as a result of heat and passage of time it decomposes releasing the volatile aldehyde saffranal.

Chemical composition of safranal: safranal is a volatile liquid oil which produces a yellow spot in water vapor and is readily soluble in ethanol, methanol and petroleum ether.When saffron is dried after its harvest, the heat, combined with enzymatic action, splits picrocrocin to yield D-glucose and a free safranal molecule Safranal, a volatile oil, gives saffron much of its distinctive aroma. Safranal is less bitter than picrocrocin and may comprise up to 70 per cent of dry saffron's volatile fraction in

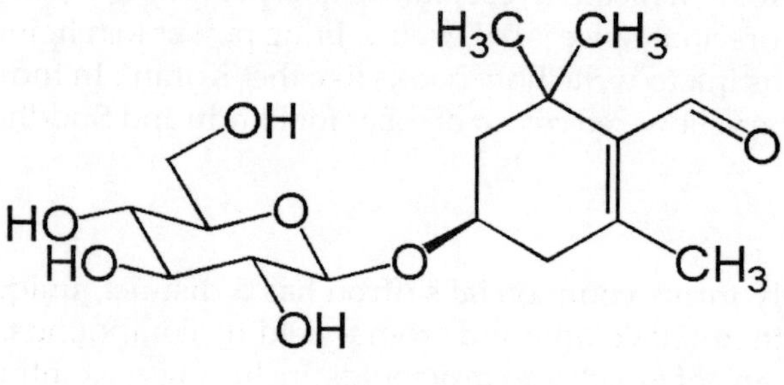

Picrocrocin

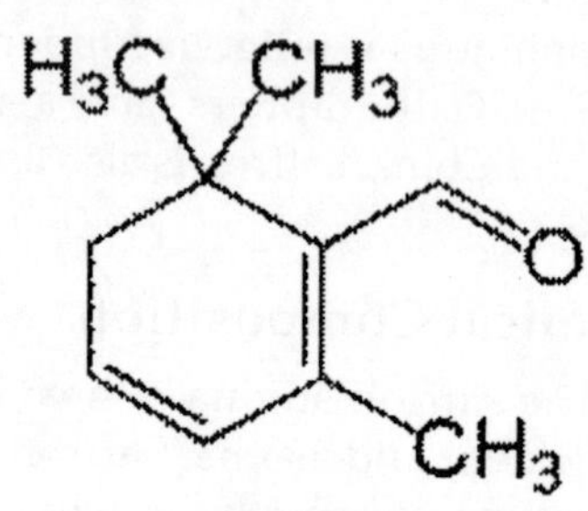

Safranal

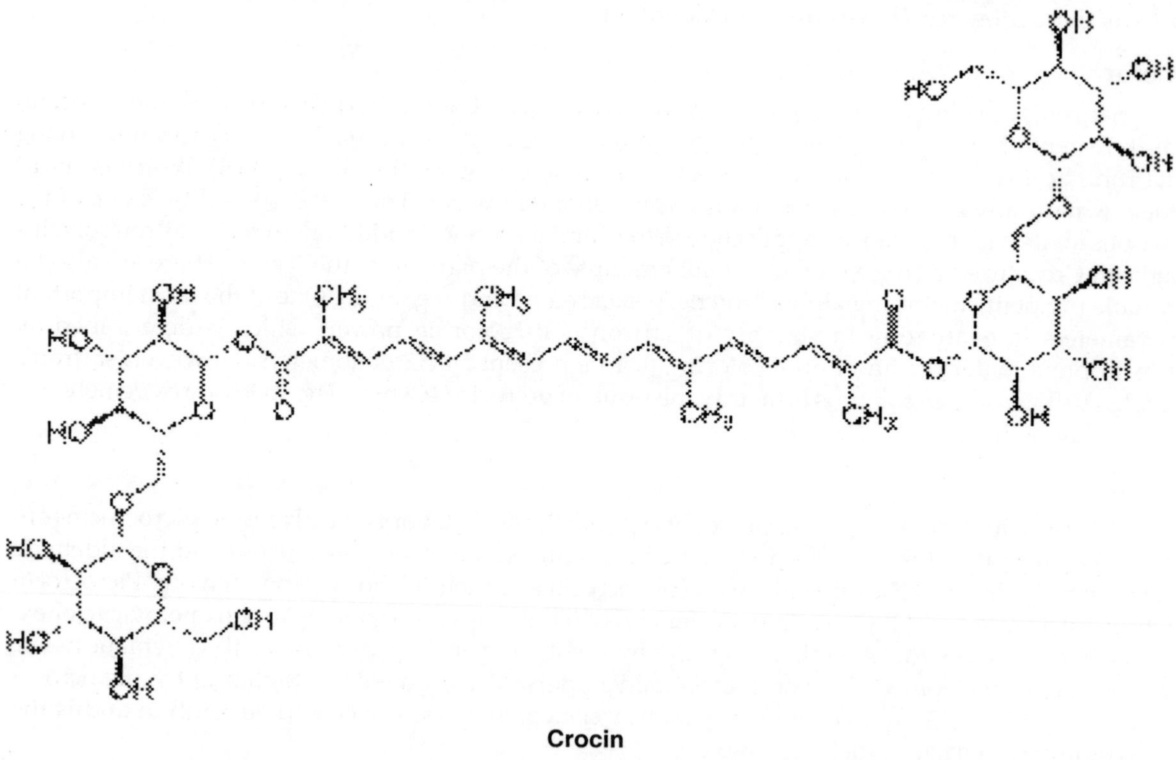

Crocin

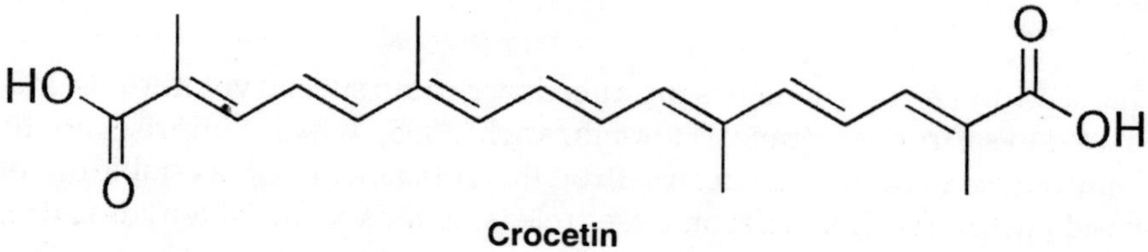

Crocetin

some samples. The essential oil derived from saffron is a complex mixture of terpenes and their derivatives (Evans, 1989). Dry saffron is highly sensitive to fluctuating pH levels, and rapidly breaks down chemically in the presence of light and oxidizing agents. It must therefore be stored away in air-tight containers in order to minimise contact with atmospheric oxygen. Saffron is somewhat more resistant to heat.

Conclusion

As in many other bulbous angiosperms, so also in *C. sativus*, triploidy has been favoured by human selection as it combines the advantages of polyploidy and hybridity. That is why triploids are generally gigantic, triploid flowers having larger floral parts including stigma. This is true of both, the densely cytoplasmic stray pollen (Chichiroicco, 1989). The stigma continues to grow in size in search of the right kind of pollen, which it never receives.

While sterility is a boon in as much as it provides sufficient time for the triploid stigmas of *C. sativus* to grow in size, it is truly a bane as it has robbed the crop of the means to generate variation on account of sterility. Saffron has been propagated through underground cormlets for centuries. It is therefore, no wonder to find huge saffron fields devoid of any significant phenotypic variation.

These are variations in flower count per corm, stigma size and the time of flowering. With respect to last character *i.e.* time of flowering, one notices within the same field plants which bear flowers and leaves together and other in which flowers are set first and leaves appear only after flowering has been completed. The pattern of resource partitioning in the two plant types should vary. Whereas all resources in the first case, termed hysteranthous type, will be chanalized towards differentiation of flower, in the second type, called sub-hysteranthous, they will get shared between flowers and foliage. Thus, the difference in flowering time should get reflected in the size of flower and individual floral parts, including stigma. But for these, variation in saffron is not of such magnitude that it can be of much consequence.

The strategy for genetic improvement of saffron has to be evolved in light of the constraint of its recalcitrance due to its triploid nature. The tragedy is that despite the economic potential of this crop, its maladies for which solutions are required have not been identified as yet. The major weakness projected is the low yield of Kashmir clones compared to Spanish strains, some of which yield as high as 16Kg of saffron per hectare. The maximum yield recorded from the valley is 5.8Kg, except for a solitary report of 12.5Kg (Mir, 1984). It is obviously no wonder that the Spanish produce takes care of 90 per cent of the world trade in saffron. This significant difference in yield is often attributed to difference in cultivation practices and agroclimate. Never have the Spanish genotypes been introduced in the valley and evaluated for their performance. Genotypic difference cannot be ruled out because the Kashmir and Spanish clones have remained isolated for centuries, during which period sufficient genetic divergence is expected to have set in. How should we go about to raise the yield and increase the production of saffron. The following action plan is proposed.

1. Extension of saffron cultivation to new areas.
2. Introduction of exotics.
3. Import of desirable genes from allies through.
   - § Hybridization
   - § Protoplast culture and its utility in genetic manipulation
   - § Development of transgenics
   - § Cell cultures for harvesting active principles

References

Abdullaev FI, Espinosa-Aguirre JJ. (2004). Biomedical properties of saffron and its potential use in cancer therapy and chemoprevention trials. *Cancer Detect Prev.*, 28:426–32.

Abdullaev FI, Riveron-Negrete L, Caballero-Ortega H, *et al.* (2003). Use of *in vitro* assays to assess the potential antigenotoxic and cytotoxic effects of saffron (*Crocus sativus* L.). *Toxicol In Vitro*, 17:731–6.

Abdullaev Jafarova F, Caballero-Ortega H, Riveron-Negrete L, *et al.* (2003) *In vitro* evaluation of the chemopreventive potential of saffron [in Spanish]. *Rev Invest Clin.*, 54:430–6.

Abe K, Saito H. (2000). Effects of saffron extract and its constituent crocin on learning behaviour and long-term potentiation. *Phytother Res.*, 14:149–52.

Akhondzadeh S, Tahmacebi-Pour N, Noorbala AA, *et al.* (2005). *Crocus sativus* L. in the treatment of mild to moderate depression: a double-blind, randomized and placebo-controlled trial. *Phytother Res.*, 19:148–51

Bouvier F, Suire C, Mutterer J, Camara B. (2003). Oxidative remodeling of chromoplast carotenoids: identification of the carotenoid dioxygenase CsCCD and CsZCD genes involved in Crocus secondary metabolite biogenesis. *Plant Cell.*, 15:47-62. 5.

Brighton, C. A. (1977). Cytology of Crocus sativus and its allies (Iridaceae). *Plant Syst. Evol.*, 128: 137-157.

Chichirocco, G. (1989). Microsporogenesis and pollen development in *Crocus sativus* L. 42: 249-257

Chichirocco, G. (1999). Sterility and perspectives for genetic improvement of *Crocus sativus* L. (In Moshe, N 1999 Saffron. *Crocus sativus* L. Harwood Acad. Publishers, Netherlands)

Deng Y, Guo ZG, Zeng ZL, Wang Z. (2002). Studies on the pharmacological effects of saffron (*Crocus sativus* L.): A review. *Zhongguo Zhong Yao Za Zhi.*, 27(8):565-8.

el Daly ES. (1998). Protective effect of cysteine and vitamin E, Crocus sativus and Nigella sativa extracts on cisplatin-induced toxicity in rats. *J Pharm Belg.*, 53:87–93.

Escribano J, Alonso GL, Coca-Prados M, Fernandez J-A. (1996). Crocin, safranal and picrocrocin from saffron (Crocus sativus L.) inhibit the growth of human cancer cells *in vitro*. *Cancer Lett.*, 100:23-30.).

Evans WC (1989). Trease and Evans' Pharmacognosy. 13th ed. London: Balliere Tindall.

Folch, R. A. (1957). A drug which is gradually disappearing from the medical armamentarium: Saffron. *Farmacognosia*, 17: 145-224.

Garcia-Olmo DC, Riese HH, Escribano J, *et al.* (2000). Effects of long-term treatment of colon adenocarcinoma with crocin, a carotenoid from saffron (Crocus sativus L.): an experimental study in the rat. *Nutr Cancer*, 35:120–6.

Ghaffari, S. M. (1986). Cytogenetic studies of cultivated Crocus sativus. *Pl. Syst. Evol.*, 153: 199-204.

Grisolia S. (1974). Letter: Hypoxia, saffron, and cardiovascular disease. *Lancet*, 2:41-42.

Hosseinzadeh H. *et al.* (2005). Safranal, a constituent of Crocus sativus (saffron), attenuated cerebral ischemia induced oxidative damage in rat hippocampus. *J Pharm Pharm Sci.*, 8(3):394-9.

Hosseinzadeh H, Younesi HM. (2002). Antinociceptive and anti-inflammatory effects of *Crocus sativus* L. *stigma* and petal extracts in mice. *BMC Pharmacol.*, 2:7.

Karasawa, K. (1940). Karyological studies in Crocus II. *Jap. J. Bot.*, 11: 129-146.

Karasawa, K. (1942). List of chromosome numbers in genus Crocus. *Proc. Imp. Acad. Japan*, 18: 117-122..

Mather, K. (1932). Chromosome variation in Crocus. *I. J. Gent.*, 26: 129-142.

Mathew, B. (1999). Botany, taxonomy and cytology of *Crocus sativus* and its allies (In Negbi, M (1999) Saffron, *Crocus sativus* L.) *Harwood Acad. Publishers, Amsterdam, the Netherland*, 19-30.

Mathew, B. (1977). *Crocus sativus* and its allies (Iridaceae). *Plant Syst. Farm.* 128: 89-103.

Mathur, S. C. (1973). *Crocus sativus* and its allies (Iridaceae) *Plant Syst. Farm.* 22: 29-31.

Mir, G. M. (1984). Saffron cultivation in Kashmir valley. A study on inter-and intra-village variation on socioeconomic development. Ph.D Thesis. University of Kashmir, India.

Moshiri E, Basti AA, Noorbala AA *et al.* (2006). *Crocus sativus* L. (petal) in the treatment of mild-to-moderate depression: A double-blind, randomized and placebo-controlled trial. *Phytomedicine*, 14

Nadkarni, A. K. (1982). Dr. K. M. Nadkarni's Materia Medica. Vol 2. Revised and enlarged by A. K. Mandkarni. Popular Prakashan, Bombay. P 391.

Noorbala AA, Akhondzadeh S, Tahmacebi-Pour N, *et al.* (2005). Hydro-alcoholic extract of Crocus sativus L. versus fluoxetine in the treatment of mild to moderate depression: a double-blind, randomized pilot trial. *J Ethnopharmacol.*, 97:281–4.

Srivastava, R. P. (1964). Saffron finds a new home in U.P. Ind. Farm. 13: 20.

Suzhou New Medical College. Dictionary of Traditional Chinese Medicine (Zhong Da Zi Dian). Shanghai: Shanghai People's Publication House, Vol. 2:pp2622–2623, 1977.

Xu GL, Yu SQ, Gong ZN, et al..(2005). Study of the effect of crocin on rat experimental hyperlipemia and the underlying mechanisms [in Chinese]. *Zhongguo Zhong Yao Za Zhi.*, 30:369–72.

Utilisation and Management of Medicinal Plants (2010) *Pages 306–318*
Editors: **V.K. Gupta, Anil K. Verma and Sushma Koul**
Published by: **DAYA PUBLISHING HOUSE, NEW DELHI**

Chapter 17

Antibacterial Activity of *Acacia daviesii* (M. Bartolome) sp. nov.: A New and Rare Species Identified in North-Eastern Victoria, Australia

Hilde Lie Kjaerstad, Allison McGill and Enzo A. Palombo*
Environment and Biotechnology Centre, Faculty of Life and Social Sciences, Swinburne University of Technology, PO Box 218, Hawthorn, Victoria 3122, Australia

ABSTRACT

The genus *Acacia* comprises over 1300 species of which nearly 1000 are found in Australia. Numerous species have been used as traditional medicines by the Aboriginal peoples of Australia, although few of the medicinal properties have been investigated. The species *Acacia daviesii* is a newly discovered plant and is reported to have oily phyllodes which emit a pungent smell. Although there is no documented medicinal use for this particular plant, the traditional use of other *Acacia* species prompted us to investigate this new species. Aqueous and organic (ethanol, acetone and petroleum ether) extracts of the phyllodes and stems of *Acacia daviesii* were tested for antibacterial activity. With the exception of the aqueous extracts, all were active against the Gram positive bacteria tested (inhibitory concentrations of 200-1600 mg/ml), while none were active against Gram negative bacteria. Preliminary phytochemical analysis indicated the presence of sugars, steroids, terpenes and flavonoids. Bioautography indicated that common antibacterial fractions were present within the active phyllode and stem extracts. Further investigation of the

* Corresponding Author: E-mail: epalombo@swin.edu.au.

extracts indicated that they exhibited activity against bacteria implicated in the development of dental caries (*Streptococcus mutans* and *S. sobrinus*). Time-kill assays showed that the extracts displayed bactericidal activity within 60 minutes, and they also inhibited glycolytic acid production over a 30 minute time period. In addition, a reduction in biofilm formation was observed at sub-MIC levels. These finding suggests that extracts, or active compounds within the extracts, may have application in the prevention of oral diseases caused by cariogenic and acidogenic bacteria.

Keywords: *Acacia daviesii, Antibacterial activity, Bioautography, Minimum inhibitory concentration, Dental caries, Phytochemicals.*

Introduction

Plant-derived medicines have been part of traditional healthcare worldwide for many years (Barnes and Prasain, 2005; Gautam *et al.*, 2007). Plants contain numerous biologically active secondary metabolites and many of these have been shown to exhibit antimicrobial properties (Cowan, 1999). Plants have been used as traditional medicines by the indigenous Aboriginal peoples of Australia (Barr *et al.*, 1993) and many have been utilised as treatments for infectious diseases because of their antiseptic and bactericidal properties (Lassak and McCarthy, 2001). With the alarming incidence of antibiotic resistance in bacteria of medical importance (Monroe and Polk, 2000; Hogan and Kolter, 2002; Alpuche *et al.*, 2007), there is increasing interest in plants as sources of agents for the treatment of microbial diseases.

The genus *Acacia* belongs to the family Mimosaceae and consists of over 1300 species, of which nearly 1000 are found in Australia (Orchard and Wilson, 2001). The acacias, commonly known as wattles, are prevalent in the arid, semi-arid and dry sub-tropical regions of Australia, although they can be found in a wide range of differing habitats from the coastal to the sub-alpine regions, including areas of high rainfall and arid inland areas. *Acacia* species are used widely as food (*e.g.* seeds are ground into flour and the gum is edible) and the wood can be made into clubs, spears, boomerangs and shields (Orchard and Wilson, 2001). With respect to medicinal uses, various species are still used as narcotics and painkillers, to treat headaches, cold and fevers, as antiseptics and bactericides and to treat skin disorders by the indigenous people of Australia (Table 17.1) (Lassak and McCarthy, 2001).

A new and rare species of *Acacia* was discovered in the sub-alpine region of north-eastern Victoria, a state in the south-east of Australia, in 1998 (Bartolome *et al.*, 2002). The plant, named *Acacia daviesii* in honour of its discoverer, has very oily phyllodes which in the hot sun, emit a very pungent smell (Figure 17.1). It has a pendulous habit and is distinguished by the resinous, glandular nature of the phyllodes which have either one or two main veins. The glands are prominent along the margins and veins of the phyllodes, are scattered over the phyllode surface and also present on stems and pods. The phyllodes have a prominent apical point and the flowers are in simple axillary, globular heads (Bartolome *et al.*, 2002).

Given that numerous *Acacia* species have been used medicinally, the aim of the current study was to determine whether extracts of this newly discovered plant exhibited antibacterial activity. In addition, activity against bacterial pathogens of the oral cavity was investigated.

Oral diseases continue to be a major health problem worldwide (Petersen *et al.*, 2005), with dental caries and periodontal diseases considered to be the most important global oral health problems

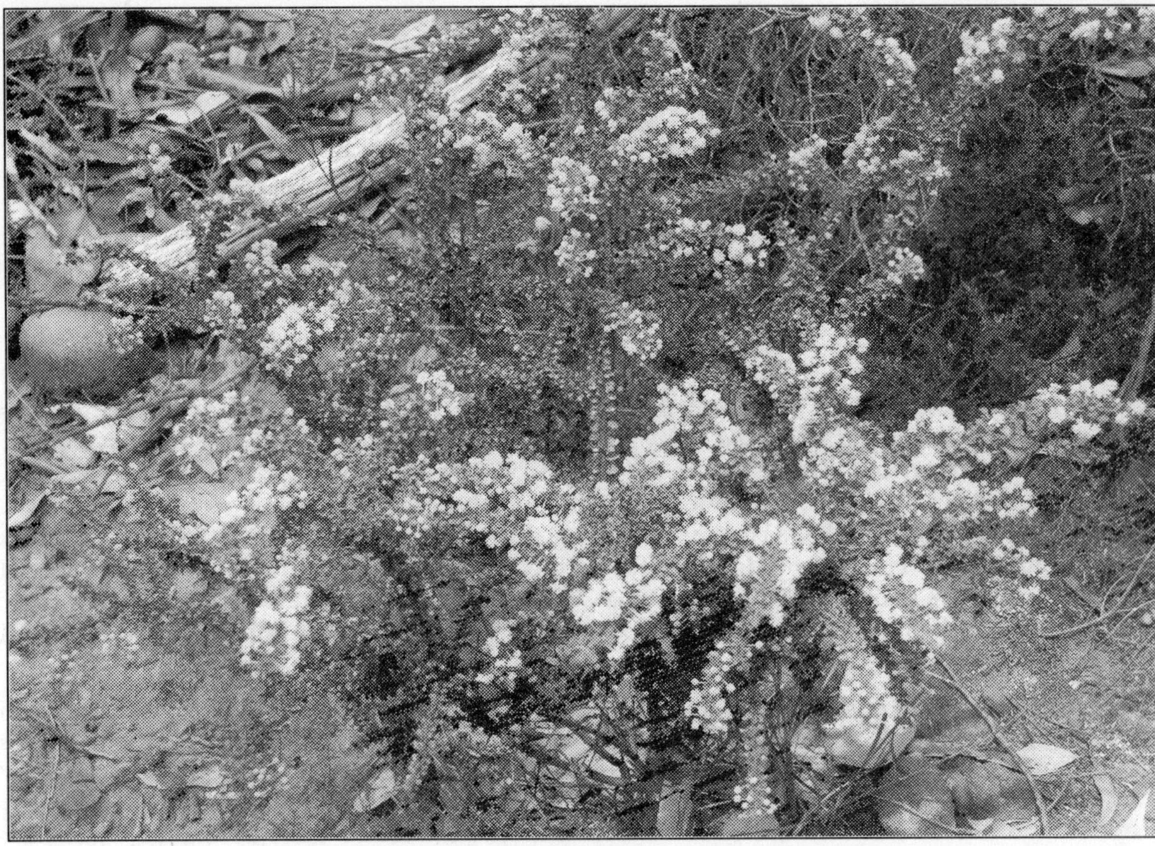

Figure 17.1: *Acacia daviesii* Growing in its Natural Habitat (Photo courtesy of Geoff Davies)

(Petersen, 2003). The link between oral diseases and the activities of microbial species that form part of the microbiota of the oral cavity is well established. The development of dental caries involves acidogenic and aciduric Gram positive bacteria, primarily the mutans streptococci (*Streptococcus mutans* and *S. sobrinus*) (Jenkinson and Lamont, 2005). The need for alternative prevention and treatment options and products for oral diseases that are safe, effective and economical comes from the rise in disease incidence in developing countries, increased resistance by pathogenic bacteria to currently used antibiotics and chemotherapeutics, opportunistic infections in immunocompromised individuals and financial considerations in developing countries (Tichy and Novak, 1998; Badria and Zidan, 2004). Despite several agents being commercially available, including sporamycin, vancomycin and chlorhexidine, these chemicals can alter oral and intestinal microbiota and have undesirable side-effects such as vomiting, diarrhoea and tooth staining (Park *et al.*, 2003; Chung *et al.*, 2006). Hence, the search for alternative products continues and natural phytochemicals isolated from plants used in traditional medicine are considered good alternatives to synthetic chemicals (Prabu *et al.*, 2006).

Dental plaque is an example of a specialised bacterial biofilm that develops on the surface of teeth, dental restorations, prostheses and implants (Bernimoulin, 2003). The colonising bacteria that make up the biofilm consortium elute lactic acid by metabolising sugars which results in the formation of dental caries (Park *et al.*, 2003). We have therefore investigated the potential use of *Acacia daviesii* in the prevention of dental diseases by assessing the antibacterial properties of extracts against oral bacterial pathogens, as well as examining the ability of the extracts to inhibit biofilm formation and acid production of these bacteria.

Table 17.1: Traditional Medicinal Uses of *Acacia* by Australian Aborigines

Species	*Traditional Medicinal Use*	*Active Constituents*
Acacia auriculoformis	As antiseptic cleanser and as a treatment for allergy rash	Possibly saponins
Acacia beaverdiana	As a narcotic, ash and small top branches mixed in equal parts of tobacco and chewed	Alkali present in ash release alkaloids in tobacco enhancing the narcotic effect
Acacia bivenosa subspecies *wayi*	Bark soaked or boiled in water and the decoction used as a cough medicine	Not known
Acacia cuthbertsonii	In conjunction with *Codonocarpus cotinifolius*, the bark was used for the relief of toothache and rheumatism	Not known
Acacia decurrens	Decoction of bark used in cases of extreme dysentery	Tannins
Acacia falcate	Embrocation of bark used to cure skin diseases	Tannins
Acacia holosericea	Mashed roots soaked in water and infusion drunk for laryngitis	Not known
Acacia implexa	Embrocation of bark used to cure skin diseases	Tannins
Acacia leptocarpa	Mashed green phyllodes soaked in water and the infusion applied to sore eyes	Not known
Acacia melanoxylum	Hot infusion of roasted bark used to bathe rheumatic joints	Bark rich in tannins
Acacia monticola	Used for coughs and colds, mashed roots soaked in water or branchlets boiled in water and solution drunk or used in bathing	Not known
Acacia tetragonophylla	Cleaned inner bark soaked in water and infusion drunk as a cough medicine; leaves chewed for dysentery; ashes from bark-free wood used as an antiseptic; points of pungent phyllodes inserted under warts	Not known
Acacia transluscens	Leaves and twigs mashed in water and the liquid used to bathe skin sores and applied to the head for headaches	Not known, probably tannins

Materials and Methods

Plant Material and Extracts

Samples of *Acacia daviesii* were collected in December 2006 from Merrijig, Victoria, Australia, and identified by Mr Geoff Davies. The samples were transported to Swinburne University of Technology and stored at –20°C. Voucher specimens are held in the School of Botany Herbarium, University of Melbourne. Extracts of phyllodes and stems were prepared by soaking the freeze-dried plant parts individually in water, ethanol, acetone and petroleum ether for 48 hours. Solvents were removed by rotary evaporation and the resultant extract yields were determined as a percentage of the mass of the dried plant material used in the solvent extraction process. The dried extracts were then re-dissolved in 1 ml of the same solvent.

Antimicrobial Testing Procedures

All extracts were tested by disc-diffusion assays (see below). The media used in this study were supplied by Oxoid Ltd. (Basingstoke, UK). The bacteria used were *Enterococcus faecalis* (ATCC 19433), *Escherichia coli* (ATCC 11775), *Pseudomonas auroginosa* (ATCC 10145) and *Staphylococcus aureus* (ATCC 12600). Bacteria were grown on nutrient agar (NA) and in nutrient broth (NB) at 37°C. *Streptococcus mutans* 969 and *Streptococcus sobrinus* 6715-247 isolates were provided by the Dental Hospital, Melbourne, and grown on de Man-Rogosa-Sharpe (MRS) agar and in MRS broth. Antibacterial activity was assessed by the disc-diffusion method (Kalemba and Kunicka, 2003) using paper discs of 6 mm diameter. Bacteria were plated onto NA or MRS plates and the inocula allowed to dry, after which discs which had been infused with 10 μL of the solvent extracts were placed on the plates and incubated at 37°C overnight. Chloramphenicol was used as a positive control and solvents were used as negative controls. A two-fold microdilution broth method was used to determine minimum inhibitory concentrations (MIC) and minimum bactericidal concentrations (MBC) (Wilkinson, 2006).

Bioautography

Bioautography was used to perform preliminary fractionation and evaluation of extracts (Shah *et al.*, 2004). Active extracts (3 ml of 1:5 dilutions) were applied 2.5 cm from the base of aluminum-backed silica plates (Sigma-Aldrich). After drying, extracts were fractionated by developing the plates using toluene:ethanol (90:10) as the solvent. After the solvent was allowed to evaporate, the plates were placed into sterile square Petri dishes. Two hundred microlitres of NB bacterial culture were added to 15 ml of molten NA, mixed well, poured over the TLC plate and allowed to set. The plate was incubated at 37°C overnight, sprayed with 2 mg/ml of MTT (3-[4,5-dimetylthiazol-2-yl]-2,5-diphenyl-tetrazolium bromide), incubated at 37°C for a further 30 minutes and examined for zones of bacterial growth inhibition (clear zones within a purple background).

Time-kill Assays

The bactericidal activities of the ethanol extracts against *S. mutans* and *S. sobrinus* were examined using time-kill curve experiments. One hundred microlitres of overnight MRS broth cultures were added to 3 ml of MRS broth containing extracts at MBC levels. The cultures were incubated at 37°C with shaking. The number of colony-forming units (cfu) (*i.e.* viable cells) was determined after 0, 60 and 120 minutes of incubation. Kill curves were constructed by plotting the $\log_{10}$ cfu/ml versus time. Control cultures without extract were incubated under the same conditions.

Glycolytic pH Drop Assays

The effects of *Acacia* extracts on glycolysis were measured by pH drop assays as described by Duarte *et al.* (2006). Cells of *S. mutans* and *S. sobrinus* from MRS broth cultures were harvested by centrifugation, washed once with salt solution (50mM KCl plus 1mM $MgCl_2$) and resuspended in salt solution with or without extracts at MIC levels. The pH was adjusted to 7.2-7.5 with 0.1M KOH solution, sufficient glucose was added to give a concentration of 1 per cent (w/v), and the decrease in pH was assessed by means of a glass electrode over a period of 30 minutes.

Biofilm Formation Assays

The ability of *Acacia* ethanol extracts to inhibit the formation of streptococcal biofilms was assessed by the method described by Yamanaka *et al.* (2004). Briefly, bacteria were grown in MRS broth in the presence (test) or absence (control) of plant extract for 1 day in wells of microtitre plates (Falcon, BD). Media and unattached cells were decanting and the wells washed twice with distilled water. Adherent cells were stained with 0.1 per cent crystal violet for 15 minutes, and bound dye extracted using 100 per cent ethanol. Biofilm formation was quantified by measuring the absorbance (optical density) of the solution at 595 nm using a microtitre plate reader (Emax, Molecular Devices).

Results and Discussion

Extracts of the phyllodes and stems of *Acacia daviesii* were prepared in water and various organic solvents. After rotary evaporation of the solvent, the mass of the residue was determined and used to calculate the yield as percentage of the original dried mass of plant material. The following yields were obtained: phyllodes (water), 15.1 per cent; stems (water), 11.9 per cent; phyllodes (ethanol), 17.8 per cent; stems (ethanol), 13.1 per cent; phyllodes (acetone), 15.0 per cent; stems (acetone), 12.0 per cent; phyllodes (petroleum ether), 7.4 per cent; stems (petroleum ether), 4.8 per cent.

Preliminary screening using disc-diffusion assays indicated that ethanol, acetone and petroleum ether extracts of phyllodes and stems of *Acacia daviesii* exhibited antibacterial activity against Gram positive bacteria (*E. faecalis* and *S. aureus*) (Table 17.2). The aqueous extracts exhibited no activity, even though this solvent produced yields equivalent to or superior to other solvents. No activity was observed against the Gram negative bacteria (*E. coli* and *P. aeruginosa*). Hence, the antibacterial activity appeared to be specific to Gram positive bacterial species.

Table 17.2: Antibacterial Activity of *Acacia daviesii* Extracts

Plant Part (solvent)	*Antibacterial Activity[a] Against*			
	E. faecalis	*S. aureus*	*E. coli*	*P. aeruginosa*
Phyllodes (water)	–	–	–	–
Stem (water)	–	–	–	–
Phyllodes (ethanol)	11	12	–	–
Stem (ethanol)	13	13	–	–
Phyllodes (acetone)	14	12	–	–
Stem (acetone)	14	14	–	–
Phyllodes (PE[b])	13	12	–	–
Stem (PE)	11	10	–	–
Chloramphenicol[c]	26	26	28	16

[a]: Antibacterial activity was determined using disk diffusion assays and is indicated by the size (mm) of zones of inhibition. A zone greater than 6 mm is considered positive. A dash indicates no activity. Results are the average of duplicate assays.

[b]: Petroleum ether

[c]: 50 mg disc.

MIC values ranged from 200-1600 mg/ml and MBC values ranged from 400 mg/ml to >1600 mg/ml (Table 17.3). Given that the MBC values were greater than the MIC values, it suggested that the extracts exerted bacteriostatic rather than bactericidal activity at inhibitory concentrations, especially against *E. faecalis*. To be considered as valuable leads, it has been suggested that the inhibitory concentrations of crude extracts should be <100 mg/ml (Cos *et al.*, 2006). While the MICs are higher for the extracts examined in this study, the values for the ethanol and acetone extracts, especially against *S. aureus*, indicate that more efficient extraction procedures may yield extracts with greater potency.

Table 17.3: MIC and MBC of *Acacia daviesii* Extracts Against Gram Positive Bacteria

Plant Part (Solvent)	*MIC (mg/ml) Against*		*MBC (mg/ml) Against*	
	E. faecalis	*S. aureus*	*E. faecalis*	*S. aureus*
Phyllodes (ethanol)	400	400	>1600	800
Stem (ethanol)	200	200	400	400
Phyllodes (acetone)	800	400	>1600	800
Stem (acetone)	400	400	>1600	800
Phyllodes (PE[a])	1600	1600	>1600	>1600
Stem (PE)	1600	1600	>1600	>1600
Chloramphenicol [b]	12.5	25	>100	>100

[a]: Petroleum ether

[b]: 50 mg disc.

Bioautography indicated that phyllodes and stems contained identical antibacterial constituents identified within three fractions (R_f = 0.36, 0.44 and 0.49) of the extracts separated by silica gel (Figure 17.2). The mobility of the active constituents suggested that these compounds were non-polar, which is supported by the observation that aqueous extracts did not exhibit activity (Table 17.2), indicating that the active compounds have limited solubility in water. The active constituents were present in lower concentrations in the petroleum ether extracts, as expected from the MIC and MBC results. TLC spray reagents specific for alkaloids, sugars, steroids, terpenes and flavonoids (Krebs *et al.*, 1969) indicated that alkaloids were absent but the other classes of phytochemicals were present in the extracts (data not shown). However, the chemical identities of active fractions are unknown. Indeed, little is known about the pytochemistry of most *Acacia* species (Seigler, 2002) making it difficult to speculate on the likely active constituents for this species. Given that tannins and saponins have previously been identified in other *Acacia* species (Lassak and McCarthy, 2001; Mandal *et al.*, 2005), further investigations will aim towards identification of the active principles of *Acacia daviesii*.

Given the promising activity against Gram positive bacteria, we were interested in whether the *Acacia* extracts were able to inhibit the growth of bacteria of importance to oral diseases. Disc-diffusion assays indicated that all but the acetone extracts were able to inhibit the growth of the oral pathogens, *S. mutans*, and all extracts inhibited *S. sobrinus* (Table 17.4). The resultant zones of inhibition were similar to those observed for other Gram positive bacteria, indicating comparable activity. Time-kill assays showed that the ethanol extracts were able to inhibit bacterial growth within 1 hour at MBC levels (Figure 17.3). The phyllodes extract completely eliminated viable *S. sobrinus* cells within 1 hour and a minimum of a 3-log reduction in viable cells was observed after 2 hours for both bacteria.

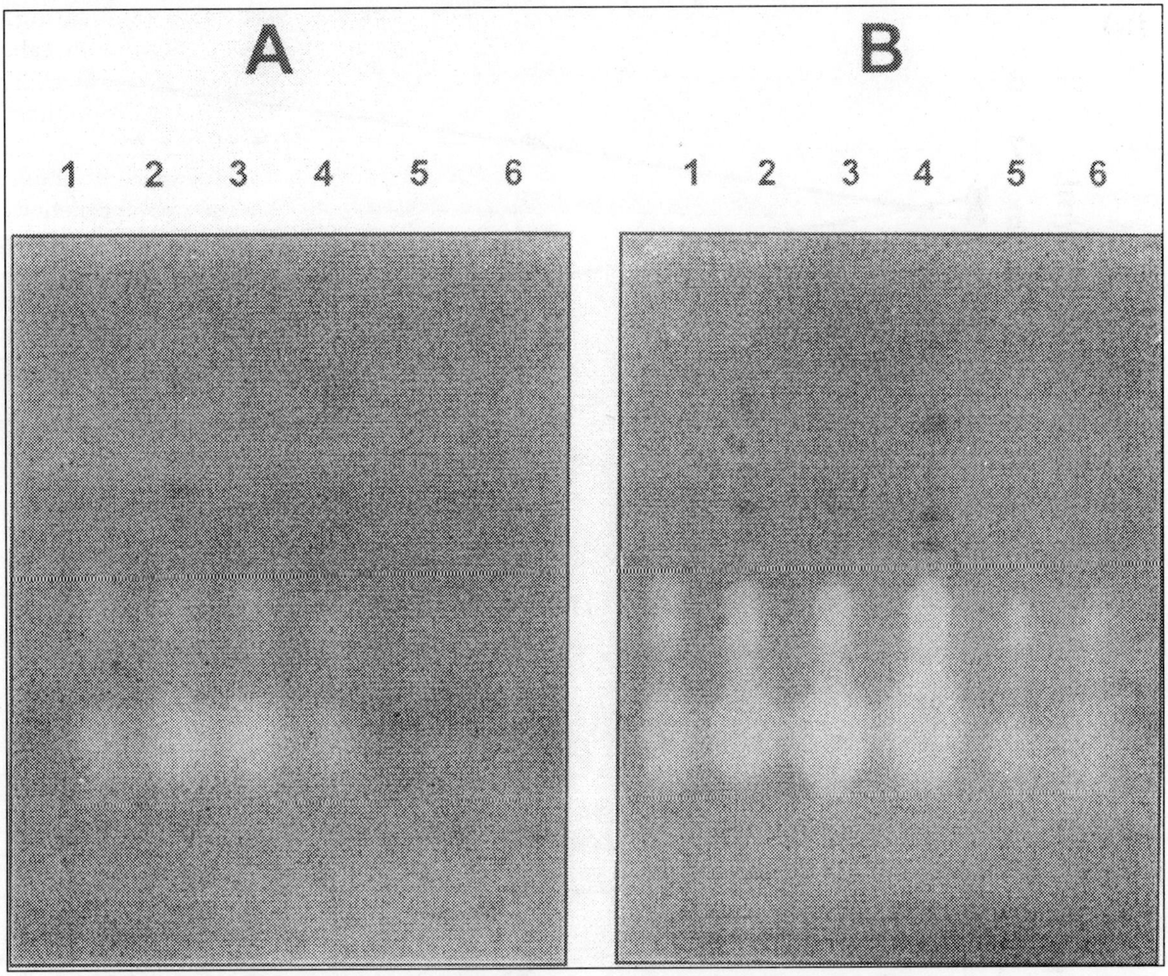

Figure 17.2: Bioautography of *Acacia daviesii* Extracts Against *Enterococcus faecalis* (A) and *Staphylococcus aureus* (B)

Ethanol, acetone and petroleum ether extracts of leaves are in lanes 1, 3 and 5, respectively. Ethanol, acetone and petroleum ether extracts of stems are in lanes 2, 4 and 6, respectively.

However, further experiments are required to determine the minimum time of exposure and the minimum concentration of extracts required for complete bactericidal effects.

Acid production is an important factor in the ability of both *S. mutans* and *S. sobrinus* to induce the formation of dental caries and extracts that can inhibit this virulence factor, and thus prevent dental caries, are of interest (Song *et al.*, 2006). Exposure of the bacteria to MIC levels of extracts resulted in a noticeable inhibition of glycolytic acid production which was obvious within five minutes for *S. sobrinus* and ten minutes for *S. mutans* (Figure 17.4). This indicated that the extracts interfered with bacterial metabolism or membrane integrity (Song *et al.*, 2006). Another important virulence factor is the ability for *S. mutans* and *S. sobrinus* to colonise the surface of teeth as the first step towards the development of dental plaque. While a reduction in biofilm development was observed for bacteria

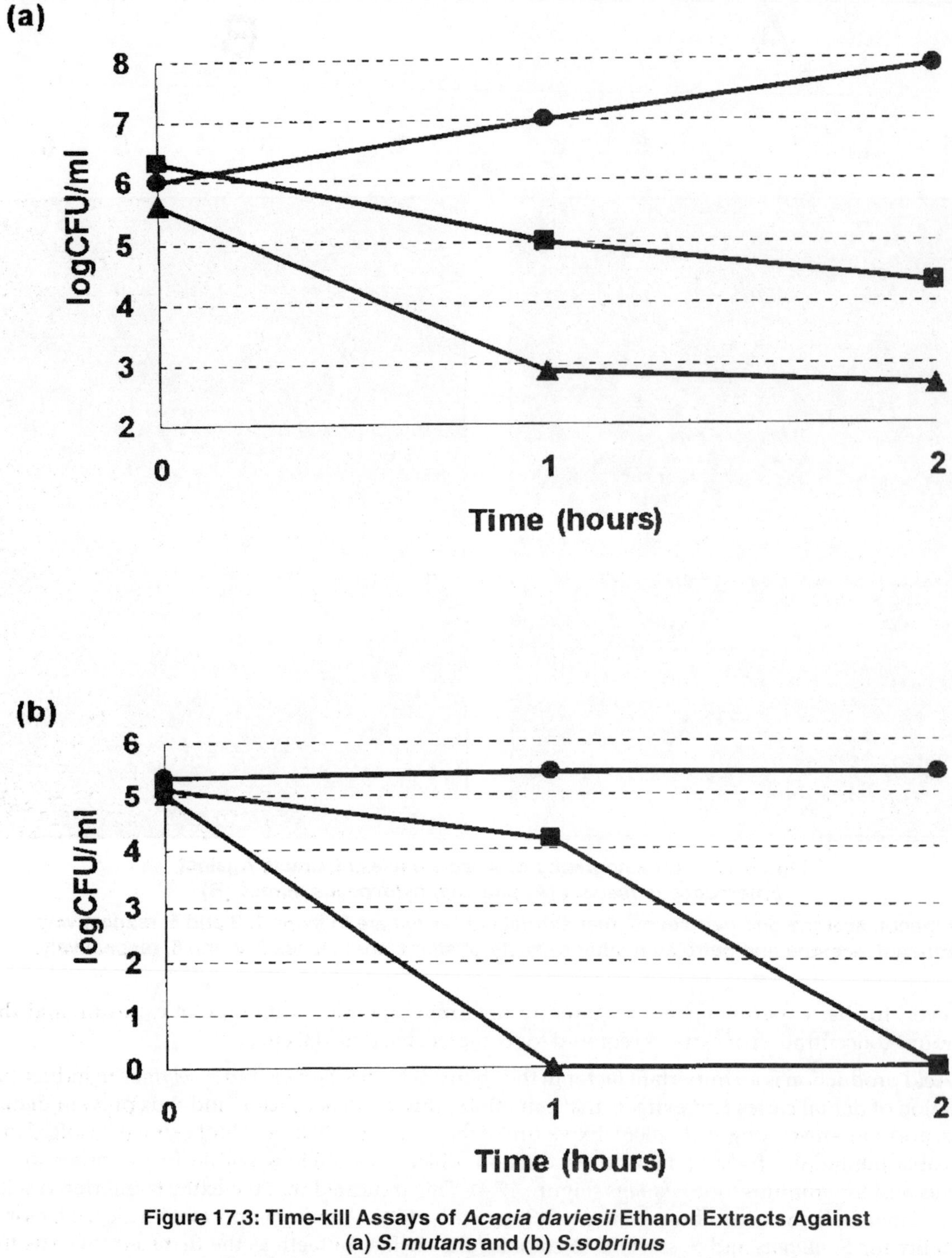

Figure 17.3: Time-kill Assays of *Acacia daviesii* Ethanol Extracts Against (a) *S. mutans* and (b) *S.sobrinus*
●: Control (no extract); ■: Stem extract; ▲: Phyllodes extract.

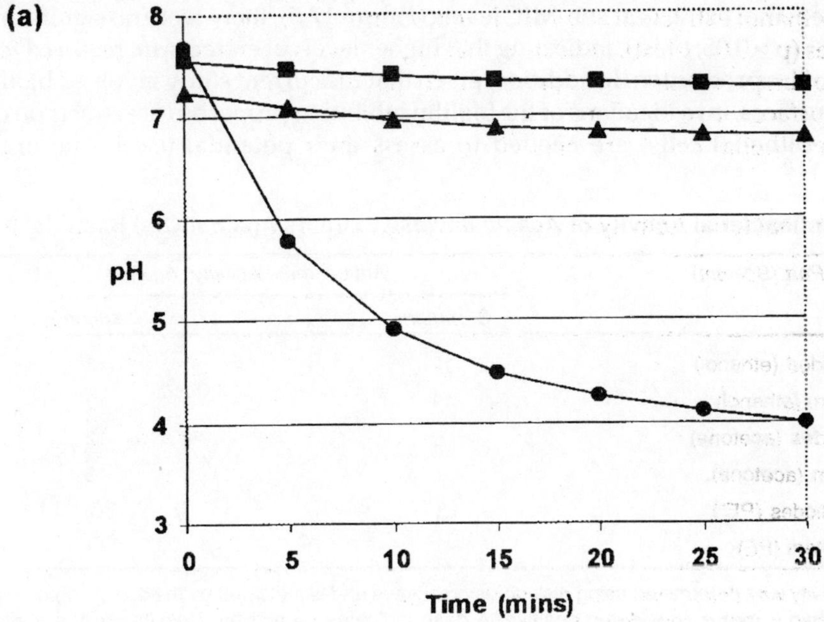

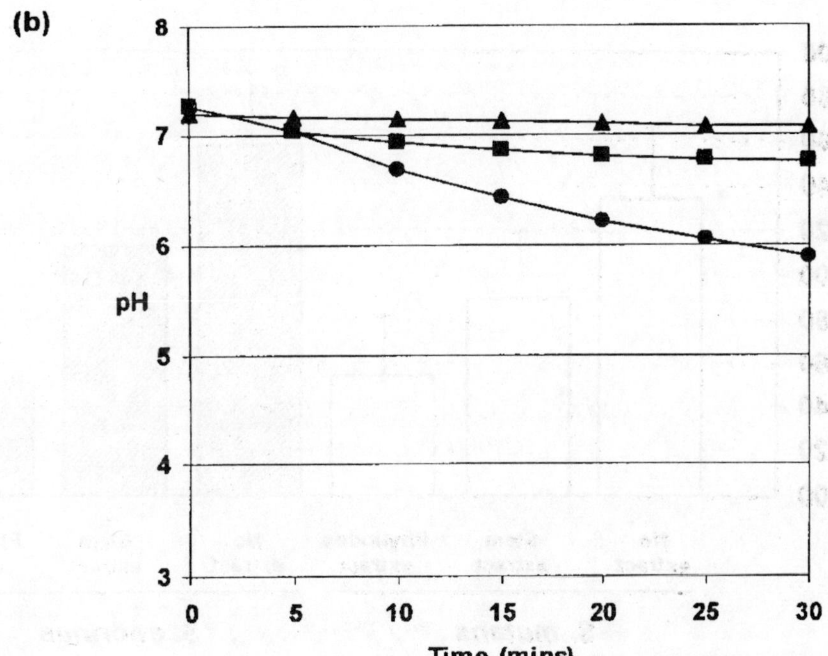

Figure 17.4: Inhibition of Glycolytic pH Drop of (a) *S. sobrinus* and (b) *S. mutans* by Ethanol Extracts of *Acacia daviesii*

●: Control (no extract); ■: Stem extract; ▲: Phyllodes extract.

treated with the ethanol extracts at sub-MIC levels (Figure 17.5), there were no significant differences to control cultures ($p > 0.05$; t-test), indicating that higher levels of extracts are required to significantly interfere with biofilm production. In addition, given that the current study involved biofilm formation on polystyrene surfaces, investigations of the biofilm inhibiting properties of extracts on other surfaces (*e.g.* glass and epithelial cells) are needed to assess their potential use in the oral and dental environments.

Table 17.4: Antibacterial Activity of *Acacia daviesii* Extracts Against Oral Bacterial Pathogens

Plant Part (Solvent)	*Antibacterial Activity[a] Against*	
	S. mutans	*S. sobrinus*
Phyllodes (ethanol)	12	16
Stem (ethanol)	11	12
Phyllodes (acetone)	-	12
Stem (acetone)	-	13
Phyllodes (PE[b])	8	12
Stem (PE)	8	11

[a]: Antibacterial activity was determined using disk diffusion assays and is indicated by the size (mm) of zones of inhibition. A zone greater than 6 mm is considered positive. A dash indicates no activity. Results are the average of duplicate assays.

[b]: Petroleum ether.

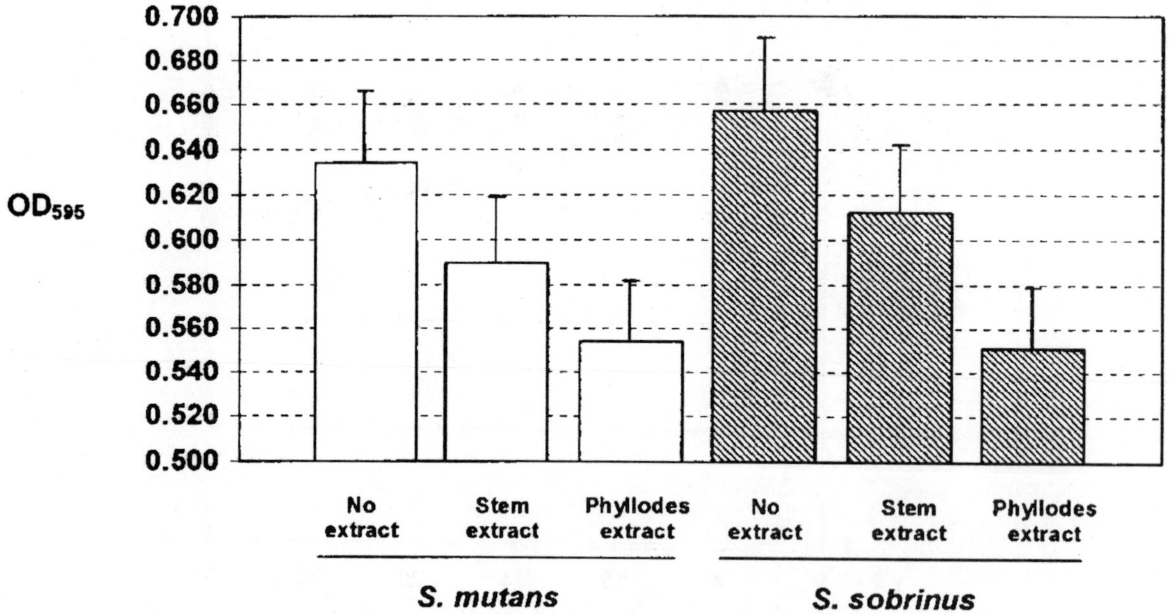

Figure 17.5: Biofilm Formation of *S. mutans* and *S. sobrinus* in the Absence and Presence of Ethanol Extracts of *Acacia daviesii*

In summary, our study has indicated that extracts of *Acacia daviesii* were able to inhibit the growth of a number of important pathogenic bacterial species and that these extracts, or compounds within them, may be useful in applications where specific inhibition of such bacteria is desired. Although there is no documented traditional medicinal use of *Acacia daviesii*, the data presented here demonstrated that specific bioactivity may be observed in plant species that have not been used previously in medical applications. Hence, investigation of plants that do not have an enthnomedical history, especially those that have been newly discovered, is warranted. However, whether such plants will yield useful bioactive compounds is yet to be determined. In addition, whether such compounds can be utilized in medical, dental or food industry applications requires assessment of their safety and tolerability.

Acknowledgements

We are grateful to Mr. Geoff Davies for providing plant material. Financial support was provided by the Sunshine Foundation and the Swinburne University Alumni and Development Office.

References

Alpuche, C., Garau, J. and Lim, V. (2007). Global and local variations in antimicrobial susceptibilities and resistance development in the major respiratory pathogens. *International Journal of Antimicrobial Agents*, 30 Suppl 2: S135-S138.

Badria, F.A. and Zidan, O.A. (2004). Natural products for dental caries prevention. *Journal of Medicinal Food*, 7: 381-384.

Barnes, S. and J. Prasain, 2005. Current progress in the use of traditional medicines and nutraceuticals. *Current Opinion in Plant Biology*, 8: 324-328.

Barr, A., Chapman. J., Smith, N., Wightman, G., Knight, T., Mills, L., Andrews, M. and Alexander, V. (1993). Traditional Aboriginal Medicines in the Northern Territory of Australia by Aboriginal Communities of the Northern Territory. Conservation Commission of the Northern Territory: Darwin.

Bartolome, M., Walsh, N.G., James, E.A. and Ladiges, P.Y. (2002). A new, rare species of *Acacia* from north-eastern Victoria. *Australian Systematic Botany*, 15: 465-475.

Bernimoulin, J.P. (2003). Recent concepts in plaque formation. *Journal of Clinical Periodontology*, 30 (Suppl 5): 7-9.

Chung, J.Y., Choo, J.H., Lee, M.H. and Hwang, J.K. (2006). Anticariogenic activity of macelignan isolated from *Myristica fragrans* (nutmeg) against *Streptococcus mutans*. *Phytomedicine*, 13: 261-266.

Cos, P., Vlietinck, A.J., Berghe, D.V. and Maes, L. (2006). Anti-infective potential of natural products: how to develop a stronger in vitro 'proof-of-concept'. *Journal of Ethnopharmacology*, 106: 290-302.

Cowan, M.M. (1999). Plant products as antimicrobial agents. *Clinical Microbiology Reviews*, 12: 564-582.

Duarte, S., Gregoire, S., Singh, A.P., Vorsa, N., Schaich, K.., Bowen, W.H. and Koo, H. (2006). Inhibitory effects of cranberry polyphenols on formation and acidogenicity of *Streptococcus mutans* bioflms. *FEMS Microbiology Letters*, 257: 50–56.

Hogan, D. and Kolter, R. (2002). Why are bacteria refractory to antimicrobials? *Current Opinion in Microbiology*, 5: 472-477.

Gautam, R., Saklani, A. and Jachak, S.M. (2007). Indian medicinal plants as a source of antimycobacterial agents. *Journal of Ethnopharmacology*, 110: 200-234.

Jenkinson, H.F. and Lamont, R.J. (2005). Oral microbial communities in sickness and in health. *Trends in Microbiology*, 13: 589-595.

Kalemba, D. and Kunicka, A. (2003). Antibacterial and antifungal properties of essential oils. *Current Medicinal Chemistry*, 10: 813-829.

Krebs, K.G., Heusser, D. and Wimmer, H. (1969). Spray reagents. *In:* Thin-layer chromatography: a laboratory handbook, Ed. by Stahl, E., Springer-Verlag: Berlin, pp. 854-905.

Lassak, E.V. and McCarthy, T. (2001). Australian medicinal plants. Reed New Holland, Sydney.

Mandal, P., Sinha Babub. S.P. and Mandal, N.C. (2005). Antimicrobial activity of saponins from *Acacia auriculiformis*. *Fitoterapia*, 76: 462-465.

Monroe, S. and Polk, R. (2000). Antimicrobial use and bacterial resistance. *Current Opinion in Microbiology*, 3: 496-501.

Orchard, A.E. and Wilson, A.J.G. (2001). Flora of Australia: *Mimosaceae*, Acacia. Environment Australia; CSIRO: Melbourne.

Park, K.M., You, J.S., Lee, H.Y., Baek, N.I. and Hwang, J.K. (2003). Kuwanon G: an antibacterial agent from the root bark of *Morus alba* against oral pathogens. *Journal of Ethnopharmacology*, 84: 181-185.

Petersen, P.E. (2003). The world oral health report 2003: continuous improvement of oral health in the 21st century–the approach of the WHO Global Oral Health Programme. *Community Dentistry and Oral Epidemiology*, 31(Suppl 1): 3-24.

Petersen, P.E., Bourgeois, D., Ogawa, H., Estupinan-Day, S. and Ndiaye, C. (2005). The global burden of oral diseases and risks to oral health. *Bulletin of the World Health Organization*, 83: 661-669.

Prabu, G.R., Gnanamani, A. and Sadulla, S. (2006). Guaijaverin–a plant flavonoid as potential antiplaque agent against *Streptococcus mutans*. *Journal of Applied Microbiology*, 101: 487-495.

Shah, A., Cross, R.F. and Palombo, E.A. (2004). Identification of the antibacterial component of an ethanolic extract of the Australian medicinal plant, *Eremophila duttonii*. *Phytotherapy Research*, 18: 615-618.

Seigler, D.S. (2002). Economic potential from Western Australian *Acacia* species: secondary plant metabolites. *Conservation Science W.A*, 4: 109–116.

Tichy, J. and Novak J.J. (1998). Extraction, assay, and analysis of antimicrobials from plants with activity against dental pathogens (*Streptococcus* sp.). *Journal of Alternative and Complementary Medicine*, 4: 39-45.

Wilkinson, J.M. (2006). Methods for testing the antimicrobial activity of extracts. *In:* Modern phytomedicine. Ed. by Ahmed, I., Aqil, F. and Owais, M. Wiley-VCH, Weinheim, pp. 157-171.

Yamanaka, A., Kimizuka, R., Kato, T. and Okuda, K. (2004). Inhibitory effects of cranberry juice on attachment of oral streptococci and biofilm formation. Oral Microbiology and Immunology 19: 150-4.

Utilisation and Management of Medicinal Plants (2010) *Pages 319–339*
Editors: **V.K. Gupta, Anil K. Verma and Sushma Koul**
Published by: **DAYA PUBLISHING HOUSE, NEW DELHI**

Chapter 18

A Review on Some Potential Anthelmintic Herbal Drugs

Ravindra G. Mali*
L.B.Rao Institute of Pharmaceutical Education and Research,
B.D.Rao College Campus, Khambhat – 388 620
Dist. Anand, Gujarat, India

ABSTRACT

Medicinal plants are of great importance in providing health care to a large portion of population in the World. Medicinal plants have contributed to a greater extent in the preservations of health and cure of human diseases at such time when no other remedies were available. With the advancement in science many of the crude drugs used in traditional system of medicine came under the phytochemical scrutiny and led to the isolation of therapeutically active constituents like digoxin, morphine, atropine, vincristine, taxol etc. Some of these phytoprinciples were synthesized and some of them served as prototypes/models for the synthesis of new drugs with similar pharmacological activity. The same later gave birth to synthetic drugs, which are mainly utilized in today's modern system of medicine. Gradually synthetic drugs replaced the traditional system of medicine and became popular throughout the world. But because of high cost and lack of availability in the rural areas, people still depend on the traditional system of medicine like Ayurveda, Siddha, Unani etc. Modern synthetic medicines are very effective in cure of diseases but also cause a number of side effects. While crude drugs are less efficient with respect to cure of diseases but are relatively free from side effects. Parasites have been of

* E-mail: ravigmali@yahoo.co.in; Phone: 02587 222678, 09275161224.

concern to the medical field for centuries and the helminths still cause considerable problems for human beings and animals. A large number of medicinal plants have been claimed to possess anthelmintic activity in traditional systems of medicine and also utilized by ethnic groups worldwide. Following the folk claims, several medicinal plants have been scrutinized for their anthelmintic activities using various *in vitro* and *in vivo* methods. The present review highlights scientific screenings on some medicinal plants, products thereof and isolated principles from them, which can be investigated further to achieve lead molecules in the search of novel anthelmintic drugs. We have reviewed the relevant literature on the plants which have been experimentally studied for anthelmintic activity.

Keywords: *Anthelmintic activity, Essential oils, Hookworms, Indian earthworms, Piperazine citrate, Phytoprinciples, Tapeworms.*

Introduction

Helminthic infections are among the most common infections in human beings, affecting a large proportion of the world's population. In developing countries they pose a large threat to public health and contribute to the prevalence of anaemia, malnutrition, eosinophilia and pneumonia. Although the majority of infections due to worms are generally limited to tropical countries, they can occur to travelers who have visited those areas and some of them can be developed in temperate climates (Bundy, 1994).The helminthes which infect the intestine are cestodes *e.g.* tapeworms (*Taenia solium*), nematodes eg.hookworm (*Ancylostoma duodenale*), roundworm (*Ascaris lumbricoids*) and trematodes or flukes *e.g. Schistosoma mansoni* and *Schistosoma hematobolium*. The diseases originated from parasitic infections causing severe morbidity include lymphatic filariasis, onchocerciasis and schistosomiasis. These infections can affect most populations in endemic areas with major economic and social consequences. Helminthes also affect millions of livestock resulting in considerable economic losses in domestic and farm yard animals. Because of limited availability and affordability of modern medicines most of the world's population depends, to a greater extent, on traditional medical remedies. The traditional medicines hold a great promise as source of easily available effective anthelmintic agents to the people, particularly in tropical developing countries, including India. It is in this context that the people consume several plants or plant-derived preparations to cure helminthic infections (Satyavati, 1990). Ideally an anthelmintic agent should have broad spectrum of action, high percentage of cure with a single therapeutic dose, free from toxicity to the host and should be cost effective. None of the synthetic drug available meets this requirement. Even most common drugs like piperazine salts have shown side effects like nausea, intestinal disturbances and giddiness (Liu and Weller, 1996). Resistance of the parasites to existing drugs (Walter and Prichard, 1985) and their higher cost warrant the search of newer anthelmintic molecules. The origin of many effective drugs is found in the traditional medicine practices and in view of this several researchers have undertaken studies to evaluate folklore medicinal plants for their proclaimed anthelmintic efficacy (Temjenmongla and Yadav, 2005).

Most of the screenings reported are *in vitro* studies using some worm samples like Indian earthworm *Pheretima posthuma*, *Ascardia galli*, *Ascaris lumbricoids* etc. Adult Indian earthworm, *Pheretima posthuma* has been used as test worm in most of the anthelmintic screenings as it shows anatomical and physiological resemblance with the intestinal roundworm parasite of human beings (Vidyarthi, 1967; Thorn *et al.*, 1977; Vigar, 1984; Chatterjee, 1967).

Because of easy availability, earthworms have been used widely for the initial evaluation of anthelmintic compounds *in vitro* (Sollmann, 1918; Jain *et al.*, 1972; Dash *et al.*, 2002; Szewezuk *et al.*, 2003; Shivkar *et al.*, 2003; Mali *et al.*, 2005). *Ascardia galli* worms are easily available from freshly slaughtered fowls and its use, as a suitable model for screening of anthelmintic drug was advocated earlier (Kaushik *et al.*, 1974; Lal *et al.*, 1976; Tandon *et al.*, 1997; Mali *et al.*, 2007a). These *in vitro* screenings of medicinal plants are important as they are platforming for further *in vivo* studies to investigate their efficacy and possible toxic effects, if any.

A survey of literatures available indicated that though the number of crude plant extracts, essential oils and isolated active principles (Figure 18.1) via bioactivity guided fractionation, have been screened

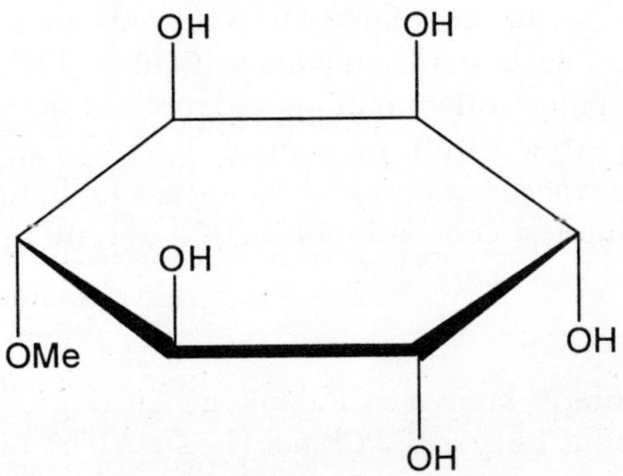

D-3-0-Methylchiroinositol

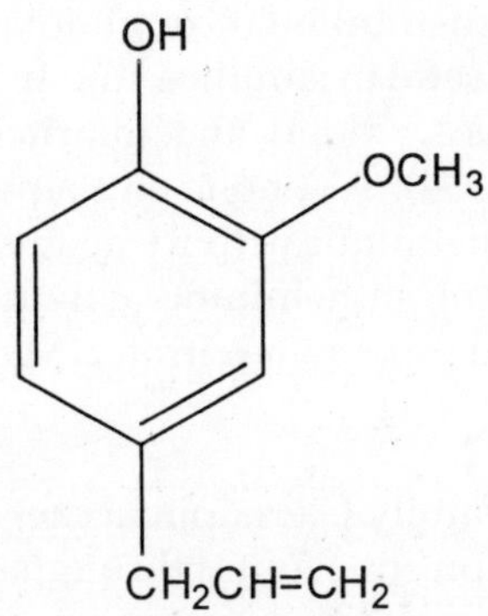

Eugenol

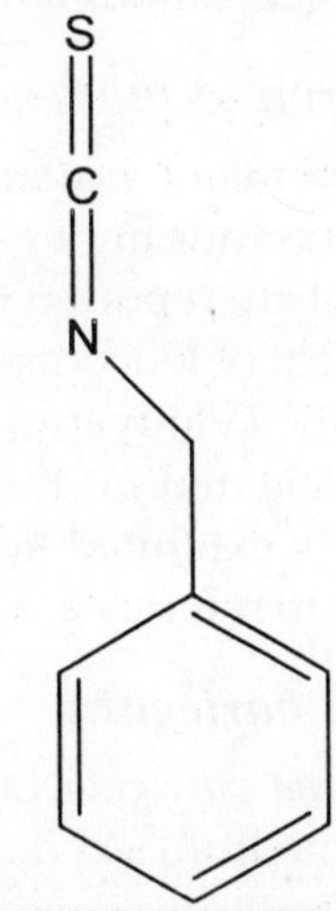

Benzyl isothiocynate

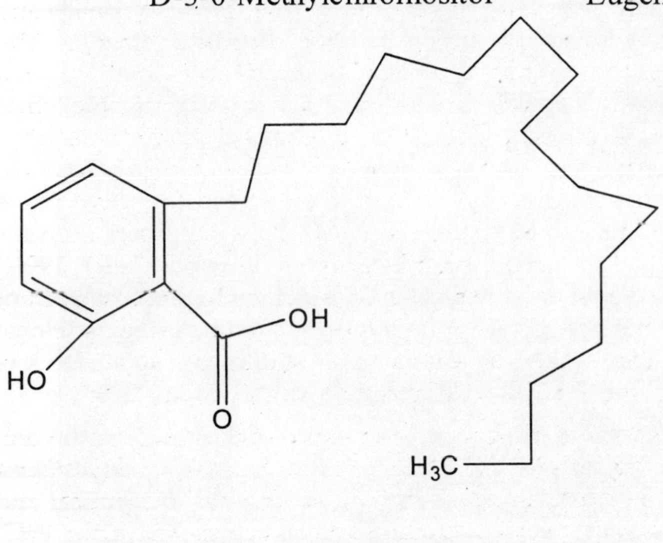

Anacardic acid

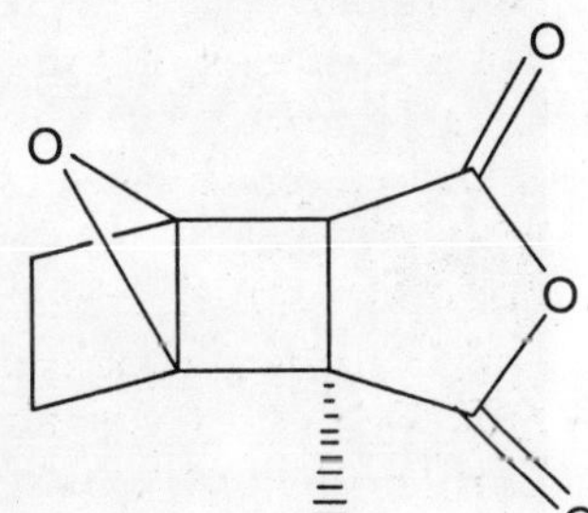

Palasonin

Figure 18.1: Isolated Phytoprinciples with Anthelmintic Potential

for *in vitro* and *in vivo* anthelmintic studies but very few of them successively turned up into effective drugs. In the present review, we have discussed the various screenings and attempts made by the researchers to evaluate the efficacy of plant-derived materials as a new possible anthelmintic molecule and to establish their possible mechanism (s) of action.

Anacardium occidentale

Garg and Kasera, (1982) have reported that the oil obtained from *Anacardium occidentale* Linn. (Anacardiaceae) possess significant anthelmintic activity against earthworms and tapeworms. The activity was found better than reference standard piperazine phosphate. The oil was also found to be effective against hookworms as compared to hexyl resorcinol.

Baliospermum montanum

Baliospermum montanum Muell. Arg (Family. Euphorbiaceae) commonly known as Danti, is a leafy monoecious under shrub distributed throughout India, Burma and Malaya. In Ayurveda, roots of the plant are reported to be useful in jaundice, and in traditional system of medicine highly valued for treatment of leucoderma, piles, wound, anaemia, itching, pains, inflammations and reputed as an anthelmintic (Vaidyaratnam, 1994). Alcoholic and aqueous extracts from the roots of *B. montanum* were investigated for their anthelmintic activity against *Pheretima posthuma* and *Ascardia galli*. Both the extracts exhibited significant anthelmintic activity at highest concentration of 100 mg/ml as compared to reference standard piperazine citrate, (Mali and Wadekar, 2008).

Bauhinia variegata

Bauhinia variegata Linn. (Family-Caesalpiniaceae) popularly known as Raktakanchan (Figure 18.2), is a medium sized deciduous tree found throughout India, Burma and China. The stem bark of

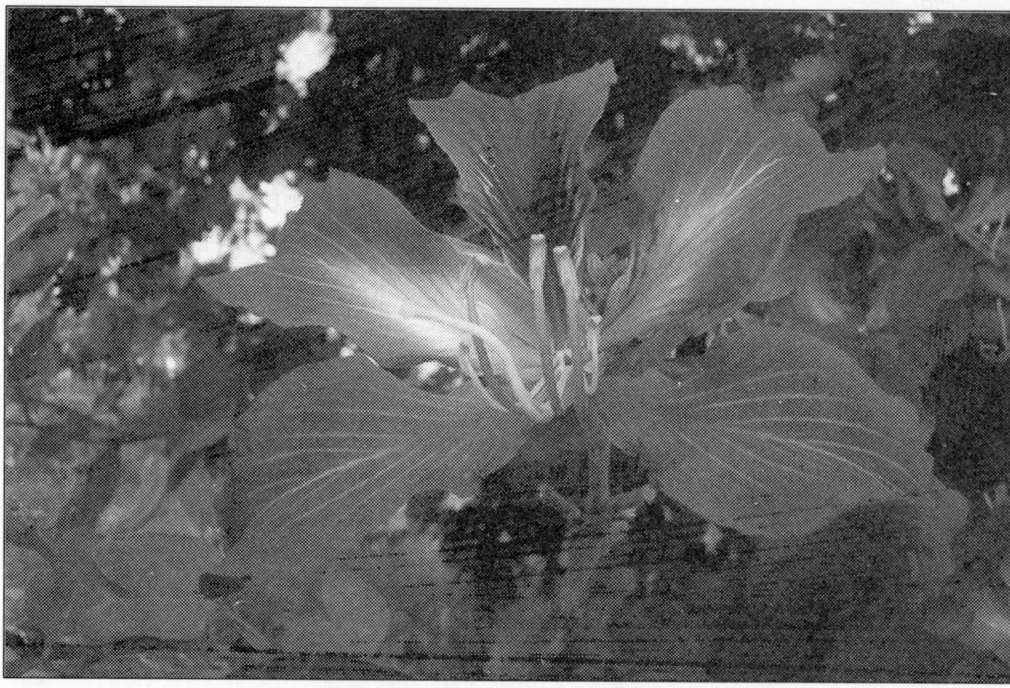

Figure 18.2: *Bauhinia variegata*

the plant is of great medicinal importance and traditionally used as astringent, liver tonic and anthelmintic (Nadkarni, 1960). The crude ethanolic extract of the plant was evaluated for anthelmintic activity using Indian earthworm *Pheretima posthuma* and *Ascardia galli* as test worms. Following the traditional claim, different concentrations (10-100 mg/ml) of ethanolic extract were tested in the bioassay using piperazine citrate (10 mg/ml) as reference standard. The ethanolic extract showed promising anthelmintic activity comparable to standard (Mali *et al.*, 2008).

Butea frondosa

Butea frondosa Koenig ex Roxb. (Leguminoceae) (Figure 18.3) seeds are known to possess anthelmintic activity and their efficacy has been reported against ascarids (Ramanan, 1960), stomach worms of the sheep (Garg and Mehta, 1958) and *Ascardia galli* (Satyanarayanrao *et al.*, 1982). The anthelmintic property of *B. frondosa* seeds was attributed to the main active principle palasonin, a lactone ($C_{16}H_{22}O_6$) compound (Raj and Kurup, 1967). Palasonin was found to be effective against *Ascaris lumbricoids* (Rao *et al.*, 1977) and *Fasciola hepatica* (Sabir *et al.*, 1977). Kumar *et al.* (1995) has investigated the biochemical mechanism of anthelmintic action of palasonin on *Ascardia galli* and concluded that palasonin inhibit the glucose uptake and deplete the glycogen content in the presence of glucose indicating that palasonin affects the energy generating mechanism of the parasite. It also significantly increased the lactic acid suggesting inhibition of ATP production. The results indicated that palasonin may act via either inhibition of energy metabolism and/or alteration in the motor activity of the parasite.

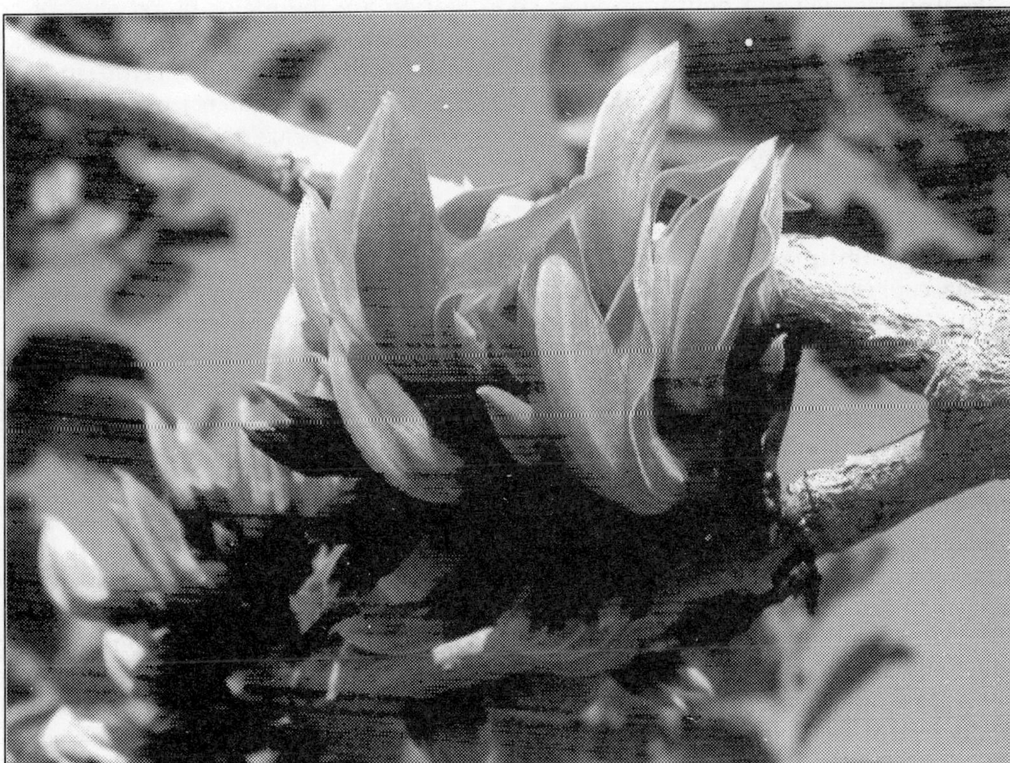

Figure 18.3: *Butea frondosa*

Calotropis procera

Calotropis procera (Ait) is a wild tropical plant (Asclepidiaceae) used in traditional system of medicine for treatment of rheumatism, lupus, eczema, helminthic infections, asthma, leprosy, and syphilis (Anonymous, 1992). The latex of *C. procera* (Figure), has been shown to possess anthelmintic activity against *Haemonchus contortus* infection in Najdi sheep in which it decreased the egg production and the number of worms in the abomasum and also *in vitro* larvicidal activity (Al-Qarawi *et al.*, 2001). Both fresh and aqueous extracts of dried latex were evaluated for their anthelmintic potential using earthworms as test worms. Both the extracts exhibited does-dependant inhibition of spontaneous motility and evoked responses to pin-prick. With higher doses (100 mg/ml of aqueous extract and 100 per cent fresh latex) the effects were comparable with that of 3 per cent piperazine.The study suggested that it might be effective against parasitic infections of both animals and humans caused by *Ostertagia, Nematodirus, Dictyocaulis, Taenia, Ascaris* and *Fasciola* (Shivkar and Kumar, 2003). The flowers of *C. procera* were evaluated for anthelmintic activity in comparison with levamisole through *in vitro* and *in vivo* studies and found to possess good activity against nematodes (Iqbal *et al.*, 2005).

Carica papaya

The anthelmintic potential of the aqueous extract of *Carica papaya* Linn. (Caricaceae) (Figure 18.4) was evaluated using roundworm *Ascaris lumbricoids* and *Ascardia galli* (Nematodes) as test parasites (Dhar *et al.*, 1965). The phytoprinciple benzyl isothiocyanate isolated from the extract was found to possess significant anthelmintic activity. The metabolic pathways in general and carbohydrate pathways in particular and neuromuscular coordination are the major target sites of action of anthelmintic compounds (Sharma, 1987). The compound benzyl isothiocyanate exerted its action by inhibiting energy metabolism and by affecting motor activity of the parasites, *in vitro* studies (Kumar *et al.*, 1991). In another study (Kermanshai *et al.*, 2001) benzyl isothiocyanate isolated from *C. papaya*, seed extracts was tested for anthelmintic activity by viability assay using *Caenorhabditis elegans* and claimed it as the chief or sole anthelmintic agent.

Capparis decidua

The anthelmintic activity of ethanolic extract of root bark of *Capparis decidua* Edgew (Capparidaceae) (Figure 18.5) was evaluated against adult Indian earthworm *Pheretima posthuma* (Annelida). The activity was found dose dependant, comparable with piperazine citrate (10 mg/ml) at the higher concentration of 100 mg/ml of the extract (Mali *et al.*, 2004). The root bark of *C.decidua* is reported to contain spermidine alkaloids (Ahmed *et al.*, 1992). Ethanolic extract of root bark of another species *Capparis spinosa* Linn. (Capparidaceae) has shown good anthelmintic activity against earthworm *Pheretima posthuma*. The activity was found dose dependant (Mali *et al.*, 2005).

Cleome viscosa

Cleome viscosa Linn (Capparidaceae) (Figure 18.6), commonly known as Hul-Hul, is an annual common weed found all over the plains of India and throughout the tropics of the world. In Ayurvedic system of medicine this plant is believed to have several medicinal properties such as stomachic, laxative, diuretic, anthelmintic, skin diseases, itching, ulcers, leprosy, malarial fevers (Chatterjee and Prakashi, 1991). The crude alcohol and aqueous extracts of the seeds of *C. viscosa* Linn. were investigated for their anthelmintic activity against *Pheretima posthuma* and *Ascardia galli.* Various concentrations (10-100 mg/ml) of each extract were tested in the bioassay, which involved determination of time of paralysis and time of death of the worms. Both the extracts exhibited considerable anthelmintic activity

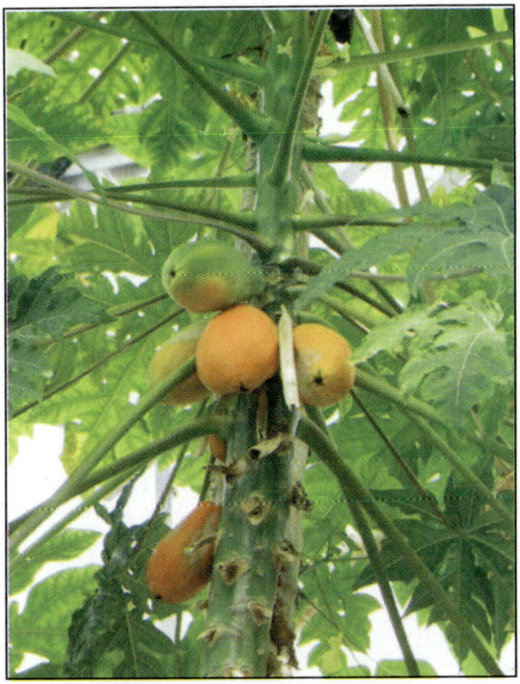

Figure 18.4: ***Carica papaya***

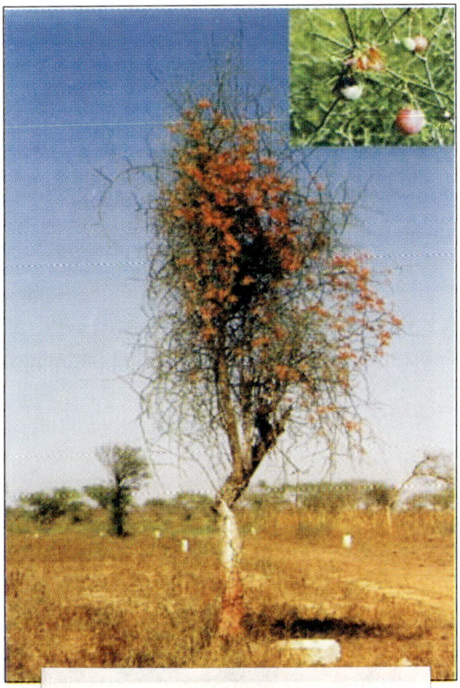

Figure 18.5: ***Capparis decidua***

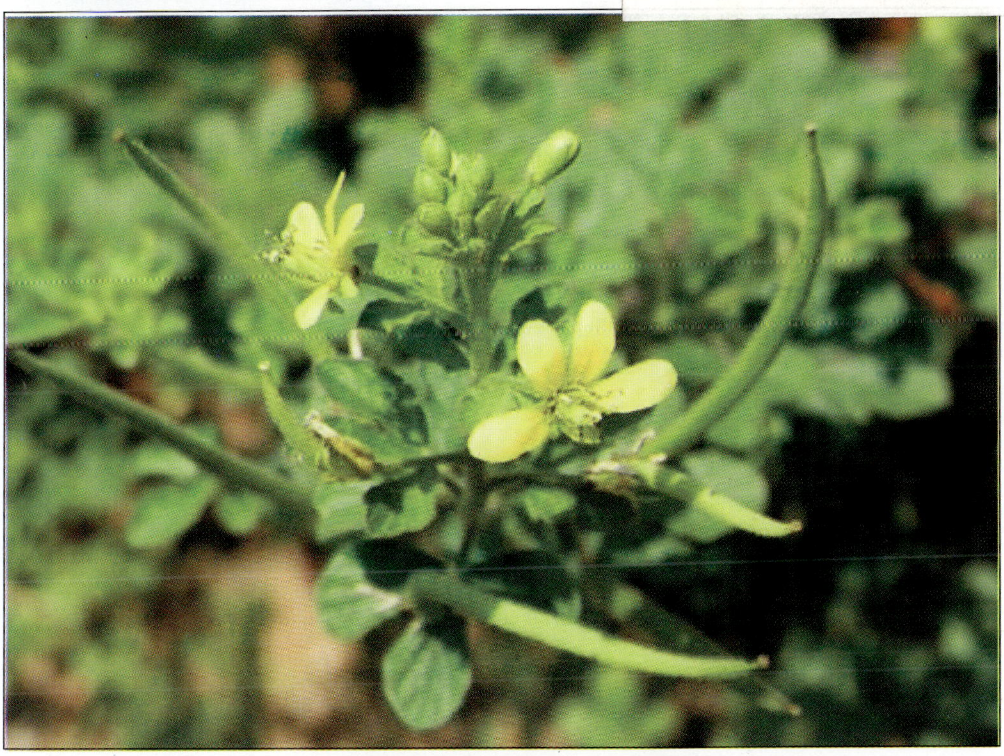

Figure 18.6: ***Cleome viscosa***

in dose dependant manner. The most significant activity was observed at 100 mg/ml concentration of against both types of worms (Mali *et al.*, 2007b).

Clitorea ternatea

In one study, Anthelmintic activity of *Clitorea ternatea* Linn (Fabaceae) (Figure 18.7) commonly known as Gokarna, has been evaluated by Khadatkar *et al.* (2008). The crude ethanolic extract of the plant and its various fractions *viz.*, petroleum ether, ethyl acetate and methanol were tested for anthelmintic potential using adult earthworm *Pheretima posthuma* as test worm. The crude extract and its ethyl acetate and methanol fraction exhibited potent activity at the concentration of 50 mg/ml as compared to the reference standard piperazine citrate.

Commiphora mukul

Guggul is one of the noted drugs from Ayurveda and Unani system. In recent times, its demand in therapeutics has been substantially increased. The essential oil obtained from oleogum resin of guggul *Commiphora mukul* Linn. has shown good anthelmintic activity against hookworms and tapeworms. The activity was comparable to that of reference standards piperazine phosphate and hexyl resorcinol used in the study (Kakrani and Kalyani, 1984).

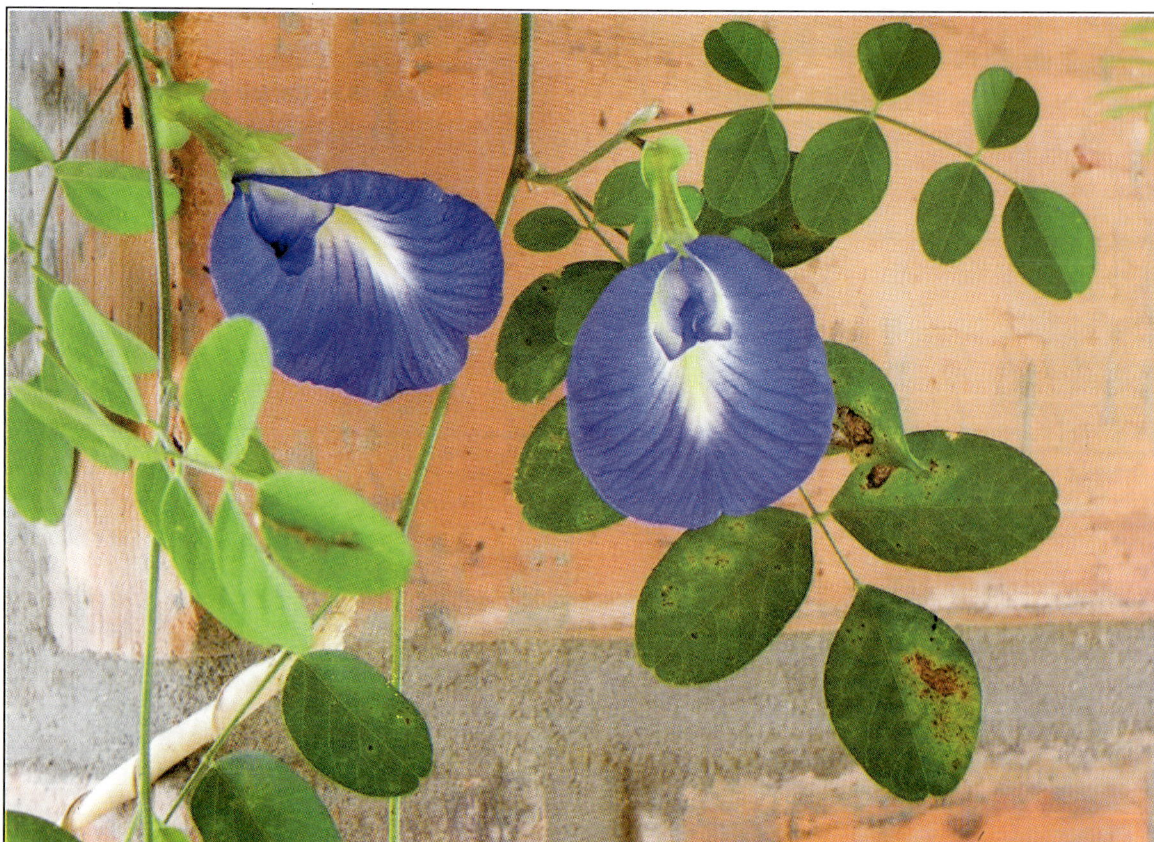

Figure 18.7: *Clitorea ternatea*

Cucurbita maxima

Cucurbita maxima Duch. ex Lam. (Family: Cucurbitaceae) (Figure 18.8) seeds are reputed in Ayurvedic system of medicine as an anthelmintic especially against tape worms. The aqueous, alcoholic and ethereal extracts of the seeds were tested *in vivo* and *in vitro* on trematodes, cestodes and nematodes. The aqueous and alcoholic extracts of the plant were found to be more potent than the ethereal extract. The kymographic studies suggested that the seed extracts acted by bringing about a decrease in the movements leading to temporary paralysis (Shrivastav and Singh, 1967).

Enicostemma littorale

Enicostemma littorale Blume (Gentianaceae) is a glabrous perennial herb distributed throughout India and found in Malaysia, Sri Lanka, Java, South Africa and West Indies. Traditionally *E.littorale* is used as an anthelmintic, carminative, stomachic and laxative. The aqueous extract of *E.littorale* and its several fractions(petroleum ether, toluene and n-butanol were screened for their anthelmintic efficacy against *Pheretima posthuma* and *Ascardia gall.*. The anthelmintic activity was carried out using different concentrations of the aqueous extract and its fractions, which involved determination of time of paralysis and time of death of the worms. Piperazine citrate was included as reference standard and distilled water as control. The results indicated that the crude aqueous extract and its toluene and n-butanol fractions, significantly, demonstrated paralysis, and also caused death of worms especially at higher concentration of 100 mg/ml, as compared to standard reference Piperazine citrate (Mali, 2007c).

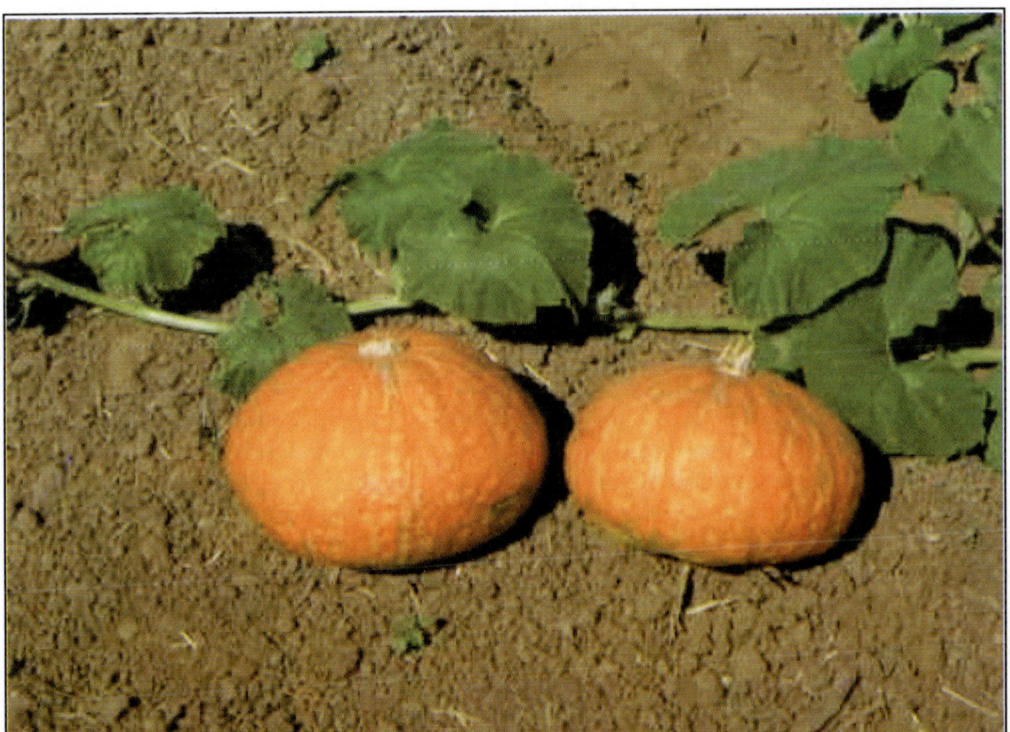

Figure 18.8: *Cucurbita maxima*

Evolvulus alsinoides

Evolvulus alsinoides Linn. (Convolvulaceae) is widely used in Ayurveda as powerful brain stimulant, aphrodisiac and anthelmintic. Ethanolic extract of whole plant material was screened for anthelmintic activity against adult Indian earthworm, *Pheretima posthuma*. The extract caused paralysis followed by death of the worms at all tested dose levels. At concentration of 100 mg/ml the ethanolic extract were found more potent than reference control piperazine citrate (Dash *et al.*, 2002).

Flemingia vestita

Flemingia vestita Benth and Hooker (Fabaceae) is a leguminous root crop commonly found in the north-eastern regions of India. Its fleshy tuberous roots along with the peel are consumed raw by the Meghalayan local tribal people to cure intestinal helminth infections. In a preliminary study the crude extract of the whole root tubers of this plant was reported to be effective against *Ascaris suum in vitro* (Yadav *et al.*, 1992). Tegumental alterations and deformity were also observed in digenean flukes treated with the crude peel extract of the roots (Roy and Tandon, 1996). Further in one of the study, root-tuber extract (50 mg/ml) and genistein (0.5 mg/ml), an active principle isolated from the root-tuber peel were tested against live parasites (Nematode: *Ascaris suum* from pigs, *A.lumbricoids* from humans, *Ascardia galli* and *Heterakis gallinarum* from domestic fowl; Cestode: *Raillietina echinobothrida* from domestic fowl; Trematode: *Paramphistomum spp.* from cattle). The crude extract and genistein revealed complete immobilization of the trematode and cestode but not against cuticle-covered nematodes. The treated parasites also showed structural alteration in their tegumental architecture. The activity of the peel extract and genistein attributed to the changes induced in the tegumental integrity of the parasite (Tandon *et al.*, 1997).

Gynandropsis gynandra

In one study, Ajaiyeoba *et al.* (2003) has investigated anthelmintic potential of methanol extracts of leaves and stems of *Gynandropsis gynandra* Merr. (Capparidaceae) using *Fasciola gigantica* (liverfluke), *Taenia solium* (Tapeworm) and *Pheretima posthuma* (Earthworm) as test worms. Both the extracts exhibited considerable activity in dose dependant manner and order of sensitivity of the extract to the worms was *P. posthuma*> *F. gigantica*> *T. solium*. The methanolic extract of stem was found more active and showed significant activity compared to piperazine citrate, standard reference used in the study

Melia azedarach

Melia azedarach Linn (Meliaceae) (Figure 18.9) is a native tree of Persia, India and China. This plant has long been recognized as an insecticidal and medicinal plant all over the world. The ethanolic extract of drupes of *M. azedarach* was tested for its anthelmintic activity against the tapeworm *Taenia solium* (Cestoda) and the earthworm *Pheretima posthuma* (Annelida) using piperazine phosphate as the standard drug. The extract was found active against both the tapeworm and the earthworm tested. But the activity was better against tapeworm *Taenia solium*, than that of piperazine phosphate (Szewezuk *et al.*, 2003). In another study, *in vitro* anthelmintic activity of the aqueous and alcoholic extracts of *Melia azedarach*, *Ananas sativus*, *Embelica ribes* and *Mucuna prurita* was evaluated against *Taenia canina* and *Phamphistomum cervi* (Neogi *et al.*, 1964). *Mucuna prurita* was found more active against the trematodes.

Millettia pachycarpa

The root bark of *Millettia pachycarpa* Bentham (Fabaceae) traditionally used as a remedy for gastrointestinal infections among the Mizo tribes of north-east India, was tested *in vitro* to evaluate its anthelmintic activity on the poultry intestinal tapeworm, *Raillietina echinobothrida*. On treatment of the parasites with varying concentrations of the plant extract, *viz*, 0.5, 1, 2, 5, 10 and 20 mg/ml, a dose dependant lethal efficacy was observed. Scanning electron microscopy revealed extensive distortion and destruction on the surface fine topography of the worm. Focal truncation with formation of pits and vacuoles on the tegument were evident. Deformities on the scolex with its suckers were particularly conspicuous at the anterior extremity (Roy *et al.*, 2008).

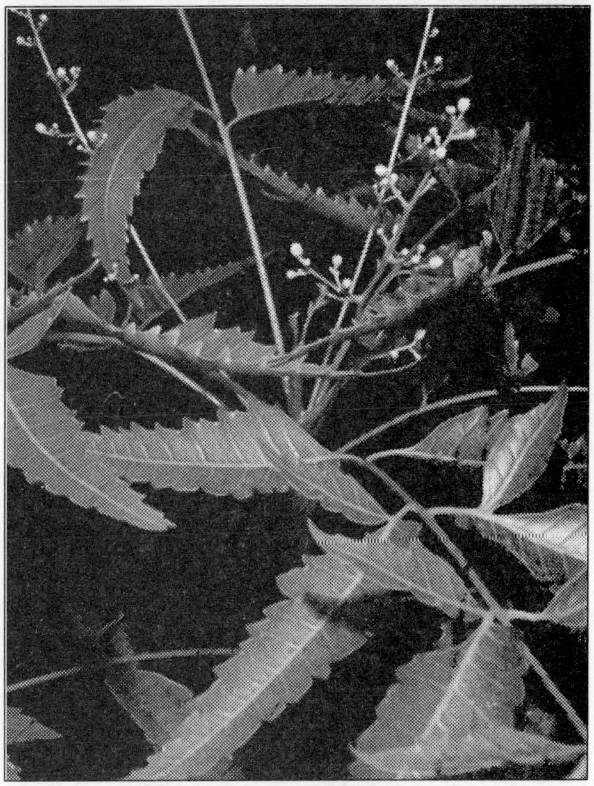

Figure 18.9: ***Melia azadirach***

Mimusops elengi

In indigenous system of medicine the bark of *Mimusops elengi* Linn. (Sapotaceae) is reported to possess various therapeutic properties as cardiotonic, stomachic, alexipharmic, anthelmintic and astringent (Kirtikar and Basu, 1935). Various phytoprinciples such as taraxerol, taraxerone, ursolic acid, betulinic acid, α-spinosterol, β-sitosterol, alkaloid isoretronecyl tiglate and mixture of triterpenoid saponins have been reported from stem bark of *M.elengi.* The crude alcoholic extract and its various fractions of the plant were evaluated for their anthelmintic potential using *Pheretima posthuma* (Annelida) and *Ascardia galli* (Nematode) as test worms. The crude alcoholic extract and its ethyl acetate and n-butanol fractions significantly demonstrated paralysis and also caused death of worms especially at higher concentration of 100 mg/ml as compared to standard reference piperazine citrate (10 mg/ml). The activity of *M.elengi* was attributed to the presence of polyphenolic compounds and tannins in the stem bark (Mali *et al.*, 2007a). Tannins are believed to interfere with energy generation in helminth parasites by uncoupling oxidative phosphorylation and can bind to glycoprotein on the cuticle of the parasite, thereby causing death (Thompson and Geary, 1995).

Neolamarckia cadamba

Neolamarckia cadamba Roxb. (Rubiaceae) is an ornamental plant traditionally used in stomatitis, eye inflammation and as an anthelmintic.It is reported to contain triterpenoids, alkaloids and saponins (Kaushik and Dhiman, 1999). Aqueous and ethanolic extracts of mature stem-bark of the plant were screened for anthelmintic potential against earthworms, tapeworms and roundworms using albendazole as reference drug. The ethanolic extract was found potent than aqueous extract and activity was comparable with the standard drug used in the study (Gunasekaran *et al.*, 2006).

Nicotiana tobacum

In vitro and *in vivo* anthelmintic activity of *Nicotiana tobacum* Linn (Solanaceae) leaves was studied to rationalize its traditional use. Live *Haemonchus contortus* were used to assess the *in vitro* anthelmintic effect of a crude aqueous extract and methanol extract of the plant. For the *in vivo* studies both the extracts were administered in increasing doses (1.0-3.0 g/kg) to sheep naturally infected with mixed species of gastrointestinal nematodes. The results of the study showed that both the extracts of *N. tobacum* exhibit dose-dependant anthelmintic activity both *in vivo* and *in vitro* justifying its use in traditional system of medicine (Iqbal *et al.*, 2006a).

Nigella sativa

Nigella sativa Linn (Ranunculaceae) commonly known as Kala Jira, is reputed plant in Indian system of medicine for its usefulness in variety of ailments and possesses carminative, digestive astringent and diuretic properties (Nadkarni, 1960). The anthelmintic activity of essential oil of *N. sativa* was evaluated against earthworms, tapeworms, hookworms and nodular worms and has exhibited fairly good activity against earthworms and tapeworms. The activity against hookworms and nodular worms being comparable with that of hexyl resorcinol (Agrawal *et al.*, 1979). The plant is reported to contain main active principles such as thymoquinone, dithymoquinone-cymene and α-pinene.

Ocimum sanctum

Ocimum sanctum Linn (Labiatae) (Figure 18.10) is an herbaceous plant found throughout India. It contains volatile oil of which chief constituents are eugenol (about 51 per cent) and β-caryophyllene (37 per cent) and number of sesquiterpenes and monoterpenes (Handa and Kapoor, 1988). The essential oil of *O.sanctum* and eugenol showed potent *in vitro* anthelmintic activity against *Caenorhabditis elegans* (Nematode).Various concentrations of essential oil and eugenol were tested using Levamisole as reference standard. The essential oil and eugenol exhibited ED50 of 237.9 and 62.1 μg/ml respectively. Eugenol being the predominant component of the essential oil was suggested as the putative anthelmintic principle (Asha *et al.*, 2001).

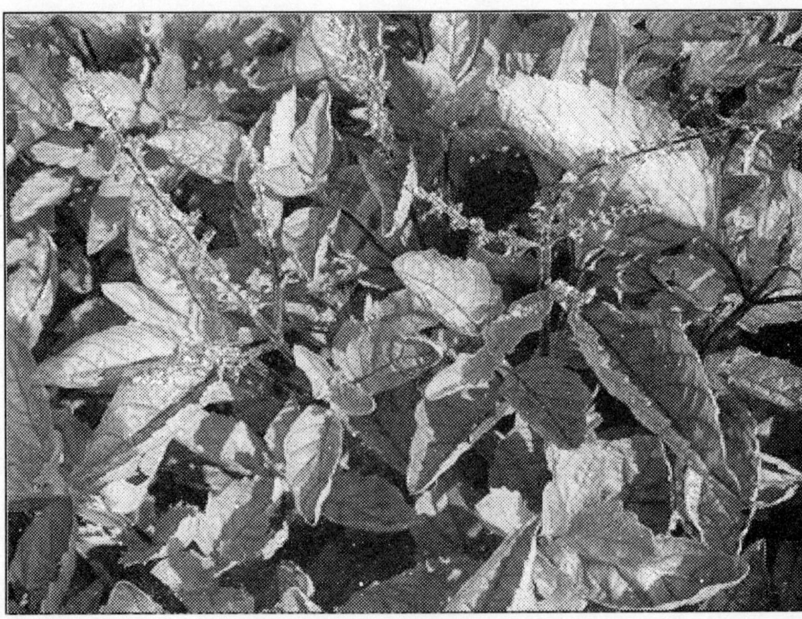

Figure 18.10: *Ocimum sanctum*

Picrolemma sprucei

Picrolemma sprucei Hook. is a small tree or low shrub which is native to and widely distributed in the Amazon region. It is used against worms in Peru, French Guyana and Brazil (Duke and Vasquez, 1994). In the Brazilian Amazon, this plant is known by the popular name *caferana.* The aqueous and ethanol extracts prepared from stems and roots of the plant were evaluated for the anthelmintic activity against a gastrointestinal nematode parasite, *Haemonchus contortus,* found in domestic and wild ruminants. Neosergeolide, Isobrucein B isolated from stems of the plant and standard Levamisole all caused comparable mortality rates (68-77 per cent) *in vitro* to *H. contortus* at similar concentrations (81-86 ppm). The study revealed the potential anthelmintic activity of water and ethanol stem and root extracts against parasite *in vitro* and suggested further *in vivo* studies as nematicides on isolated phytoprinciples from stem of the plant (Nunomura *et al.,* 2006)

Piliostigma thonningii

Piliostigma thonningii Schum. (Caesalpiniaceae) stem bark traditionally used to treat dysentery, snake-bite, toothache and as anthelmintic (Lewis and Elvin, 1979). The ethanolic extract of the plant exhibited a potent dose dependant anthelmintic activity in *Ascardia galli* infected cockrels by stimulating the neuromuscular junction principally and the ganglion to a lesser degree (Asuzu and Onu, 1994). Following its traditional claim, an active principle D-3-*O*-Methylchiroinositol was isolated by bioassay-guided chromatographic separation technique from methanolic extract of stem bark of the plant and screened for anthelmintic activity by larval paralysis using Levamisole as a reference drug. Third stage larvae (L3) of *Haemonchus contortus* from faecal samples of infected lambs were used in the study. D-3-*O*-Methylchiroinositol of *P. thonningii* stem bark induced approximately 60 per cent larval paralysis within 24 h. of contact with *H. contortus* larvae at 4.4 mg/ml concentration (Asuzu *et al.,* 1999).

Piper betle

The essential oil of *Piper betle* Linn (Piperaceae) (Figure 18.11) has revealed *in vitro* anthelmintic activity against the earthworm *Pheretima posthuma* (Ali and Mehta, 1970). The anthelmintic activity of the essential oil obtained from *P. betle* cultivar Sagar Bangla was tested against tapeworms and found better than the standard piperazine phosphate and activity against hookworm found greater than the reference drug hexyl resorcinol (Garg and Jain, 1992).

Piper longum

The essential oil from the fruits of *Piper longum* Linn (Piperaceae) was screened for the anthelmintic activity against *Ascaris lumbricoids.*The experiment revealed that oil of *P. longum* had a definite paralytic action the nerve-muscle preparation of *Ascaris lumbricoids.*The activity of oil was found more than the piperazine citrate used as standard in the study (D´Cruz *et al.,* 1980).

Punica granatum

Punica granatum Linn (Punicaceae) (Figure 18.12) locally known as Anar is cultivated in all parts of India. The root and stem bark of the plant is used as astringent and anthelmintic in indigenous system of medicine. The alcoholic extract of *P.granatum* stem bark was evaluated for its proclaimed anthelmintic potential. The activity was found dose dependant, inhibiting transformation of eggs to filariform larvae of *Haemonchus contortus* (Prakash *et al.,* 1980). In clinical studies, the plant showed efficacy in nematodiasis in calves (Pradhan *et al.,* 1992). The stem bark of *P.granatum* is reported to contain an alkaloid, pelletierine. The molluscicidal activity of bark *Punica granatum* and *Canna indica* against the snail *Lymnaea acuminata* was studied. The activity was found to be both time and dose

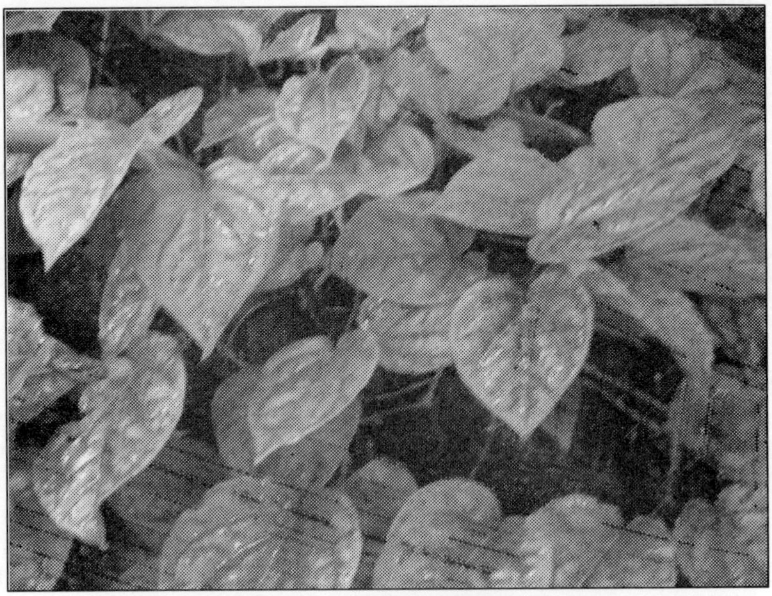

Figure 18.11: *Piper betle*

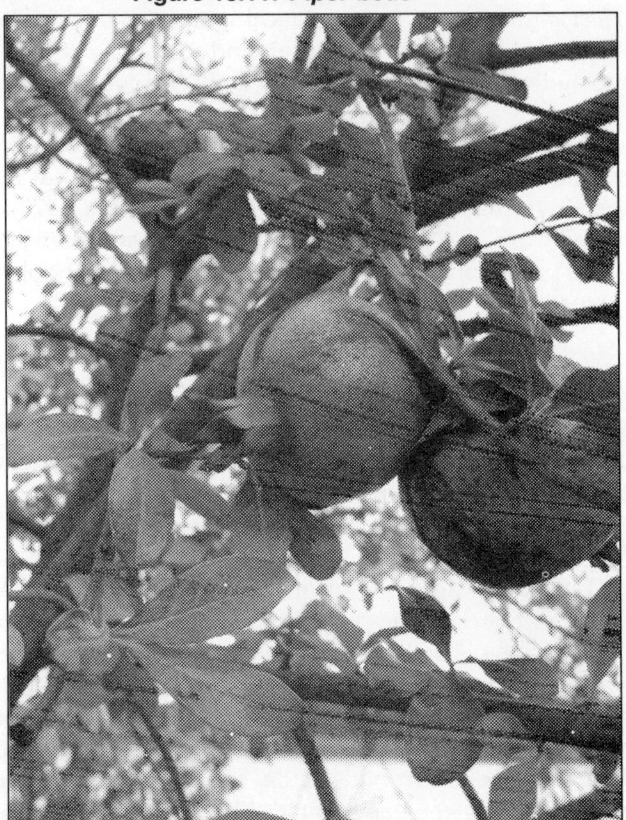

Figure 18.12: *Punica granatum*

dependant. The ethanol extract of *P.granatum* (24 h, LC_{50}: 22.42 mg/l) was more effective than the ethanol extract of *C.indica* in killing the test animals (Tripathi and Singh, 2000).

Semecarpus anacardium

The nuts of *Semecarpus anacardium* Linn (Anacardiaceae) commonly known as Bhilawa found throughout the hotter parts of India. The various concentrations of oil, anacardic acid isolated from the oil of nuts of *Semecarpus anacardium* and its sodium salt were tested for anthelmintic activity. The anacardic acid and its sodium salt have been found to be potent anthelmintic agent than piperazine citrate in the same concentration (Chattopadhyaya and Khare, 1969).

Trachyspermum ammi

The seeds of *Trachyspermum ammi* Linn (Umbelliferae) commonly known as Ajowan, are used as diuretic, analgesic, anthelmintic and in the treatment of asthma. The seed extract was screened for its anthelmintic activity in sheep (Lateef *et al.*, 2006).The crude aqueous and methanol extract of seeds of *T. ammi* was also evaluated for the ovicidal efficacy by egg hatch test (EHT) on *Haemonchus contortus* ova. Lethal concentrations (LC_{50}) values were found 0.1698 and 0.1828 mg/ml, respectively (Jabbar *et al.*, 2006).

Veronia anthelmintica

Veronia anthelmintica Roxb (Asteraceae), commonly known as Kali Jiri is reputed in Ayurvedic system of medicine as anthelmintic. Various extracts of seeds of *V.anthelmintica* have been evaluated for their proclaimed anthelmintic activity by *in vivo* and *in vitro* methods (Iqbal *et al.*, 2006b).

A study was conducted using *Fasciolopsis buski* and *Ascaris lumbricoides* and *Hymenolepsis nana* as test worms. Alcoholic extract of the plant was found to possess maximum anthelmintic activity followed by ether extract, while aqueous extract found almost with no anthelmintic activity (Singh *et al.*, 1985). A comparative study was reported for *in vivo* and *in vitro* anthelmintic screening of *V.anthelmintica* seeds and levamisole. *In vitro* studies revealed higher anthelmintic effects of methanolic extract as compared to aqueous extract on live *Haemonchus contortus* as evident from their mortality. *In vivo*, maximum reduction (73.9 per cent) in faecal egg counts per gram was recorded with crude aqueous extract, in sheep naturally infected with gastrointestinal nematodes (Iqbal *et al.*, 2006 b).

Xylopia aethiopica

Xylopia aethiopica Rich (Annonaceae) is used commonly in Nigeria by traditional herbalists to control gastrointestinal helminth parasites. To verify the claim, anthelmintic effect of the crude methanol extract of seeds was evaluated in rats experimentally infected with the rat hookworm *Nippostrongylus brasiliensis*. The plant exhibited activity at doses between from 1.2 to 2.0 g/kg as measured by reduction in worm counts at necropsy (Suleiman *et al.*, 2005). Tannins, flavonoids or terpenoids present in the crude extract of *X.aethiopica* were claimed to be responsible for the anthelmintic activity as these phytochemicals reported to have an anthelmintic effect (Thompson and Geary, 1995; Lahlou, 2002).

Miscellaneous

Seed oils of *Gynandropsis gynandra, Impatiens balsamina, Celastrus paniculata, Embelica ribes* and *Mucuna pruriens* were investigated for their anthelmintic property against *Pheretima posthuma*. Three concentrations (10, 50 and 100 mg/ml) of each oil were studied in the bioassay. *Embelica ribes* seed oil showed the best activity as compared to piperazine citrate (10 mg/ml) included as reference standard (Jalalpure *et al.*, 2007). Different parts of ten indigenous medicinal plants were screened for their *in vitro* anthelmintic activity against *Ascardia galli* worms of the birds. Preparations from *Carica papaya, Sapindus trifoliatus, Butea frondosa* and *Momordica charantia* were found more effective than piperazine hexahydrate (Lal *et al.*, 1976). In another study, the essential oil of *Gardenia lucida* Roxb was evaluated for anthelmintic activity and showed better efficacy against *Taenia solium* at higher concentration (Girgune *et al.*, 1979).

Conclusion

Herbal medicines have been the oldest form of healthcare. For centuries, natural products have been a major source of new drugs and drug leads. By the middle of the 19th century at least 80 per cent of all medicines were derived from herbs. According to a recent survey by Newman *et al.* (2003), 61 per cent of the 877 small-molecule new chemical entities introduced as drugs worldwide during 1981–2002 can be traced to or were inspired by natural products. During the last one decade or two, there has been revival in the use of herbal products in their crude form (botanicals), a revival which is so dramatic that the annual global sale of herbal products is over US $ 100 billions. According to WHO estimates over three-quarters of world population depends on botanicals for prevention and cure of all kinds of diseases.

Parasites have been of concern to the medical field for centuries and the helminths still cause considerable problems for human beings and animals. During the past few decades, despite numerous advances made in understanding the mode of transmission and the treatment of these parasites, there are still no efficient products to control certain helminths and the indiscriminate use of some drugs has generated several cases of resistance (Coles, 1999; Geerts and Gryseels, 2000; Sangster, 1999). Furthermore, it has been recognized recently that anthelmintic substances having considerable toxicity to human beings. Consequently, the discovery and development of new chemical substance for helminth control is greatly needed and has promoted studies of traditionally used anthelmintic plants, which are generally considered to be very important sources of bioactive substance (Hamond *et al*, 1997). Plants are recognized for their ability to produce a wealth of secondary metabolites and mankind has used many species for centuries to treat a variety of diseases (Cragg *et al.*, 1999). Secondary metabolites are biosynthesized in plants for different purposes including growth regulation, inter and intra-specific interactions and defense against predators and infections. Many of these compounds from natural sources have been shown to present interesting biological and pharmacological activities and are used as chemotherapeutic agents or serve as the prototypes or models for synthetic drugs possessing physiological activities similar to the originals (Verpoorte, 1998). The present review is an attempt to highlight some of the interesting screenings of various organic and aqueous extracts of medicinal plants, their products (latex, essential oils) and isolated phytoprinciples which can serve as a vast resource to search for and also to prepare best alternative anthelmintic formulations, which can replace or complement the anthelmintic drugs which are currently in use.

In conclusion, all the investigations discussed here may be explored further to reach upto novel lead anthelmintic molecule with establishment of their molecular mechanism of action (s) and also for preparation of best herbal formulation.

References

Agrawal, R., Kharya, M.D., and Shrivastava, R. (1979). Antimicrobial and anthelmintic activities of the essential oil of *Nigella sativa* Linn. *Indian Journal of Experimental Biology*, 17: 1264-1265.

Ahmed, V.U., Ismail, N., Arif, S., and Amber, A. (1992). Two new N-acetylated spermidine alkaloids from *Capparis decidua*. *Journal of Natural Products*, 55: 1509-1512.

Ajaiyeoba, E.O., Onocha, P.A., and Olarenwaju, O.T. (2001). *In vitro* anthelmintic properties of *Buchholzia coriaceae* and *Gynandropsis gynandra* extracts. *Pharmaceutical Biology*, 39: 217-220.

Ali, S.M., and Mehta, R.K. (1970). Preliminary pharmacological and anthelmintic studies of the essential oil of *Piper betle* Linn. *Indian Journal of Pharmacy*, 32: 132-133.

Al-Qarawi, A.A., Mahmoud, O, M., Sobaih, Haroun, E.M., and Adam, S.E. (2001). A preliminary study on the activity of *Calotropis procera* latex against *Haemonchus contortus* infection in Najdi sheep. *Veterinary Research Communication*, 25: 61-70.

Anonymous, (1992). The Wealth of India, Raw Materials. Publication and Information Directorate, CSIR, New Delhi.

Asha, M.K., Prashant, D., Murali, B., Padmaja, R., and Amit, A. (2001). Anthelmintic activity of essential oil of *Ocimum sanctum* and Eugenol. *Fitoterapia*, 72: 669-670.

Asuzu, I.U., and Onu, O.U. (1994). Anthelmintic activity of the ethanolic extract of *Piliostigma thonningii* bark in *Ascardia galli* infected chickens. *Fitoterapia LXV* 4: 291-297.

Asuzu, I.U., Gray, A.I., Waterman, and P.G. (1999). The anthelmintic activity of D-3-*O*-methylchiroinositol isolated from *Piliostigma thonningii* stem bark. *Fitoterapia*, 70: 77-79.

Bundy, D.A.P. (1994). Immunoepidemiology of intestinal helminthic infection. *Transactions of the Royal Society of Tropical Medicine and Hygiene*, 8: 259-261.

Chatterjee, A. and Prakashi, S.C. (1991). The Treatise on Indian Medicinal Plants. Vol. I, Council for Scientific and Industrial Research, New Delhi.

Chatterjee, K.D. (1967). Parasitology, Protozoology and Helminthology. Guha Ray Sree Saraswaty Press Ltd, Calcutta.

Chattopadhyaya, M.K., and Khare, R.L. (1969). Isolation of anacardic acid from *Semicarpus anacardium* Linn and study of its anthelmintic activity. *Indian Journal of Pharmacy*, 31: 104-105.

Coles, G.C. (1999). Anthelmintic resistance and the control of worms. *Journal of Medical Microbiology*, 48: 323-325.

Cragg, G.M., Boyd, M.R., Khanna, R., Kneller, R., Mays, T.D., Mazan, K.D., Newman, D.J., and Sausville, E.A. (1999). International collaboration in drug discovery and development: the NCI experience. *Pure Applied Chemistry*, 71: 1619-1633.

D'Cruz, J.L., Nimbkar, A.Y., and Kokate, C.K. (1980). Evaluation of fruits of *Piper longum* L. and leaves of *Adhatoda vasica* Nees. for anthelmintic activity. *Indian Drugs* 17: 99-101.

Dash, G.K., Suresh, P., Sahu, S.K., Kar, D.M., Ganapaty, S., and Panda, S.B. (2002) Evaluation of *Evolvulus alsinoides* Linn for anthelmintic and antimicrobial activities. *Journal of Natural Remedies*, 2: 182-185.

De Morin, A., Borba, H.R., Carauta, J.P., Lopes, D., and Kaplan, M.A. (1999). Anthelmintic activity of the latex of Ficus species. *Journal of Ethnopharmacology*, 64: 255-258.

Dhar, R.N., Garg, L.C., and Pathak, R.D. (1965). Anthelmintic activity of *Carica papaya* seeds. *Indian Journal of Pharmacy*, 27: 335-336.

Duke, J.A., and Vasquez, R. (1994). Amazonian ethnobotanical dictionary. CRC Press, Boca Raton.

Garg, L.C., and Mehta, R.K. (1958). *In vitro* studies on anthelmintic activity of *Butea frondosa* and *Embelica ribes*. *Journal of Animal Husbandry Research*, 3: 28-32.

Garg, S.C., and Kasera H.L. (1982). *In vitro* anthelmintic activity of the essential oil of *Anacardium occidentale*. *Indian Perfumery*, 26: 239-140.

Garg, S.S., and Jain R. (1992). Biological activity of the essential oil of *Piper betle* Linn cultivar Sagar Bangla. *Journal of Essential Oil Research*, 4: 601-606.

Geerts, S., and Gryseels, B. (2000). Drug resistance in human helminths: current situation and lessons from the livestock. *Clinical Microbiology Reviews*, 13: 207-222.

Girgune, J.B., Jain, N.K., and Garg, B.D. (1979). Antimicrobial and anthelmintic activity of essential oil from *Gardenia lucida* Roxb. *Indian Perfumery*, 23: 213-215.

Gunasekaran, R., Senthilkumar, K.L., and Gopalkrishnan, S. (2006). Anthelmintic activity of bark of *Neolamarckia cadamba*. *Indian Journal of Natural Products*, 22: 11-13.

Hamond, J.A., Fielding, D., and Bishop, S.C. (1997). Prospects for plant anthelmintics in tropical veterinary medicine. *Veterinary Research Communications*, 21: 213-228.

Handa, S.S. and Kapoor, V.K. (1988). Pharmacognosy, Vallabh Prakashan, New Delhi.

Hansson, A., Zelada, J.C., and Noriega, H.P. (2005). Reevaluation of risks with the use of *Ficus insipida* latex as a traditional anthelmintic remedy in the Amazon. *Journal of Ethnopharmacology*, 98: 251-257.

Iqbal, Z., Lateef, M., Jabbar, A., Muhammad, G., and Gilani H.A. (2006a). *In vitro* and *in vivo* anthelmintic activity of *Nicotiana tobacum* L. leaves against gastrointestinal nematodes of sheep. *Phytotherapy Research*, 20: 46-48.

Iqbal, Z., Lateef, M., Jabbar, A., Muhammad, G., and Khan, M.N. (2006b). Anthelmintic activity of *Veronia anthelmintica* seeds against Trichostrongylid nematodes of sheep. *Pharmaceutical Biology*, 44: 563-567.

Iqbal, Z., Lateef, M., Jabbar, A., Muhammad, G., and Khan, M.N. (2005). Anthelmintic activity of *Calotropis procera* (Ait) flowers in sheep. *Journal of Ethnopharmacology*, 102: 256-261.

Jabbar, A., Iqbal, Z., and Khan, M.N. (2006). *In vitro* anthelmintic activity of *Trachyspermum ammi* seeds. *Pharmacognosy Magazine*, 2: 126-128.

Jain, M.L., and Jain, S.R. (1972). Therapeutic utility of *Ocimum basilicum* var. *album*. *Planta Medica*, 22: 66-70.

Jalalpure, S.S., Alagawadi, K.R., Mahajanshetti, C.S., Shah, B.N., Singh V., and Patil, J.K. (2007). *In vitro* anthelmintic property of various seed oils against *Pheretima posthuma*. *Indian Journal of Pharmaceutical Sciences*, 69: 158-160.

Kakrani, H.K., and Kalyani, G.A. (1984). Anthelmintic activity of the essential oil of *Commiphora mukul*. *Fitoterapia*, 55: 232-234.

Kaushik, P. and Dhiman, A. (1999). Medicinal Plants and Raw Drugs of India, New Delhi.

Kaushik, R.K., Katiyar, J.C., and Sen, A.B. (1974). Studies on the mode of the action of Anthelmintics with *Ascardia galli* as a test parasite. *Indian Journal of Medical Research*, 62: 1367-75.

Kermanshai, R., Brian, E., Rosenfeld, J., Summers, P.S., and Sorger, G.J. (2001). Benzyl isothiocyanate is the chief or sole anthelmintic in papaya seed extracts. *Phytochemistry*, 57: 427-435.

Khadatkar, S.N., Manvar, J.V., and Bhajipale, N.S. (2008). *In vitro* anthelmintic activity of roots of *Clitorea ternatea* Linn. *Pharmacognosy Magazine*, 4: 148-150.

Kirtikar, K.R. and Basu, B.D. (1935). Indian Medicinal Plants, 2nd Edn. M/S Bishensingh Mahendra Palsingh, Dehradun.

Kumar, D., Mishra, S.K., Tandan, S.K., and Tripathi, H.C. (1991). Mechanism of anthelmintic action of benzyl isothiocyanate. *Fitoterapia* LXII 5: 403-410.

Kumar, D., Mishra, S.K., Tandan, S.K., and Tripathi, H.C. (1995). Possible mechanism of anthelmintic action of palasonin on *Ascardia galli*. *Indian Journal of Pharmacology*, 27: 161-166.

Lahlou, M. (2002). Potential of *Origanum compactum* as a cercaricide in Moracco. *Annuals of Tropical Medical Parasitology*, 96: 587-593.

Lal, J., Chandra, S., Raviprakash, V., and Sabir, M. (1976). *In vitro* anthelmintic action of some indigenous medicinal plants on *Ascardia galli* worms. *Indian Journal of Physiology and Pharmacology*, 20: 64-68.

Lateef, M., Iqbal, Z., Akhtar, M.S., Jabbar, A., Khan, M, N., and Gilani, A.H. (2006). Preliminary screening of *Trachyspermum ammi* (L) seeds for anthelmintic activity in sheep. *Tropical Animal Health Products*, 38: 491-496.

Lewis, W.H. and Elvin-Lewis M.P.F. (1979). Medical Botany. John Wiley and Sons, New York.

Liu, L.X., and Weller, P.F. (1996). An update on Antiparasitic drugs. *New England Journal of Medicine*, 334: 1178

Mali, R.G. (2007c). Anthelmintic activity of *Enicostemma littorale*. *Journal of Medicinal and Aromatic Plant. Sciences*, 29: 209-211.

Mali, R.G., and Wadekar, R.R. (2008). *In Vitro* Anthelmintic Activity of *Baliospermum montanum* Muell. Arg roots. *Indian Journal of Pharmaceutical Sciences*, 70: 131-133.

Mali, R.G., Hundiwale, J.C., Sonawane, R.S., Patil, R.N., and Hatapakki, B.C. (2004). Evaluation of *Capparis decidua* for anthelmintic and antimicrobial activities. *Indian Journal of Natural Products*, 20:10-13.

Mali, R.G., Mahajan, S., and Patil, K.S. (2005). Anthelmintic activity of root bark of *Capparis spinosa*. *Indian Journal of Natural Products*, 21: 50-51.

Mali, R.G., Mahajan, S.G., and Mehta, A.A. (2007a). *In vitro* anthelmintic activity of stem bark of *Mimusops elengi* Linn. *Pharmacognosy Magazine*, 3: 73-76.

Mali, R.G., Mahajan, S.G., and Mehta, A.A. (2007b). *In vitro* anthelmintic screening of *Cleome viscosa* extract for anthelmintic activity. *Pharmaceutical Biology*, 45: 766-768.

Mali, R.G., Mahajan, S.G., and Mehta, A.A. (2008). Evaluation of *Bauhinia variegata* Linn. stem bark for anthelmintic and antimicrobial properties. *Journal of Natural Remedies*, 8: 39-43.

Nadkarni, A.K. (1960). Indian Materia Medica, Vol.I, Popular Book Depot, Bombay.

Neogi, A.C.,Baliga, P.A.C., and Srivastava, R.K. (1964). Anthelmintic activity of some indigenous drugs. *Indian Journal of Pharmacy*, 26: 37-40.

Newman, D.J., Cragg, G.M., and Snader, K.M. (2003). Natural products as a source of new drugs over the period 1981-2002. *Journal of Natural Products*, 66: 1022-1037.

Nunomora, R.S., Costa Da Silva, E.C., Oliveira, D.F., and Pohlit, A.M. (2006). *In vitro* studies of the anthelmintic activity of *Picrolemma sprucei* Hook. (Simaroubaceae). *Acta Amazonica*, 36: 327-330.

Phillips, O. (1990). *Ficus insipida*: Ethnobotany and ecology of an Amazonian anthelmintic. *Economic Botany*, 44: 534-536.

Pradhan, K.D., Thakur, D.K., and Sudhan, N.A. (1992). Therapeutic efficacy of *P.granatum* and *C.maxima* against clinical cases of nematodiasis in calves. *Indian Journal of Indigenous Medicine*, 9: 53-54.

Prakash, V., Singhal, K.C., and Gupta, R.R. (1980). Anthelmintic activity of *Punica granatum* and *Artemisia silversiana*. *Indian Journal of Pharmacology*, 12: 62.

Raj, R.K., and Kurup, P.A. (1967). Isolation and characterization of palasonin, an anthelmintic principle from the seeds of *Butea frondosa*. *Indian Journal of Chemistry*, 5: 86-87.

Ramanan, M.V. (1960). *Butea frondosa* seeds in round worm infestation. *Antiseptic*, 57: 927-928.

Rao, K.S., Raviprakash, V., Chandra, S., and Sabir, M. (1977). Anthelmintic activity of *Butea frondosa* against *Ascaris lumbricoids*. *Indian Journal of Physiology and Pharmacology*, 21: 250.

Roy, B., and Tandon, V. (1996). Effect of root-tuber extract of *Flemingia vestita*, a leguminous plant, on *Artyfechinostomum sufratyfex* and *Fasciolopsis buski*: a scanning electron microscopy study. *Parasitological Research*, 82: 248-252.

Roy, B., Lalchhandama K., and Dutta, B.K. (2008). Scanning electron microscopic observations on the *in vitro* anthelmintic effects of *Millettia pachycarpa* on *Raillietina echinobothrida*. *Pharmacognosy Magazine*, 4: 20-26.

Sabir, M., Lal, J., Raviprakash, V., Chandra, S., and Rao, K.S. (1977). Anthelmintic effect of *Butea frondosa* seeds. *Proceedings of Decennial Conference of Indian Pharmacological Society*. 103.

Sangster, N.C. (1999). Anthelmintic resistance: past, present and future. *International Journal of Parasitology*, 29: 115-124.

Satyanarayanrao, V., and Krishnaiah, K.S. (1982). Note on comparative efficacy of some indigenous anthelmintics against *A. galli* infection in chicks. *Indian Journal of Animal Sciences*, 52: 485-486.

Satyavati, G.V. (1990). Use of plant drugs in Indian Traditional System of Medicine and their relevance to primary health care. *In:* Economic and Medicinal Plant Research, Vol.4, Ed. By Farnworth, N.R. and Wagner, H, Academic Press Ltd., London, pp. 190.

Sharma, S. (1987). Treatment of helminth diseases–Challenges and achievements. *In:* Progress in Drug Research., Ed. By Jucker, E, Birdhauser Verlag, Boston, pp. 69-100.

Shivkar, Y.M., and Kumar, V.L. (2003). Anthelmintic activity of latex *Calotropis procera*. *Pharmaceutical Biology*, 41: 263-265.

Singh, S., Ansari, N.A., Srivastava, M.C., Sharma, M.K., and Singh, S.N. (1985). Anthelmintic activity of *Veronia anthelmintica*. *Indian Drugs*, 22: 508-511.

Sollmann, T. (1918). Anthelmintics: Their efficiency as tested on earthworms. *Journal of Pharmacology and Experimental Therapeutics*, 12: 129-170.

Srivastava, M.C., and Singh, S.W. (1967). Anthelmintic activity of *Cucurbita maxima* (kaddu) seeds. *Indian Journal of Medical Research*, 55: 629-632.

Suleiman, M.M., Mamman, M., Aliu, Y.O., and Ajanusi, J.O. (2005). Anthelmintic activity of the crude methanol extract of *Xylopia aethiopica* against *Nippostrongylus brasiliensis* in rats. *Veternairy Archives*, 75: 487-495.

Szewezuk, V.D., Mongelli, E.R., and Pomilio, A.B. (2003). Antiparasitic activity of *Melia azadirach* growing in Argentina. *Molecular Medicinal Chemistry*, 1: 54-57.

Tandon, V., Pal, P., Roy, B., Rao, H.S.P., and Reddy, K.S. (1997). *In vitro* anthelmintic activity of root-tuber extract of *Flemingia vestita*, an indigenous plant in Shillong, India. *Parasitological Research*, 83: 492-498.

Temjenmongla., Yadav, A. (2005). Anticestodal efficacy of folklore medicinal plants of naga tribes in north-east India. *African Journal of Traditional CAM*, 2: 129-133.

Thompson, D.P. and Geary, T.G. (1995). The structure and function of helminth surfaces. *In:* Biochemistry and Molecular Biology of Parasites, Ed. By Marr, J.J, Academic Press, New York, pp. 203-232.

Thorn, G.W., Adams, R.D., Braunwald, E., Isselbacher, K.J., and Petersdorf, R.G. (1977). Harrison's Principals of Internal Medicine. McGraw Hill Co, New York.

Tripathi, S.M., and Singh, D.K. (2000). Moluscicidal activity of *Punica granatum* bark and *Canna indica* root. *Brazilian Journal of Medical Biology Research*, 33: 1351-1355.

Vaidyaratnam, P.S.V. (1994) Indian medicinal plants-a compendium of 500 species. Vol II, Orient Longman Ltd., Madras.

Verpoorte, R. (1998). Exploration of nature's chemodiversity: the role of secondary metabolites as leads in drug development. *Drug Development Trends*, 3: 232-238.

Vidyarthi, R.D. (1977). A Textbook of Zoology. S.Chand and Co, New Delhi.

Vigar, Z. (1984). Atlas of Medical Parasitology. P G Publishing House, Singapore.

Walter, P.J., and Prichard, K.K. (1985). Chemotherapy of parasitic infections. Plenum, New York.

Yadav, A.K., Tandon, V., and Rao, H.S.P. (1992). *In vitro* anthelmintic activity of fresh tuber extract of *Flemingia vestita* against *Ascaris suum*. *Fitoterapia*, 63: 395-398.

Utilisation and Management of Medicinal Plants (2010) *Pages 340–347*
Editors: **V.K. Gupta, Anil K. Verma and Sushma Koul**
Published by: **DAYA PUBLISHING HOUSE, NEW DELHI**

Chapter 19

Variations in Tannin and Oxalic Acid Content in *Terminalia arjuna* (Arjuna) Bark

A.K. Pandey* and D.C. Kori
Tropical Forest Research Institute,
(Indian Council of Forestry Research and Education)
P.O. RFRC, Mandla Road, Jabalpur – 482 021, India

ABSTRACT

Terminalia arjuna (Arjuna), belonging to family combretaceae, grows along the streams or rivers and often in the shallow streambeds and riverbeds in central India. It has been considered by the Ayurvedic physicians as well as by the modern practitioners as a cardiac tonic. Clinical evaluation indicated that it has been found beneficial in the treatment of coronary artery disease, heart failure and possibly hypercholesterolemia. It has also been found to possess antibacterial, antimutagenic and antioxidant activities. Demand for *T. arjuna* bark, both in India and abroad has been increasing rapidly for over a decade. About 95 percent of the requirement is met from the wild and collected in a pattern that is not concomitant with sustainable harvesting practices. The quality of the bark is directly dependent on harvesting technique and time. There is also a clear relationship between the part of the plant harvested, harvesting method used and the impact of these on the plant. Keeping above into consideration it has been planned to carry out systematic study on phytochemical investigation of Arjuna bark collected from various parts of the tree at different harvesting time. The bark samples were analyzed for tannin and oxalic acid. The tannin and oxalic acid content varied from 6.75 to 14.82 per cent and 7.66 to 20.05 per cent respectively in various samples of *T. arjuna* bark collected from various places of Madhya Pradesh.

* Corresponding Author: E-mail: akpandey10@rediffmail.com.

The middle-aged trees having GBH around 130 cm were found to contain more amount of tannin. The study gives important information to obtain better quality of *T. arjuna* bark on sustainable basis.

Keywords: *Terminalia arjuna, Sustainable harvesting, Tannin, Oxalic acid.*

Introduction

Terminalia arjuna L. (Combretaceae) is a large deciduous tree found throughout India growing to a height of 20-25 meters. It commonly grows on banks of rivers, streams and dry watercourses in sub-Himalayan tract, Central and South India and West Bengal. It is also planted for shade or as ornamental tree in avenues and parks. It has been a common observation that the Arjun tree thrives better in areas with sandy or shallow soil layer. Therefore ecologically it can be said that the natural abundance of Arjun is due to higher water table in the area. Our inquiries with the local people revealed that no one has planted Arjun specifically. Also there has not been any religious reason for abundance of Arjun trees. Nevertheless people are aware about its medicinal properties. Local people use the fallen leaves as manure and the woody fruits as a fuel. In addition Arjun serves as minor timber in making agricultural implements. In the case of Arjun trees on tank bunds and field bunds, it was the local people who planted them. Profuse seeding is another character of the Arjun tree. The seeds are wind dispersed. Farmers replant the germinated seedlings and saplings growing in their cultivation lands onto the bunds.

Bark of *T. arjuna* is flat or slightly curved, external surface pink or flesh colored with a mealy coating; inner surface reddish brown, finely striated, peeling out in thin flakes, odorless, gritty and astringent. The bark has been used in India's native Ayurvedic medicine for centuries, primarily as a cardiac tonic. Clinical evaluation of this botanical medicine indicates that it can be beneficial in the treatment of coronary artery disease, heart failure, and possibly hypercholesterolemia (Alpana *et al.*, 1997; Chander *et al.*, 2004). It has also been found to possess antibacterial, antioxidant and antimutagenic activities. The pharmacology of *T. arjuna* have been discussed by Kumar and Prabhakar (1987) and pharmacological activities are mainly due to the tannins present in their barks.

Demand for *T. arjuna* bark, both in India and abroad has been growing rapidly for over a decade. Presently the bark of *T. arjuna* is being extracted through unscientific and destructive harvesting practices. Presently the collectors harvest the bark by making a blaze too deep and wide, damaging the cambium and ray cells responsible for the transport of nutrient and water from the roots to other parts of the tree. This is evident by many injured trees in natural habitat. About 95 percent of the requirement is met from the wild and collected in a pattern that is not concomitant with sustainable harvesting practices. Harvesting commercial quantity of bark can also affect tree population.

Although it is commonly believed that most tree species completely regenerate their bark after it has been damaged. *T. arjuna* trees are thick-barked and withstand fire damage, but are vulnerable to fungal or borer attack once their bark is removed. The ability to withstand bark damage offered the potential for sustainable harvesting of *T. arjuna* bark.

A fair amount of chemical work has been done on this plant. The major active constituents include tannins, triterpenoid saponins (arjunic acid, arjunolic acid, arjungenin, arjunglycosides), flavonoids (arjunone, arjunolone, luteolin), oxalic acid, gallic acid, ellagic acid, oligomeric proanthocyanidins (OPCs), phytosterols, calcium, magnesium, zinc, and copper (Dwivedi and Udupa,

1989; Ali *et al.*, 2003). It contained unusually, large quantities of calcium salts with small amounts of aluminum and magnesium salts; about 12 per cent of tannins, consisting mainly pyrocatechol tanning; an organic acid with a high melting point and a phytosterol; some coloring matters, and sugars, etc. *T. arjuna* bark has been found to be a potent source of oxalic acid (Bhatia *et al.*, 1977; Bhatia and Ayyar, 1980). Many factors such as soil composition, water stress, temperature and humidity can affect levels of phenolics present in plants (Kouki and Manetas, 2002). Tannin content alter during the development of the plant and also as a response to the environmental changes (Hatano *et al.*, 1986; Santos *et al.*, 2002; Salminen *et al.*, 2001). These variations influence directly the quality of the plant for medicinal use.

The quality of the bark is directly dependent on harvesting technique and time. There is also a clear relationship between the part of the plant harvested, harvesting method used and the impact of these on the plant. Keeping above into consideration this study was carried out to find out the variation in tannin and oxalic acid content in *T. arjuna* bark.

Materails and Methods

The surveys were conducted in different areas of Madhya Pradesh to select Arjun growing areas. Arjun trees of different age group and girth size were selected for extraction of bark. The experiments were laid out in the forest areas of Balaghat and Jabalpur as well as in the farmer's field on randomized block design for the extraction of bark. The girth of selected trees at breast height (GBH) ranged between 77-228 cm. Trees of less than 60 cm GBH were rejected. Care was taken not to include trees with pollarded crown, broken branches or those infected with fungi and insects.

Bark Harvesting

The bark of Arjuna was harvested by putting blazes of different sizes *e.g.*, 19x30, 24x30, 30x30, 22.5x45, 25x45, 30x45, 32x45, 28x60, 30x60, 37.5x60, 41x60, 45x60, 38x90, 42x90, 57x90, 31x120, 45x120 and 46x120 cm. The sizes of blaze were according to GBH and age of tree. The breadth of the blaze was ¼ or $1_{/3}$ of the girth of the trunk at breast height. However, the length of the blazes was 30,45,60,90 and 120 cm. The harvested bark was brought to laboratory for chemical analysis. The Fresh and dry weights of the bark were recorded. Data on regrowth (regeneration of bark) was recorded on quarterly basis. The physical appearance of bark regrowth was also recorded. The bark's regenerative properties were determined by the time taken to regenerate the bark.

Chemical Analysis

Tannin content in the bark was estimated by Folin-Denis Method (Schanderi, 1970) and oxalic acid content by using methods of Bhatia *et al.*, 1977.

Estimation of Tannins by Folin-Denis Method

0.5 g of the powdered bark was taken in a 250 ml conical flask. 75-ml distilled water was added in it. The flask was gently heated and boiled for 30 minutes. Centrifuged at 2000 rpm for 20 minutes and filtered. The supernatant liquid was collected in 100 ml volumetric flask and the volume was made up 100 ml. 1ml of the sample extract was transferred to a 100ml volumetric flask containing 75-ml distilled water. Added 5 ml of Folin-Deins reagent, 10 ml of 35 per cent sodium carbonate solution and diluted to 100 ml with distilled water. The solution was shaken well and the absorbance was read at 700 nm after 30 minutes. Blank was prepared with water instead of the sample. Standard graph was also prepared by using 0–100µg tannic acid. The tannin content of the samples as tannic acid equivalents from the standard graph was calculated.

Determination of Oxalic Acid

One part of the air-dried, water-extracted *T. arjuna* bark was treated with three parts of 20 per cent H_2SO_4 acid at boiling temperature for one hour. After acid treatment the material was filtered while hot and the bark chips washed with hot water till free of acid (usually 3-4 washings). The filtrate was left overnight at room temperature till most of the calcium sulphate with some quantity of oxalic acid separated which was isolated by filteration. The filtrate was concentrated over a water-bath to a density of 1.15 or when the colour of the liquor just changed from red to dark red. At this stage oxalic acid crystals started appearing. The liquid was allowed to cool and oxalic acid crystals appeared in bulk. These crystals were separated by filtration and the filtrate was further concentrated to obtain a second crop of the oxalic acid crystals. A subsequent crop was also likewise obtained. The material obtained in the beginning with calcium sulphate and in 1st, 2nd and 3rd crops was dissolved in water; a pinch of activated carbon was added to the solution and the solution was warmed over water-bath. The solution was filtered and concentrated to obtain crystals of oxalic acid. Total oxalic acid was recrystallized using distilled water.

Results and Discussion

The bark of *T. arjuna* was analysed for their tannin and oxalic acid content. The data pertaining to tree, blaze size, tannin and oxalic acid content is depicted in Table 19.1. Minimum and maximum girth of the trees selected for study was 77 cm and 228 cm respectively. Bark thickness at breast height ranged from 8.12 to 20.96 mm. Mean bark thickness at breast height in Arjuna trees was 15 mm. Mean thickness of bark varied from tree to tree. It is irrespective from the age/girth of tree. Mean bark yield per square centimeter ranged between 0.22 g to 1.14 g and varies from tree to tree. The tannin content ranged from 6.75 to 14.82 g per 100 g. The amount of oxalic acid in the bark ranged between 7.66 g to 20.05 g per 100 g. The variation was observed in tannin and oxalic acid content with season and age of the tree. The variation in protein, phenol, tannin, nitrate, oxalate in addition to vitamin C, anthocyanin and chlorophyll in the leaves was reported by Srivastava *et al.* (1997). Seasonal variations in leaf tannins have already been reported for deciduous trees such as: *Quercus robur* (Feeny, 1970) and *Betula pubescens* (Salminen *et al.*, 2001). These variations occurred during leaf growth and development, from spring to fall and were related with herbivore resistance of plants. In the present study only bark tannins were evaluated and they also showed seasonal variations. Inner bark is the potent part, and contains more tannin in comparison to dry inactive outer portion to the bark. Variation in tannin and oxalic acid content may be due to variation in climatic conditions (rainfall, humidity and mean temperature). Barks collected in the March contained higher amount of tannins (14.82 per cent) followed by the bark collected in November.

Tannin and oxalic acid content in terms of girth/age of the tree is depicted in Table 19.2. The data revealed that there is direct relationship between tannin and oxalic acid content in terms of the girth of the tree. The trees of girth size 40 cm contained minimum amount of tannin (7.56 per cent) and oxalic acid (11.54 per cent) while trees of girth size 116 cm and 100 cm contained higher tannin (14.25 per cent) and oxalic acid (20.05 per cent).

Barks of different plant parts *e.g.* trunk, branch and twigs were also analysed for tannin and oxalic acid content. The data presented in Table 19.3 revealed that the trunk bark contains maximum amount of tannin (13.03 per cent) and oxalic acid (18.46 per cent), whereas lowest tannin (6.32 per cent) and oxalic acid (10.08 per cent) content was determined from the bark of the twigs.

Table 19.1: Tannin and Oxalic Acid Content in *Terminalia arjuna* Bark

Date of Collection	*Location*	*GBH cms*	*Blaze Size cm*	*Thickness of Bark (mm)*	*Bark wt. per cm²*	*Tannin %*	*Oxalic Acid %*
6.11.2004	Chillod, Balaghat	97	24x30	09.80	0.40	7.68	7.66
6.11.2004	Chillod, Balaghat	77	19x30	12.53	0.57	7.56	17.55
6.11.2004	Chillod, Balaghat	97	24x30	12.12	0.38	10.73	12.30
6.11.2004	Chillod, Balaghat	97	24x30	10.12	0.69	12.08	11.40
6.11.2004	Chillod, Balaghat	130	32x45	11.60	0.33	14.17	18.66
6.11.2004	Chillod, Balaghat	120	30x45	11.64	0.35	11.32	10.99
6.11.2004	Chillod, Balaghat	120	30x45	20.96	1.03	10.99	13.61
6.11.2004	Chillod, Balaghat	120	30x45	08.70	0.38	12.33	12.87
7.11.2004	Chikhlabaddi, Balabhat	152	38x90	15.68	0.78	11.70	13.47
7.11.2004	Chikhlabaddi, Balabhat	228	57x90	13.11	0.51	11.34	12.77
7.11.2004	Chikhlabaddi, Balabhat	172	42x90	20.94	1.14	10.55	14.51
7.11.2004	Chikhlabaddi, Balabhat	185	46x120	18.75	0.96	12.98	12.58
7.11.2004	Chikhlabaddi, Balabhat	125	31x120	10.80	0.40	13.65	13.69
7.11.2004	Chikhlabaddi, Balabhat	180	45x120	13.66	0.40	12.54	11.72
7.11.2004	Chikhlabaddi, Balabhat	144	30x60	16.18	0.58	12.43	13.40
7.11.2004	Chikhlabaddi, Balabhat	165	41x60	18.60	0.87	11.58	12.39
7.11.2004	Chikhlabaddi, Balabhat	112	28x60	13.12	0.27	7.31	13.52
28.7.2005	Dokarbandi, Karanjia	100	25x45	11.20	0.56	11.80	12.40
28.7.2005	Dokarbandi, Karanjia	95	30x45	9.32	0.44	11.24	13.68
28.7.2005	Dokarbandi, Karanjia	105	35x65	11.20	0.51	10.11	14.13
28.7.2005	Dokarbandi, Karanjia	115	37.5x60	10.65	0.42	12.12	13.57
28.7.2005	Karajiya, Balaghat	100	25x45	11.03	0.555	11.8	13.01
28.7.2005	Karajiya, Balaghat	90	30x45	9.40	0.444	11.24	14.3
28.7.2005	Karajiya, Balaghat	105	35x60	11.21	0.511	12.91	10.98
28.7.2005	Karajiya, Balaghat	115	37.5x60	10.40	0.422	12.12	16.66
28.7.2005	Chillod, Balaghat	120	30x30	10.00	0.611	11.56	7.66
28.7.2005	Chillod, Balaghat	90	22.5X45	11.00	0.790	12.31	17.55
28.7.2005	Chillod, Balaghat	130	45X60	13.00	0.814	8.11	12.30
28.7.2005	Chillod, Balaghat	92	30X45	13.02	0.370	10.28	11.40
28.7.2005	Chillod, Balaghat	144	36X60	12.13	0.687	8.82	18.66
28.7.2005	Chillod, Balaghat	130	30X60	10.00	0.527	6.75	10.99
01.9.2005	Kanjai, Balaghat	134	30x60	10.00	0.517	12.44	16.02
01.9.2005	Kanjai, Balaghat	130	30.5x60	12.00	0.589	14.24	13.19
01.9.2005	Kanjai, Balaghat	124	31x60	11.25	0.645	12.34	11.76
01.9.2005	Kanjai, Balaghat	90	22x45	12.00	0.5m95	11.76	14.52

Contd...

Table 19.1–Contd..

Date of Collection	*Location*	*GBH cms*	*Blaze Size cm*	*Thickness of Bark (mm)*	*Bark wt. per cm²*	*Tannin %*	*Oxalic Acid %*
01.9.2005	Kanjai, Balaghat	110	27.5x45	12.50	1.030	7.74	16.00
01.9.2005	Chillod, Balaghat	120	30x30	10.23	0.61	11.56	13.56
01.9.2005	Chillod, Balaghat	90	22.5x45	11.31	0.80	12.31	14.57
01.9.2005	Chillod, Balaghat	135	45x60	13.25	0.81	8.16	14.26
01.9.2005	Chillod, Balaghat	92	30x45	13.12	0.37	10.28	12.87
01.9.2005	Chillod, Balaghat	144	36x60	12.09	0.79	8.82	13.40
01.9.2005	Chillod, Balaghat	130	30x60	8.12	0.53	6.76	12.56
02.9.2005	Bhandaruri, Balaghat	134	33x60	10.12	0.58	12.46	16.02
02.9.2005	Bhandaruri, Balaghat	130	32.5x60	12.30	0.59	14.29	13.01
02.9.2005	Bhandaruri, Balaghat	124	31x60	11.13	0.65	12.34	13.19
02.9.2005	Bhandaruri, Balaghat	90	22.5x45	12.14	0.66	13.36	11.76
02.9.2005	Bhandaruri, Balaghat	110	27.5x45	12.15	0.53	7.74	14.52
02.9.2005	Bhandaruri, Balaghat	137	32x45	15.23	0.74	12.13	16.00
02.9.2005	Bhandaruri, Balaghat	172	43x45	14.33	0.62	11.84	10.55
02.9.2005	Bhandaruri, Balaghat	210	70x45	14.20	0.49	12.54	18.46
02.9.2005	Bhandaruri, Balaghat	170	60x45	13.18	0.58	12.44	13.40
13.1.2006	Barha, Jabalpur	280	70x70	8.12	0.549	11.81	16.62
13.1.2006	Barha, Jabalpur	150	40x45	11.00	0.638	13.37	18.08
13.1.2006	Barha, Jabalpur	80	20x45	7.15	0.222	13.66	12.88
13.1.2006	Barha, Jabalpur	140	36x45	10.21	0.570	12.15	14.66
13.1.2006	Barha, Jabalpur	131	36x60	10.18	0.497	9.98	16.00
03.3.2006	Dokarbandi, Balaghat	97	25x75	10.00	0.613	12.08	12.40
03.3.2006	Dokarbandi, Balaghat	98	30x80	9.50	0.500	11.69	13.68
03.3.2006	Dokarbandi, Balaghat	80	25x50	11.00	0.460	14.82	14.13
03.3.2006	Dokarbandi, Balaghat	150	50x100	12.20	0.325	13.79	13.51
03.3.2006	Dokarbandi, Balaghat	110	40x90	8.33	0.319	12.86	13.26

Table 19.2: Tannin and Oxalic Acid Content in *Terminalia arjuna* bark

Sl.No.	*Girth (cm)*	*Blaze Size (cm)*	*Tannin Content %*	*Oxalic Acid % (gm/100 gm)*
1.	40	10X25	7.56	11.54
2.	50	12.5X25	8.25	15.23
3.	60	15X25	8.56	13.52
4.	100	25X30	13.59	20.05
5.	116	29X40	14.25	18.55
6.	117	29X40	13.85	16.55

Table 19.3 Tannin and Oxalic Acid Content in Different Parts of *Terminalia arjuna* Bark

Date of Collection	*Location*	*Plant Parts*	*Blaze Size cm*	*Bark wt. per cm²*	*Tannin %*	*Oxalic Acid %*
13.01.06	Barha, Jabalpur	Trunk	35x60	0.523	13.03	18.46
13.01.06	–do–	Branch	30x12	0.347	8.52	15.52
13.01.06	–do–	Twig	30x12	0.152	6.32	10.08

Sustainable Harvest

Remove only ¼ or $^1/_3$ of the mature bark on total girth of the tree. Remove only outer and middle bark leaving the inner bark for regeneration. The bark should be dried in sun before storage.

Regular field observations were taken on the recovery of bark. The stage of bark recovery (regrowth) varied from tree to tree. After one year, the stripped trees exhibited an average of 42 per cent recovery based on surface area covered with fresh bark. Findings of studies conducted elsewhere indicated that some other factors like temperature, relative humidity and time of stripping influences wound healing in woody species. The trees in which the bark was harvested on 25th December 2003 by putting blaze size (30X30cm) showed almost complete bark recovery nearly after two years. However, few trees showed partial recovery of bark. The study shows that the technique of making of blaze on the tree also plays an important role in the recovery of bark. If the blaze is sharp the recovery is faster whereas if the blaze (cut) is not sharp the recovery is slow. The study shows that bark regeneration in Arjuna depends on the extent of damage on the cambium layer. With damaged cambium when the wound extends beyond the cambium and into the wood, the cut may not heal or if it does, very slowly, exposing it to fungal and insect attack. Some insect and fungal infestations were observed on the blazes. Exposed part of the trunk was attached by the insects, but the damage was not severe. In some trees gums oozed out from the blazes. We did not observe any adverse trend on the overall development of tree. No tree was found to die after harvesting of bark. Although Arjuna shows remarkable bark regrowth in moist sites but this would be very early to predict at this stage of study.

Acknowledgements

Authors are thankful to Dr.A.K.Mandal, Director, Tropical Forest Research Institute, Jabalpur for providing necessary facilities to carry out work and M.P. M.F.P. Federation, Bhopal for financial assistance.

References

Ali, A., Abdullah, S.T., Hamid, H., Ali, M. and Alam, M.S. (2003). Two new pentacyclic triterpenoid glycosides from the bark of *Terminalia arjuna*. *Indian Journal of Chemistry*, 42B(11):2905-2908.

Alpana, R., Laurai, P., Gupta, R., Kumar, P. and Sharma, V.N. (1997).Hypochesreloamic effects of *Terminala arjuna* tree bark, *Journal of Ethnopharmacology*, 55:65-67.

Bhatia, K. and Ayyar, K.S. (1980). Barks of Terminalia species-A new source of oxalic acid. *Indian Forester*, 106(5):363-367.

Bhatia, Kundip, Jia Lal and Swalesh, Mohd. (1977). Utilization of barks of *Terminalia* species from Uttar Pradesh. *Indian Forester*, 103:273-280.

Chander, R., Singh, K., Khanna, A.K., Kaul, S.M., Puri, A., Saxena, R., Bhatia, G., Rizvi, F. and Rastogi, A.K. (2004). Antidyslipidemic and antioxidant activities of different fractions of *Terminalia arjuna* stem bark. *Indian Journal of Clinical Biochemistry*, 19(2): 41-148.

Dwivedi S, Udupa, N. (1989). *Terminalia arjuna*: Pharmacognosy, Phytochemistry, Pharmacology and clinical use. A review. *Fitoterapia*, 60:413-420.

Feeny P. (1970). Seasonal changes in oak leaf tannins and nutrients as a cause of spring feeding by winter moth caterpillar. *Ecology*, 51: 565-581.

Hatano, T., Kira, R., Yoshizaki, M. and Okuda, T. (1986). Seasonal changes in the tannins of *Liquidanbar formosana* reflecting their biogenesis. *Phytochemistry*, 25:2787-2789.

Kouki, M. and Manetas, Y. (2002). Resource availability affects differentially the levels of gallotannins and condensed tannins in *Ceratonia siliqua*. *Biochem Syst. Ecol.*,30:631-639.

Kumar DS, Prabhakar YS. (1987). On the ethnomedical significance of the Arjun tree, *Terminalia arjuna* (Roxb.) Wight and Arnot. *J Ethnopharmacol.* 20(2):173-90.

Salminen, J.P., Ossipov, V., Haukioja, E. and Pihlaja, K. (2001). Seasonal variation in the content of hydrolysable tannins in the leaves of *Betula pubescens*, *Phytochemistry*, 57(1):15-22.

Santos, S.C., Costa, W.F., Ribeiro, J.P., Guimarães, D.O., Ferri, P.H., Ferreira, H.D. and Seraphin, J.C. (2002). Tannin composition of barbatimao species. *Fitoterapia*, 73: 292-299.

Schanderi, S.H. (1970). Methods in Food Analysis, Academic Press. New York, p. 709.

Srivastava N, Prakash D, Behl HM. (1997). Biochemical contents, their variation and changes in free amino acids during seed germination in *Terminalia arjuna*. *Int J Food Sci Nutr.*, 48(3):215-9

Utilisation and Management of Medicinal Plants (2010) *Pages 348–360*
Editors: **V.K. Gupta, Anil K. Verma and Sushma Koul**
Published by: **DAYA PUBLISHING HOUSE, NEW DELHI**

Chapter 20

Natural Sweetening Agents: A Review

Annie Shirwaikar[1]*, Arun Shirwaikar[2], Richard Lobo[1] and Kirti S. Prabhu[1]
[1]Department of Pharmacognosy, Manipal College of Pharmaceutical Sciences, Manipal, India
[2]Dean, Gulf Medical College, Ajman, U.A.E

ABSTRACT

Thirteen species of plants accumulating non-saccharides as their sweet principles have been identified in India. The active sweet principles stored in these plants can be grouped under the terpenoids, steroidal saponins, dihydroisocoumarins, dihydrochalcones, proteins, etc. These sweeteners are not only low in calorific values but are also health compatible. Almost all of them are 100–10,000 times sweeter than sucrose on a unit weight basis. Scientific names of plants containing these natural sweetening agents along with the corresponding chemical structures of the sweet principles have been presented in this paper.

Keywords: Natural sweetening agents, Source, Sweeteners-saccharides, Non-saccharides.

Introduction

Our quality of life is highly dependent on our taste sensory system. Taste is the final check used to evaluate the quality of a food. Research on taste indicates that "sweet" is an innately preferred sensation; infants favor sweetness when presented with the other basic tastes (salty, bitter, sour) or

* Corresponding Author: E-mail: annieshirwaikar@yahoo.com.

even umami, the so-called fifth basic taste, characterized as "savory." This recognition of the importance of sweetness confirms why sweet foods are by far the most popular treats (Saulo, 2005).

Approximately 150 million people in the United States use sugar-free low-calorie products, with their use having tripled over the last 20 years. It has been estimated that the consumption of both nutritive and non-nutritive sweeteners will increase by about 3 per cent per year over the next few years, with the market value of food additives inclusive of artificial sweeteners accounting for about $1.5 billion in the United States. All of the currently approved "high-intensity" sweeteners in the United States are synthetic substances (aspartame, acesulfame K, saccharin, and sucralose). Thus far, there are about 80 sweet compounds exclusive of monosaccharides, disaccharides, and polyols obtained from natural sources, with all of these from vascular plants. These plant-derived compounds mainly belong to three major structural classes, namely, the terpenoids, flavonoids, and proteins. At present, none of these highly sweet compounds has been approved for use as a "high-intensity" sweetener in the United States, although plant derived compounds such as glycyrrhizin, neohesperidin dihydrochalcone and stevioside are used commercially in some other countries for sweetening purposes (Kinghron and Soejarto, 2002).

Sweetening agents are the substances that impart sweetness to the preparation in which they are incorporated. They are incorporated into the formulation to mask the objectionable taste of the drug and to make the preparation sweet in taste.

They are obtained from both synthetic and natural sources.

Synthetic Sweetening Agents

Sweeteners obtained from synthetic sources are called artificial sweetening agents.

There are two kinds of artificial sweeteners:

1. Low calorie sweeteners: Low calorie sweeteners are the euphemism for synthetic chemical sweeteners such as aspartame.
2. Reduced calorie sweeteners: Reduced calorie sweeteners are known as polyols. The polyols are sugar alcohols, and are referred to as reduced calorie sweeteners because they contain less calories per gram than sugar.

Natural sweetening agents are preferred over their artificial counterparts as they are not known to cause any adverse reactions in the human body. As many artificial sweetening agents have proved carcinogenic, there is a great demand for natural sweetening agents. Modern analytical techniques have developed to isolate the exact active principle of sweetening agents.

Ideal Requirements for Sweetening Agents

An ideal sweetening agent should be non carcinogenic, stable at a wide range of temperature, have very low calorific values, should impart specific taste in minute quantities and should be effective, when used in small concentrations.

Natural Sweetening Agents

Natural sweetening agents are obtained from plant and animal sources.

e.g. Honey, Fructose.

Classification of Natural Sweetening Agents

The natural sweetening agent can be classified as

1. Saccharide Sweetening Agents–*e.g.*: Glucose, Honey
2. Non Saccharide Sweetening Agents

- ☆ Terpenoids–*e.g.*: Trans anethole. Glycyrrhizin
- ☆ Steroidal saponins–*e.g.*: Polypodoside, Oslandin
- ☆ Dihydrochalcones–*e.g.*: Glycyphyllin, Trilobatin
- ☆ Dihydroisocoumarin–*e.g.*: Phyllodulcin.
- ☆ Proteins–*e.g.*: Monellin, Miraculin, Thaumati
- ☆ Flavanol sweeteners

Saccharide Sweetening Agents

These are the sugars obtained from sacchariferous sweet plants and include sucrose, glucose, fructose, dextrose etc. They have high calorific values of 3600-4000 cal/g. Regular usage of these sugar leads to many diseases like dental caries, diabetes, obesity etc.

Honey

Honey is a saccharine substance deposited by the hive bee, *Apis mellifera, Apis dorsata* and other species of *Apis* in the cells of honeycomb, Family Apidae, Order Hymenoptera.

In most honeys, fructose predominates and tends to make its taste slightly sweeter than sugar. On an average, honey is 1 to 1.5 times sweeter (on a dry weight basis) than sugar.

It consists mainly of invert sugar and water. Honey is basically a solution of levulose (40-50 per cent), dextrose (30-&70 per cent), sucrose (0.2 per cent) and water (13-20 per cent).Its properties vary with the floral source and on the activity of invertase present therein.

It is used as a demulcent and a sweetening agent. It is also used in the preparation of creams, lotions and as a component of linctuses and cough mixtures (Evans, 1996; Dwivedi, 1999).

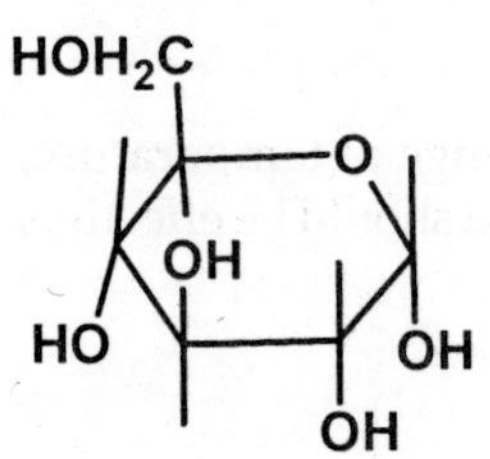

Glucose

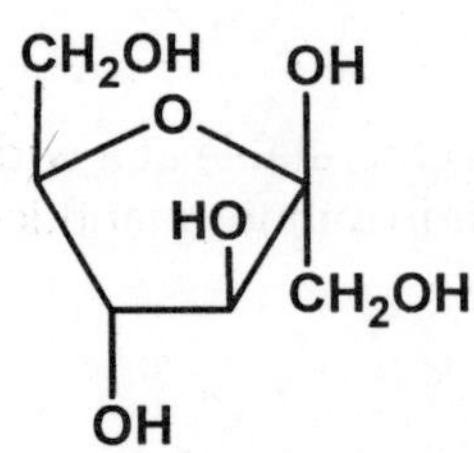

Fructose/levulose

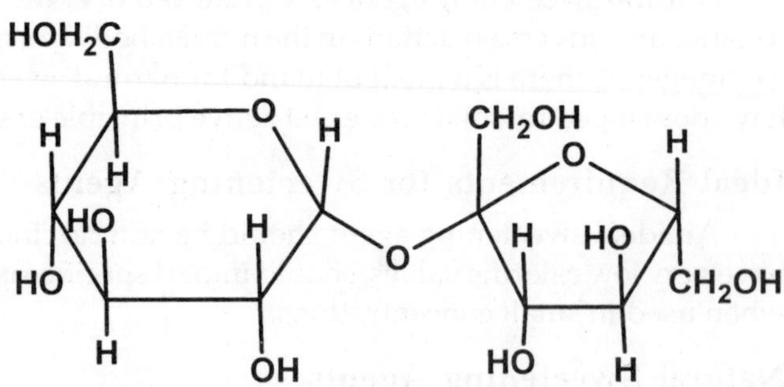

Sucrose

Sucrose

Sucrose is a disaccharide sugar obtained from sugar cane juice *Saccharum officinarum.* Family Graminae and from the roots of *Beta vulgaris,* Family Chenopodiaceae. It is used for making syrups and lozenges. It imparts viscosity and consistency to fluids (Dwivedi, 1999).

Non-Saccharide weetening Agents

These are substances, which contain terpenoids, proteins, steroidal saponins etc as sweet principles. Plants that contain non-saccharide sweetening agents are known as non-sacchariferous sweet plants. They are advantageous over saccharide sweeteners as they are non-carcinogenic potent sweeteners (1000 times sweet than sucrose) which have little or no calorific value. Hence they are useful for diabetic patients and do not pose any effect on the prevalence of diseases.

Terpenoids

Glycyrrhizin

Glycyrrhizin is a pentacyclic triterpenoid saponin glycoside obtained from the roots and rhizomes of the plant *Glycyrrhiza glabra* commonly known as liquorice, Family Leguminosae,

A non-calorific sweetener, extracted from the root, licorice is 50 to 100 times sweeter than sucrose. However because of its pronounced licorice flavor, its uses are limited. It is used as a flavoring in tobacco, pharmaceuticals and for some confectionary products. It is also used as a foaming agent in some non-alcoholic beverages. Glycyrrhizin is approved for use in the United States as a flavor and flavor enhancer. Glycyrrhizin is found in the form of potassium and calcium salts of glycyrrhizic acid with different varieties containing different concentrations of glycyrrhizin e.g, *G. glabra* var. *violacea* commonly known as Persian liquorice contains approximately 7.5-13 per cent.of glycyrrhizin, *G. glabra* contains approximately 5-10 per cent of glycyrrhizin while *G. glabra* var. *glandulifera* commonly

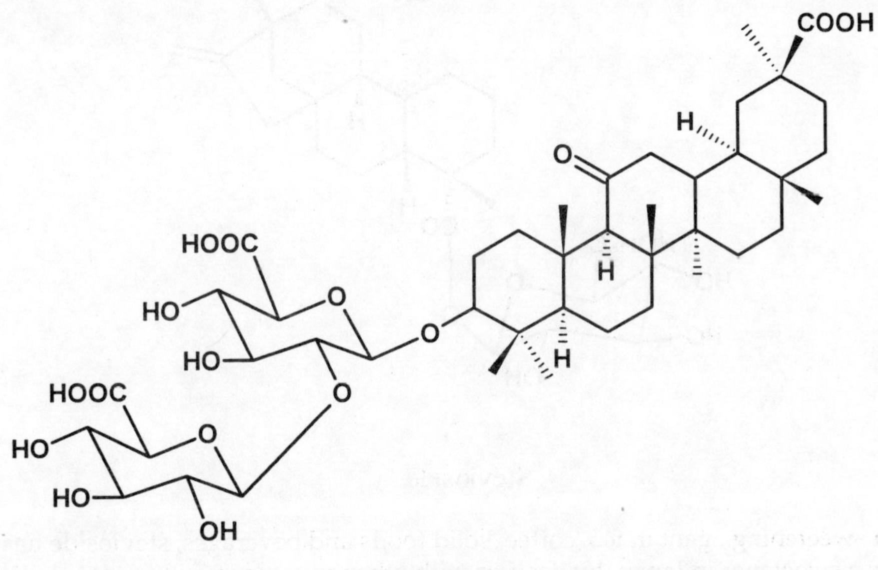

Glycyrrhizin

known as Russian liquorice contains 10 per cent. of glycyrrhizin. In addition licorice also contains glucose (upto 4 per cent), sucrose (2.5-4.5 per cent), resin, bitter principles, glycyramerin, asparagin (2-4 per cent) fats, flavonoids, liquertin and isoliquirtin. In the United States there is an increasing use of plant extractives known to contain highly sweet terpenoids. An ammoniated derivative of the oleanane-type triterpene glycoside, glycyrrhizin, has been available for several years on the generally recognized as safe (GRAS) list of approved natural flavors (Saulo, 2005)

Stevioside

Stevioside belongs to the group of ent-kaurane glycosides. It is obtained from *Stevia rebaudiana* Family Compositae. It is a tricyclic diterpenoid glycoside. It contains rebaudiosides A, B, C, D, E and dulcoside A. Stevioside is 100-400 times sweeter than sucrose. A low-calorie sweetener. It is approved for use as a sweetener in South Korea and Brazil. A subsequent review by Joint FAO/WHO Expert Committee on Food Additives (JECFA) in 2004 granted a temporary designation for stevioside of an acceptable daily intake of 2 mg/kg body weight. Citing insufficient testing, the Food Drug Administration (FDA) has not allowed the use of stevioside in the United States as a sweetener food additive, but it may be sold as a dietary supplement without any reference to sweetness.

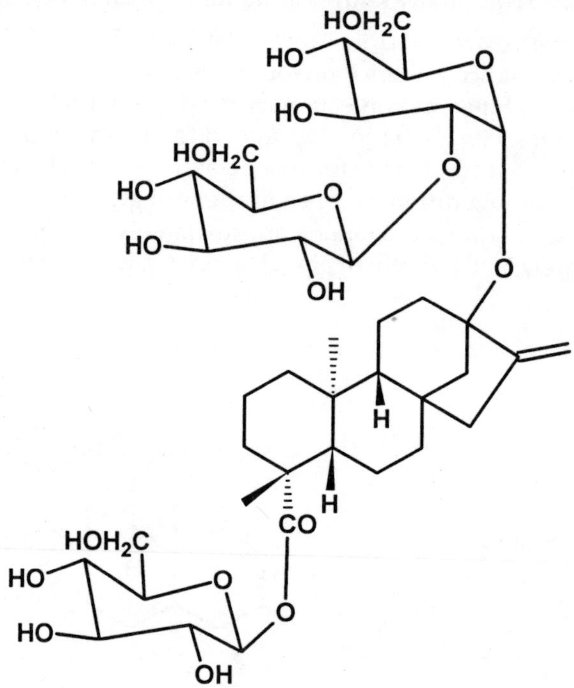

Stevioside

Used as a sweetening agent in tea, coffee, solid foods and beverages, stevioside has been used since 1970's as a sweetener in Japan, by itself or with other sweeteners in beverages, pickles, dried seafoods, flavorings, confections, chewing gum, and table-top sweeteners. (Saulo, 2005)

Trans-Anethole

Trans-anethole is a phenyl propanoid sweet principle present in high concenteration in the volatile oil obtained from the leaves of *Piper marginatum* (Family Piperaceae); from the fresh roots of *Myrrhis odorata* (Family Apicaeae); from the fresh aerial parts of *Foeniculum vulgare* (Family Apicaeae) and the dried fruits of *Illicium verum* (Family Illiciaceae). It is used as a sweetener in beverages, candy, chewing gums etc.(Hussain, 1988)

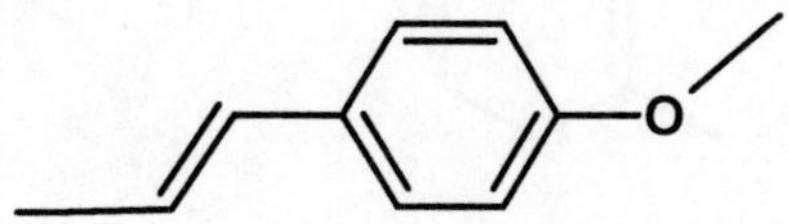

Anethole

Perillartine

Perillartine is a monoterpene volatile oil obtained from the leaves, seeds and flowering tops of *Perilla frutescens*, belonging to the family Labiatae. Perillartine, also known as perillartin and perilla sugar, is about 2000 times as sweet as sucrose and is mainly used in Japan. Perillartine, a type of monoterpenoid is the oxime of perillaldehyde (Dwivedi, 1999).

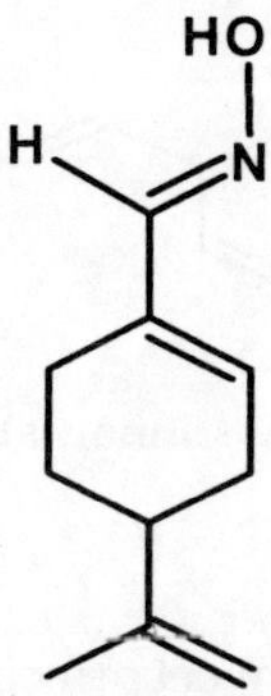

Perillartine

It is used as a flavoring agent in confectioneries and in the preparation of sauces.

Hernandulcin

Hernandulcin is a sesquiterpene volatile sweet principle obtained from the leaves and flowers of the plant *Lippia dulcis* (Family Verbenaceae) grown in Mexico.

This new bisabolane sesquiterpene was determined to be about 1000 times sweeter than sucrose on a molar basis. This constituent was named after the Spanish physician Francisco Hernández. Although, hernandulcin has been patented as a potential noncaloric sweetener,the compound does have disadvantages as a sweetener. It is not highly water soluble and decomposes to ketones on heating. Moreover, the compound exhibits definite off–and after taste as well as some bitterness when tasted.

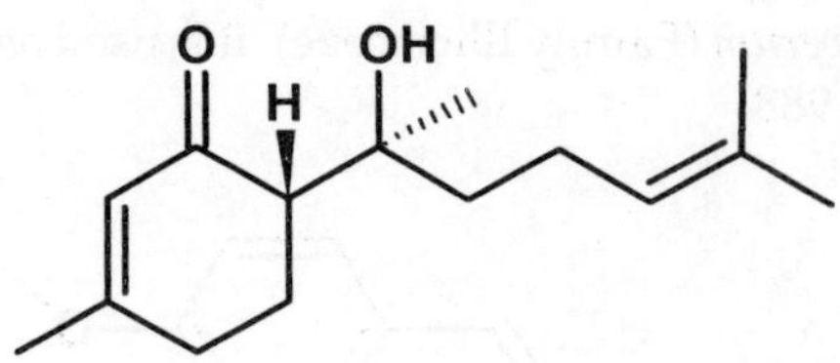

Hernandulcin

This sweet compound may be suitable for use in oral dentifrices when formulated with *l*-menthol and the ketones menthone, isomenthone, and piperitone.(Compadre *et al.*, 1985)

Trans-Cinnamaldehyde

Trans cinnamaldehyde is a highly sweet phenyl propanoid obtained from the leaves of the Taiwan species of *Cinnamomum osmophloeum*,Family Lauraceae. It is the major volatile oil constituent of the plant and is used as a sweetener in preparations of chewing gums(Hussain *et al.*, 1986).

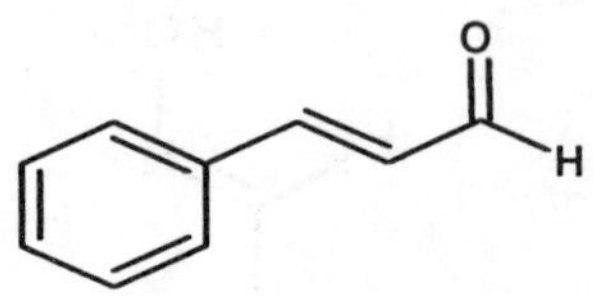

Trans cinnamaldehyde

Periandrin

Periandrin is a triterpenoid glycoside, a sweet principle obtained from the rhizomes of *Periandra dulcis*. Family Leguminosae. It is commonly known as Brazilian Licorice. The constituents periandrin-I-IV were found to be 90-100 times sweeter than sucrose, while periandrin V was found to be 200 times sweeter than 2 per cent sucrose. Its relative sweetness is similar to that of glycyrrhizin (Kinghorn and Soejarto, 2002; Hashimoto *et al.*, 1983).

Steroidal Saponins

Polypodoside A

This sweet principle is obtained from the rhizomes of *Polypodium glycyrrhiza* (Family Polypodiaceae). Polypodoside A is 600 times sweeter than 60 per cent w/v aqueous sucrose solution.

Polypodoside A is a mixture of D-glucose, L-rhamnose and Polypodogenin (aglycone). The rhizomes have a strong licorice flavor due to the presence of a compound, Polypodoside A, which was evaluated in one study as being 600 times sweeter then sugar. The rhizomes are chewed as an appetite

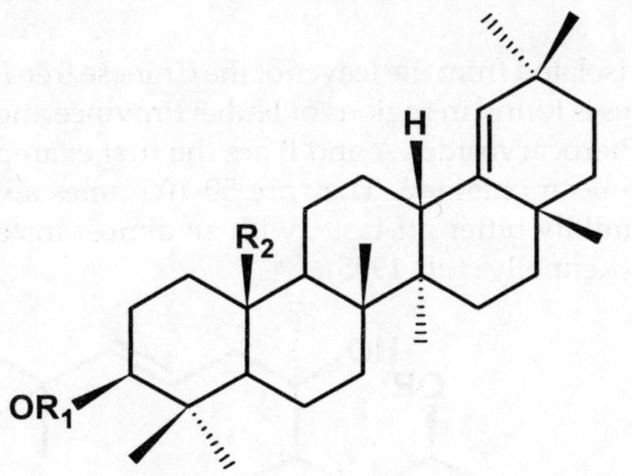

Periandrin

Periandrin I–R_1 =β-glcA^2-β–glcA, R_2=CHO
Periandrin V–R_1=β-glcA^2-β-xyl, R_2=CHO

stimulant and a mouth sweetener by most of the Northwest coast groups. They are known to make water taste sweet if chewed just before drinking (Nishizawa *et al.*, 1994).

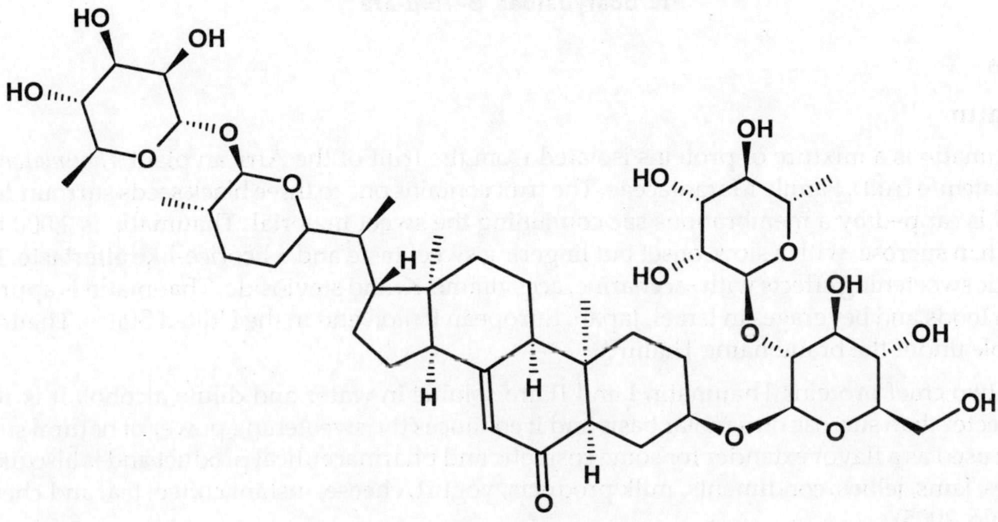

Polypodoside A

They are also used to flavour foods. The rhizomes are used in medicine for sore throat, cold and sometimes used in cough syrups.

Oslandin

Oslandin is obtained from the rhizomes of the European polypody fern *Polypodium vulgare* (family Polypodiaceae). It is 300-3000 times sweater than sucrose (Jizba *et al.*, 1981).

Pterocaryoside A and B

Pterocaryoside A and B are isolated from the leaves of the Chinese tree *Pterocarya paliurus* (Family Juglandaceae). *Pterocarya paliurus* is found in regions of Hubei Province and the People's Republic of China call it "sweet leaf tree". Pterocaryosides A and B are the first examples of highly sweet seco-dammarane glycosides to have been obtained. They are 50-100 times sweeter than sucrose. Both compounds have a persistent, mildly bitter off-taste, with an almost instantaneous onset of sweet taste. It is used to sweeten food (Kennelly *et al.*, 1995).

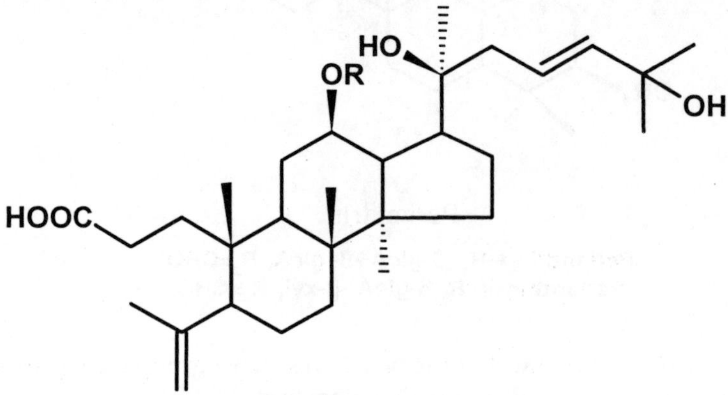

Pterocaryosides A–R=β-qui
Pterocaryosides B–R=α-ara

Proteins

Thaumatin

Thaumatin is a mixture of proteins isolated from the fruit of the African plant *Thaumatococcus danielli* (katemfe fruit), Family Marantaceae. The fruit contains one to three black seeds surrounded by a gel and is capped by a membranous sac containing the sweet material. Thaumatin is 2,000 times sweeter than sucrose, with a slow-onset but lingering sweet taste and a licorice-like aftertaste. It has synergistic sweetening effects with saccharine, acesulfame-K, and stevioside. Thaumatin is approved for use in foods and beverages in Israel, Japan, European Union and in the United States. Thaumatin is available under the brand name Thalin™.

The two chief proteins Thaumatin I and II are soluble in water and dilute alcohol. It is 10,000 times sweeter than sucrose on a molar basis and it enhances the sweetening power of natural sugars. It may be used as a flavor extender for some cosmetic and pharmaceutical product and is also used in beverages, jams, jellies, condiments, milk products, yogurt, cheese, instant coffee, tea, and chewing gum (Saulo, 2005).

Monellin

Monellin is present in the fruit pulp of the tropical western African plant *Dioscoreophyllum cuminsii* (Family Menispermaceae). Monellin is a protein that elicits a flavor approximately 100,000 times sweeter than sugar on a molar basis. The protein exists naturally as a heterodimer, with its sweet flavor lost upon denaturation. Its toxicological data limits its use. It is used mainly to enhance the flavour of beverages and foodstuffs (Kohmura *et al.*, 2002)

Miraculin

This sweetener is obtained from the miracle fruits of the western African shrub, *Synsepalum dulcifucum* (Family Sapotaceae). This sweetening principle is a glycoprotein which has the ability to modify taste. Miraculin was denied approval by the Food and Drug Administration (FDA) and has also no legal status in the European Union. However it is approved in Japan as a harmless additive, according to the List of Existing Food Additives published by the Ministry of Health and Welfare. It is used to enhance the flavour of beverages and foodstuffs

Cynarin

Cyanarin is present in the leaves and flowers of the plant *Cynara scolymus* (Family Asteraceae). The plant contain cynarin and chlorogenic acid as sweetening principles. It is used for imparting a sweet taste to the water (Dwivedi, 1999).

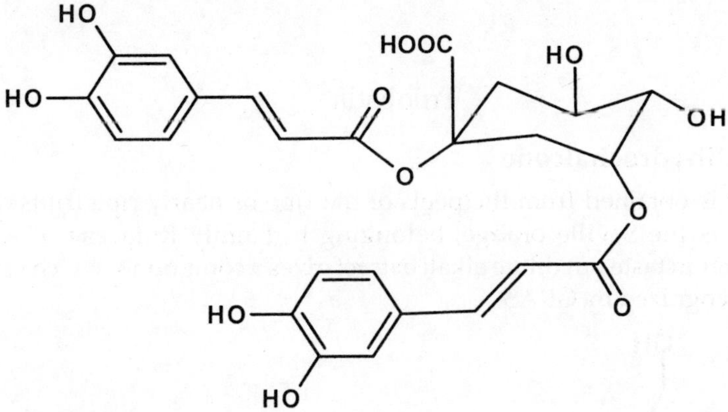

Cynarin

Dihydrochalocones

Glycyphyllin

Glycyphyllin is present in the whole plant of *Smilax glycyphylla* (Family Liliaceae), a plant found in the Himalayas and in Assam. A dihydrochalcone glycoside glycyphillin is 100-200 times sweeter than sucrose (Dwivedi, 1999).

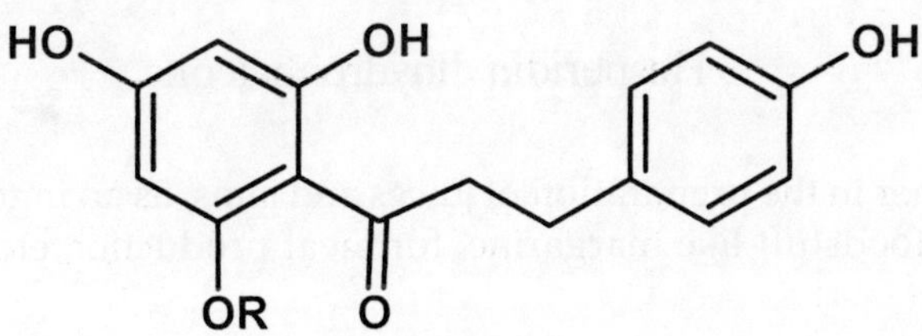

Glycyphyllin

Trilobatin

Trilobatin is obtained from the plant *Symplococcus paniculata* belonging to the Family Symplocaceae and is commonly known as sweet leaf. Mainly propagated through seeds, it is 400–1000 times sweeter than sucrose (Dwivedi, 1999).

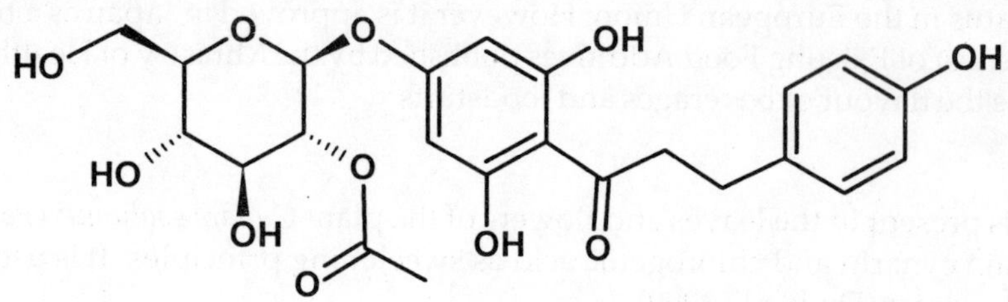

Trilobatin

Neohesperidin Dihydrochalcone

This sweetener is obtained from the peels of the ripe or nearly ripe fruits of *Citrus aurantium* commonly known as the Seville orange, belonging to Family Rutaceae. Flavonoid compound neohesperidin is bitter in taste but dilute alkali extract gives a compound, which is 1000 times sweeter than sucrose. It is recognized by GRAS.

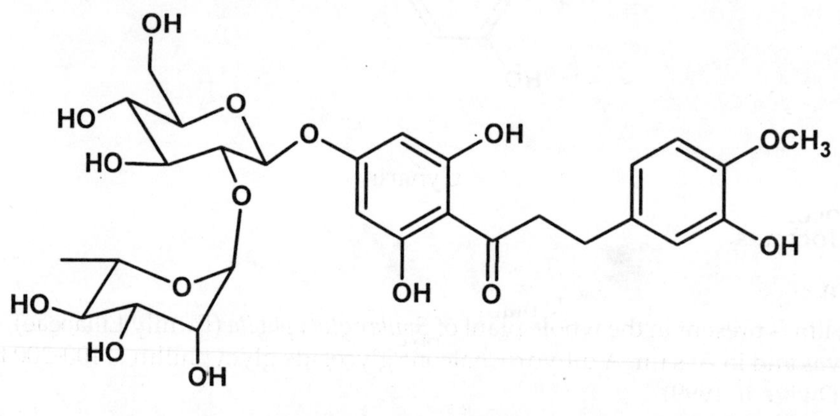

Hesperidin dihydrochalcone

It is used as a sweetener in the preparation of juices and jams, as an ingredient in new feeds for cultured fish and also in foodstuff like margarine, for meat production etc.(Handro and Ferreira, 1989).

Dihydro Iso Coumarins

Phyllodulcin

Phyllodulcin is obtained from *Hydrangea macrophylla* (Family Saxifragaceae) and commonly known as amancha. The sweet principle phyllodulcin is 300-400 times sweeter than sucrose.It exhibits a delay in the onset of sweetness and has a licorice–like after-taste.

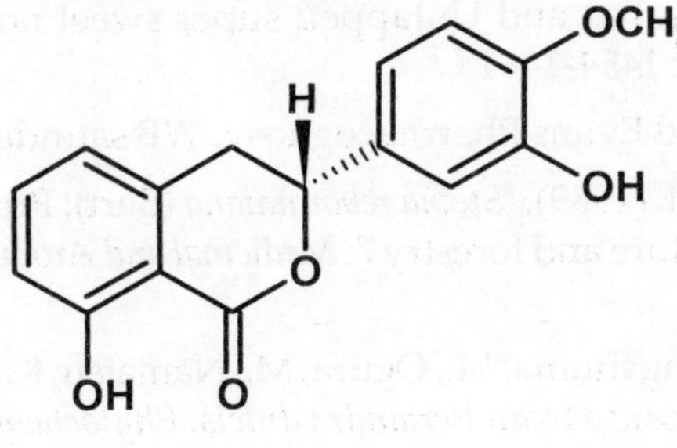

Phyllodulcin

As phyllodulcin has a lingering taste, it is used in the manufacture of hard candies and confectionaries, chewing gums and in oral hygiene products (Asahina andUeno, 1916).

Miscellaneous

Flavonol Sweetening Agents

Two dihydro flavanol sweeteners are found in the plant *Eremophila glutinosa* (Family Alaudidae). The genus Eremophila is restricted to Australia.

The two sweeteners are 2p, 3R, 3-acetoxy 4,5-dihydroxy, 7-methoxy flavanone and 2R, 3R, 3-acetoxy–4,5,7 _ trihydroxy–6-methoxy flavanone. They are 400 times sweeter than sucrose.

Conclusion

More than 180 million adult Americans now consume low-calorie or sugar-free foods and beverages. This number has doubled within the last decade. Calorie-consciousness is part of today's lifestyle, and reduced-calorie, low-calorie, and non-caloric sweeteners are a major component of this lifestyle. The growing consumer demand challenges food manufacturers to provide a wider selection of good tasting, more stable, more economically available, and safe foods and beverages.

Natural sweeteners like sucrose, honey and glycyrrhizin are very familiar to man from ancient times. Sucrose is an important energy source, but its regular use may pose several health problems due to its high calorific value. Artificial sweetening agents though low calorific and more potent sweeteners than natural sweetening agents have been found to be carcinogenic. The use of non-saccharide natural sweeteners, which are low calorific, non-toxic and super sweet in nature can overcome the problems of sucrose and synthetic sweeteners. Ammoniated glycyrrhizin, thaumatin, stevioside, phyllodulcin, and monellin are commercially available super sweeteners of this type and could be useful sugar substitutes for diabetic patients.

References

Asahina, Y. and Ueno, E. (1916). Phyllodulcin, a chemical constituents of Amacha (*Hydrangea thunbergii*). *Chemical Abstracts*, 10:1524.

Compadre, C.M., Pezzuto, J.M., Kinghorn, A.D. and Kamath, S.K.(1985). Hernandulcin: an intensely sweet compound discovered by review of ancient literature. *Science*, 227:417-419.

Dwivedi, S.R. (1999). Unnurtured and Untapped super sweet non-sacchariferous plant species in India. *Current Science*, 76: 1454-1461.

Evans,W.C. (1996). Trease and Evans Pharmacognosy. WB saunders Company Ltd, London

Handro, W. and Ferreira, C.M. (1989). '*Stevia reboundiana* (Bert): Production of natural sweeteners', in Biotechnology in Agriculture and forestry 7: *Medicinal and Aromatic Plan II.* Springer Verlag, Berlin, pp-468-482.

Hashimoto, Y., Ishizone, H., Suganuma, M., Ogura, M., Namatsu, K. and Yoshika, H. (1983). Periandrin I, a sweet triterpene glycoside from *Periandra dulcis*. *Phytochemistry*, 22: 259-264.

Hussain, R.A., Kim, J., Hu, T.W., Pezzuto, J.M. and Soejarto, D.D. (1986). Isolation of a highly sweet constituents from *Cinnamomum osmophloeum* leaves. *Planta Medica*, 52: 403-404.

Hussain, R.A., Kinghorn, A.D. and Soejarto, D.D. (1988). Sweetening agents of plant origin:literature search for candidate sweet plants. *Economic Botany*, 42:267.

Jizba, J., Dolejs, S., Herout, V. and Sorm, F. (1981). The structure of oslandin, the sweet principle of the rhizomes of *Polypodium vulgare.* Tetrahedron Letters, 1329.

Kennelly, E.J., Cai, L., Long,L., Shamon, L., Zaw, K., Zhou, B.N., Pezzuto, J.M. and Kinghorn, A.D. (1995). Novel highly sweet secodammarane glycoside from *Pterocarya paliurus*. *J. Agric. Food Chem.* 43: 2602–2607.

Kinghorn, A.D. and Soejarto, D.D. (2002). Discovery of terpenoids and phenolic sweeteners from plants. *Pure Appl. Chem*, 74: 1169-1179.

Kohmura M., Mizukoshi, T., Nio, N., Suzuki, E. and Ariyoshi, Y. (2002). Structure-taste relationships of the sweet protein monellin. *Pure Appl. Chem.* 74: 1235-1242.

Nishizawa, M., Yamada,H., Yamaguchi, Y., Hatakeyama, S., IK-Soo, Lee., Jinwoong, Kim. and Kinghorn, A. D.(1994) Structure revision of polypodoside A. Major sweet principle of *Polypodium glycyrrhiza*. *Chemistry Letters*, 8: 1555-1558.

Saulo, A.A. (2005). Sugars and Sweeteners in Foods. *Food Safety and Technology*, 16: 1-7.

www.caloriecontrol.org.

Utilisation and Management of Medicinal Plants (2010) *Pages 361–375*
Editors: V.K. Gupta, Anil K. Verma and Sushma Koul
Published by: DAYA PUBLISHING HOUSE, NEW DELHI

Chapter 21

Pseudomonas fluorescens as Microbial Pesticides in Black Pepper: Their Mechanisms of Action

Diby Paul[1]* and Y.R. Sarma[2]
[1]Department of Environmental Engineering, Konkuk University, Seoul 143-701, South Korea
[2]FAO Consultant and Team Leader (Black Pepper), Former Director, Indian Institute of Spices Research, Calicut, Kerala, India

ABSTRACT

Foot rot of black pepper caused by *Phytophthora capsici* is the major production constraint. Chemical control measures, even though effective are not a healthy practice due to the residual effect of the same in the produce. Biological control measures have been experimented with Plant Growth Promoting Rhizobacteria (PGPR) for disease suppression. Five strains of *Pseudomonas fluorescens* have been demonstrated to aid in suppression of root rot up and also enhanced the growth parameters in the host plant (Paul, 2004). The mechanisms by which these strains bring about the beneficial properties in the host plant are discussed. The different modes by which these bacterial strains acted were found to be through the production of inhibitory metabolites, antibiotics *viz.* pyoluteorin, pyrrolnitrin, mycolytic enzymes *viz.* b-1,3 glucanases, b-1,4 glucanases and lipases. Siderophore mediated inhibition existed between *P. fluorescens–P. capsici* antagonistic system. The *P. fluorescens* strains also induced systemic resistance in the plant as evidenced by the enhanced levels of defence enzymes in the phenyl propanoid pathway, *viz.*

* Corresponding Author: E-mail: dibypaul@konkuk.ac.kr.

Phenylalanine Ammonia Lyase (PAL), Peroxidases (PO) and Polypheol Oxidases (PPO) upon root bacterization. This lead to the accumulation of lignin in the vascular region, causing cell wall thickening and thereby increased protection against the pathogen.

Keywords: *Antibiosis, Black pepper, Disease suppression, Phenolics, Pseudomonas fluorescence, Root rot, Siderophore.*

Introduction

Black pepper (*Piper nigrum* L.) 'King of Spices' has its origin in the western ghats of Kerala (the ancient Malabar coast). In earlier times pepper in India was valued not so much for its qualities as spice but for its medicinal properties. Foot rot caused by *Phytophthora capsici* is one of the major production constraints (Sarma *et al.*, 1992). Globally this disease causes an annual loss of 4.5–7.5 million dollars. Integrated Pest Management (IPM) constituting of phytosanitation, cultural practices, chemical and biological control continues to be the major strategy. In way of export nature of the commodity, the exporters shun pesticide residue in the produce. In view of this, biocontrol strategies as component of IPM have been found highly effective. Fluorescent pseudomonads are some of the effective candidates for biological control of soil borne plant pathogens owing to their rhizosphere competence (Kloepper *et al.*, 1980a, 1981; Loper *et al.*, 2007). These bacteria are also termed as Plant Growth Promoting Rhizobacteria (PGPRs) because of their ability to improve plant growth through suppression of deleterious root colonizing microorganisms and by production of plant growth regulators (Suslow *et al.*, 1982). Strains of fluorescent pseudomonads have been demonstrated to reduce plant diseases by suppressing soil borne pathogens through different mechanisms in many different crops including spices (Sarma *et al.*, 2000; Pieterse *et al.*, 2000). Five strains of *P. fluorescens* isolated from black pepper rhizospheres were found to be very effective in disease suppression and plant growth promotion in black pepper in the field (Paul, 2004). They also induced systemic resistance to the host plant in the green house (Paul, 2004). The present study dealt with the different modes through which these strains of *P. fluorescens* act in antagonism against *Phytophthora capsici* in order to suppress root rot in black pepper.

Materials and Methods

The Microorganisms Used

P. fluorescens strains *viz.* IISR-6, IISR-8, IISR-11, IISR-13 and IISR-51 used in the study had been isolated from black pepper roots and rhizosphere soil collected from different locations in South India and they were characterized and identified. The strains were shortlisted based on antibiosis against fungal pathogens and also by their ability to induce ISR in host plants. The strains were also found to be very effective in disease suppression and plant growth promotion in black pepper (Paul, 2004). The strains were maintained in glycerol at–80°C for long-term storage. The *Phytophthora capsici* isolate 99-101 used for the present study was obtained from the National Repository of *Phytophthora* (NaRPh) maintained at the Indian Institute of Spices Research, Calicut. *P. capsici* was maintained in Carrot Agar (CA) plates for routine use.

Action of Metabolites of *P. fluorescens* on the Different Stages in the Life Cycle of *P. capsici*

The *P. fluorescens* strains were cultured separately in minimal medium (Elad *et al.*, 1982) amended with the live mycelium of *P. capsici* in order to get their *P. capsici*-induced metabolites. The *P. capsici* mycelium was prepared in Glucose Yeast Peptone (GYP) medium. The Cell Free Culture Filtrate (CFCF) was collected and concentrated to 5ml in a flash evaporator at 28°C. This CFCF was filter sterilized and tested for inhibition of different stages in the lifecycle of *P. capsici viz.* Sporangial formation, Release of zoospores, and Germination of zoospores. Appropriate controls were maintained.

Effect on Mycelial Growth

The effect of metabolites produced by the strains of *P. fluorescens* was studied by dual culture assay (Dennis and Webster, 1971) wherein both the organisms were grown in a PDA plate and inhibition of growth of *P. capsici* was measured.

Effect on Sporangia Production

Ten disks (3mm) of *P. capsici* cut from the growing edge of a CA plate were placed in sterile micro petriplate (5cm). The concentrated CFCF (1ml) was added to the plate, sealed with cling film and placed in fluorescent light for 48h to induce sporulation. The plates were observed under an inverted microscope and the number of sporangia developed per disc of *P. capsici* were counted.

Effect on Release of Zoospores

The sporulated discs of *P. capsici* were placed in micropetriplate with 1ml of the concentrated CFCF of the bacterial strains and induced for release of the zoospores by giving them cold shock for 15min at 4°C. The opened and un-opened sporangia were counted separately per disc under an inverted microscope.

Effect on Germination of Zoospores

50ml of the CFCF was taken in a sterile cavity slide and 10ml of the *P. capsici* zoospore suspension was incorporated to it. The cavity slides were kept in a moisture chamber prepared using a petriplate. The slides were observed after 24h under microscope for germination of the zoospores.

Detection of the Antibiotics by Thin Layer Chromatography (TLC)

The *P. fluorescens* strains were tested for the production of antibiotics *viz.* Pyoluteorin (Plt) (Howell and Stipanovic, 1980) and Pyrrolnitrin (Prn) (Howell and Stipanovic, 1980) by thin layer chromatography (Kraus and Loper, 1992). Extraction of the antibiotic was done from bacterial cells and spent media of bacterial cultures by a modification of published procedures.

Siderophore Mediated Antagonism in *P. fluorescens–P. capsici* System

The iron-regulated production of siderophore by *P. fluorescens* IISR-6 was studied by growing it in a medium amended with a range of concentration of iron. The involvement of siderophore mediated antagonism in *P. fluorescens–P. capsici* antagonistic system was studied by testing the response of *P. capsici* to simulated iron-depleted conditions.

The estimation of siderophores was performed as per the method described by Sneh *et al.* (1984). Relative concentration of siderophores in the supernatant was read in the spectrophotometer (VARIAN-Cary–50 Bio. UV-Visible) at 366 nm. Also the growth of *P. capsici* at iron-depleted conditions (under conditions of siderophore production) was studied. The iron-limited/regulated conditions were simulated *in vitro* by adding different concentrations of EDTA (100-1000mg/ml) or $FeCl_3$ (20-80mM) to CA plates thus getting a range of iron concentration in the media. The plates were incubated for 72h and the diameter of the colony was measured.

Production of Mycolytic Enzymes by the *P. fluorescens* Strains

The ability of the *P. fluorescens* strains in lysing the cell wall components of *P. capsici* was studied by estimating the mycolytic enzymes produced by the bacteria in presence of *P. capsici* mycelium. Further, microscopic observations were made on the fate of the mycelium upon co-habitation with the bacterial strains. Log phase culture (100ml) of the *Pseudomonas* strain was pippeted to MM, incorporated with live mycelium of *P. capsici* and incubated in an orbital shaker at 150 rpm at 28°C for 72h. The culture was centrifuged at 7,000 rpm for 10min at 10°C. The CFCF was collected and concentrated to 10ml in a flash evaporator (HEIDOLPH-Laborota-4001) at 28°C. The total protein in the crude samples was estimated by the method of Lowry *et al.* (1951). b-1,3 glucanase, b–1,4 glucanase and lipases was estimated by methods reported by Pan *et al.* (1991), Miller (1959), Elad *et al.* (1982) respectively. After co-culturing with *Pseudomonas*, the live mycelium of *P. capsici* was observed under the microscope. The integrity of cytoplasmic contents was compared with the normal mycelium.

Induction of Defence Related Enzymes and Phenolics in Black Pepper upon Treatment with *P. fluorescens*

Black pepper plants were treated at the roots with IISR-6, IISR-8, IISR-11, IISR-13 and IISR-51 separately and looked for induction of defence enzymes in the leaves. Assay of PAL, PPO and PO were performed with leaves of the root-bacterized plants from 0 to 14 days after treatment. The PAL assay was carried out by the method of Brueske *et al.* (1980), PO by Rathmell and Sequiera (1974) and PPO by Mayer *et al.* (1965).

Root bacterized black pepper cuttings were up rooted after two weeks of treatment and the total phenolics present in roots were estimated by Folin-Ciocalteau method. The relative lignification in the vascular region of plants also was studied adopting the protocol of Doster *et al.* (1988).

Results

Action of Metabolites of *P. fluorescens* on the Different Stages in the Life Cycle of *P. capsici*

The CFCF of IISR-6 completely inhibited (100 per cent) the sporangia production in *P. capsici* (Table 21.1). The sporangia production was inhibited by the CFCF of other strains in varying degrees (92.3 per cent–99.5 per cent). The CFCF of all the strains inhibited the indirect germination of sporangia (release of zoospores) considerably. When 102 numbers of sporangia per disk liberated zoospores in the sterile water control, only 2–16 numbers of sporangia released their zoospores in the CFCF treated plates. The percent inhibition of release of zoospores varied from 89–98 per cent. Only few zoospores germinated due to the inhibitory action of metabolites in the CFCF treated sets (2–8 numbers in a microscopic field) while there were 33 numbers of zoospores germinated in the sterile water control. Based on the reduction in the colony diameter of *P. capsici*, the metabolites of all the strains inhibited the mycelial phase of *P. capsici* in varying degrees (61 per cent–72 per cent). IISR-51 inhibited *P. capsici* to the highest percentage followed by IISR-6 and IISR-13.

Detection of the Antibiotics by Thin Layer Chromatography (TLC)

All the strains *viz.* IISR-6, IISR-8, IISR-11, IISR-13 and IISR-51 produced pyrrolnitrin (Rf: 0.86). Even though pyrrolnitrin was not detected in the CFCF of IISR-8, it was observed in the cell extract of the same. The fluorescent band for pyrrolnitrin appeared in the cell extraction of IISR-6 and IISR-8. The band at Rf: 0.36 (Pyoluteorin) appeared in the CFCF of only IISR-11 and IISR-51. Pyoluteorin was detected in the cell extracts of all the strains. So it was found that all the strains produced plt and prn, which were detected either in CFCF or in cell extractions.

Table 21.1: Inhibitory Effect of the Bacterial Strains on Different Stages in the Life Cycle of *P. capsici*

Treatment	*% Inhibition of Sporangia Production by CFCF*	*% Inhibition of Zoospore-Release by the CFCF*	*% Inhibition of Germination of Zoospores with CFCF*	*% Inhibition of Mycelial Growth of P. capsici by the Bacteria*
IISR-6	100.0 [a]	92.15 [ab]	90.90 [a]	64.06 [b]
IISR-8	97.6 [c]	90.2 [ab]	84.84 [b]	60.93 [d]
IISR-11	97.6 [c]	89.22 [b]	84.84 [b]	62.50 [c]
IISR-13	99.5 [b]	97.70 [a]	93.03 [a]	64.06 [b]
IISR-51	92.3 [d]	89.22 [b]	75.75 [c]	71.87 [a]

CFCF: Cell Free Culture Filtrate.

Values followed by same letters in a column do not differ significantly at p=0.05.

Siderophore mediated antagonism in *P. fluorescens–P. capsici* System

Production of siderophores by bacteria reduced as the concentration of $FeCl_3$ increased in the growth medium as shown in Figure 21.1. At 300mM of $FeCl_3$, IISR-6 released only half the quantity of siderophores with respect to the media without any addition of $FeCl_3$ (Optical density of 0.7 and 1.44 respectively at A_{420}).

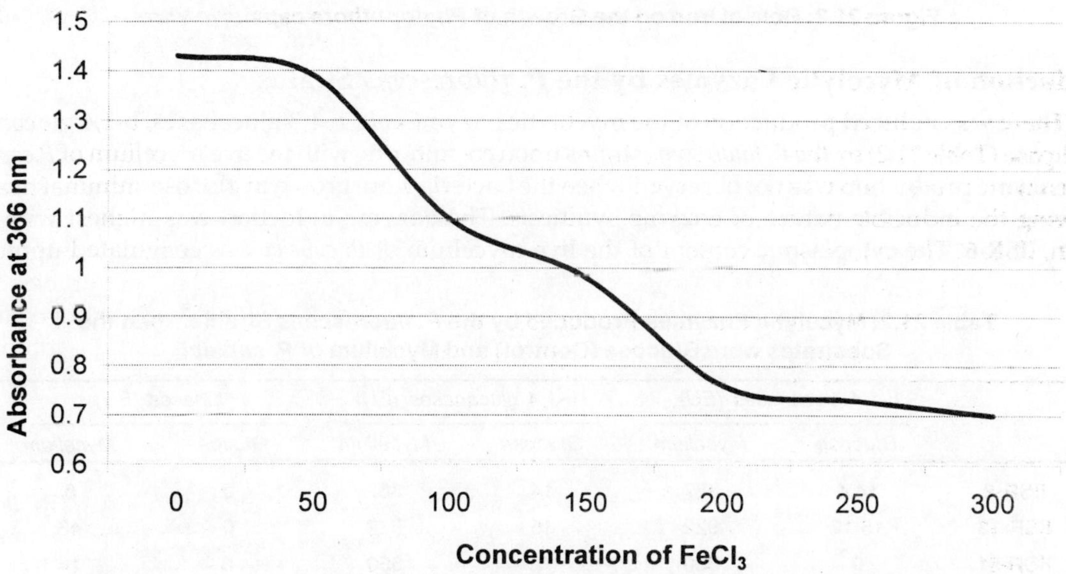

Figure 21.1: Iron Regulated Production of Siderophores by *P. fluorescens* IISR-6

With the addition of 100-1000 mg/ml of EDTA, the growth of *P. capsici* reduced drastically (colony diameter of 0.8cm to 1cm) and at 1000 mg/ml of EDTA, the growth was completely inhibited (Figure 21.2) due to the deficiency of available iron. The increased production of siderophores by the *P. fluorescens* strains as well as the limited growth of *P. capsici* at lower concentrations of iron in the medium could be extrapolated to the involvement of siderophores in *Pseudomonas–P. capsici* antagonistic system.

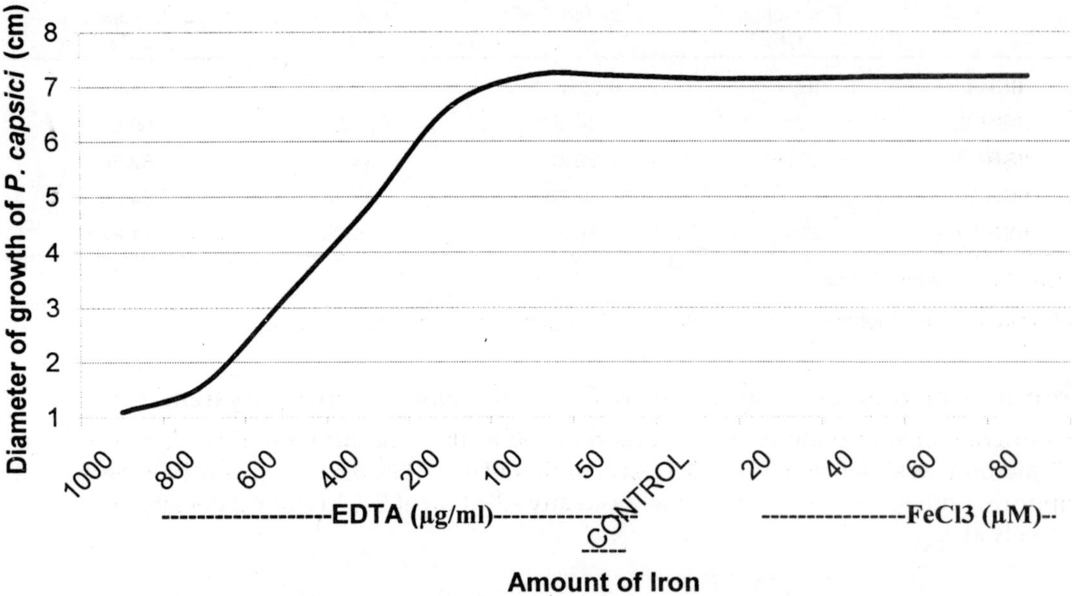

Figure 21.2: Role of Iron on the Growth of *Phytophthora capsici in vitro*

Production of Mycolytic Enzymes by the *P. fluorescens* Strains

There was induced production of the mycolytic enzymes *viz.* b-1,3 glucanases, b-1,4 glucanase and lipase (Table 21.2) by the *P. fluorescens* strains upon co-culturing with the live mycelium of *P. capsici*. The enzyme production was not observed when the bacteria were grown in glucose-minimal media, showing the inducible nature of enzyme synthesis. The enzyme induction was highest with the strain, IISR-6. The cytoplasmic content of the live mycelium of *P. capsici* was coagulated upon co-

Table 21.2: Mycolytic Enzymes Produced by the *P. fluorescens* Strains when the Substrates were Glucose (Control) and Mycelium of *P. capsici*

	b-1,4 glucanases (EU)		*b-1,4 glucanases (EU)*		*Lipases (EU)*	
	Glucose	*Mycelium*	*Glucose*	*Mycelium*	*Glucose*	*Mycelium*
IISR-8	14.4	367	14	367	0	6
IISR-13	15.12	922	15	922	0	43
IISR-51	0	350	0	350	0	14
IISR-6	0	1500	0	1500	0	62
IISR-11	0	385	0	385	0	3

culturing with the *P. fluorescens* strains (Figure 21.3). Further, co-culturing of the mycelia with the antagonists resulted in complete disintegration of the cytoplasmic contents. The cytoplasmic contents were intact in the glucose amended MM (Figure 21.4).

Induction of Defence Related Enzymes and Phenolics in Black Pepper upon Treatment with *P. fluorescens* Strains

Bacterial treatments increased the amount of peroxidase in the plant significantly over time (Figure 21.5). Significantly higher quantities were observed on the second day itself, except for IISR-8, for which it was on the 6th day of bacterization. Even though not significant after 4th days, a higher level of PO was maintained in bacterized roots unlike in the non-bacterized. PO activity remained constant in the untreated plants. All the strains induced significant quantities of PAL in the treated black pepper roots over the period of time, wherein the untreated plants did not show any significant change in the pattern of PAL production (Figure 21.6). IISR-51 induced highest production of the

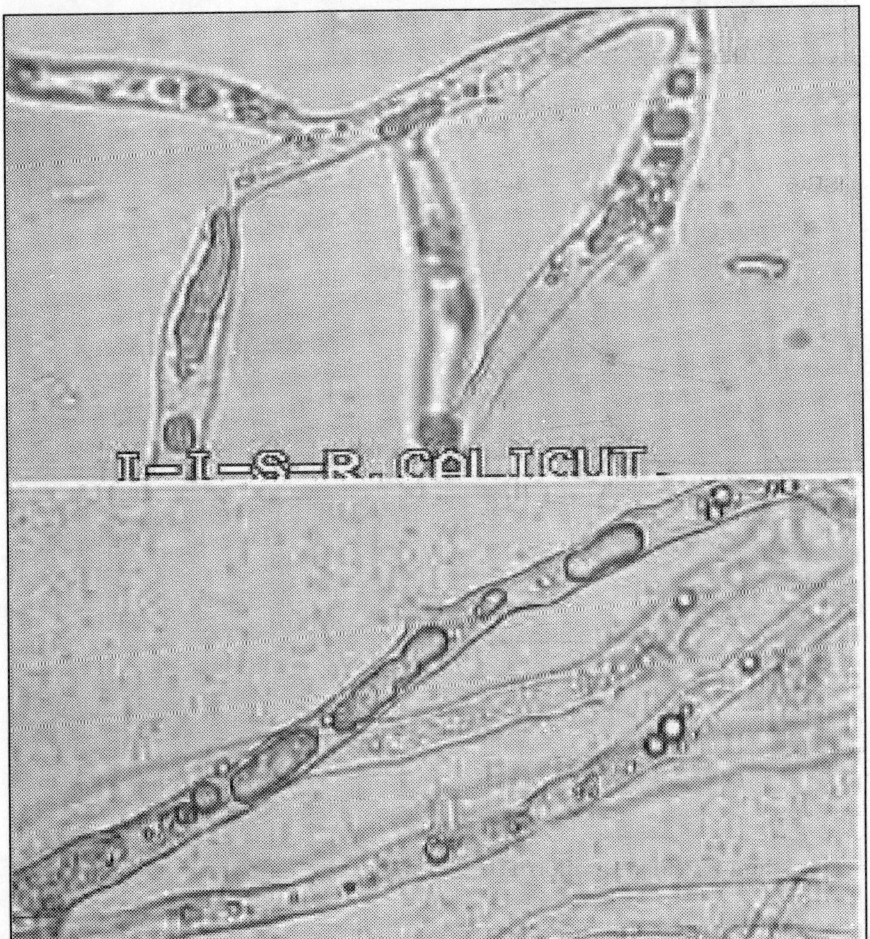

Figure 21.3: Coagulation of Cytoplasmic Contents of *P. capsici* by the Action of *P.fluorescens*

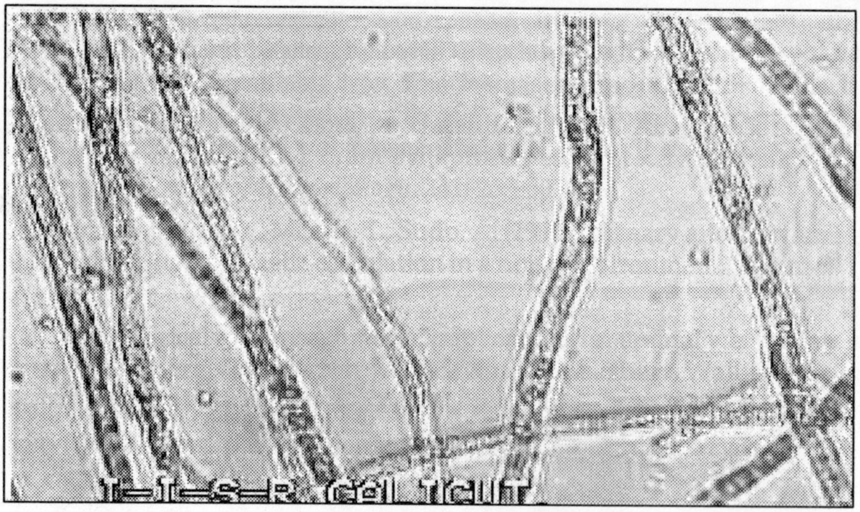

Figure 21.4: Normal Mycelium

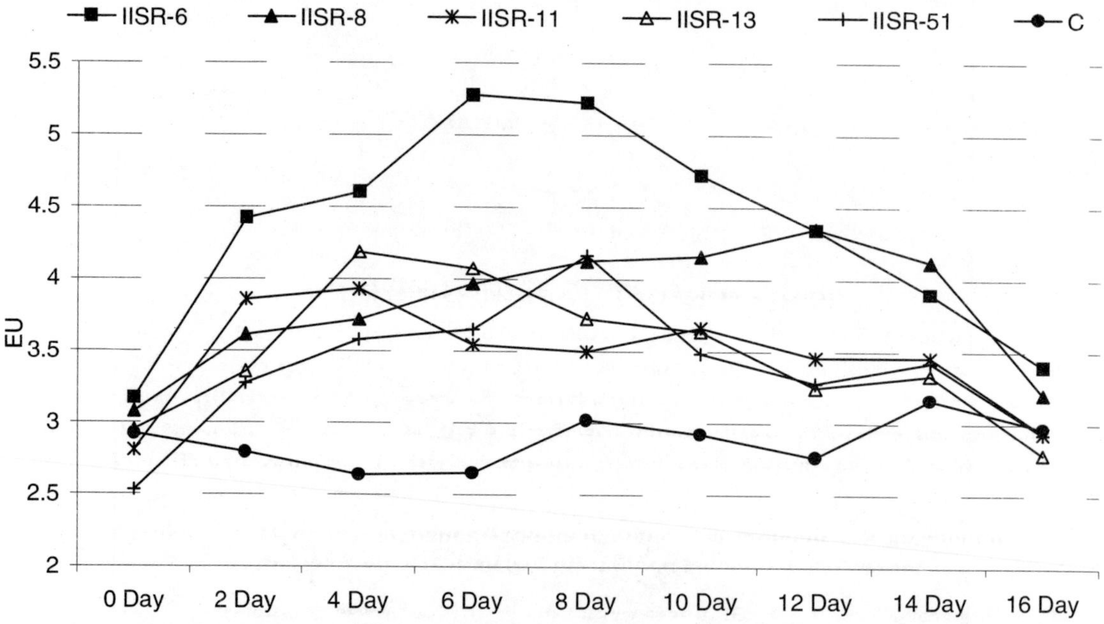

Figure 21.5: Induction of PO in the Leaf of Root-bacterized Plants

enzyme in roots on the 4th day and for other strains it was on the 2nd day of bacterization itself. Unlike the other enzymes studied, the highest peak with PPO level upon bacterization of the black pepper roots occurred only on a later stage, which is 8 days after bacterization (Figure 21.7). Untreated plants did not show any significant fluctuations in PPO activity in the study period.

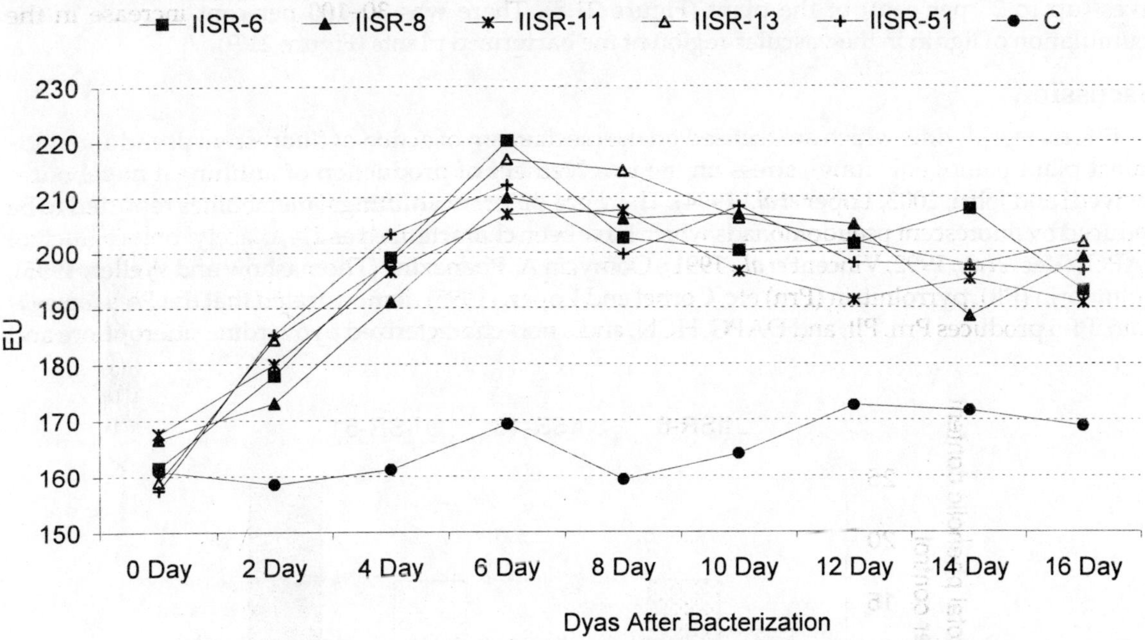

Figure 21.6: Induction of PAL in the Leaf of Root-bacterized Plants

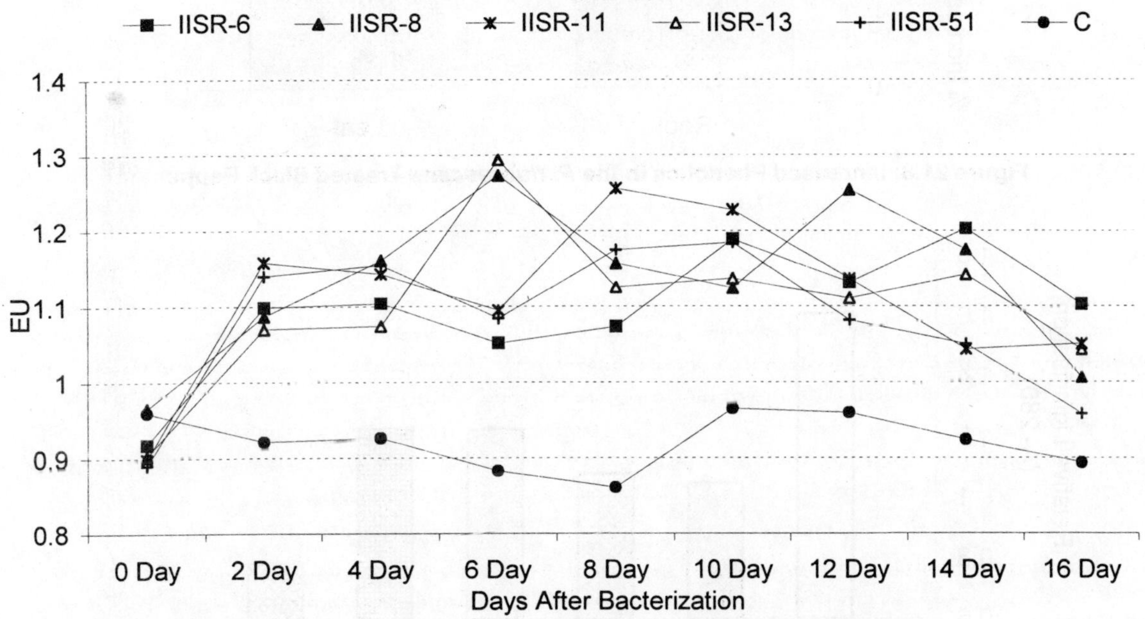

Figure 21.7: Induction of PPO in the Leaf of Root-bacterized Plants

There was an increase in the levels of total phenolics in the plant upon root bacterization of the plant. The enhanced quantity was observed not only in the roots (up to 17 per cent) but also in the leaves (up to 25 per cent) of the plant (Figure 21.8). There was 30–100 per cent increase in the accumulation of lignin in the vascular region of the bacterized plants (Figure 21.9).

Discussion

Efforts worldwide, which are focused on the mechanism of action of fluorescent pseudomonads against plant pathogenic fungi, stress on the involvement of production of antifungal metabolites (Dwivedi and Johri, 2003; Loper *et al.*, 1994). There are different antifungal metabolites reported to be produced by fluorescent pseudomonads which have been characterized as 2, 4, diacetyl phloroglucinol (DAPG) (Keel *et al.*, 1992; Vincent *et al.*, 1991), Oomycin A, Phenazine (Thomashow and Weller, 1995), pyoluteorin (Plt), pyrrolnitrin (Prn) etc. Corbel and Loper, (1995) demonstrated that the *Pseudomonas* strain, Pf-5 produces Prn, Plt, and DAPG, HCN, and a non-characterized pyoverdine siderophore and

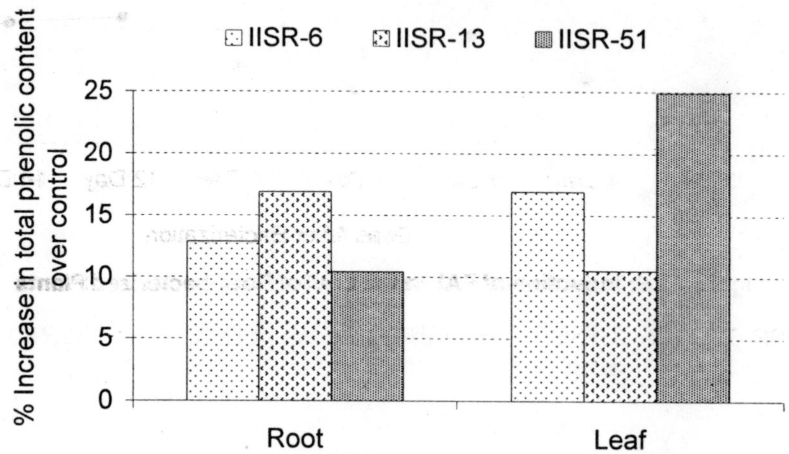

Figure 21.8: Increased Phenolics in the *P. fluorescens* Treated Black Pepper

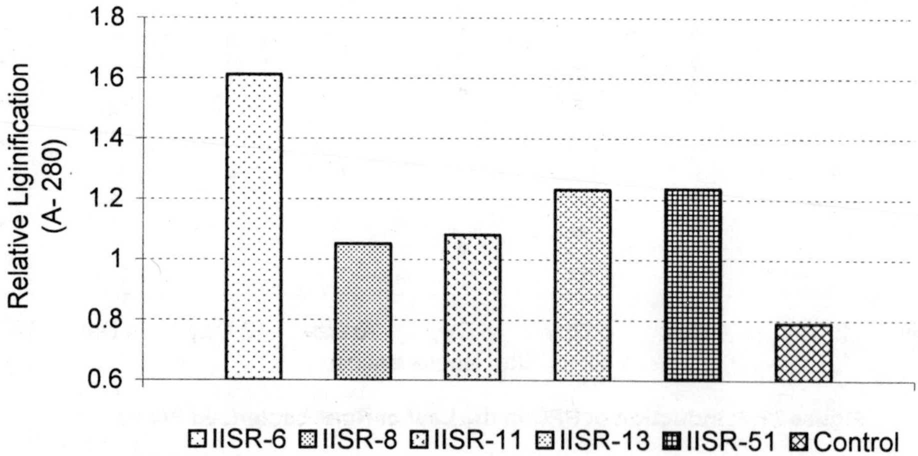

Figure 21.9: Induced Accumulation Lignin in PGPR Treated Plants

each of the antibiotic has a unique spectrum of activity against fungal pathogens *viz.* Pyrrolnitrin inhibits *R. solani* and *Pyrenophora tritici-repentis*, Pyoluteorin inhibits *Pythium ultimum*, and 2,4-diacetylphloroglucinol inhibits all three fungi (Loper and Gross, 2007). Pyrrolnitrin (Prn) and pyoluteorin (Plt) are broad-spectrum antibiotics produced by several strains of *Pseudomonas* and *Burkholderia* species. Both antibiotics play important roles in the suppression of multiple plant pathogenic fungi (Jorge *et al.*, 2003). All the strains under the present study were found producing Prn. Whereas IISR-6 and IISR-8 produced Plt. The antifungal activity of Plt and Prn has been proved in many cropping systems in the field wherein the negative mutants failed to protect the crop from the soil borne fungal pathogen.

The inhibitory metabolites produced by the *Pseudomonas* spp. strains inhibited the different stages in the lifecycle of *P. capsici viz.* mycelial growth, sporangial formation, release of zoospores, and germination of zoospores. This clearly makes it evident the potency of the strains to antagonize all the reproductive phases of the pathogen thus effectively preventing its growth and proliferation. These attribute of the *Pseudomonas* strains makes it effective candidates in suppressing *P. capsici* in all seasons of plant growth and especially in rainy season to take care of the zoospore mediated spread of the pathogen to the adjacent vines. However the population of *Pseudomonas* in the rainy season and the level of inhibitory principles in the soils need study in depth.

Siderophore mediated antagonism in biocontrol of plant pathogens has been well proved (Loper *et al.*, 2007). The iron dependent production of siderophores by the fluorescent pseudomonad isolates was found to be in agreement with the findings of Kloepper *et al.* (1980b). In the present study, as the concentration of iron increased, the production of siderophores by the strains was less (Figure 3). Current studies on the effect of iron chelation on the growth of *P. capsici* revealed that at 1000 mg/ml of EDTA, the growth was completely inhibited due to the deficiency of available iron. The increased production of siderophores by *Pseudomonas* as well as the limited growth of *P. capsici* at lower concentrations of iron in the medium indicated the involvement of siderophores in *Pseudomonas–P. capsici* antagonistic system.

Mycolytic enzymes have been reported to play an important role in the degradation of the target pathogen and consequent mycoparasitism (Ajit *et al.*, 2004). In the present study, the mycolytic enzymes *viz.* b-1,3 glucanase, b-1,4 glucanase and lipase, produced by the bacterial strains lysed the cell wall of *P. capsici*. Since 80-90 per cent the cell wall of *P. capsici* consisted largely of cellulose (Ribeiro, 1978), it could be inferred that b-1,3 glucanase and b-1,4 glucanase produced by the antagonists were involved in pathogen suppression. Coagulation of cytoplasmic contents of *P. capsici*, upon co-culturing with the *Pseudomonas* strains, as observed in the present study, can also be attributed to the hydrolytic enzymes produced by the antagonists and consequent leakage of electrolytes from the mycelium. Paulitz *et al.* (1998) observed cytoplasmic damage in *Pythium ultimum* colonizing the roots of cucumber when roots were treated with *Pseudomonas aureofaciens*. The cell membrane with increased permeability might be allowing the other inhibitory metabolites to act upon the cytoplasmic contents leading to coagulation and further disintegration.

The current study also dealt with the induction of PGPR mediated defence enzymes in black pepper *viz.* Phenyl alanine Ammonia Lyase, Peroxidases and Poly phenol oxidases which are involved in the defence mechanism in the plant to resist the invading pathogen. Similar induction has been reported in many different cropping systems (Ahn *et al.*, 2002, Silva *et al.*, 2004). All the 5 strains used in the study induced defence enzymes in leaves of black pepper when the plants were root-bacterized, which in turn reflected in the reduced root rot when the plants were challenge inoculated with the root rot pathogen. The synthesis of the defence enzymes even in the distal end of the plant upon root treatment shows the systemic nature of protection that the strains offered. An early induction of PAL is very important as the biosynthesis of lignin originates from L-phenyl alanine. General phenyl propanoid metabolism is defined as the sequence of reactions involved in the conversion of L-phenyl alanine to activated cinnamic acids (Hahlbrock and Scheel, 1989). The first enzyme of this path way is PAL, catalyze the trans–elimination of ammonia from L-phenyl alanine to form trans cinnamic acid which in turn enter different biosynthetic path ways leading to lignin. Studies in cucumber revealed that PAL is a key enzyme in the production of Phenolics and phytoalexin (Daayf *et al.*, 1997).

Peroxidase (PO) is involved in lignification leading to disease resistance and polymerization of cinnamyl alcohols to lignin is catabolised by PO (Lagrimini *et al.*, 1987). For lignification, specific cell wall peroxidases are thought to be required to generate H_2O_2 and monolignol radicals (van Huystee, 1987). The present study revealed over three-fold increase in the peroxidase level within two days of bacterial treatment and continues to be synthesized throughout the study period. The increased peroxidase activity in the present study was correlated with increased lignification in treated plants. The induction of polyphenol oxidases (PPO) was found to be gradual in the bacterized plants unlike the other defence enzymes studied. The accumulation of PPO occurs usually upon wounding in plants. Constabel and Ryan, (1998) proved that PPO could be induced upon induction by jasmonic acid.

The defence proteins induced while treatment with PGPR reinforces the cell wall structure by lignification and accumulates the phenolic compounds including phytoalexin in the phenyl propanoid pathway. The enhanced quantity of phenolics produced in black pepper is supposed to contribute to the disease suppression obtained. Ongena *et al.* (2000) found that several inducible root phenolic conjugants are involved in the protective effect observed in cucumber, by PGPR.

Lignin play important roles in plant defence against several pathogens. Accumulation of lignin and thereby cell wall thickening was observed in *Pseudomonas* spp. treated black pepper cuttings. In the present study, a relatively higher quantity of lignification (30–100 per cent) in the bacterized roots was found as compared to the untreated plants. Lignin is supposed to restrict fungal growth in a number of ways. Primarily it make cell walls more resistant to fungal penetration and to dissolution by fungal enzymes. Second, lignin restricts the translocation of water and nutrients from plant tissue to the fungus and with the movement of toxin and enzymes from the fungus to the plant. Fungal penetration may be stopped due to lignification of hyphal tips, and low molecular weight phenolic precursors of lignin may inactivate certain fungal metabolites. Finally, lignification and other cell wall modifications may decelerate fungal development, allowing phytoalexins to accumulate to effective levels. Phytoalexins also retard fungal growth, providing enough time for cell wall modifications to become effective (van Peer *et al.*, 1991).

As the strains performed various mechanisms to prevent pathogen proliferation in the plant and also showed direct antagonistic potential, the strains could bring about significant disease suppression in the host plant.

Acknowledgements

The financial support from the Department of Biotechnology, Government of India is gratefully acknowledged.

References

Ahn, I. P., Park, K., and Kim, C. H. (2002). Rhizobacteria-induced resistance perturbs viral disease progress and triggers defense related gene expression. *Mol. Cells.*, 13: 302–308.

Ajit, N. S., Verma, R. and Shanmugam, V. (2006). Extracellular Chitinases of Fluorescent Pseudomonads Antifungal to *Fusarium oxysporum* f. sp. dianthi Causing Carnation Wilt *Current Microbiology*, 52: 310–316

Brueske, C. H. (1980). Phenyl alanine ammonia lyase in tomato roots infected and resistant to the root knot nematode *Meloidogyne incognita*. *Physiol. Plant. Pathol.*, 16: 409-414.

Constabel CP and Ryan CA (1998). A survey of wound–and methyl jasmonate-induced leaf polyphenol oxidase in crop plants. *Phytochemistry*, 47: 507-511.

Corbell, N. and Loper, J. E. (1995). A Global Regulator of Secondary Metabolite Production in *Pseudomonas fluorescens* Pf-5 *J. Bacteriol.*, p. 6230–6236.

Daayf, F., Bel-Rhlid, R. and Belanger, R. R. (1997). Methyl ester of P–coumaric acid: A Phytoaelxin-like compound from long English cucumber leaves. *J. Chem. Ecol.*, 23:1517-1526.

Dennis, C. and Webster, J. (1971). Antagonistic properties of species groups of *Trichoderma* I: The production of non-volatile antibiotics. *Trans. Brit. Mycol. Soc.*, 57 : 25-39

Doster, M. A. and Bostoc R. M. (1988). Quantification of lignin formation in almond bark in response to wounding and infection by *Phytophthora* sp. *Phytopathol.*, 473-477.

Dwivedi, D and Johri B. N. (2003). Antifungals from fluorescent pseudomonads:Biosynthesis and regulation. *Current Science*, 85(12) 1693-1703

Elad, Y., Chet, I. and Henis, Y. (1982). Degradation of plant pathogenic fungi by *Trichoderma harzianum*. *Can. J. Microbiol.*, 28: 719–725.

Hahlbrock, K., Scheel, D. (1989). Physiology and molecular biology of the phenylpropanoid metabolism. *Ann. Rev. Plant. Physiol. Plant Mol. Biol.*, 40: 347-369

Howel, C. R. and Stipanovic, R. D. (1980). Suppression of *Pythium ultimum* induced damping off of cotton seedlings by *Pseudomonas fluorescens* and its antibiotic pyoluteorin. *Phytopathology*, 70: 712–715.

Jorge, T., de Souza and Raaijmakers, J. M. (2003) Polymorphisms within the *prnD* and *pltC* genes from pyrrolnitrin and pyoluteorin-producing *Pseudomonas* and *Burkholderia* spp. *FEMS Microbiology Ecology*, 43 (1) pp. 21-34.

Keel, C., Schnider, V., Maurhofer, M., Voisard, C., Laville, J., Burger, U., Wirthner, P., Haas, D. and Defago, G. (1992). Suppression of root diseases by *Pseudomonas fluorescence* CHAO: Importance of the bacterial secondary metabolite 2,4 diacetyl phloroglucinol. *Mol. Plant. Microbe Interact.*, 5: 4–13.

Kloepper, J. W. and Schroth, M. N. and Miller, T. D. (1980a). Effect of rhizosphere colonization by plant growth promoting rhizobacteria on potato development and yield. *Phytopathology*, 70: 1078-1082.

Kloepper, J. W., Leong, J., Teintze, M. and Schroth, M. N. (1980b). *Pseudomonas* siderophores: A mechanism explaining disease suppressive soils. *Current Microbiology*, 4: 317-320.

Kraus, J. and Loper, J. E. (1992). Lack of evidence for a role of antifungal metabolite production by *Pseudomonas fluorescens* Pf-5 in biological control of *Pythium* damping-off of cucumber. *Phytopathology*, 82:264-271.

Loper, J. and Gross, H. (2007). Genomic analysis of antifungal metabolite production by *Pseudomonas fluorescens* Pf-5 *European Journal of Plant Pathology*, 119 (3) :265–278

Loper, J. E., Kobayashi, D. Y. and Paulsen, I. T. (2007). The Genomic Sequence of *Pseudomonas fluorescens* Pf-5: Insights In to Biological Control, 97(2): 233-238

Loper, J. E., Kraus, J. and Henkels, M. (1994). Antagonism of soil borne Plant Pathogens by rhizosphere pseudomonads. In. *Biotechnology and Plant protection*. Bills, D. D. and Kung, S. (Eds) World Scientific Publishing Company Co. Singapore.

Mayer, A. M., Harel, E. and Shaul, R. B. (1965). Assay of catechol oxidase, a critical comparison of methods. *Phytochemistry*, 5:783-789.

Miller, G. L. (1959). Use of dinitro salycilic acid reagent for the determination of reducing sugars. *Anal. Chem.*, 31: 426.

Ongena, M; Daayl, F; Jcques, P; Thonart, P; Behmon, N; Panlitz, T.C and Belanger, R.R (2000). Systemic induction of phytoalexins in cucumber in response to treatments with fluorescent pseudomonads. *Plant Pathology*., 49: 523-530.

Pan, S. Q., Ye, X. S. and Kuc, J. (1991). Association of b-1,3 glucanase activity and isoform pattern with systemic resistance to blue mold in tobacco induced by stem injection with *Peronospora tabacina* or leaf inoculation with tobacco mosaic virus. *Physiol. Mol.Pl. Pathol.*, 39: 25–39

Paul, D. (2004). Physiological, Biochemical, and Molecular Studies on the Root Rot (Caused by *Phytophthora capsici*) Suppression in Black Pepper (*Piper nigrum* Linn) by Rhizosphere Bacteria. PhD Thesis. Calicut University, India

Paulitz, T. C., Chen, C., Belanger, R and Benhamou, N. (1998). Induced systemic resistance by *Pseudomonas* spp. against *Pythium* root rot. http://www.ag.auburn.edu/argentina/pdfmanuscripts/paulitz.pdf

Pieterse, C. M. J., Van Pelt, J. A., Parchmann, S., Mueler, M. J., Buchela, A. J. Metaux, J. P. and Van Loon, L. C. (2000) Rhizobacteria mediated induced systemic resistance (ISR) in *Arabidopsis* requires sensitivity to jasmonate and ethylene but is not accompanied by an increase in their production. *Physiological and Molecular Plant Pathology*, 57: 123-134.

Rathmell. W. G. and Sequira, L. (1974). Soluble peroxidase in fluid from the intercellular spaces of tobacco leaves. *Plant Physiol.*, 53:317-318.

Ribeiro, O. K. (1978). *A source book of the genus. Phytohthora.* J. Cramer, Germany.

Sarma, Y. R., Anandaraj, M. and Ramachandran, N. (1992). Recent advances on *Phytophthora* foot rot research in India and the need for holistic approach. In Proceedings International Workshop on Black Pepper Diseases, Bandar Lampung, Indonesia. Wahid.P., Sitepu.D., Deciyanto.S and Suparman.U (eds.) pp. 133-143.

Sarma, Y. R., Rajan, P. P., Paul, D., Beena, N., and Anandaraj, M. (2000). Role of Rhizobacteria on disease suppression in spice crops and future prospects. In: *Seminar on Biological Control with Plant Growth Promoting Rhizobacteria for sustainable* agriculture. University of Hyderabad, Hyderabad.April.3-4.

Silva HAS, Romeiro RS, Macagnan D, Halfeld-Vieira BA, Pereira MCB, Mounteer A (2004). Rhizobacterial induction of systemic resistance in tomato plants: Non-specific protection and increase in enzyme activities. *Biol. Control*, 29:288–295

Sneh, B., Dupler, M., Elad, Y., and Baker, R. (1984). Chlamydospore germination of *Fusarium oxysporum* f. sp. *cucumerinum* as affected by fluorescent and lytic bacteria from a *Fusarium* suppressive soil. *Phytopahtology*,74: 1115–1124.

Suslow, T. V. and Schroth, M. N. (1982b). Rhizobacteria of sugar beets: effects of seed application and root colonization on yield. *Phytopathology,* 72:199-206.

Thomashow, L. S. and Weller, D. M. (1995). Current concepts in the use of introduced bacteria for biological control: mechanisms and anti-fungal metabolites. Pages 187-235. *Plant microbe interactions,* Vol. 1. G. Stacey and N. Keen (Eds) Chapman and Hall, New York.

van Huystee, R. B. (1987). Some molecular aspects of Plant Peroxidases: Biosynthetic studies. Annual Review of *Plant Physiology,* 38: 205-219.

van Peer, R., Neemann, G. J. and Schippers, B. (1991). Induced resistance and phytoalexin accumulation in biological control of *Fusarium* wilt of Carnation by *Pseudomonas* spp. strain WCS 417r. *Phytopathology,* 81: 728–734.

Vincent, M. N., Arrison, L. A. Brackin, J, Kovacevich, P. A., Mukerji, P., Weller, D. M. and Pierson, E. A. (1991). Genetic analysis of the antifungal activity of a soil borne *Pseudomonas aureofacience* strain. *Appl. Environ. Microbiol.,* 57: 2928-2934.

Index

B

D